N

Basic Pharmacology

D0316468

Book No. **02722740**

30121 0 02722740

Basic Pharmacology

Fourth edition

Editor
R.W. Foster, BSc, MB, BS, PhD

Authors
The pharmacologists of the School of Biological Sciences, University of Manchester, UK, and their teaching collaborators:

A.J.M. Boulton, MD, FRCP
J.R. Carpenter, BSc, PhD
B. Clarke, BSc, MD, FRCP
M.J. Dascombe, BPharm, PhD
J.F.W. Deakin, PhD, MRCPsych
Caroline Dive, BPharm, PhD
A.J. Duxbury, MSc, PhD, DDS, FDS RCPSGlas
R.W. Foster, BSc, MB, BS, PhD
C.C. Hardy, MD, FRCP
Ariane L. Herrick, MD, MRCP
M. Hollingsworth, PhD, DSc
Alison S. Johnson, MB, ChB, MSc
G.E. Mawer, BSc, MB, ChB, PhD, FRCPEd

I.D. Morris, BPharm, PhD, DSc
F. Owen, BSc, PhD
Barbara J. Pleuvry, BPharm, MSc, PhD, MRPharmS
A.K. Scott, MD, FRCP
J.L. Shaffer, MB, BS, MRCP
P. Slater, BPharm, PhD
R.C. Small, PhD, DSc, FRPharmS
D.G. Thompson, MD, FRCP
Mary P. Tully, MSc, MRPharmS
R.D.G. Tunbridge, MD, FRCP
Janet Vale, MSc, MRPharmS
A.H. Weston, PhD, DSc
P.M. Wilkinson, MB, ChB, MSc, FRCP, FRCR

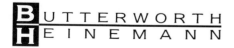

BUTTERWORTH
HEINEMANN

STAFFORDSHIRE
UNIVERSITY
LIBRARY

Butterworth-Heinemann
Linacre House, Jordan Hill, Oxford OX2 8DP
225 Wildwood Avenue, Woburn, MA 01801-2041
A division of Reed Educational and Professional Publishing Ltd

A member of the Reed Elsevier plc group

OXFORD   AUCKLAND   BOSTON
JOHANNESBURG   MELBOURNE   NEW DELHI

First published 1980
Reprinted 1983, 1985
Second edition 1986
Reprinted 1990
Third edition 1991
Reprinted 1994, 1995
Fourth edition 1996
Reprinted 1997, 1999

STAFFORDSHIRE
UNIVERSITY
LIBRARY

SITE: Nelson

-9 SEP 1999

CLASS No.
615.1024613 (Iwl)

© Reed Educational and Professional Publishing Ltd 1996

All rights reserved. No part of this publication
may be reproduced in any material form (including
photocopying or storing in any medium by electronic
means and whether or not transiently or incidentally
to some other use of this publication) without the
written permission of the copyright holder except in
accordance with the provisions of the Copyright,
Designs and Patents Act 1988 or under the terms of a
licence issued by the Copyright Licensing Agency Ltd,
90 Tottenham Court Road, London, England W1P 9HE.
Applications for the copyright holder's written
permission to reproduce any part of this publication
should be addressed to the publishers

British Library Cataloguing in Publication Data
A catalogue record for this book is available from the British Library

Library of Congress Cataloguing in Publication Data
A catalogue record for this book is available from the Library of Congress

ISBN 0 7506 2198 2

Composition by Scribe Design, Gillingham, Kent
Printed and bound in Great Britain by MPG Books Ltd, Bodmin, Cornwall

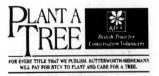

PLANT A
TREE

British Trust for
Conservation Volunteers

FOR EVERY TITLE THAT WE PUBLISH. BUTTERWORTH-HEINEMANN
WILL PAY FOR BTCV TO PLANT AND CARE FOR A TREE.

Contents

02722740

STAFFS UNIVERSITY LIBRARY

9   Pharmacotherapeutics   **457**

STAFFS UNIVERSITY LIBRARY

Preface

This fourth edition of *Basic Pharmacology* retains the overall objectives of the first. It aims to present accounts of drug actions and their mechanisms in compact, inexpensive and up-to-date form. The book is therefore designed to help students of medicine, and subjects allied to medicine, to appreciate the rationale underlying the uses of drugs in therapeutics.

The authors of this book, the pharmacologists of the School of Biological Sciences at Manchester University and their teaching colleagues, have been able to draw on experience developed during many years of teaching pharmacology to students of several different disciplines within changing curricula. Such experience is tempered by other aspects of their work with drugs, such as prescribing, dispensing, and conducting laboratory-based and clinical research.

The book is divided into sections. Each section follows a particular theme and is introduced by the relevant pharmacological general principles. Prompts to revise the relevant anatomical, biochemical or physiological concepts and data are also given. In each section the major groups of drugs relevant to the theme are discussed with detailed expositions of the important <u>type substances</u>. Drugs of lesser importance are placed in proper context or have been excluded.

As outlined in the *Introduction*, this book is addressed to a wide spectrum of readers. We hope that no reader who intends to exploit the properties of drugs will fail to appreciate two key notions:

(1) Selectivity (the ability to influence chemically one kind of biological activity without modifying another) is the central theme of pharmacology.
(2) Pharmacological selectivity is relative, rather than absolute. This places the onus of responsibility for safe usage firmly on the intending exploiter of the properties of drugs.

The principal changes that this fourth edition of *Basic Pharmacology* shows from the third are:

(1) Updating (as of 1995) of the accounts of mechanisms of drug action.
(2) Updating (after *British National Formulary* [*BNF*] September 1995, Number 30) of the selection of drugs for discussion – this encompasses

not only the inclusion of new drugs and new mechanisms of drug action, but also the deletion of drugs that have become obsolete.

(3) Renaming the section previously entitled *Clinical pharmacology* as *Pharmacotherapeutics* and moving some material from the *General pharmacology* section to a newly developed *Clinical pharmacology* section.

(4) Provision of new chapters on openers (activators) of potassium channels, immunosuppressive drugs, principles of prescribing, prescribing for special groups, legal aspects of prescribing, practical problems of compliance with the prescription, the process of rational therapeutics, analgesia.

(5) Significant rewriting of parts of the chapters on targets of drug action, antagonists at adrenoceptors, local anaesthesia, cardiac antidysrhythmic drugs, cardiac glycosides, blockers of calcium channels, anticoagulant, antiplatelet and fibrinolytic compounds, angiotensin, chemical transmission in the CNS, antidepressant drugs, biochemical selectivity, acquired drug resistance in parasites, chemotherapy of bacterial infections, hypertension and antihypertensive drugs, asthma, headache and migraine, depressive illness, epilepsy, haematinic drugs and the cellular elements of blood.

(6) Rewording of the explanations of drugs properties for improved clarity – no part of the book remains untouched.

(7) Inclusion of more summaries at the ends of chapters.

(8) Provision of additional figures.

(9) Redrawing of some of the existing figures to improve the way they convey their message.

Introduction

This book is intended for all who are embarking on the study of pharmacology. Most of its readers will be students of medicine, or of subjects allied to medicine (pharmacy, dentistry, nursing). These students will be studying pharmacology as a subsidiary subject and will require emphasis on the therapeutic exploitation of the properties of drugs. However, other students will regard pharmacology as their main or second subject in biological science. We teach all such students ourselves and have attempted to satisfy their varied needs in a single text. The text is broadly introductory, supporting the first and second years of study by any of the above student groups.

Our various readers will have two things in common: an interest in the uses to which drugs are put, and the fact that they are embarking on the study of pharmacology. Thus, we have provided a textbook that begins at the beginning, assuming only a modicum of chemistry, biology and physiology as prerequisites. The book proceeds in the direction of paramedical or therapeutic, rather than chemical, pharmacology, and it is assumed that the student will still be developing his/her knowledge of biology or physiology.

The principal aim is to explain the basis of the current therapeutic exploitation of drugs. Although some large reference texts already achieve this aim at an advanced level (the most eminent and highly recommended bears the title that most succinctly expresses this aim – *The Pharmacological Basis of Therapeutics* – see Gilman et al. (1992) in Suggested further reading and study), this book is offered to fill the need for a comprehensive yet simple and concise student text.

Drug names

A major problem encountered in the learning of pharmacology is the large and ever-increasing number of drug names. Certainly new students often complain of this. The complaint is not simply about weight of numbers but also about the apparent similarity in the names of drugs from different pharmacological groups. For the inexperienced (for whom drug names are invested with no 'personality') this can lead to misunderstanding and confusion. Therefore, in this book we have defined a rigorous policy on drug names (see below). We have limited the number of drugs included, and have attempted an approach to the teaching of pharmacology that places a premium on understanding, clothing drug names with personality and reducing rote memorization to the essential minimum.

Policy on drug names

We have used the non-proprietary names approved by the British Pharmacopoeial Commission and have largely excluded trade names. For readers who are more familiar with North American terminology, the US Pharmacopoeial name has been included in square brackets in the text after the first occurrence of the name. However, only significant Anglo-American differences have been declared; we have not bothered to draw special attention to systematic differences arising from different spelling conventions (-ph- [-f-], -oe- [-e-]). Neither did -trophin [-tropin] nor -barbi-tone [-barbital] seem likely to mystify our readers.

We were pleasantly surprised by the currently small number of significant differences, for there was formerly an era of fundamental differences, witness pethidine [meperidine], paracetamol [acetaminophen] and salbutamol [albuterol]. Modern drugs are deliberately being assigned the same name on both sides of the Atlantic.

Policy on which drugs to include

We have actively sought to limit the number of different drugs described because our primary objective has been to teach the principles of the pharmacological basis of therapeutics rather than familiarity with all drugs. We have therefore a narrower scope than the *BNF* or the Monthly Index of Medical Specialties (*MIMS*), which seek coverage of all available drugs – we describe a limited selection of the most useful drugs. We have followed the advice offered in the *Notes for prescribers* sections of the *BNF* on the selection of drugs with maximum available therapeutic effectiveness and minimal contaminating unwanted effects. Where that authoritative source describes a drug first and out of the otherwise alphabetical sequence, that drug is an acknowledged reference drug and an obvious choice for one of our type substances (see (2) below). This policy produces a very similar result to that adopted by the World Health Organization (WHO) Expert Committee reporting on The Use of Essential Drugs.

Drugs have been categorized according to two criteria:

(1) Drugs listed in *BNF* (1995) and printed in bold type in one of its *Notes for prescribers* sections are italicized (e.g. *non-proprietary name*).
(2) From each pharmacological group of drugs we have, if possible, chosen one that typifies the group. If its actions are understood the rest of the group, too, has been comprehended. We show these substances in bold type (e.g. **non-proprietary name**).

The plan of the book

Each of the nine sections of the book is a reasonably self-contained unit that expounds a particular pharmacological theme. We have tried to limit the presentation of material to a single occasion, in its most appropriate location. Cross-references are provided, when material is relevant to more than one theme, in preference to succumbing to the temptation to repeat it. Book use that follows the order of the sections will therefore result in minimal following of cross-references, leading to new material but, for the reader intent on acquiring all the contained information on one drug or group of drugs, the index will be an essential resource.

The book opens with a section, the theme of which is those general principles that need no specific drug group, physiological system or disease state for their discussion but that can be exemplified from any or all of the other sections. Unifying concepts within pharmacology, targets of drug action, interaction between drugs and the earlier phases of the process of drug discovery and development are considered as *General pharmacology*. Classical phenomena in General pharmacology (and also Drug disposition and Clinical pharmacology) are, in other books, often illustrated using the drugs (now obsolete) that led to their discovery. We have been careful to illustrate them, instead, with current pharmacotherapeutic agents.

The drugs that act on peripheral excitable tissues by modulating signalling and transduction mechanisms directly related to receptors for the neurotransmitters acetylcholine and noradrenaline impinge on so many physiological systems that they are most efficiently dealt with as a theme, and comprise our second section. This is a theme presented early in the book, because it is in this area that mechanisms of drug action are probably best understood. Also, the system can be used as a model to predict or infer the mechanism of action of drugs in other less well understood areas (e.g. the central nervous system, CNS).

The third section collects together groups of drugs that also act on peripheral tissues but by modulating signalling and transduction mechanisms other than those directly related to receptors for neurotransmitters and hormones. Drug targets including ion channels in the cytoplasmic membranes and enzymes of peripheral cells are brought together here.

The fourth and fifth sections – *Endocrine pharmacology* and *Drug action on the central nervous system* – correspond with the system-based subdivision of the subject common in therapeutic texts, although the former section includes local hormones. Our understanding of drug action in the CNS leans heavily on the concepts of specific interaction with physiological chemical mediators developed in the preceding sections. A second important principle, that of non-specific depressant action on biological function, also emerges.

So far the section themes have been drug interactions with targets in endogenous systems of the human or mammalian body but, in the fifth section, consideration is given to the mechanism of drug action on parasites, be they metazoa, micro-organisms or human neoplastic cells. The emphasis is now on mechanisms by which parasitic cell growth or survival is selectively inhibited.

By now the student has been provided with sufficient information on pharmacodynamics for the name of a drug to be invested with a character that concentrates on the bodily changes induced by drug action. The theme of the seventh section therefore changes from drug action to drug disposition and metabolism – from what drugs do to the body to what the body does to drugs – so that an appreciation of how these factors influence drug action can be gained.

Our eighth section – *Clinical pharmacology* – draws together principles, within the craft of drug treatment of human disease, that are not specific to a disease or symptom. Such issues relate to drug disposition, to social, legal and health-policy considerations and to the unwanted effects of drug therapy.

Our final section – *Pharmacotherapeutics* – illustrates, at least for certain carefully selected disease states, how the principles and concepts of mechanistic pharmacology are exploited in the rational selection of drugs for practical therapeutics. Some other disease states have been dealt with in previous sections, when almost all of the drugs rational for their treatment are described in that section (e.g. Parkinson's disease, infections, cancer).

Policy on unfamiliar words

Words that are unfamiliar to the reader may be part of the technical language of pharmacology or medicine, and all such words we have defined or explained on their first occurrence and represented by underlining (technical term). A second category exists in the ordinary stock of the English language – definitions are not provided in the text and the reader is advised to consult a dictionary.

Text revision

Pharmacology, like most other scientific disciplines, develops rapidly and the perennial problem of any text is that of keeping up to date. We have so far managed to make regular revisions of this book at intervals of approximately 5 years and hope to be able to continue so to do.

We thank all our students, colleagues and correspondents who have explicitly or unconsciously suggested improvements. The editor remains happy to receive suggestions for further improvements from any user of the book.

Acknowledgements

The editor wishes especially to thank Dr Roger Small for preparing the new and altered diagrams, Mrs Beryl Foster for typing the new sections of manuscript, staff at Butterworth-Heinemann for their care and attention in guiding this book through to publication and all of the co-authors for the time invested in evolving common policies and in proof reading.

Aims and objectives

Overall aim

The aim of this book is to provide the sound pharmacological basis on which could be built a rational approach to therapeutics.

Knowledge and understanding objectives

By the end of the book the reader should:

(1) recognize all the therapeutic groups of drugs that form part of the rational management of common diseases;
(2) recognize a selection of the British Pharmacopoeia Commission Approved names of drugs appearing in bold type in the *Notes for prescribers* sections of the *BNF* (latest edition) and be able to group together those drugs that share common pharmacological properties;
(3) know the site and understand the mechanism of action of the members of each pharmacological group of drugs;
(5) know the pharmacological properties of each drug group that are relevant to its therapeutic uses and unwanted effects, with special emphasis on those that can be deduced from a knowledge of the site and mechanism of action.

Skill and competency objectives

By the end of the book the student should be able, knowing:

(1) the primary mechanism of action of a drug, to deduce its pharmacodynamic properties – its actions on cells, tissues, organs, systems and the whole organism;
(2) the physicochemical properties of a drug, to deduce its pharmacokinetic properties;
(3) the general principles of the subject, to assess the described properties and therapeutic claims made for any new drug or group of drugs.

STAFFS UNIVERSITY LIBRARY

List of abbreviations

These abbreviations are used in multiple locations in the book; there are others, just used in a single chapter, that are defined where first used.

ACE	angiotensin converting enzyme
ACh	acetylcholine
ACTH	adrenocorticotrophic hormone, corticotrophin
ADH	antidiuretic hormone
ATP	adenosine triphosphate
AV	atrioventricular
BNF	*British National Formulary*
BP	blood pressure
cAMP	cyclic 3'5'-adenosine monophosphate
cf.	(lit. *confer*) compare
cGMP	cyclic 3'5'-guanosine monophosphate
Cl.	*Clostridium*
CL	clearance
CNS	central nervous system
CoA	coenzyme A
CMPM	Committee on Proprietary Medicinal Products
COMT	catechol-*O*-methyl transferase
CSF	cerebrospinal fluid
CTZ	chemosensitive trigger zone
d-	deci (10^{-1})
Da	Dalton(s)
DAG	diacylglycerol
DHF	dihydrofolate
DNA	deoxyribonucleic acid
dopa	dihydroxyphenylalanine
E.	*Escherichia*
EC_{50}	concentration of drug evoking a half maximal effect
ECF	extracellular fluid
e.g.	(lit. *exampli gratia*) for example
epp	end-plate potential
epsp	excitatory postsynaptic potential
FEV_1	forced expiratory volume in one second

FSH	follicle stimulating hormone
g	gram(s)
GABA	gamma-aminobutyric acid
GFR	glomerular filtration rate
GH	growth hormone
GMP	guanosine monophosphate
GTP	guanosine triphosphate
H.	*Haemophilus*
h	hour(s)
HCG	human chorionic gonadotrophin
HMG	human menopausal gonadotrophin
Hz	Hertz (1 Hertz is 1 cycle per second)
Ig-	immunoglobulin-
i/m	intramuscular(ly)
IP$_3$	inositol 1,4,5-trisphosphate
i/v	intravenous(ly)
k-	kilo- (10^3)
L	litre(s)
LH	luteinizing hormone
lit.	literally
log	logarithm
LT	leukotriene
μ	micro- (10^{-6})
M.	*Mycobacterium*
m	metre(s)
m-	milli- (10^{-3})
MAC	minimum alveolar concentration for anaesthesia
MAO	monoamine oxidase
MFO	mixed function oxidase
MIC	minimum inhibitory concentration
min	minute(s)
mole	gram molecular weight
mRNA	messenger ribonucleic acid
MW	molecular weight
N.	*Neisseria*
n-	nano- (10^{-9})
NA	noradrenaline
NADPH	nicotinamide adenine nucleotide phosphate (reduced)
NSAID	non-steroidal anti-inflammatory drug
p-	pico- (10^{-12})
P.	*Plasmodium*
P-	partial pressure
Pa-	partial pressure in arterial blood
PG	prostaglandin
qv.	(lit. *quod vide*) which see
REM	rapid eye movement
RNA	ribonucleic acid
s	second(s)
SA	sinoatrial
s/c	subcutaneous(ly)

SG	specific gravity
SSRI	selective serotonin re-uptake inhibitor
Staph.	*Staphylococcus*
Str.	*Streptococcus*
$t_{1/2}$	half-time, half-life
THF	tetrahydrofolate
tRNA	transfer RNA
TSH	thyroid stimulating hormone, thyrotrophin
UK	United Kingdom
V	apparent volume of distribution
viz.	(lit. *vide licet*) namely
v/v	volume per unit volume
w/v	weight per unit volume

1

General pharmacology

Aims

- To introduce terminology, such as potency and selectivity, that can be applied to all classes of drugs.
- To illustrate how the three-dimensional structures of most drugs are key to their interaction with their cellular targets.
- To describe the kinds of cellular targets with which drugs interact.
- To provide a mechanistic basis for drug actions and interactions.
- To outline the processes by which new drugs are developed.

Unifying concepts

A drug produces its effects by interacting with biological targets that are chemical components of the body. These chemical components of the body are commonly:

(1) receptors for neurotransmitters, autacoids or hormones;
(2) enzymes;
(3) transport carriers;
(4) membranes.

In most cases ((1)–(3) above) the chemical interaction involves the reversible association of drug with target, based on a complementary relationship between the structure of the drug and the structure of the target.

Dose and concentration

The <u>dose</u> of drug is an amount and has the dimension mass (e.g. units ng, μg, mg, pmole, nmole, μmole). A <u>concentration</u> of drug is an amount per unit volume and has the dimension mass/volume (e.g. units ng/mL, µmole/L). People and animals are given doses of drugs and concentrations are achieved in bodily fluids (see Chapter 7).

The relationship between drug concentration and effect

The magnitude of the effect of a drug is usually related to its concentration at its site of action (within certain limits) in a smoothly graded manner. For example, a piece of intestinal smooth muscle in an organ bath may shorten progressively as the concentration of a spasmogenic drug in the bathing medium is increased. The relationship between the effect and the drug concentration is generally hyperbolic (Figure 1.1a). For convenience, pharmacologists generally relate effect to the logarithm of the drug concentration (Figure 1.1b), which results in log concentration/effect curves that are sigmoid ('S'-shaped) and contain a useful central portion (between approximately 20 and 80% of the maximal effect) where effect is approximately linearly related to the logarithm of the drug concentration.

$EC_{`N'}$ notation

The concentration (or dose) of a drug that evokes a biological effect equivalent to N% of the maximal effect is known as the $EC_{`N'}$ ($ED_{`N'}$), for example, $\underline{EC_{50}}$ means the concentration of drug evoking a half maximal effect (Figure 1.1a).

Potency

The potency of a drug is a measure of the dilution in which it causes a specified effect; thus a drug that evokes the specified effect when present in great dilution (i.e. small concentration) is said to be highly potent.

Most commonly the specified effect used in assessment or comparison of drug potencies is the half maximal effect, thus potency = $1/EC_{50}$. The rank order of potency within a series of drugs is therefore the reverse of

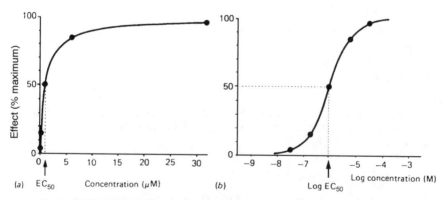

Figure 1.1 Relationship between drug concentration and effect: (a) effect versus concentration; (b) effect versus $\log_{10}$ concentration (the same data are used in both graphs; M = mole/L)

the rank order of their EC_{50} values and is independent of the absolute magnitude of their maximal effects. As drugs commonly have EC_{50} values in the nmole/L range or less, a convenient way of expressing potency uses the pD scale (cf. pH, pK_a). The pD_2 (or pEC_{50}) is defined as the negative $\log_{10}$ of the molar EC_{50} and is 6.0 calculated from the data in Figure 1.1b.

Sensitivity

This is the tissue or target equivalent of potency (see above). In other words, potency is the property of the drug that describes how little of it is needed. Sensitivity is the property of the responding system that describes the concentration at which it responds to a drug. The units of measurement are the same in both cases (e.g. nmole/L). Desensitization or loss of sensitivity is represented by a shift of the concentration/effect relationship towards larger concentrations, not a reduction in the maximum. Thus in Figure 1.17, a shift from curve B to curve A represents the occurrence of desensitization. A change from curve C to curve A does not (it represents the occurrence of reduced responsiveness with slight potentiation).

Maximal response

Drugs can differ in the maximal effect they produce. Thus in Figure 1.2 **morphine** is more potent than **aspirin** as an analgesic but also produces a greater maximal effect.

Selectivity

Selectivity is the central theme of pharmacology and is the phenomenon that allows drugs to be useful. No drug is absolutely specific – that is produces only one (desirable) effect at very high potency. Selectivity is

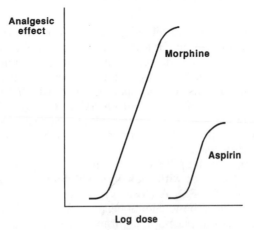

Figure 1.2 Relationships between log dose and pain relief for two drugs to illustrate differing maximal responses

the term used to describe the ability of a given dose or concentration of a drug to produce one effect rather than another. In quantitative terms, selectivity is expressed as the ratio of the potency for effect A to the potency for effect B.

$$\text{Selectivity} = \frac{\text{potency for effect A}}{\text{potency for effect B}}$$

If effect A is the desired (therapeutic) action of the drug and effect B an undesired (adverse) effect, then the selectivity is equivalent to the therapeutic index (see pp. 268, 372).

Theories of drug action

Drugs may be divided into two general classes on the basis of their mechanism of action:

(1) structurally non-specific;
(2) structurally specific.

By structure we mean the distribution of charge within a molecule and the spatial distribution of these potential binding sites.

Structurally non-specific drugs

Certain chemically dissimilar drugs can affect biological activity in a similar manner. The action of these drugs is not related to their precise three-dimensional structure. These drugs are said to be structurally non-specific. It is the characteristic of structurally non-specific drugs that:

(1) small (or even large) changes in structure may have negligible effects on activity;
(2) they do not display stereoselectivity;
(3) drugs with widely different structure share a common pharmacological action.

The only examples of structurally non-specific drugs of profound pharmacological interest are the general anaesthetic agents. General anaesthesia may be brought about by a wide variety of chemically dissimilar compounds, including inert gases (xenon), halogenated hydrocarbons (**halothane**, *isoflurane*), cyclic hydrocarbons (cyclopropane), ethers (diethyl ether), alcohols (ethanol), and oxides of nitrogen (**nitrous oxide**) (Figure 1.3).

The pharmacological activity of the general anaesthetic agents is not attributable to a common three-dimensional structure but rather to a common physical property.

Figure 1.3 compares the potency of a range of anaesthetic agents having widely different structures with their lipid solubility expressed as a partition coefficient (see p. 330). A close correlation exists, implying that the drugs are general anaesthetic agents because they are lipophilic. The site of this lipid phase is the plasma membranes of neurones within the brain and it represents a target for interaction with these structurally non-specific drugs.

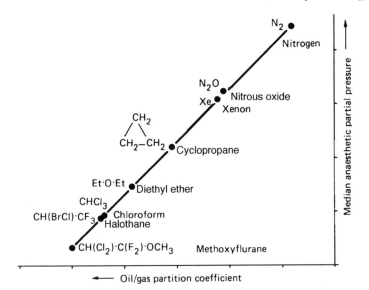

Figure 1.3 The high correlation in mice between potency as a general anaesthetic agent and oil/gas partition coefficient despite very varied structure (both scales are logarithmic)

Structurally specific drugs

Structurally specific drugs have the following characteristics:

(1) they produce their effects at small concentrations;
(2) minor changes in structure have major effects on activity;
(3) they commonly show stereoselectivity.

The pharmacological activity of structurally specific drugs results from an interaction between drug molecules and targets, both of which have precise three-dimensional structures. Drug molecules must satisfy different structural requirements for each kind of target. The interaction between drug and target must be considered from two aspects:

(1) the distribution of charge within the molecule;
(2) the spatial distribution of these centres of charge.

Charge distribution

Structural components that convey centres of charge in drug molecules are ions and dipoles.

The majority of ions result from the weakly acidic or basic nature of drugs, usually in the form of charged $-NH_3^+$ and $-COO^-$ substituents. Note the importance of pH and pK_a. Less common are the quaternary nitrogen compounds, $-NR_4^+$.

Dipoles arise because there is an uneven electron distribution in chemical bonds between atoms of different electronegativities. The greater the difference in electronegativities, the greater the dipole moment. Common atoms in drug molecules (and their targets) in ascending order of electronegativity are H, P, C, S, N, Cl, O, F. Thus the –OH group has a strong dipole moment, whereas –CH has a weak dipole moment.

The same principles must be applied to the structure of the target of drug action – revise the structures of proteins, sugars, lipids and nucleic acids.

The complementary structures of drug and target then result in the formation of various kinds of bond.

Polar bonds

Ion–ion bonds

This kind of bond has a strength of the same order (approximately 500 kJ/mole) as that of a covalent bond.

Ion–dipole, dipole–dipole

Such bonds are very common in the interaction between drugs and their cellular targets. They are weaker (approximately 150 kJ/mole) than ion–ion bonds.

Covalent bonds

The familiar covalent bond is unusual in drug/target interactions. It is a very strong bond (approximately 500 kJ/mole). Examples are the covalent bond formed in alkylation of DNA by some cytotoxic drugs, and the phosphorylation of the cholinesterase enzyme. Since the process is irreversible, such bonds are relatively unimportant in therapeutics but are of importance in toxicology.

Hydrogen bonds

The hydrogen bond is an electrostatic attraction between a proton and the unshared electrons of an atom (usually O). It is a weak bond (approximately 30 kJ/mole) but of enormous biochemical importance. Without the hydrogen bond water would not exist as a liquid and it is the bond largely responsible for determining the shape of proteins and nucleic acids. Only the hydrogen atom can be involved in such a bond because it possesses no inner electron shell, which would otherwise contribute a repulsive influence. Common substituents that may be involved in hydrogen bonding are –OH and –NH–.

Coordinate bonds

Chelates

Chelates result from a coordinate bond between electron donor atoms (commonly N, O and S) and a metal. Two or more atoms donate pairs of electrons holding the metal ion in a ring. Chelate formation is important in drugs used to treat metal poisoning (e.g. **desferrioxamine**) and in drug toxicity (e.g. the binding of tetracyclines with Ca^{2+}).

Van der Waals forces

In neutral molecules (hydrocarbon chains, phenyl substituents), centres of positive and negative charge do not always correspond and the substituent behaves like a little magnet. Typical attraction might occur between a benzene ring of a drug and a benzene ring of an amino acid component of the target. The bond is highly dependent on very close proximity of the participating substituents and is a weak bond (approximately 2 kJ/mole).

Drug shape

The preceding section explains why parts of molecules carry charge, and therefore how drugs can associate with their targets. The other consideration is the shape that holds these centres of charge in a conformation that complements that of the target.

Many drug molecules have rigid frameworks that carry essential substituents in key positions. Good examples of rigid frameworks include the phenanthrene structure of **morphine**, the steroid nucleus and the phenothiazine ring structure.

Exercise: Study the shape of the steroid nucleus. Compare the structures of oestradiol and testosterone (see Figure 4.7).

Note that many neurotransmitters are flexible structures on which essential substituents are arranged. A single neurotransmitter can therefore adopt different conformations and can consequently interact with closely related targets with different stereochemical structures.

Exercise: Write down the structures of acetylcholine and 5-hydroxy-tryptamine (5-HT). Identify the important parts of the molecule that could be involved in association with its targets. Note how these centres of charge can be arranged in different conformations.

Although a flexible neurotransmitter may be able to effect transmission at more than one target, more selective agonist activity can often be achieved by synthesizing stereochemically more rigid derivatives. One such derivative may hold the essential components of the neurotransmitter in one fixed conformation, a different rigid analogue holding the same components in a different shape.

Exercise: Compare the structures of acetylcholine, nicotine and muscarine (Figure 1.4).

Isomerism

Optical Isomerism

If the four substituents around a carbon atom differ, they can be arranged in one of two ways (two enantiomers) that are mirror images of each other. If all three of these substituents are involved in target binding, it is clear that only one of these mirror-image conformations can associate with a rigid target (Figure 1.5).

Laevo and dextro Such isomers are distinguished by their ability to rotate the plane of polarization of light to the right (+), or to the left (−).

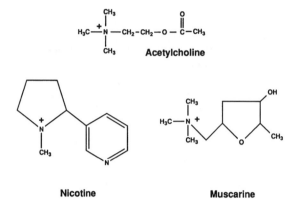

Figure 1.4 The structures of acetylcholine, nicotine and muscarine

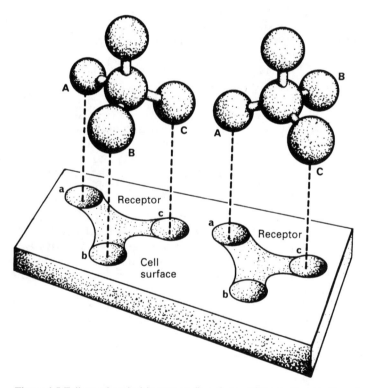

Figure 1.5 Failure of optical isomer to fit a three-point receptor binding site

Note that this terminology only distinguishes isomers on the basis of their ability to rotate the plane of polarization of light but does not describe the absolute configuration of a structure. At one time the D-, L- system was used to describe absolute configuration, but this has been largely replaced by the *R*-, *S*- system. A 50 : 50 mixture of the two enantiomers is called a racemate.

Rectus and sinister   The *R*- and *S*- configuration system of nomenclature enables one to write out the configuration of a drug given its name, or vice versa (neither of the other systems permits this directly). To determine the configuration of a molecule, first identify the <u>chiral</u> (asymmetric) carbon atom (i.e. that with four different substituents). Now assign an order of <u>priority</u> to the four atoms attached to the chiral carbon atom. Priority is based upon atomic number – the higher the atomic number, the higher is the priority. If two atoms are the same, go to the next atom of the attached group until a difference is found. If there is a double or triple bond, double or triple the atomic number. (The atomic numbers of the commoner elements in drug molecules are: H = 1, C = 6, N = 7, O = 8, F = 9, P = 15, S = 16, Cl = 17, Br = 35.)

Now arrange the molecule so that it can be viewed from opposite the atom with the lowest priority (commonly –H). If the priority of the three remaining atoms descends in a clockwise manner, the configuration is designated *R*- (Latin *rectus* = right). If the priorities descend anticlockwise, the configuration is *S*- (Latin *sinister* = left).

For *isoprenaline* (Figure 1.6a), the order of priority of the four groups attached to the chiral carbon is: –OH > catechol > –CH$_2$– > –H. The structure shown in Figure 1.6a is rearranged with the –H away from the eye (Figure 1.6b). The priorities can then be seen to fall in a clockwise direction. The conformation of *isoprenaline* shown in Figure 1.6a is therefore *R*-isoprenaline. In fact, this isomer rotates plane-polarized light to the left, so its full description is *R*-(–)-isoprenaline. This isomer is a potent agonist at β-adrenoceptors as there is an appropriate contact with the protein of the receptor. *S*-(+)-isoprenaline is much less potent. Increasingly, only the

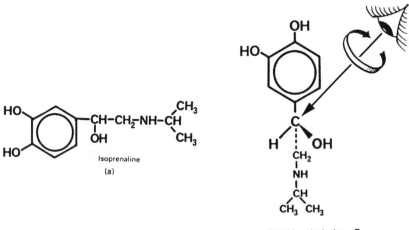

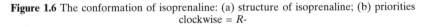

Figure 1.6 The conformation of isoprenaline: (a) structure of isoprenaline; (b) priorities clockwise = *R*-

active enantiomers are used as therapeutic agents, rather than the racemate.

If a drug has more than one chiral centre (*ephedrine* has two), the *R/S* configuration at each centre must be defined.

Reminder: There is no correlation between the *R*- and *S*-, and (+) and (-) systems. They tell you different things about the molecule.

Cis–trans *isomerism*

Two pairs of similar substituents can be arranged about a double bond in one of two ways. When the same (or similar) substituents are on the same side of the bond, the isomer is designated *cis*, when on opposite sides, *trans*.

Exercise: Compare the structures of the two isomers of *stilboestrol* (Figure 1.7).

Similar isomers can occur about a cyclopropane ring (e.g. *tranylcypromine*).

Preferred conformation

Although flexible molecules can theoretically exist in a wide range of conformations, a molecule is most stable in one, preferred, conformation. An indication of preferred conformation has been achieved by X-ray crystallography but nowadays can be computed.

Generally, the preferred conformation of a drug is in a fully extended shape. The shape of *isoprenaline* as drawn in Figure 1.6a is extended. (A non-preferred conformation would be with the side-chain rotated so that the amino group lies above the benzene ring.) The long side-chain of a tricyclic antidepressant drug (see p. 233) would lie distant from the rings.

Steric hindrance

The substitution of a group (usually bulky) close to a critical part of a drug molecule can have a profound effect on the stability and/or pharmacological properties of a drug.

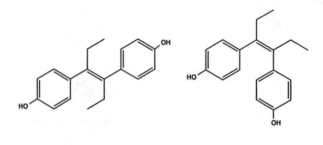

Trans - stilboestrol   *Cis* - stilboestrol

Figure 1.7 The two isomers of *stilboestrol*

Such substitution may:

(1) Render a drug resistant to enzymic breakdown (cf. acetylcholine and methacholine; **benzylpenicillin** and **flucloxacillin**).
(2) Turn a substrate for an enzyme into an inhibitor of the enzyme (cf. phenylethylamine and **phenelzine** or *tranylcypromine*).
(3) Alter the selectivity of an agonist (cf. noradrenaline and *isoprenaline*).
(4) Turn an agonist into an antagonist (cf. *adrenaline* and **propranolol** (the bulky substituent is the second benzene ring); **morphine** and **naloxone**).

Chemical structure and drug disposition

Changes in drug structure also alter the disposition of drugs (see p. 328). For example, the removal of the hydroxyl substituents from a catecholamine results not only in a drug (amphetamine) that cannot interact directly with adrenoceptors but also in a drug that can enter the central nervous system (CNS) easily as it is more lipid-soluble. The quaternization of **atropine** confers some activity at nicotinic acetylcholine receptors but also restricts it to the periphery as it renders the drug more water-soluble.

Summary

(1) The effect of a drug usually exhibits a sigmoidal relationship to the logarithm of its concentration.
(2) The effect of a drug can be measured by its potency and maximal response.
(3) Selectivity is the ratio of potencies for two effects.
(4) Structurally non-specific drugs share the common physical property of lipophilicity; general anaesthetic agents are examples.
(5) For most drugs their three-dimensional structure is crucial and complimentary to that of a part of their target macromolecule.
(6) Important bonds between drug and target molecules, in descending order of strength, are: ion–ion = covalent > ion–dipole, dipole–dipole > hydrogen bond > Van der Waals forces.
(7) The stereochemistry of a drug can be defined by optical isomerism, *R*- and *S*- configuration and *cis–trans* isomerism.

Targets of drug action

A drug-induced response can be considered at its simplest level as consisting of three stages:

(1) The combination of the drug with a target molecule (the binding or occupation process).

STAFFS UNIVERSITY LIBRARY

(2) The presumed change in the conformation of the target molecule plus the initial biochemical or electrical events (the transduction process); the transduction process includes the initial ion channel opening and ion movements (for ligand-gated ion channels) and G-protein translocation and coupling to the effector protein (for G-protein coupled receptors) (see below).

(3) Subsequent biological effects (the effector processes).

Techniques of molecular biology have revealed the precise structures of many kinds of drug targets. Most are proteins, although a few are lipids or nucleic acids. The location of these targets includes the cell plasma membrane, the cytoplasm and the nucleus. The natures of the drug target molecule, the transduction and effector processes provide a rational basis for features of the drug response such as time to onset and offset. Transduction results in amplification of the original stimulus. One way of classifying targets is illustrated in Figure 1.8 and listed below:

Ligand-gated and voltage-sensitive ion channels

These targets are part of *trans*-plasma membrane ion-selective channels. Binding of some drugs to the target protein causes a change in the conformation of the channel that increases its permeability to a particular ion (e.g. Na^+, Ca^{2+}, K^+, Cl^-). Large numbers of ions rapidly move down an electrochemical gradient and initiate a response in that cell. Hence the time between drug binding to the target and the initial biological response is in milliseconds. Well-understood examples of this kind of target are acetylcholine (or nicotine) at the nicotinic acetylcholine receptor (see p. 52) and γ-aminobutyric acid (GABA) at the $GABA_A$ receptor on Cl^--channels (see p. 223).

Alternatively, a drug may bind to part of an ion channel and so prevent it increasing its permeability when a naturally occurring stimulus is

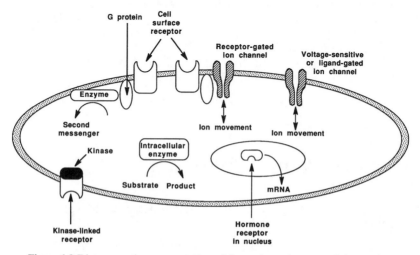

Figure 1.8 Diagrammatic representation of the variety of targets of drug action

applied. For example, local anaesthetic agents (see p. 105) and blockers of L-type Ca^{2+} channels (see p. 127) prevent voltage-sensitive Na^+ channels and Ca^{2+} channels respectively opening in response to depolarization.

Cell-surface receptors, G-protein coupled

These targets generally have highly conserved structures, the amino acid sequences of which includes seven highly lipophilic segments that span the cell membrane. Combination of the appropriate drug with specific amino acids in the target causes it to change its conformation. The receptor is now able to bind to one of a family of guanosine triphosphate-dependent proteins known as G-proteins.

These G-proteins are in turn secondarily linked to activation or inhibition of a cell membrane or intracellular enzyme. Examples of these enzymes are adenylyl cyclase that converts ATP to cyclic AMP (cAMP), and phospholipase C that converts phosphatidyl inositol (4,5) bisphosphate to inositol (1,3,5) trisphosphate (IP_3) and diacylglycerol (DAG). These second messengers form part of a cascade of intracellular events, usually leading to a change in the cytoplasmic Ca^{2+} concentration.

Alternatively, the secondary linkage of the G-protein can be to an ion channel, increasing its permeability to a particular ion (e.g. Na^+, Ca^{2+}, K^+, Cl^-).

The time to onset of drug response is slower than with drug action at ligand-gated ion channels, due to the need to initiate a cascade of biochemical processes, and is generally a few seconds.

Drugs interacting with this kind of target include agonists at β_2-adrenoceptors (see p. 91), agonists at muscarinic acetylcholine receptors (see p. 68) and agonists at H_1 histamine receptors (see p. 200).

Kinase-linked receptors

These targets are proteins embedded in the cell membrane with a linked kinase enzyme as an integral part of the same protein on the intracellular side. The targets for insulin and many growth factors are of this kind and are linked to tyrosine kinase and serine/threonine kinases respectively. There are few drug examples. Binding of insulin to its target activates the tyrosine kinase to phosphorylate itself, which in turn activates many intracellular enzymes. Time to onset of effect for insulin is measured in seconds. However, the onset and offset of action of growth factors can be hours or days.

Pumps and carrier molecules

These targets are proteins embedded in the cell membrane that aid transportation of ions or organic molecules into and out of cells. Drugs, when they combine with recognition sites on the proteins, modify (usually depress) the pump or carrier function. The onset of effect is rapid, within seconds, but many minutes or hours may be needed for the full effect of the drug if this depends on the changed distribution of the carried molecule. Drug examples include the tricyclic antidepressant agents and cocaine inhibiting the noradrenaline pump into neurones (see p. 87), and **digoxin** inhibition of the Na^+/K^+-ATPase pump of cardiac cells (see p. 122).

Enzymes

The normal and abnormal functioning of cells requires enzymes. It is, therefore, not surprising that the targets for many drugs are enzymes. Most drugs inhibit enzyme function. The pharmacological effect is, therefore, a consequence of an increased concentration of substrate (e.g. acetylcholine with inhibitors of acetylcholinesterase, see p. 71) or a decreased concentration of product (e.g. angiotensin II with inhibitors of angiotensin-converting enzyme, see p. 196; eicosanoids with **aspirin**-related drugs, see p. 213).

Inhibitors of enzymes can be classified by the mechanism of their inhibition:

(1) Competitive reversible inhibitors – the inhibitor and substrate reversibly compete for the active site of the enzyme. Examples include *ibuprofen* and cyclo-oxygenase; **captopril** and angiotensin-converting enzyme; **trimethoprim** and bacterial dihydrofolate dehydrogenase; *moclobemide* and monoamine oxidase; **allopurinol** and xanthine oxidase.

(2) Competitive irreversible inhibitors – these compounds can be of two kinds:
  (a) active-site-directed irreversible inhibitors in which the drug binds by covalent binding to part of the active site of the enzyme. Examples include acetylation of cyclo-oxygenase by **aspirin**; phosphorylation of acetylcholinesterase by organophosphorus compounds; acylation of bacterial glycopeptide transpeptidase by penicillins;
  (b) mechanism-based irreversible inhibitors, also called 'suicide' inhibitors, where the enzyme converts the drug to another compound that irreversibly binds to its active site. Examples include *clavulanic acid* and bacterial β-lactamase; **phenelzine** and monoamine oxidase.

(3) Non-competitive reversible inhibitors – the drug interacts with a site on the enzyme that is not the active centre, or alters the enzyme indirectly. An example is **paracetamol** and cyclo-oxygenase.

The time to onset for a significant drug effect varies considerably, depending on the rate of conversion of substrate to product. The offset of effect may be rapid if the drug is a competitive inhibitor, as the effect declines once the drug is removed from the target enzyme. However, if a drug is an irreversible inhibitor then the effect could be prolonged, only terminating when new enzyme is synthesized.

There are but few examples of drugs that are activators of enzymes, either by direct or indirect means. An example is the nitrovasodilator group (**glyceryl trinitrate**, *sodium nitroprusside*). These drugs are metabolized to release nitric oxide which in turn activates the enzyme guanylyl cyclase.

Nuclear hormone receptors

The targets for most steroid hormones, and drugs that are close analogues, are large soluble proteins found in the nucleus. Binding of the appropriate steroid drug causes it to change shape. The protein–steroid complex can now bind to defined regions of DNA, causing an increase in transcribing RNA-polymerase activity and messenger RNA (mRNA) production. The subsequent cellular response, due to altered protein synthesis, may take hours or days to occur. Drugs that act via this kind of target include glucocorticosteroid (see p. 181), oestrogenic (see p. 163) and androgenic (see p. 171) agents.

The term receptor is sometimes used to encompass all drug targets or recognition sites. However, receptor is better restricted to those protein molecules that, when an appropriate drug (an agonist see below) combines with them, initiate a response. Hence pumps, carriers and enzymes are not strictly receptors for drugs.

Drug/target interactions and response magnitude

Active and passive biological responses: agonists and antagonists

A drug-induced response from a living cell is said to be an active response if the drug produces the change in ongoing activity even when the cell is isolated from all external biological control factors, such as neurotransmitters and hormones. Active responses may be either excitatory (depolarization of the membranes of excitable cells, muscle contraction, increased glandular secretion, growth) or inhibitory (hyperpolarization of the membranes of excitable cells, muscle relaxation, reduced pacemaker frequency).

In contrast, the response is said to be a passive one if the drug acts to remove the effects of some endogenous or external biological factor regulating cellular function (e.g. an antagonist acting at an inhibitory synapse at which there is a basal release of neurotransmitter).

A drug that induces an active response by activating receptors is known as an agonist, whether the response is an increase or decrease in cellular activity. Some drugs behave like agonists but act through an intermediary and do not themselves activate the receptor responsible for the response. They are commonly referred to as indirectly acting agonists (e.g. tyramine, see p. 82).

Of the drugs that attach to a particular receptor site:

(1) Agonists form a drug/receptor complex that triggers an active response from the cell.
(2) Antagonists form a drug/receptor complex that does not evoke an active response from the cell. Antagonists simply prevent attachment of agonists to the receptor. The response to the antagonist is therefore passive – blockade of the effects of an agonist.

The binding of drugs to receptor sites

The following text concentrates upon drug/plasma membrane receptor interactions, but similar principles apply to drug interaction with the other biological targets described above.

The binding of drugs to their receptor sites can be described in terms of the law of mass action:

$$\text{drug} + \text{receptor} \underset{k_{-1}}{\overset{k_{+1}}{\rightleftharpoons}} \text{drug/receptor complex}$$

Association rate constant $= k_{+1}$
Dissociation rate constant $= k_{-1}$

When a drug is added to the system, the initial concentration of the drug/receptor complex is zero but increases as the association reaction progresses. As the concentration of the drug/receptor complex increases, the rate at which dissociation occurs also increases until the rates of dissociation and association are equal, i.e. the system comes to an equilibrium. The occupancy of receptors is frequently a rapid, reversible and dynamic process. The actual time that an individual receptor is occupied by a drug molecule is measured in milliseconds. What are the concentrations of each of the reactants when the reaction is at equilibrium?

Let us assume that:

(1) The concentration of the drug is so great that it is not significantly reduced by maximal formation of the drug/receptor complex.
(2) One molecule of drug combines with one molecule of receptor.
    Molar concentration of free drug $= [D]$
    Initial (that is, total) concentration of receptors $= R$
    Concentration of occupied receptors $= r$
    Concentration of unoccupied receptors $= R - r$

According to the law of mass action:
    the rate of association (the forward reaction) $= k_{+1}[D](R - r)$
    the rate of dissociation (the backward reaction) $= k_{-1}r$

When equilibrium is reached these two rates are equal:

$$k_{+1}[D] (R-r) = k_{-1}r$$

Rearranging:

$$\frac{k_{-1}}{k_{+1}} = K_d = [D] \frac{(R-r)}{r} \tag{1.1}$$

where K_d is known as the equilibrium dissociation constant.

The equation is often rearranged and presented in terms of receptor occupation:

$$r = \frac{[D] R}{(K_d + [D])}$$

Both of these are equations for a rectangular hyperbola, that is, a curve relating two variables (in the case of Equation 1.1, $[D]$ and $(R - r) / r$)

that vary in such a way that their product (K_d) is constant (noting that R is constant as well). All rectangular hyperbolas can in fact be described by just two parameters:

(1) The maximal value of the dependent variable (r).
(2) A constant, called the location parameter, that fixes the position of the curve on the axis of the independent variable ($[D]$).

In this case, the maximal value that r can have is R, i.e. when all the receptors are occupied. The value of the location parameter is K_d, the equilibrium dissociation constant, which has the same units as $[D]$, that is, those of concentration: mole/L.

Some pharmacologists use the equilibrium association constant (K_a) or affinity constant instead of the dissociation constant. This term is simply the reciprocal of K_d:

$$K_a = \frac{1}{K_d}$$

The units of K_a are L/mole (dilution rather than concentration).

It can easily be shown that K_d is the concentration of drug ($[D]$) that causes half the receptors to be occupied, that is, when $r = R/2$.

Radioligand binding

Radioligand binding is a powerful technique that enables the direct measurement of drug occupancy of receptors.

The technique involves homogenization of tissues to prepare membranes containing receptors. These membranes are incubated with varying concentrations of radioactively (e.g. ^{3}H, ^{125}I) labelled drug for sufficient time to allow equilibration between drug and receptors. In this context, drugs are also called ligands. The membranes containing bound drug are separated from unbound drug by filtration or centrifugation and counted for radioactivity. As some drug may bind also to non-receptor sites in the membranes (non-specific binding), the experiment is repeated in the presence of a saturating concentration of a second compound that prevents binding to the specific receptor sites. Hence, by difference, the specific binding can be determined. The data can then be drawn as shown in Figure 1.9.

From such an experiment the following can be calculated:

B_{max} = number of receptors in the membrane (units mole/mg of tissue)

K_d = concentration of drug to occupy 50% of the receptors (units mole/L)

The K_d is, therefore, a reciprocal measure of the ability of the drug to bind to its target, which is called the affinity. If a drug requires only a very small concentration to occupy 50% of the receptors, it is said to have high affinity. By contrast, if a large concentration is needed, then it has low affinity. K_d (mole/L) can be converted to a pK_d ($-\log_{10}K_d$; *note* analogy with pD_2).

Note: both agonists and antagonists have affinity for their receptors.

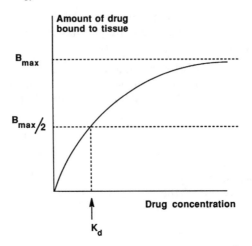

Figure 1.9 Saturation curve for a drug binding to receptors in membranes

The triggering of responses by agonists: intrinsic efficacy

Our knowledge of the mechanism by which an agonist triggers an active biological response is still incomplete. However, it is likely that occupancy of a receptor by an agonist causes a change in the conformation of the protein of the receptor molecule (transduction). This transduction in turn triggers the effector processes. Modern receptor occupancy theories propose that drugs have a property that governs their ability to trigger an active biological response once they have combined with a receptor. Different terms for this property have been used in the past, but the most useful term now is <u>intrinsic efficacy</u>. It is envisaged that agonist drugs with high intrinsic efficacy can evoke the maximal effect of which the biological system is capable. Such drugs are known as full agonists and may even be able to elicit the maximum possible effect without occupying all the receptors if the efficiency of coupling to the effector processes is high. In such circumstances, the fraction of receptors not occupied by the drug is known as <u>receptor reserve</u> (or <u>spare receptors</u>), and the EC_{50} of the agonist can be smaller than its K_d.

A pure antagonist can occupy receptors but does not trigger a response. Hence, it has a reasonable affinity (measured by K_d) for the receptors but zero intrinsic efficacy.

There are drugs that are intermediate between full agonists and antagonists – they are called <u>partial agonists</u>. When given by themselves they can evoke an active response but cannot evoke the maximal response of which the biological system is capable, despite occupying all available receptors. They have reasonable affinity but low intrinsic efficacy. The magnitude of the maximal effect of a partial agonist is lesser in tissues with a smaller receptor reserve. When given with a full agonist they reduce the response to that agonist by competing for the same receptors. Partial agonists that are therapeutically exploited include those acting at β-adrenoceptors (see p. 96) and at opioid receptors (see p. 242).

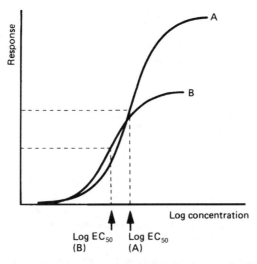

Figure 1.10 Drug B is more potent than drug A but has smaller intrinsic activity

The term intrinsic activity is used simply to describe the maximal effect an agonist can produce as a fraction (or %) of the maximum that can be produced by a full agonist. Thus in Figure 1.10, if drug A is a full agonist, i.e. has an intrinsic activity of 1.0 (100%), drug B has an intrinsic activity of 0.6 (60%). Intrinsic activity, which is a descriptive property within one tissue, should not be confused with intrinsic efficacy, which is a property of a drug and is independent of tissue properties.

The concentration of a drug needed to evoke an agonist action is dependent upon its affinity, its intrinsic efficacy and the total concentration of receptors.

Clinical or therapeutic effectiveness is often abbreviated to efficacy, when it needs to be clearly distinguished from intrinsic efficacy.

Identification and classification of drugs and their targets

Historically, drug groups and their targets have been identified and named in relation to the activity of naturally occurring agonists for receptors (e.g. noradrenaline acts at adrenoceptors, oestradiol at oestrogen receptors) or substrates for enzymes (e.g. angiotensin I is metabolized to angiotensin II by angiotensin-converting enzyme).

However, most major receptor types and enzymes comprise a number of subtypes. Among the criteria that have been used to support the idea of subtypes of receptors have been the existence of more than one:

(1) rank order of relative potency of agonists (comparison of pD_2 values);
(2) rank order of relative potency of antagonists (comparison of pA_2 values; see p. 24);

Table 1.1 Subgroups of drug targets

Target designation	Cross reference
Skeletal muscle and neural nicotinic acetylcholine receptors	Tables 2.2 and 2.4
Monoamine oxidase	Page 85
β_1- and β_2-adrenoceptors	Table 2.13
Phosphodiesterase	Page 131
H_1 and H_2 histamine receptors	Table 4.16
Angiotensin converting enzyme	Page 196
5-Hydroxytryptamine receptors	Page 203
Opioid receptors	Page 242

(3) rank order of affinity of compounds measured by ligand binding (comparison of pK_d values).

Similar criteria of more than one rank order of rate of metabolism of substrates or rank order of potency for inhibitors of an enzyme have been used to suggest the idea of isoenzymes.

Examples of subdivision of drug targets that have been identified in this way are presented in Table 1.1.

The reasoning has been that differences in order of potency or affinity must relate to differences in target structure. These conventional pharmacological methods of classifying targets are now combined with techniques drawn from molecular biology. The exact amino acid sequences of most of the common targets are now known, and the kind of target in any particular tissue can now be determined almost as conveniently by the techniques of molecular biology as by the older conventional techniques. However, molecular biology has revealed kinds of target with no known function and targets with small differences in their amino acid sequences, which appear not to differ in their sensitivities to drugs. Furthermore, techniques of molecular biology cannot yet be relied upon to give a true estimate of the potency or intrinsic efficacy of a drug. Consequently, conventional pharmacological techniques must still be employed at some stage in the development of new drugs.

Selectivity is used to describe properties of individual drugs within groups of drugs (in parallel with the use of the term on page 3). Thus, the antagonists at β-adrenoceptors (**propranolol, atenolol**) are highly selective for β-adrenoceptors; that is, they act at β-adrenoceptors at concentrations several orders of magnitude lower than that at any other kind of receptor, including α-adrenoceptors. Therefore, they are called selective antagonists at β-adrenoceptors. However, **propranolol** is sometimes described also, confusingly, as a non-selective antagonist at β-adrenoceptors because it acts at two subtypes of adrenoceptors, namely β_1- and β_2-adrenoceptors, at similar concentrations. **Atenolol**, on the other hand, is 10–100 times more potent at β_1- than at β_2-adrenoceptors and is hence described as a selective antagonist at β_1-adrenoceptors.

The connection between the primary mechanism of action of a drug and its pharmacodynamic properties

The molecular mechanism of action (e.g. of some agent acting at a molecular target in vascular smooth muscle) leads to:

(1) Direct and immediate consequences:
   (a) change in cellular function (e.g. contractile state of smooth muscle cells of arterioles);
   (b) change in tissue function (e.g. radius of lumen of arterioles);
   (c) change in organ function (e.g. resistance to blood flow of vascular bed).
(2) Indirect and delayed consequences:
   (a) change in organ function (e.g. modulation of change in vascular bed resistance by homeostatic reflexes);
   (b) change in system function (e.g. modulation of cardiac and integrated cardiovascular function by homeostatic reflexes);
   (c) change in whole organism function (e.g. those of brain function arising from changed perfusion).

In particular disease states, these changes could be:

- beneficial (e.g. hypertension, angina pectoris);
- unwanted (e.g. orthostatic hypotension).

Summary

(1) An active biological response induced by a drug is a consequence of its binding to a target molecule, transduction to an initial biochemical or electrical event and the effector process.
(2) Targets of drug action include ligand-gated and voltage-sensitive ion channels, G-protein-coupled cell-surface receptors, kinase-linked receptors, pumps and carrier molecules, enzymes and nuclear hormone receptors.
(3) The time to onset and offset of drug effect is determined by the molecular mechanism of action.
(4) Agonists occupy receptors and induce active responses.
(5) Antagonists occupy receptors and prevent attachment of agonists; they may evoke passive responses.
(6) The technique of radioligand binding enables the determination of the number of receptors (B_{max}) and the drug concentration to occupy one half of the receptors (K_d).
(7) Affinity is a measure of the ability of a drug to bind to its target.
(8) Intrinsic efficacy is a measure of the ability of a drug to evoke an active response.
(9) Subdivision of drug targets can be achieved by molecular structure or functional criteria.

Interactions between drugs

Antagonism

Antagonism is the name given to the interaction between two drugs when the biological effect of the two drugs together is smaller than the expected sum of their individual effects (Figure 1.11).

The many mechanisms by which antagonism can occur may be divided into two principal kinds:

(1) Where the concentration of agonist at its site of action is reduced by the antagonist (i.e. it alters agonist disposition (pharmacokinetic antagonism, discussed on page 440)).

(2) Where the concentration of agonist at its site of action is not reduced by the antagonist. This kind (pharmacodynamic antagonism) may be due to direct or indirect mechanisms.

Direct mechanisms of pharmacodynamic antagonism

The agonist and antagonist share the same receptors. Antagonists, by occupying the receptors themselves, prevent the attachment of agonist

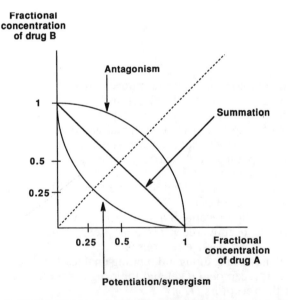

Figure 1.11 The method of mixtures used to reveal interactions between two drugs having qualitatively similar effects. An equi-effective concentration (1) of each drug (A, B) acting alone is determined. Mixtures are assayed to determine at what fractions (or multiples) of these concentrations equi-effectiveness occurs. The coordinates of equi-effective mixtures are joined by a line (isobole) that is straight under addition; the more strongly concave the greater is the potentiation and the more strongly convex the greater is the antagonism.

molecules to the receptors. There are two main kinds of pharmacody-namic antagonism: competitive and non-equilibrium (or irreversible).

Competitive antagonism

The agonist and antagonist compete for the same receptors. Both agents combine with the receptor in a readily reversible fashion, so the propor-tion of receptors occupied by each agent at equilibrium is determined by their concentrations and their K_d values. The proportion of receptors occupied by the competitive antagonist at equilibrium can be reduced by increasing the concentration of agonist. This means that, in the continued presence of the antagonist, the same response can be achieved by provid-ing a larger concentration of agonist.

The effects of a competitive antagonist on the shape and position of the log concentration/effect curve of an agonist are shown in Figure 1.12. Increasing the concentration of antagonist causes progressive parallel shifts of the log concentration/effect curve of the agonist to the right along the log concentration axis. The central slope of the curve is unchanged and the maximal effect is undiminished.

The magnitude of the antagonism is expressed as the antilog of the rightward displacement of the curve: that is, the equi-effective agonist concentration ratio. As the concentration of the competitive antagonist is increased, the shift in the agonist log concentration/effect curve increases. The increment in shift is a simple function of the increment in concen-tration of the competitive antagonist.

Competitive antagonism is sometimes described as <u>surmountable</u> antag-onism, a term that implies that both the antagonist dissociates from the receptors and the full maximal response can be restored. However, note that even when the response has been restored by increasing the concen-tration of agonist (that is the antagonism has been surmounted), the antag-onism is still present and its extent can be expressed by the increase in

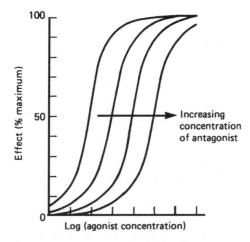

Figure 1.12 Competitive antagonism

concentration of agonist needed to cause the same response as in the absence of antagonist.

There are many therapeutically important competitive antagonists, including: **atropine** antagonism of acetylcholine at muscarinic acetylcholine receptors; **tamoxifen** antagonism of oestradiol at oestrogen receptors; **naloxone** antagonism of **morphine** and β-endorphin at opioid receptors; **cimetidine** antagonism of histamine at H_1 receptors; **propranolol** antagonism of adrenaline at β-adrenoceptors.

Measuring potency is more difficult for a competitive antagonist than for an agonist, as these antagonists do not cause active responses. However the potency of an antagonist, as for an agonist (see p. 2), is still a dilution. The specified effect is the rightward shift in the agonist concentration/effect curve (equi-effective concentration ratio). A plot of the log (equi-effective concentration ratio –1), which is the extent of antagonism, against the –log molar concentration of antagonist (Figure 1.13) summarizes a log concentration/effect relationship for an antagonist. The pA scale for expressing the potency of antagonists is analogous to the pD scale for agonists. The pA_2 is defined as the negative $\log_{10}$ of the molar concentration of antagonist that causes a two-fold rightward shift of the agonist concentration/effect curve (that is, an equi-effective concentration ratio of two). The $\log_{10}$ of a concentration ratio of 2–1 (i.e. 1) is zero. Hence the pA_2 is where the straight line crosses the abscissa and is 9 in the example in Figure 1.13. Under certain circumstances the pA_2 is the $\log_{10}$ of the K_d for the antagonist.

Non-equilibrium antagonism

In this form of direct antagonism, the agonist and antagonist occupy the same receptors but the antagonist forms a chemical (usually covalent)

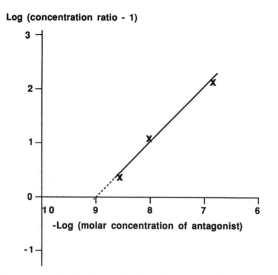

Figure 1.13 The extent of antagonism (ordinate) versus the log concentration of a competitive antagonist (abscissa) – the Schild plot

bond with the receptor that is not easily disrupted. As time passes, more and more of the receptors become inactivated in this fashion. Increasing the concentration of the agonist may delay the onset of the antagonism but cannot prevent the eventual outcome – the total inactivation of all the receptors.

As there is effectively no dissociation reaction, equilibrium kinetic analyses cannot be applied to antagonists of this kind. This has led to the term non-equilibrium antagonists.

In a biological system that is only modestly endowed with receptors, even agonists with high intrinsic efficacy need to occupy all the receptors to produce a maximal response. Figure 1.14a shows a biological system where no spare receptors exist. Increasing the concentration of the non-equilibrium antagonist (or increasing exposure time to a single concentration of the antagonist) results in a progressive proportional depression of the agonist log concentration/effect curve, without changing its position on the log concentration axis.

However, in a system in which a drug with high intrinsic efficacy can elicit a maximal response when occupying only a small fraction of the receptors, non-equilibrium antagonists cause at first a parallel, rightward shift of the curve that cannot be reversed by even prolonged washing. This is eventually followed by depression of the maximum effect, once the spare receptors have been inactivated (Figure 1.14b). This behaviour gives the illusion of non-equilibrium antagonists being competitive at first but then becoming non-equilibrium.

Providing no spare receptors are available, a non-equilibrium antagonist reduces the maximal response that can be attained, no matter what agonist concentration is used. The antagonism is therefore said to be insurmountable. The reversibility of non-equilibrium antagonism depends on the kind of chemical bond that is formed between the receptor and the

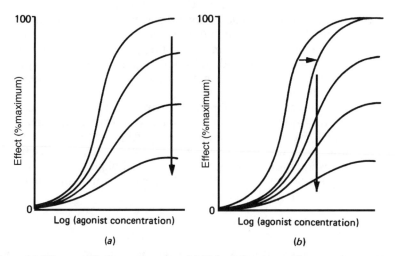

Figure 1.14 Non-equilibrium antagonism: (a) biological system with no spare receptors; (b) biological system having spare receptors

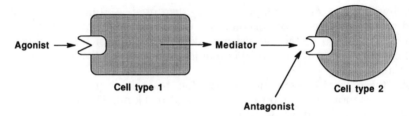

Figure 1.15 Mechanism by which an antagonist indirectly inhibits the effect of an agonist

antagonist. Some non-equilibrium antagonists can be removed from the receptor by prolonged washing. Others have truly irreversible actions (e.g. **phenoxybenzamine** at α-adrenoceptors).

No convenient scale exists for expressing the potency of non-equilibrium antagonists as so many patterns of antagonism exist.

Indirect mechanisms of pharmacodynamic antagonism

The agonist acts indirectly to cause the release of or to potentiate a second agent, this second agent acting as the final mediator of the observed response (Figure 1.15). The antagonist (which can be of the competitive or non-equilibrium kind) occupies the same receptor as the mediator.

Examples of indirect antagonism include: **atropine** antagonism of nicotine on the guinea-pig ileum (contraction mediated by acetylcholine released from postganglionic parasympathetic nerves); **propranolol** antagonism of tyramine on the isolated heart (stimulation mediated by noradrenaline released from postganglionic sympathetic nerves).

Functional opposition

This term describes the situation in which two different agonists evoke opposing responses from a single biological system by activating different receptors (Figure 1.16). For example, one agonist causes active contraction of a piece of smooth muscle and a second agonist causes active relaxation. If two such agonists are administered together then the responses tend to nullify each other and the net response is intermediate between their individual effects.

Some examples of this phenomenon represent the mere algebraic summation of the individual agonist actions while others do merit the antagonism label. Examples of functional opposition include: reversal of histamine-induced contraction of bronchial smooth muscle by **salbutamol**; reversal of vasodilatation induced by acetylcholine by *adrenaline*. Functional opposition has also been called functional antagonism and, less satisfactorily, 'physiological antagonism'.

Summation

Summation is the term used to describe the phenomenon in which two drugs acting together produce a predictable response. If a concentration

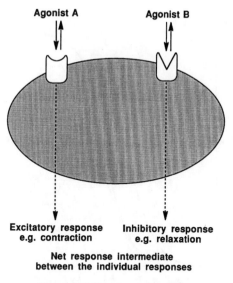

Figure 1.16 Functional opposition

or dose, x, of drug A produces the same response as a concentration or dose, y, of drug B, then summation of drug A and B is said to occur when the response to ½x + ½y is the same as that to either x or y (Figure 1.11). This phenomenon occurs with full agonists acting at the same receptor.

Potentiation

This is the phenomenon in which one drug (sometimes devoid of activity itself) makes another drug more potent (Figure 1.11). In Figure 1.17 the change from curve A to curve B represents the occurrence of potentiation. Potentiation is measured as the leftward shift in the log concentration/effect curve. Examples of potentiation are: acetylcholine by the inhibitor of acetylcholinesterase **neostigmine** (which inhibits metabolism of acetylcholine) and noradrenaline/5-hydroxytryptamine by the antidepressant agent **amitriptyline** (which inhibits their uptake into neurones). The change from curve A to curve C represents the occurrence not of potentiation but of an enhancement of maximal effect.

Summary

(1) Antagonism occurs when the effect of two drugs is smaller than the expected sum of their individual effects; one reduces the potency of the other.
(2) Competitive antagonists compete reversibly for occupancy of receptors with agonists. Their potency can be measured by the concentration halving the potency of an agonist.

STAFFS UNIVERSITY LIBRARY

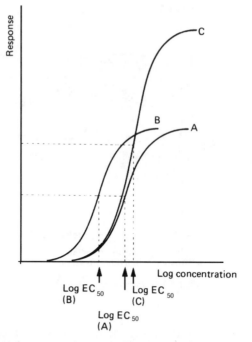

Figure 1.17 A change from curve A to curve B represents the occurrence of potentiation. A change from curve A to curve C represents the occurrence of increased responsiveness. A change from curve B to curve A represents the occurrence of either antagonism or desensitization

(3) Non-equilibrium antagonists form strong bonds with receptors preventing agonist occupancy. The extent of antagonism increases with time of exposure.
(4) Functional opposition occurs when two different agonists evoke opposing responses from a single biological system by activating different receptors.

Drug design, development and testing – preclinical phases

Most new drugs are discovered and all are developed by pharmaceutical companies. The vast financial investments that these companies must make in order to develop a new drug is protected by a 20-year patent. During this time only the patent-holding company or other agreed licensed companies can make and sell the drug. Such patents cover only a family of particular chemical structures and not a general principal of drug action. It currently takes approximately 10 years from first synthesis of a new drug until its appearance on the market with a Product Licence issued by the Licensing Authority (in the UK = the Ministers of Health) advised by the Committee on the Safety of Medicines (CSM). Its European counterpart is the Committee on Proprietary Medicinal Products (CPMP). The average research and development costs for a new drug are of the order of £120m (£200m if expenditure on failures is included), all of which must be recouped in the remainder of the patent-protected life of the drug. A company will only decide to embark upon a research programme if sufficient sales to cover the research and development costs can be predicted. Most rewarding are those programmes leading to the development of a drug to treat a relatively common condition for which no other successful treatment exists – filling a gap in the therapeutic armamentarium. Another approach is to develop another drug to treat a condition for which other treatments already exist. This is more likely to be profitable if the new drug has a novel mechanism of action, although often 'me too' drugs are developed by modifying the molecular structure of existing drugs until a novel structure is found that still has the desired pharmacological properties. To succeed, such a drug must have certain advantages. Higher potency alone is not an advantage. A better drug must show one or all of the following features:

(1) Increased selectivity, i.e. a higher therapeutic index, which is achieved either by increasing therapeutic potency or by reducing toxic potency or both.
(2) Decreased selectivity; the introduction of a second desirable property, e.g. neuromuscular blocking action in a general anaesthetic agent.
(3) Better pharmacokinetic properties, e.g. longer or shorter duration of action, depending upon the indications for use.
(4) More convenient formulation – tablets for oral dosing are usually preferable to a solution for injection.
(5) Price advantage.

This approach has been called molecular roulette and has led to the introduction of many very similar drugs. For example, there are now approximately 20 antagonists at β-adrenoceptors on the UK market sold under some 40 or so tradenames. This excludes preparations that contain more than one drug and different formulations of the same product. Despite unnecessary replication, many novel drugs have been discovered accidentally (by serendipity) during games of molecular roulette.

Initial research is directed at detecting new potential targets of drug action and lead compounds (the first chemicals showing activity at the target).

Pharmacological activity is detected by means of batteries of pharmacological tests commonly known as screens. Preliminary screens are intended to identify all the chemical compounds that have the desired action. These chemical compounds are provided by organic chemists (medicinal chemists) working to synthesize new structures according to a systematic plan based upon a set of theories about the required structures for a particular pharmacological activity. Such screens should ideally produce more <u>false-positive</u> than <u>false-negative</u> results. Promising compounds then pass to a series of more detailed pharmacological tests intended to confirm and extend the findings of the preliminary screen.

Once promising activity has been found in a compound many lines of attack are followed simultaneously. These centre around the medicinal chemistry laboratory, which studies the relationships between chemical structure and pharmacological activity. The hope is that the ideal structure can be predicted, synthesized, tested and eventually sold as an effective drug. Additional studies involve full pharmacological evaluations, both quantitative and qualitative, dispositional and metabolic studies in animals and preliminary toxicological evaluation both in vitro and in experimental animals.

Once preliminary toxicity tests show that the compound is unlikely to be toxic in man, short-term, healthy volunteer (Phase I) studies are carried out. These are intended to provide quantitative and qualitative information on the absorption, metabolism and excretion of the drug and its pharmacological effects. The volunteers are young and healthy, and able to give their informed consent to participate. They are usually men as this eliminates the risk of damaging the fetus in an unrecognized pregnancy (see p. 433). Volunteers are usually paid for their services but it is considered bad practice to offer such large sums that caution is outweighed by financial considerations. The risk of death or serious harm occurring to the volunteer in such studies is comparable to that involved in flying with a commercial airline.

From healthy volunteer studies, likely dosage regimens in clinical practice can often be predicted. Major differences in metabolism between experimental animals and man may also be detected.

When healthy volunteer studies and more detailed pharmacological and toxicological tests have produced favourable results, application can be made to the CSM (or CPMP) for a <u>clinical trials certificate</u>. Only when the clinical trials and detailed toxicity tests have been successfully completed and confirm that the drug has the intended therapeutic efficacy and is acceptably safe, can application be made to the CSM (or CPMP) for a <u>product licence</u>. Once granted, this enables the manufacturer to promote and sell the new compound under its tradename, for use in certain specified conditions. The UK Medicines Control Agency (a Department of Health bureaucracy serving the Licensing Authority) attempts to monitor the occurrence of adverse effects and the evidence of therapeutic efficacy for the whole of a product's life on the market. The most critical phase in this postmarketing (that is postproduct licence) surveillance is the first few years, when sales are expected to be highest. Should unacceptable adverse effects be detected, the CSM (or CPMP) can modify either the indications for use of the drug, the contraindications to the use of the drug or its recommended dose. They may even recommend withdrawal of the product licence.

Toxicity testing

Testing new drugs for adverse effects begins with toxicity tests in animals. Whenever possible, however, non-animal tests replace those in animals, both on humane grounds and because it is usually possible to reduce the variability associated with tests not based on whole animals. However tests designed to detect unforeseeable toxicity generally require that the drug be given to intact animals. Such preclinical predictive toxicity tests of new drugs fall into three major categories:

(1) acute toxicity evaluation;
(2) subacute toxicity evaluation;
(3) chronic toxicity evaluation.

Acute toxicity tests ask the questions how poisonous (lethal) is the drug in the short term and by what mechanisms does it kill? The best known acute toxicity parameter is the LD_{50} – the median lethal dose. In addition to providing information about the dosage levels needed for other toxicity tests, acute toxicity testing provides information about the likely effects of accidental or self-administered overdoses once the drug is marketed. Few licensing authorities still require LD_{50} tests to be carried out on new drugs. Subacute toxicity tests are of intermediate duration, usually around 12 weeks, and involve giving animals doses that are near the limits of tolerance on the assumption that the frequency of occurrence of a rare adverse effect increases with the cumulative dose given to the test population. Chronic toxicity tests involve giving doses of the new drug for prolonged periods of time, often near the whole lifetime of the test species. Rodents are the most widely used species for such lifetime tests, which commonly run for 2 years. The dose levels are chosen to be representative of normal (and likely maximal) therapeutic doses in man.

All three kinds of test are performed using at least two species of animals, typically rats, mice, guinea-pigs or rabbits. Other species (dogs, cats, monkeys) are employed when the chemical fate of the drug in these species more closely resembles that in man than in the smaller species. Throughout toxicity tests, animals are examined frequently for behavioural changes, assessment of many body functions and general well-being. At intervals, sample groups of animals are killed and examined post-mortem in detail. This includes biochemical analysis of body fluids and histological examination of every organ and tissue. At the end of the tests, all surviving animals are subjected to this procedure. A prime concern is to detect toxicity that is selective for a particular organ (bone marrow, kidney, liver).

Special testing techniques are used to detect adverse effects on reproductive function in both male and female animals and particularly the effects of the drug on embryonic and fetal growth and development – teratogenicity testing. Testing for carcinogenicity forms part of the chronic toxicity trial but is backed up by non-animal tests, most of which are based upon the ability of known carcinogens to cause mutations in certain strains of bacteria (e.g. Ames test).

Summary

(1) New drug development involves identification of targets and lead compounds, synthesis of many analogues, determination of candidate

compound(s) to progress, toxicity tests, healthy volunteer (Phase I) studies and clinical trials.

(2) The Committee on the Safety of Medicines regulates the use of new drugs in patients by issuing clinical trials certificates and product licences.

2

Drug action on peripheral excitable tissues – drugs acting on signalling mechanisms directly related to receptors for the neurotransmitters acetylcholine and noradrenaline

Aims

For each drug mentioned you should understand:

- Its mechanism of action and the changes it evokes in effector cell activity, both in vitro and in vivo.
- Its interactions with other pharmacological agents.
- Its principal therapeutic or scientific usage – and the rationale behind that usage.
- Its principal undesirable effects.

Introduction

Studies of drug effects exerted upon the peripheral nervous system or the cells that it innervates can provide an excellent introduction to mechanisms of drug action, the rationale behind the use of drugs as investigative tools or as therapeutic agents and the methods by which the properties of drugs are measured. Furthermore, such studies provide a working base from which to approach the pharmacology of other body systems.

Clinical applications

Most of the drugs described in this section are clinically useful. They may be used:

(1) To modify physiological processes and thus permit or facilitate an operative or other procedure, for example, **tubocurarine** used to paralyse skeletal muscle during surgery (see p. 56).
(2) As aids in the diagnosis of disease, for example, *edrophonium* used in the diagnosis of myasthenia gravis (see p. 74).
(3) In the symptomatic treatment of disease, for example, **propranolol** used in the treatment of essential hypertension (see p. 101).

It is important to realize that most agents mentioned in this section cannot be used to effect radical cure of disease.

Anatomy and physiology of the efferent peripheral nervous system and its effectors

Before you can understand how drugs produce their effects in the body, you must have a reasonable understanding of the anatomy and physiology of the relevant organ systems.

The nervous system can be subdivided as shown in Figure 2.1.

The central nervous system (CNS) comprises the brain and spinal cord. The peripheral nervous system lies outside the skull and vertebral column

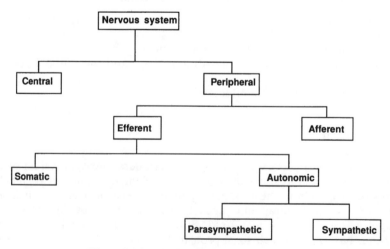

Figure 2.1 Subdivision of the nervous system

and comprises 12 pairs of nerves that emerge from the brain stem (cranial nerves) plus 31 pairs of nerves that emerge from the spinal cord (spinal nerves).

Peripheral neurones that carry impulses towards the CNS are called afferent neurones. Those that carry impulses away from the CNS are called efferent neurones.

Some cranial nerves consist only of afferent neurones, some of both afferent and efferent neurones and some only of efferent neurones. For the major part of their length, the spinal nerves consist of both afferent and efferent neurones and are thus called mixed spinal nerves. However, between its main trunk and the spinal cord, each spinal nerve breaks into a dorsal and a ventral root. Afferent neurones enter the spinal cord via the dorsal root whilst efferent neurones emerge via the ventral root (Figure 2.5).

The efferent peripheral nervous system can be subdivided into somatic and autonomic components.

The somatic division of the efferent peripheral nervous system comprises neurones that emerge from the spinal cord (via the ventral roots of spinal nerves) to provide excitatory innervation of skeletal muscle (Figure 2.5). The region where a somatic motor neurone closely approaches a skeletal muscle cell is known as the skeletal neuromuscular junction. Acetylcholine (ACh) is the chemical transmitter at this junction (Figure 2.2).

The autonomic division of the efferent peripheral nervous system provides excitatory or inhibitory innervation to cardiac muscle, smooth muscle and exocrine glands (its effector cells). The autonomic nervous

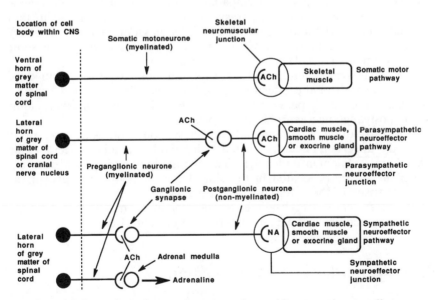

Figure 2.2 Comparison of a somatic motor pathway with autonomic neuroeffector pathways. Neurotransmitters are acetylcholine (ACh) or noradrenaline (NA)

pathway between the CNS and the effector cells comprises two neurones. The axon of the first neurone in the pathway emerges from the CNS (either in the course of a cranial nerve or via the ventral root of a spinal nerve) and terminates a short distance from the cell body of the second neurone in the pathway.

The region where an axon terminal of the first neurone closely approaches a dendrite or cell body of the second neurone is called a synapse. In many cases the synapses of autonomic pathways occur together in the course of a peripheral nerve. The collection of cell bodies in this region gives rise to a swelling of the nerve known as a ganglion. Hence the first neurone in an autonomic pathway is called the preganglionic neurone and the second cell is called the postganglionic neurone. Acetylcholine is the chemical transmitter at all autonomic ganglionic synapses (Figure 2.2).

The region where the axon of the postganglionic neurone closely approaches its effector cell is called a neuroeffector junction. The chemical transmitter at this junction may be acetylcholine or noradrenaline (NA [norepinephrine]), depending on the particular pathway under consideration (Figure 2.2).

The autonomic division of the efferent peripheral nervous system is subdivided into parasympathetic and sympathetic components according to the point of outflow of preganglionic neurones from the CNS.

The parasympathetic nervous system

A plan of the parasympathetic nervous system and its effectors is presented in Figure 2.3. Parasympathetic outflow comprises both cranial and sacral elements. Cranial parasympathetic outflow is carried in four cranial nerves (III oculomotor, VII facial, IX glossopharyngeal, X vagus). Sacral parasympathetic outflow is carried in the spinal nerves of some sacral segments (2, 3, 4) of the spinal cord.

Many parasympathetic ganglia are located close to, or are embedded within, the wall of the effector organ. Such ganglia are called terminal ganglia. In general, parasympathetic preganglionic neurones are long, while postganglionic neurones are short.

The distribution of parasympathetic innervation in the body is relatively limited – to certain effectors located within the head and to viscera within the thorax, abdomen and pelvis. The parasympathetic system does not innervate effectors located in the skin, limbs or body wall (except the erectile tissue of the external genital organs).

In every case acetylcholine is the chemical transmitter between postganglionic parasympathetic neurones and their effector cells.

The sympathetic nervous system

A plan of the sympathetic nervous system and its effectors is presented in Figure 2.4 and a transverse section of the spinal cord in Figure 2.5.

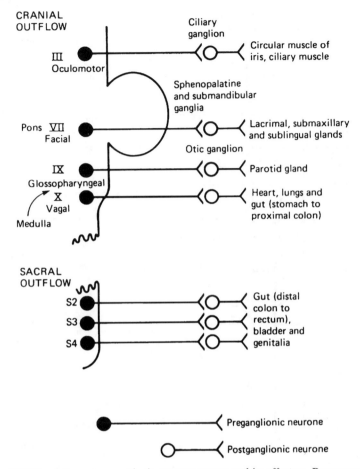

CRANIAL
OUTFLOW

III
Oculomotor

Ciliary
ganglion

Circular muscle of
iris, ciliary muscle

Sphenopalatine
and submandibular
ganglia

Pons VII
Facial

Lacrimal, submaxillary
and sublingual glands

Otic ganglion

IX
Glossopharyngeal

Parotid gland

X
Vagal

Heart, lungs and
gut (stomach to
proximal colon)

Medulla

SACRAL
OUTFLOW

S2

S3

S4

Gut (distal
colon to
rectum),
bladder and
genitalia

Preganglionic neurone

Postganglionic neurone

Figure 2.3 Plan of the parasympathetic nervous system and its effectors. Parasympathetic
outflow from the CNS is bilaterally paired; only one side is illustrated

Sympathetic outflow from the CNS is thoracolumbar – the preganglionic neurones emerge from the CNS in the ventral roots of the spinal
nerves of the first thoracic to third lumbar segments of the spinal cord
inclusive (Figure 2.4).

Sympathetic preganglionic fibres briefly join the course of the mixed
spinal nerve but soon branch away to form white communicating rami
(side branches of the spinal nerve), which enter the chains of paravertebral ganglia. These chains of ganglia lie on either side of the vertebrae.
There are 22 ganglia in each chain. Each ganglion in a paravertebral chain
is connected to the ones above and below by nerve trunks.

Only 15 of the ganglia in each chain are supplied by white communicating rami. The three cervical ganglia at the top of the chain and the four
sacral ganglia at the bottom of the chain only receive input from the CNS
by neurones running upwards or downwards through the chain of ganglia
by way of the interconnecting nerve trunks.

STAFFS UNIVERSITY LIBRARY

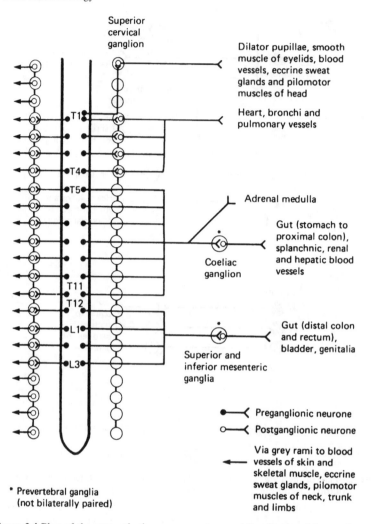

Figure 2.4 Plan of the sympathetic nervous system and its effectors. Most pathways illustrated are bilaterally paired (exceptions – coeliac and mesenteric ganglia)

   The ganglionic synapse of the sympathetic pathways supplying effectors located in the head and thorax occurs within the chain of paravertebral ganglia.

   In the sympathetic pathways supplying effectors located in the abdomen and pelvis, the preganglionic fibre enters the chain of paravertebral ganglia but passes straight through without synapsing. The synapse with the postganglionic neurone occurs in a prevertebral ganglion. In contrast to the paravertebral ganglia, the prevertebral ganglia are not bilaterally paired. They are ill-defined structures that form part of a neural plexus ventral to the abdominal aorta and its major branches. The coeliac and mesenteric ganglia are major components of this plexus. The adrenal

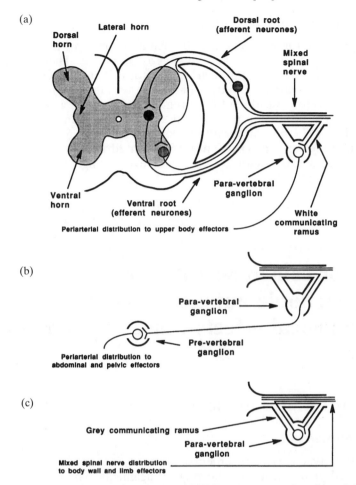

Figure 2.5 Sympathetic outflow from the CNS in transverse section. (b) and (c) show alternative arrangements to (a) of the transit of the sympathetic pathway through the paravertebral ganglia, dependent on their destination

medullae are embryologically and functionally equivalent to sympathetic prevertebral ganglia (Figure 2.2).

The preganglionic neurone of the sympathetic pathways supplying the blood vessels of skin and skeletal muscle, and the eccrine sweat glands and pilomotor muscles of the neck, trunk and limbs form a synapse with the postganglionic neurone within a paravertebral ganglion. The postganglionic neurone rejoins the course of the mixed spinal nerve (via the grey communicating ramus) for distribution to the effectors.

In contrast to the parasympathetic system, postganglionic sympathetic neurones are distributed almost universally throughout the body. With only a few exceptions (see p. 48), noradrenaline is the transmitter substance between postganglionic sympathetic neurones and their effector cells.

Autonomic neuroeffector junction

Postganglionic autonomic neurones branch and ramify within the effector organ to form a complex autonomic ground plexus. The number of autonomic neurones that approach an effector cell and the closeness of their approach varies greatly. Furthermore, the membranes of autonomic effector cells do not have regions that are specialized for the neuroeffector transmission process – the entire cell surface is sensitive to the action of the neurotransmitter (contrast with the motor end-plate of skeletal muscle, see p. 53). Hence it is often difficult to pinpoint sites of autonomic neuroeffector transmission, even using electron micrography.

Effector cells innervated by postganglionic autonomic neurones: physiological effects caused by nervous activity

Structures related to the eye

Ciliary muscle

The ciliary muscle may be regarded as a ring of smooth muscle. The lens is suspended at the centre of the ring by ligaments. The ciliary muscle receives only parasympathetic innervation. When action potential traffic in the parasympathetic pathway is increased, the acetylcholine released from postganglionic neurones evokes ciliary muscle contraction. Tension in the suspensory ligaments is reduced and, acting under its own internal pressure, the lens adopts a more spherical shape. The eye is thus accommodated for near vision (Figure 2.6). Accommodation can be altered voluntarily. Normally, however, the ciliary muscle is automatically regulated to keep the most distinct image of the object of fixation imposed on the retina.

Production and drainage of aqueous humour

Aqueous humour is produced mainly by the activity of the epithelial cells that cover the processes of the ciliary body. These epithelial cells secrete Na^+ into that part of the posterior chamber of the eye between the iris and lens. Cl^- and HCO_3^- (rapid generation catalysed by carbonic anhydrase) follow the movement of Na^+ to maintain electrical neutrality and water follows it to maintain isotonicity. The secretion of aqueous

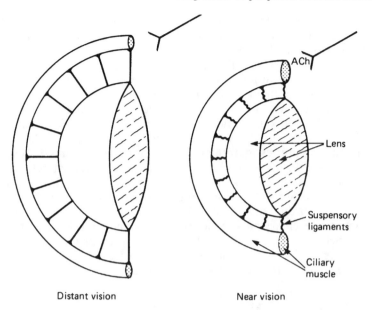

Distant vision   Near vision

Figure 2.6 Control of accommodation by the ciliary muscle; oblique view of sagittal section through ciliary muscle, suspensory ligament and lens

humour is modulated by adrenoceptors on the ciliary epithelium. In addition, the ciliary body is highly vascular and ultrafiltration is a source of some of the aqueous humour.

Aqueous humour flows forward through the pupil into the anterior chamber. It then flows into the filtration angle between the base of the iris and the inner surface of the cornea (Figure 2.7) and enters the trabecular mesh-work. It finally enters the canals of Schlemm which empty into

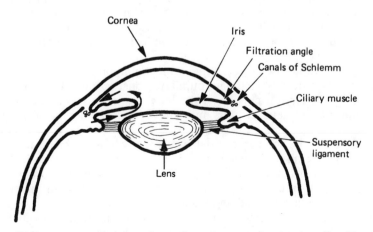

Figure 2.7 Transverse section through eye; flow of aqueous humour from the ciliary body, through the anterior chamber of the eye

the episcleral veins. Intra-ocular pressure is maintained by a balance between the production of aqueous humour in the ciliary body and its drainage via the canals of Schlemm.

When drainage is reduced, either by blockage of a narrow filtration angle (which occurs rather readily, e.g. by a relaxed iris) or by impaired movement through the trabecular mesh-work in people with an open angle, a rise in intraocular pressure ensues. The increased hydrostatic pressure of the aqueous humour in the anterior chamber of the eye is directly transmitted to the vitreous humour. The increased hydrostatic pressure there compresses retinal blood vessels and, if this is severe or prolonged enough, may cause ischaemic damage to retinal cells (loss of visual fields and cupping of the optic disc; glaucoma) and, if untreated, blindness. There are two major forms of glaucoma – acute closed-angle glaucoma and chronic open-angle glaucoma.

Activity of the ciliary muscle aids pumping of aqueous humour from the canals of Schlemm into the veins. Interference with ciliary muscle control may thus not only paralyse accommodation (cycloplegia) but may also predispose to an increased intra-ocular pressure.

The iris

The iris contains pigment cells that give the eye its characteristic colour and render the iris opaque. The iris contains two layers of smooth muscle – the sphincter pupillae (fibres arranged concentrically around the pupil) and the dilator pupillae (fibres arranged radially).

The sphincter pupillae receives only parasympathetic (acetylcholinergic) innervation and acetylcholine released from the postganglionic neurones causes contraction of the muscle fibres. The pupil thus constricts (miosis).

The dilator pupillae receives only a sympathetic innervation and noradrenaline released from the postganglionic neurones causes contraction of the muscle fibres. The pupil thus dilates (mydriasis).

Changes in the activity of the parasympathetic pathway supplying the sphincter pupillae are responsible for the pupil diameter changes associated with the light reflex. An increase in the intensity of light falling on the retina induces a reflex increase in parasympathetic discharge to the sphincter pupillae. The pupil constricts and reduces the amount of light entering the eye.

Parasympathetic discharge to the sphincter pupillae is also increased when viewing a near object. The pupillary constriction results in utilization of only the central portion of the lens. The spherical and chromatic aberration of the lens is thus minimized and its depth of focus is increased.

Relaxation of the sphincter pupillae causes mydriasis, which can lead to photophobia and also a restriction of the filtration angle. In a patient with an already narrow angle, this may rarely cause impaired drainage of aqueous humour into the canals of Schlemm and result in an increase in intra-ocular pressure (closed-angle glaucoma) (Figure 2.7).

The dilator pupillae plays little part in the light reflex. Sympathetic discharge in response to fright or other emotional states may evoke mydriasis.

The eyelids

The eyelids are largely controlled by skeletal muscle but also contain some smooth muscle, which receives only sympathetic innervation. The release of noradrenaline from the postganglionic neurones evokes contraction of the smooth muscle and the eyelids retract (that is, the palpebral fissure widens).

Paralysis of either the skeletal muscle or the smooth muscle of the eyelids allows the upper eyelid to droop (ptosis) – the palpebral fissure narrows.

The heart

The heart receives both parasympathetic and sympathetic innervations.

Parasympathetic neurones in the vagus nerve innervate the sinoatrial (SA) node (the cardiac pacemaker). The release of acetylcholine from parasympathetic nerve terminals reduces the discharge rate of the node and the heart rate decreases (bradycardia or negative chronotropic effect).

Parasympathetic neurones also innervate the atrioventricular (AV) node. This is located on the right side of the interatrial septum and gives rise to a bundle of specialized conducting cells (Purkinje fibres), which carry the cardiac excitation wave across the AV septum and distribute the excitation wave to the ventricles. The release of acetylcholine from parasympathetic neurone terminals depresses conduction through the AV node.

The ventricular myocardium (which performs most of the cardiac pumping work) does not receive a parasympathetic innervation.

Sympathetic neurones innervate all regions of the heart. The release of noradrenaline from these neurones augments the discharge rate of the SA node and the heart rate increases (tachycardia or positive chronotropic effect). It also increases conduction through the AV node and its associated Purkinje fibres and increases the force of contraction (positive inotropic effect) of the ventricular myocardium.

In a healthy young adult person heart rate is normally dominated by vagal (acetylcholinergic) tone when the subject is at rest. With increasing age, vagal tone becomes less dominant. During heavy exercise, sympathetic (noradrenergic) tone may dominate the heart, irrespective of the age of the subject.

Respiratory smooth muscle

The smooth muscle of the respiratory tract receives both parasympathetic and (sparse) sympathetic innervation. Acetylcholine release from parasympathetic neurone terminals evokes contraction of respiratory smooth muscle (bronchoconstriction), while noradrenaline release from sympathetic neurones evokes relaxation (bronchodilatation).

In a healthy young subject the bronchial airways are almost maximally dilated, even when the subject is at rest. The activation of sympathetic pathways during exercise does not therefore evoke much more bronchodilatation. The parasympathetic pathway to respiratory smooth muscle is reflexly activated in response to the inhalation of irritant substances or particles.

Gastrointestinal smooth muscle

The propulsive smooth muscle of the gut receives both parasympathetic and sympathetic innervation. The release of acetylcholine from parasympathetic neurones causes smooth muscle contraction (stimulates propulsive activity), whilst noradrenaline release from sympathetic neurones causes relaxation (inhibits propulsive activity).

Under normal circumstances the propulsive smooth muscle of the gut is dominated by parasympathetic (acetylcholinergic) tone.

The genitourinary system

The juxtaglomerular apparatus of the kidney

The juxtaglomerular apparatus comprises groups of granulated endocrine gland cells that surround afferent arterioles close to the point of their entry into the renal glomerulus (Figure 2.8). These cells are innervated by

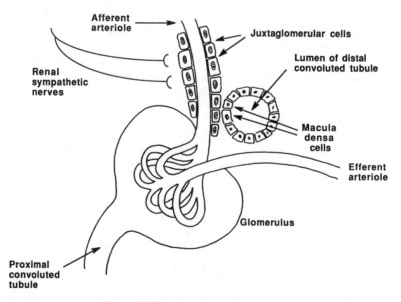

Figure 2.8 The juxtaglomerular apparatus

postganglionic sympathetic neurones carried in the renal nerves. Noradrenaline release augments the actions of other factors that promote the secretion of renin into the afferent arteriole (see p. 197).

Smooth muscle of the urinary bladder

The urinary bladder comprises a capsule of smooth muscle whose function is the storage and periodic evacuation of urine. The smooth muscle of the bladder comprises the detrusor (the greater part of the capsule) and the trigone (that part bounded by the ureteric orifices and the bladder neck). An external sphincter of skeletal muscle surrounds the bladder neck (Figure 2.9).

The detrusor receives parasympathetic innervation only. Bladder distension is the normal stimulus for micturition (passage of urine), which is normally started at will. The release of acetylcholine from parasympathetic

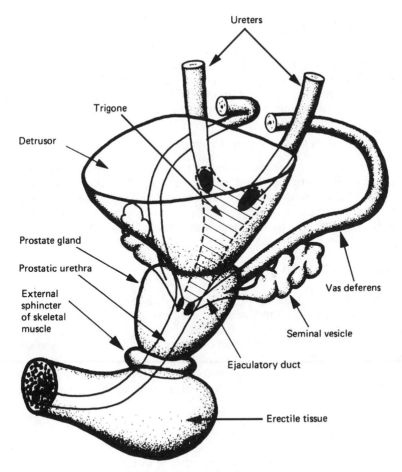

Figure 2.9 Male genitourinary tract

neurone terminals causes contraction of the detrusor and closure of the ureteric orifices. The bladder neck is shortened and widened as it is pulled upwards. This causes a reduction in the resistance of the urethra and allows the passage of urine.

The activity of skeletal muscle is involved to a variable degree in voluntary micturition. The first event may be a relaxation of the external sphincter round the bladder neck, accompanied by contraction of the diaphragm and abdominal muscles. As intra-abdominal pressure increases, urine may start to flow before detrusor activity reaches its peak. However, continence and voluntary micturition are possible in the absence of skeletal muscle activity.

The trigone and bladder neck receive only sympathetic innervation but the role of this sympathetic innervation in continence and micturition is negligible.

In males the release of noradrenaline from sympathetic nerve terminals during ejaculation causes a contraction of the trigone and bladder neck that prevents the reflux of seminal fluid into the bladder.

Seminal vesicle and vas deferens

The seminal vesicle and vas deferens (Figure 2.9) receive only sympathetic innervation. Noradrenaline release evokes contraction of the smooth muscle of these organs and hence ejaculation of spermatozoa into the prostatic urethra. Ejection of seminal fluid from the urethra (emission) is dependent on the clonic contraction of skeletal muscle.

Arterioles of external genital organs

The arterioles of the erectile tissue of the external genital organs receive only parasympathetic innervation. The release of acetylcholine from the parasympathetic neurone terminals causes relaxation of the vascular muscle, with resultant engorgement of the organ with blood (aided by reduced drainage due to venous compression).

Vascular smooth muscle

The smooth muscle of blood vessels is arranged circularly around the lumen. Most arterioles and veins receive sympathetic innervation only. The release of noradrenaline from the sympathetic neurone terminals causes contraction of vascular smooth muscle and hence vasoconstriction. The brain stem vasomotor centre governs the tonic discharge of the sympathetic neurones innervating blood vessels and the resultant vascular muscle tone is one of the factors responsible for the maintenance of BP.

Arterioles of skeletal muscle

The arterioles of skeletal muscle receive a noradrenergic, sympathetic innervation controlled by the vasomotor centre, as described for other vascular muscle. In addition, they receive a second sympathetic innervation. The postganglionic neurones in this pathway, although anatomically sympathetic, release acetylcholine as their transmitter, which causes vasodilatation of the skeletal muscle arterioles. The receptor sites for the acetylcholine are located not on the vascular smooth muscle cells but on the endothelial cells which line the vessel lumen. Activation of the receptors for acetylcholine induces the production of nitric oxide. This gaseous local hormone diffuses to the vascular smooth muscle cells and evokes their relaxation and hence dilatation of the arteriole (see p. 133). This sympathetic vasodilator pathway is activated in response to emotional shock (and so produces fainting) or in response to exercise (anticipated or current).

Effectors in the skin

Pilomotor muscles

Pilomotor muscles are responsible for the attitude of the hair shaft. They receive only a sympathetic innervation. Noradrenaline release from the sympathetic neurone terminals evokes muscle contraction and the hair shaft erects. In furry animals the pilomotor muscles play an important role in thermoregulation. In man their role is vestigial (gooseflesh).

Eccrine sweat glands

The eccrine sweat glands receive only a sympathetic innervation. The postganglionic neurones of this pathway, although anatomically sympathetic, release acetylcholine as their transmitter and thereby evoke sweat secretion. The eccrine sweat glands play an important role in thermoregulation by removing excess body heat as the latent heat of vaporization of sweat.

Apocrine sweat glands

The apocrine sweat glands are located mainly in the skin of the palms of the hands and axillae. They produce the nervous sweating associated with circulating hormonal adrenaline.

Other exocrine glands

The lacrimal glands, salivary glands, mucous glands of the respiratory tract, gastric oxyntic glands and digestive glands of the alimentary canal in general receive parasympathetic innervation. The release of acetylcholine from parasympathetic neurone terminals in each case stimulates glandular secretion.

Table 2.1 summarizes the autonomic effectors and the important effects on them of nervous activity.

STAFFS UNIVERSITY LIBRARY

Table 2.1 Some effector cells innervated by postganglionic autonomic nerves: the physiological effects on them of nervous activity

Sympathetic nervous activity	Organ	Parasympathetic nervous activity
	Eye	
No effect	Ciliary smooth muscle	Contracted
No innervation	Circular smooth muscle of iris	Contracted
Contracted	Radial smooth muscle of iris	No innervation
Contracted	Smooth muscle of eyelids	No innervation
No effect	*Lacrimal and salivary glands*	Secretion
	Heart	
Increased firing rate	SA node	Reduced firing rate
Reduced refractory period	AV node	Increased refractory period
Reduced refractory period and increased automaticity	Conducting tissue	No innervation
Increased contractile force	Ventricular myocardium	No innervation
	Respiratory tract	
Relaxed	Airway smooth muscle	Contracted
No innervation	Bronchial glands	Secretion
	Gut, stomach to rectum	
Inhibited	Propulsive smooth musculature	Stimulated
No innervation	Alimentary and pancreatic exocrine glands	Secretion
	Kidney	
Renin release	Juxtaglomerular cells	No innervation
	Urinary system smooth muscle	
No innervation	Detrusor	Contracted
Contracted	Bladder neck and trigone	No innervation
	Genital apparatus	
Contracted	Smooth muscle of seminal vesicles and vas deferens	No innervation
No effect	Blood vessels of erectile tissue of external genital organs	Dilated
	Blood vascular system smooth muscle	
Constricted	Arterioles and veins	No innervation
Dilated*	Those arterioles in skeletal muscle involved in fainting and exercise	No innervation
	Skin	
Contracted	Pilomotor smooth muscles	No innervation
Secretion*	Eccrine sweat glands	No innervation

*Acetylcholinergic transmission occurs at this site.

The pharmacology of acetylcholinergic axons and their terminals

Revise

- The anatomy of somatic motor neurones (see p. 35) and anatomy of parasympathetic nerves (see pp. 35, 36)
- The effects of stimulating parasympathetic nerves (Table 2.1).

Acetylcholinergic neurones synthesize, store and release acetylcholine as their transmitter. They include:

(1) All preganglionic autonomic neurones (parasympathetic and sympathetic).
(2) All postganglionic parasympathetic neurones.
(3) A few postganglionic sympathetic neurones.
(4) All somatic (lower) motor neurones.
(5) Some neurones lying entirely within the CNS.

Acetylcholinergic transmission

This process is basically similar at all sites in the body. It can be represented by Figure 2.10.

Drugs that act on acetylcholinergic axons and their terminals (drugs that interfere with stages A, B, F, G and H in Figure 2.10) modify acetylcholinergic transmission similarly at all sites. The clinical usefulness of such agents is thus limited by the diversity of their effects. Nevertheless, some drugs in this group (e.g. botulinum A toxin) remain useful because their sphere of action in the body can be restricted by the method of administration

Neuronal action potential conduction

Action potential conduction down the acetylcholinergic axon may arbitrarily be regarded as the first stage in the transmission process.

Release of acetylcholine from axon terminals

In the absence of action potential traffic in acetylcholinergic nerves, the random migration of storage vesicles to the axon surface occasionally results in the release of acetylcholine into the cleft. Although the amount of transmitter released spontaneously is small, it can still influence the membrane of the postjunctional cell if the cleft is narrow. The miniature end-plate potentials of twitch skeletal muscle (Figure 2.12) and the spontaneous postsynaptic potentials of ganglia (Figure 2.18) result from the spontaneous release of acetylcholine.

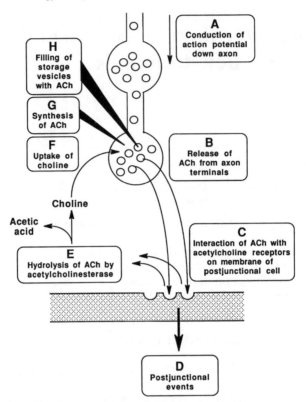

Figure 2.10 Acetylcholinergic neurotransmission (ACh = acetylcholine)

When action potentials invade terminal axons, membrane permeability changes occur, resulting in Na^+, Cl^- and Ca^{2+} entering the cells and K^+ emerging. The voltage-sensitive Ca^{2+} channels that are activated are of the N-type (see p. 127). The influx of Ca^{2+} triggers migration of many transmitter storage vesicles to the cell surface and release of acetylcholine by exocytosis. The empty vesicular membranes are recycled within the cell and refilled with newly synthesized transmitter.

As transmitter release by this mechanism requires influx of Ca^{2+}, it is reduced if the extracellular fluid (ECF) is deficient in this ion or contains a large concentration of Mg^{2+}.

After treatment of a tissue with triethylcholine, action potentials release acetyltriethylcholine (a <u>false transmitter</u>) from acetylcholinergic axon terminals (see p. 51). Acetyltriethylcholine is less potent than is acetylcholine in evoking a response from the postsynaptic or postjunctional cell.

Botulinum A toxin is an exotoxin produced by *Clostridium* (*Cl.*) *botulinum*, which also prevents both action potential-induced and spontaneous release of acetylcholine from all acetylcholinergic axons. The mechanism of the toxin action may involve inhibition of actin, an enzyme involved in exocytosis. Ingestion of foodstuffs (meat, fish and nut extracts) contaminated with *Cl. botulinum* gives rise to the condition of botulism. Death in botulism results from respiratory paralysis.

Botulinum A toxin (as a complex with haemagglutinin) may be administered by local injection in the control of hemifacial spasm or blepharospasm (persistent and disabling spasm of the eyelids). The injection is made into the affected facial muscles or upper eyelid.

Interaction of acetylcholine with postsynaptic or post-junctional acetylcholine receptors

Acetylcholine in the cleft reversibly forms complexes with receptors (acetylcholine receptors) on the outer surface of the postsynaptic or postjunctional membrane.

There are several kinds of acetylcholine receptor, which differ in their affinities for drugs, in their anatomical location and in the signal transduction process initiated by their activation. Hence this is the stage in the transmission process that offers the pharmacologist the greatest opportunity for selective interference (see pp. 52–71).

Hydrolysis of acetylcholine

The enzyme acetylcholinesterase can hydrolyse (and thus inactivate) acetylcholine to form choline and acetic acid. Drugs that inhibit the activity of acetylcholinesterase are the anticholinesterase agents (see p. 73).

Uptake of choline

Choline (dietary, synthesized from ethanolamine and methionine or formed from the hydrolysis of acetylcholine) is taken up actively by neurones. The transport of choline from the ECF into the neuronal cytoplasm is the rate-limiting step in the neuronal synthesis of acetylcholine.

Hemicholinium is a competitive inhibitor of the choline pump, but is not itself transported by the pump. It produces delayed block of acetylcholinergic transmission (preformed acetylcholine must be used up). Hemicholinium has no clinical application. Triethylcholine competes with choline for transport into the neurone.

Synthesis of acetylcholine

Some newly synthesized acetylcholine (Figure 2.11) is immediately hydrolysed by acetylcholinesterase of the axonal membrane. The acetylcholine taken up into the membrane-bound storage vesicles is protected from hydrolysis, and then stored in the vesicles as a concentrated solution.

Triethylcholine competes with choline for the synthetic mechanism and acetyltriethylcholine is synthesized and stored. Since acetyltriethylcholine can be released from the nerve terminal but is much less potent on acetylcholine receptors than acetylcholine, it is said to function as a false transmitter. Triethylcholine thus produces delayed block of acetylcholinergic transmission. Triethylcholine has no clinical application.

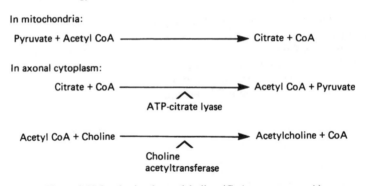

Figure 2.11 Synthesis of acetylcholine (CoA = coenzyme A)

Summary

(1) All somatic motor neurones, all preganglionic autonomic neurones and all postganglionic parasympathetic neurones are acetylcholinergic.

(2) Some CNS neurones and a few postganglionic sympathetic neurones are acetylcholinergic.

(3) The synthesis of acetylcholine can be inhibited by drugs that inhibit the neuronal uptake of choline.

(4) A non-physiological substrate leads to the synthesis, storage and release of a false transmitter.

(5) Drugs are available (botulinum A toxin) that inhibit the neuronal release of acetylcholine.

(6) Several kinds of acetylcholine receptor exist that differ in their affinities for drugs and in their anatomical location.

Pharmacology of the acetylcholine receptors of skeletal muscle

The receptors were originally designated <u>nicotinic</u> since nicotine could readily mimic the action of acetylcholine at these sites. Nicotinic acetylcholine receptors of skeletal muscle are characterized by the orders of drug potency shown in Table 2.2.

The nicotinic acetylcholine receptor is an example of a ligand-gated ion channel. It contains four kinds of membrane-spanning subunit (α, β, γ, δ). These subunits surround a central pore that acts as a cation (Na^+, K^+ and Ca^{2+}) channel. The receptor contains two of the α-subunits and each of these must bind an acetylcholine molecule for receptor activation (opening of the cation channel) to occur.

Table 2.2 Orders of drug potency at the nicotinic acetylcholine receptor of skeletal muscle

Agonists		
Acetylcholine	>>	Methacholine
Nicotine		Muscarine
Suxamethonium		
Antagonists		
Tubocurarine	>>	**Atropine**
Atracurium		Hexamethonium
Vecuronium		Trimetaphan
α-Bungarotoxin		

Note: Compounds to the left of the >> symbol are potent but not equally so; those to the right are of such low potency that they may be regarded as inactive at this site.

How do these agonists or antagonists (see p. 15) at the nicotinic acetylcholine receptor influence the development of tension by skeletal muscle? The answer depends to a certain extent upon the kind of muscle cell considered.

Focally innervated (twitch) skeletal muscle

The majority of mammalian skeletal muscle cells are of this kind. Each muscle cell forms only one region of close association with a somatic motor neurone terminal. Here the muscle cell membrane is thrown into a series of folds to form the motor end-plate. Under normal circumstances this is the only part of the muscle cell membrane that has nicotinic acetylcholine receptors. These are found on the exterior of the muscle cell membrane and are concentrated at the crests of the junctional folds.

The motor neurone axon branches near its terminal and each branch innervates a single muscle cell. The group of muscle cells innervated by a single axon is termed the motor unit and the whole motor unit responds when an action potential is transmitted down the axon.

Functionally, the skeletal muscle cells may be subdivided into fast, fatiguable (white or glycolytic) and slow, fatigue-resistant (red or oxidative) kinds. There may also be intermediate kinds. Most muscles contain some of both kinds of muscle cell. However, the neuromuscular transmission process and its susceptibility to drugs do not appear to differ significantly between these kinds of muscle cell.

Although the end-plates depolarize in a graded manner in response to increasing concentrations of acetylcholine, the muscle cells exhibit threshold behaviour. That is, if the end-plate depolarizes rapidly through a threshold of excitability, an action potential is triggered and this potential normally propagates to the cell extremities without decrement. It is the electrical event that is associated with the Ca^{2+} fluxes necessary for shortening of the myofibrils. Action potential firing (and the presence of a well-developed T-tubule system and sarcoplasmic reticulum) allows the cell to develop tension quickly (twitch).

Normal sequence of events during neuromuscular transmission

(1) Arrival of action potential in the nerve terminal.
(2) Release of acetylcholine into the junctional cleft (width 20 nm).
(3) Diffusion of acetylcholine down a concentration gradient towards the motor end-plate.
(4) Association of acetylcholine with the nicotinic acetylcholine receptors.
(5) Depolarization of the motor end-plate to give an end-plate potential (epp).
(6) When the epp crosses the threshold potential of excitability, an action potential is triggered and this travels out from the end-plate to the muscle cell extremities.
(7) Passage of the action potential into the T-tubules and triggering of release of Ca^{2+} from intracellular sites causes shortening of myofibrils and the development of tension.
(8) Dissociation of the acetylcholine/receptor complex.
(9) Hydrolysis of acetylcholine by acetylcholinesterase.
(10) Transport of choline back into the nerve terminal.
(11) Resynthesis of acetylcholine.
(12) Storage of acetylcholine in vesicles.

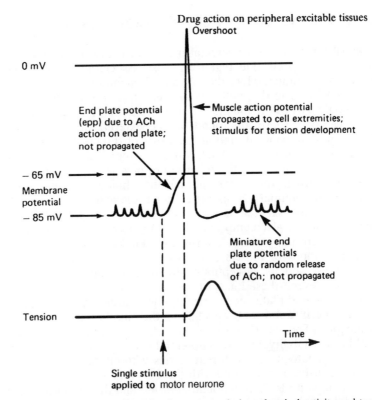

Figure 2.12 Twitch skeletal muscle: the motor end-plate electrical activity and tension development of a single fibre evoked by stimulation of its nerve supply

Under normal circumstances, a single nerve action potential releases more than sufficient acetylcholine to depolarize the end-plate to threshold; that is, a safety factor exists for transmission. Normally only one muscle action potential is generated per nerve action potential since the transmitter is hydrolysed within the refractory period of the muscle cell (Figure 2.12).

Effects of agonists at nicotinic acetylcholine receptors on neuromuscular transmission

These agonists, which include acetylcholine, nicotine and **suxamethonium** (succinyldicholine) (Figure 2.13), activate nicotinic acetylcholine receptors of the end-plate and evoke depolarization. If this depolarization is large enough to cross the threshold of excitability, and does so rapidly enough, the muscle cell generates an action potential and contracts. Since these drugs are not readily hydrolysed by acetylcholinesterase (with the exception of acetylcholine), the muscle cell often generates several action potentials and then enters a state where its end-plate membrane remains depolarized at a level less inside-negative than the threshold of excitability. Under such circumstances no further action potential can be evoked by transmitter action at the motor end-plate. The muscle cell no longer responds to stimulation of its nerve supply by contraction for it is the action potential that triggers the necessary Ca^{2+} fluxes. This is the state of depolarizing blockade of neuromuscular transmission (Figure 2.14). Blockade persists until such time as the end-plate has repolarized to a level more inside-negative than the threshold of excitability. Depolarizing blockade of neuromuscular transmission can also be caused by inhibition of cholinesterases (see p. 74).

The only agonist at nicotinic acetylcholine receptors shown in Table 2.2 that is useful for its action on skeletal muscle is **suxamethonium**. The molecule of **suxamethonium** contains two quaternary N atoms. These simultaneously interact with the binding sites on the two α-subunits of the nicotinic receptor and receptor activation can therefore be achieved by a single molecule of **suxamethonium**. This drug is used in brief surgical or diagnostic procedures to produce brief (5 min) periods of paralysis. It is also used to control the muscle spasm evoked by electroconvulsive therapy (a treatment for depression). Intravenous injection causes asynchronous twitches of individual fibres in the bodies of muscles (fasciculation) due to the early phase of action potential firing. Then a phase

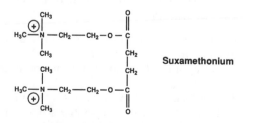

Figure 2.13 The structure of **suxamethonium** (succinyldicholine), an agonist at nicotinic acetylcholine receptors. Compare it with the structure of acetylcholine (see Figure 1.4)

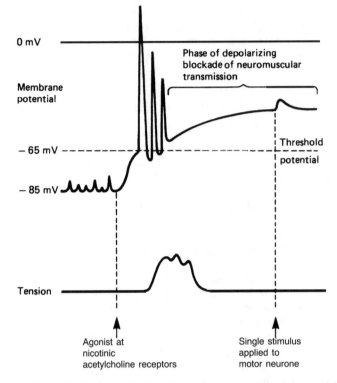

Figure 2.14 Twitch skeletal muscle: the effects of agonists at nicotinic acetylcholine receptors on the motor end-plate electrical activity and tension development of a single fibre

of flaccid paralysis ensues due to depolarizing blockade of neuromuscular transmission.

Suxamethonium-induced paralysis is short lived due to rapid hydrolysis of the drug by cholinesterase. Patients genetically deficient in this enzyme (see pp. 73 and 430) suffer prolonged paralysis after **suxamethonium** injection.

The effects of antagonists at the nicotinic acetylcholine receptors of skeletal muscle

Competitive antagonists (for definition of competitive antagonism, see p. 23) – **tubocurarine**, *atracurium*, *vecuronium*.

Non-equilibrium antagonists (for definition of non-equilibrium antagonism, see p. 24) – α-bungarotoxin.

Any of the antagonists listed above decreases the number of transmitter/receptor interactions and hence reduces the size of the epp. If the epp no longer crosses the threshold of excitability, neuromuscular transmission to that cell fails (Figure 2.15).

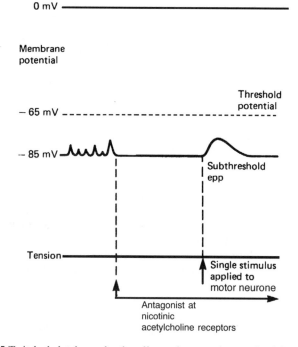

Figure 2.15 Twitch skeletal muscle: the effects of antagonists at nicotinic acetylcholine receptors on the motor end-plate electrical activity and tension development of a single twitch fibre

When the effects of a competitive antagonist are followed in vitro or in vivo, a gradual depression of the twitch of the whole muscle is seen. Since transmission to a single cell is an all-or-none process, this gradual onset of effect represents the successive inactivation of individual muscle cells.

The competitive antagonists are useful for producing muscle paralysis during surgery; they allow the anaesthetist to employ a relatively light level of anaesthesia and yet have adequate muscle relaxation (see p. 258). They are also useful in tetanus or strychnine poisoning (see p. 224). In all cases where tubocurarine-like drugs are used, there is a need to ventilate the lungs. The effects of the competitive antagonists can be terminated by an anticholinesterase drug, which increases the number of transmitter/receptor interactions by increasing the concentration of transmitter in the neuromuscular junction.

Tubocurarine causes histamine release (Table 4.12) and ganglion block-ade and hence reduces BP. These unwanted effects of **tubocurarine** are leading to its abandonment in favour of more modern derivatives. Histamine release and ganglion blockade are not problems with *vecuronium*. *Atracurium* is particularly useful in patients with impaired liver or kidney function, since its inactivation is largely brought about by spontaneous (non-enzymatic) cleavage of the molecule into inactive products (takes approximately 15 min).

Table 2.3 Clinically relevant interactions with neuromuscular blocking agents

	Competitive (tubocurarine)	Depolarizing (suxamethonium)
General anaesthetic agents; **halothane**, *enflurane*, diethyl ether	+	0
Antibiotic agents; aminoglycoside **gentamicin**	+	0
Anticholinesterase agents; **neostigmine**	–	+
Hypothermia	–	+

+ = increases neuromuscular blocking activity; – = decreases neuromuscular blocking activity; 0 = no pronounced effect on neuromuscular blocking activity.

α-Bungarotoxin is a component of the venom of a snake (the Taiwan banded krait, *Bungarus multicinctus*). It binds irreversibly and very selectively to the nicotinic acetylcholine receptors of skeletal muscle. It is not clinically useful but is a very valuable research tool, for example in the localization and isolation of nicotinic acetylcholine receptors of muscle.

Clinically relevant interactions with neuromuscular blocking agents are shown in Table 2.3.

Multiply innervated (slow) skeletal muscle

In this kind of muscle each muscle cell has several neuromuscular junctions but there is no specialized muscle membrane (end-plate) at these sites. This kind of muscle is relatively common in birds and amphibians but is uncommon in mammals. It should not be confused with the slow (red) focally innervated twitch fibres, which form a component of most mammalian muscles.

One site where multiply innervated muscle is found in mammals is in the intrafusal muscle fibres. These form part of the muscle spindles, the stretch receptors that are present within skeletal muscles. The muscle spindle consists of a central nuclear bag region, containing the sensory receptors. When stimulated these initiate the action potentials in afferent nerves that convey information about the degree and rate of stretch to the spinal cord and brain. The intrafusal muscle fibres are found at either end of the nuclear bag. The intrafusal fibres are themselves innervated by the small γ-efferent motor neurones in the motor nerve. Increasing the activity of the γ-efferent neurones leads to contraction of the intrafusal fibres with consequent stretch of the nuclear bag region and increased activity of its sensory receptors, resulting in a reflex contraction of the contractile extrafusal fibres in the muscle concerned.

The fibres of multiply innervated slow muscles have nicotinic acetylcholine receptors, which respond to the same agonists, acetylcholine and **suxamethonium**, as the acetylcholine receptors of twitch muscle but the response evoked is a slow graded depolarization associated with a slow graded contraction of the muscle. Stimulation of the nerve supply during such a response has an additive effect on both the depolarization and the tension development (Figure 2.16). Note that the phenomenon of depolarizing blockade of transmission cannot occur in these muscle cells since they do not exhibit threshold behaviour. The soreness of muscles reported by patients after **suxamethonium** is probably due to excitation of the intrafusal fibres with consequent prolonged reflex activation of the skeletal muscles.

Antagonists at the nicotinic acetylcholine receptors of twitch fibres reduce the graded depolarization and graded contraction evoked in multiply innervated skeletal muscle by nerve stimulation or the administration of agonists at the nicotinic acetylcholine receptor (Figure 2.17).

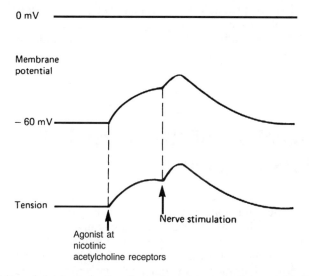

Figure 2.16 Slow skeletal muscle: the effects of agonists at nicotinic acetylcholine receptors on the electrical activity and tension development of a single fibre

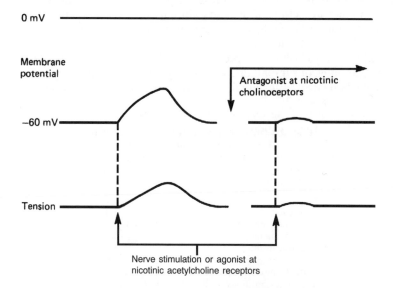

Figure 2.17 Slow skeletal muscle: the effects of antagonists at nicotinic acetylcholine receptors on the electrical activity and tension development of a single fibre

STAFFS UNIVERSITY LIBRARY

Summary

(1) The nicotinic acetylcholine receptors found on skeletal muscle cells comprise ligand-gated Na^+ channels.

(2) Agonists are available (**suxamethonium**) that paralyse skeletal muscle by mimicking the action of acetylcholine on the nicotinic receptor, causing depolarizing blockade of neuromuscular transmission.

(3) Antagonists are available (e.g. **tubocurarine**, *vecuronium*) that paralyse skeletal muscle by occupying the nicotinic receptors without causing their activation, causing competitive blockade of neuromuscular transmission.

Pharmacology of the acetylcholine receptors of ganglia

The sympathetic and parasympathetic ganglia are relay stations in autonomic efferent neural pathways. In most ganglia marked divergence occurs, that is the number of postganglionic fibres greatly exceeds the number of preganglionic fibres. However each preganglionic axon divides into many terminal branches so that each ganglion cell receives many synaptic contacts. In both the sympathetic and parasympathetic ganglia the transmitter released from the presynaptic terminals is acetylcholine.

The receptors were originally designated nicotinic, since nicotine could readily mimic the action of acetylcholine at these sites. Nicotinic acetylcholine receptors of ganglia are characterized by the orders of drug potency shown in Table 2.4.

Nicotinic acetylcholine receptors of ganglia are located over the whole of the cell bodies of sympathetic and parasympathetic ganglia (particularly numerous beneath the terminal boutons of preganglionic fibres).

Table 2.4 Orders of drug potency at the nicotinic acetylcholine receptor of ganglia

Agonists		
Acetylcholine	>>	Methacholine
Nicotine		Muscarine
Antagonists		
Hexamethonium	>>	**Atropine**
Trimetaphan		α-Bungarotoxin
Tubocurarine		

Note: Compounds to the left of the >> symbol are potent but not equally so; those to the right are of such low potency that they may be regarded as inactive at this site.

Nicotinic acetylcholine receptors of ganglia compared with those of skeletal muscle

The nicotinic acetylcholine receptors in both locations form integral parts of a ligand-gated Na^+ channel. Interaction of an agonist with nicotinic acetylcholine receptors, either in ganglia or in skeletal muscle cells, induces cellular depolarization. The nicotinic acetylcholine receptor in ganglia does not differ from that in skeletal muscle in the rank order of potency of agonists (compare Tables 2.2 and 2.4). However, among antagonists, trimetaphan shows selectivity for the nicotinic acetylcholine receptor of ganglia while α-bungarotoxin shows selectivity for the nicotinic acetylcholine receptor of skeletal muscle. This suggests that the molecular structure of the nicotinic acetylcholine receptor in ganglia differs from that of the nicotinic acetylcholine receptor in skeletal muscle.

Normal sequence of events during ganglionic transmission

(1) Simultaneous arrival of action potentials at a sufficient number (see below) of preganglionic nerve terminals.
(2) Release of acetylcholine into synaptic cleft (width 20 nm).
(3) Diffusion of acetylcholine down a concentration gradient towards the ganglion cell body.
(4) Association of acetylcholine with nicotinic acetylcholine receptors.
(5) Depolarization of the ganglion cell body (excitatory postsynaptic potential, epsp).
(6) If the epsp crosses the threshold of excitability (see below) an action potential is triggered and this moves down the postganglionic axon (Figure 2.18).
(7) Dissociation of acetylcholine/acetylcholine receptor complex.
(8) Hydrolysis of acetylcholine.
(9) Transport of choline back into the preganglionic nerve terminals.
(10) Resynthesis of acetylcholine.
(11) Storage of acetylcholine in vesicles.

Compare and contrast the above sequence of events with those occurring during neuromuscular transmission in twitch muscle fibres (see p. 54).

Note that for effective ganglionic transmission (that is, production of an epsp big enough to cross threshold) an appreciable number of preganglionic terminals must discharge transmitter in a synchronous fashion. Discharge of one terminal bouton would not normally evoke an action potential in the postganglionic cell body.

Effects of agonists at nicotinic acetylcholine receptors on ganglionic transmission

Acetylcholine, nicotine

These activate nicotinic acetylcholine receptors of the ganglion cell body and evoke depolarization. If this depolarization is sufficiently large to cross the threshold of excitability, and does so sufficiently rapidly, the ganglion cell body generates an action potential.

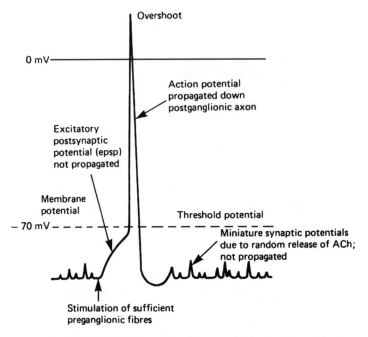

Figure 2.18 The electrical activity of an autonomic ganglion cell body

Agonists at the acetylcholine receptors of ganglia exert indirect effects on the acetylcholine receptors and adrenoceptors of smooth muscle, cardiac muscle and exocrine glands because they trigger a burst of action potential discharge by the ganglion cell body (Figure 2.19). The action on effector cells is said to be indirect, since the agonist at nicotinic acetylcholine receptors affects those cells by causing the release of a neurotransmitter. Where acetylcholine is released the effect on effector cells may be termed an indirect parasympathomimetic effect. Where noradrenaline or adrenaline is released the effect on effector cells may be termed an indirect sympathomimetic effect.

Since these drugs (even acetylcholine, if in great excess) are not readily inactivated by acetylcholinesterase, the ganglion cell body generally generates a burst of action potentials and then enters a state where its membrane potential is less inside-negative than the threshold of excitability. This is the stage of depolarizing blockade of ganglionic transmission (Figure 2.20). Under such circumstances the ganglion cell body becomes refractory (as regards action potential generation) to stimulation of the preganglionic neurones. Blockade of transmission persists until such time as the membrane of the ganglion cell body has repolarized to a level more inside-negative than the threshold of excitability. Note the analogy with the actions of these drugs on neuromuscular transmission in twitch skeletal muscle fibres (see p. 55).

If an agonist at the nicotinic acetylcholine receptors of ganglia is administered repeatedly at short intervals, then the indirect sympathomimetic

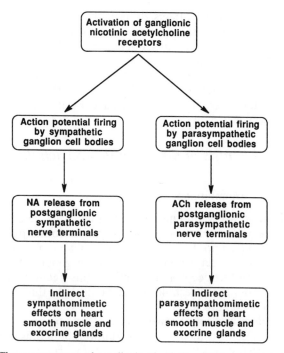

Figure 2.19 The consequences of ganglionic stimulation (ACh = acetylcholine, NA = noradrenaline)

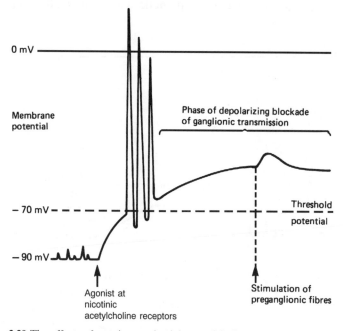

Figure 2.20 The effects of agonists at nicotinic acetylcholine receptors on the electrical activity of an autonomic ganglion cell body

and parasympathomimetic effects described above exhibit <u>tachyphylaxis</u> (that is, response amplitude declines rapidly with successive doses). The explanation is probably that subsequent doses of the agonist reach the ganglion cell body while it is still in the phase of depolarizing blockade.

Since these agents activate all sympathetic and parasympathetic ganglia, their injection into the whole animal has very diverse effects. For this and other reasons, these agents are not used clinically for their action on ganglion cell bodies.

Effects of antagonists at the nicotinic acetylcholine receptors of ganglia

Hexamethonium, trimetaphan

Like the nicotinic acetylcholine receptor found in skeletal muscle, the nicotinic acetylcholine receptor found in ganglia forms part of a ligand-gated ion channel (see pp. 12 and 52). Trimetaphan is a competitive antagonist at the nicotinic acetylcholine receptors of ganglia. By reducing the number of transmitter/receptor interactions this agent reduces the epsp until it fails to cross the threshold of excitability. At this point ganglionic transmission fails (Figure 2.21).

Hexamethonium and **tubocurarine** have effects on ganglionic transmission similar to those of trimetaphan. In addition to binding to the nicotinic acetylcholine receptor on the ganglion cell, they also act to block the ion channel that is normally gated by the acetylcholine receptor.

Trimetaphan, hexamethonium and **tubocurarine** block transmission through all ganglia (both parasympathetic and sympathetic) and at the

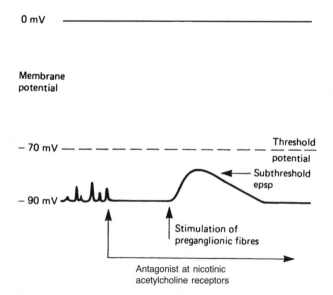

Figure 2.21 The effects of antagonists at nicotinic acetylcholine receptors on the electrical activity of an autonomic ganglion cell body

Table 2.5 Some effects of ganglion blockade (e.g. by trimetaphan, a competitive antagonist at nicotinic acetylcholine receptors of ganglia)

Sympathetic interruption	Organ	Parasympathetic interruption
	Eye	
	Ciliary smooth muscle	Relaxed
	Pupil	Dilated
Relaxed	Smooth muscle of lids	
	Lacrimal and salivary glands	Reduced secretion
	Heart	
	SA node	Tachycardia, mild
	Gut, stomach to rectum	
	Propulsive smooth musculature	Reduced motility and constipation
	Alimentary and pancreatic exocrine glands	Reduced secretion
	Bladder	Retention of urine
	Genital apparatus	
Failure of ejaculation	Smooth muscle of seminal vesicles and vas deferens	
	Blood vessels of erectile tissue of external genital organs	Impotence
	Blood vascular system smooth muscle	
Dilated; postural hypotension		
	Skin	
Reduced secretion	Eccrine sweat glands	

adrenal medulla. They competitively antagonize acetylcholine or nicotine applied to these sites. Table 2.5 shows their effects in the whole animal, from which you can deduce whether an organ is normally dominated by parasympathetic or sympathetic tone.

These agents have little therapeutic application because their effects in the whole body are so diverse. Trimetaphan is occasionally given by i/v injection to reduce BP and thereby minimize bleeding at the site of surgery ('bloodless' field). In addition to ganglion blockade, trimetaphan can reduce BP by directly relaxing vascular smooth muscle and by evoking histamine release.

Summary

(1) The nicotinic acetylcholine receptors found on autonomic ganglion cell bodies, like those in skeletal muscle, comprise ligand-gated Na^+ channels.
(2) The nicotinic acetylcholine receptors found in autonomic ganglia differ from those found in skeletal muscle, principally in their affinities for antagonists.

STAFFS UNIVERSITY LIBRARY

(3) Agonists at the nicotinic acetylcholine receptors in ganglia evoke a wide variety of changes in effector cell activity (indirect sympathomimetic and indirect parasympathomimetic effects) attributable to their provoking the release of noradrenaline and acetylcholine from post-ganglionic noradrenergic and acetylcholinergic neurones.
(4) Antagonists at the nicotinic acetylcholine receptors in ganglia (e.g. trimetaphan) interrupt ganglionic transmission in all efferent autonomic neural pathways, and thereby produce a wide variety of changes in effector cell activity.

Pharmacology of the acetylcholine receptors of smooth muscle, cardiac muscle and exocrine glands

The receptors were originally designated muscarinic since muscarine could readily mimic the action of acetylcholine at these sites. Muscarinic acetylcholine receptors of smooth muscle, cardiac muscle and exocrine glands are characterized by the orders of drug potency shown in Table 2.6.

Anatomy of parasympathetic neuroeffector junctions

Those smooth muscle, cardiac muscle and exocrine gland cells that receive an acetylcholinergic innervation are supplied by postganglionic acetylcholinergic neurones. Most neurones of this kind belong anatomically to

Table 2.6 Orders of drug potency at the muscarinic acetylcholine receptor

Agonists		
Acetylcholine	>>	Nicotine
Methacholine		
Muscarine		
Pilocarpine		
Antagonists		
Atropine	>>	**Tubocurarine**
Hyoscine	>>	Trimetaphan
		α-Bungarotoxin

Note:
(1) Compounds to the left of the >> symbol are potent but not equally so; those to the right are of such low potency that they may be regarded as inactive at this site.
(2) Muscarinic acetylcholine receptors differ from nicotinic acetylcholine receptors both in the order of potency of agonists and order of potency of antagonists (Tables 2.2 and 2.4).

Table 2.7 Some effects of acetylcholine mediated by muscarinic acetylcholine receptors

Eye	
Ciliary smooth muscle	Contracted
Circular smooth muscle of iris	Contracted
Lacrimal and salivary glands	Secretion
Heart	
SA node	Reduced firing rate
AV node	Increased refractory period
Ventricular myocardium	Reduced contractile force*
Respiratory tract	
Airway smooth muscle	Constricted
Bronchial glands	Secretion
Gut, stomach to rectum	
Propulsive smooth musculature	Contracted
Alimentary and pancreatic exocrine glands	Secretion
Urinary system smooth muscle	
Detrusor	Contracted
Genital apparatus	
Blood vessels of erectile tissue	Dilated
Blood vascular system smooth muscle	
All arterioles	Dilated*
Those arterioles in skeletal muscle involved in fainting and exercise	Dilated
Skin	
Eccrine sweat glands	Secretion

*Two effects of administered acetylcholine that cannot be mimicked by autonomic nerve stimulation. Muscarinic acetylcholine receptors are not restricted to cells receiving an acetylcholinergic nerve supply. In blood vessels muscarinic acetylcholine receptors lie on endothelial cells rather than smooth muscle cells and modulate the release of the intermediate vasodilator substance nitric oxide (see p. 133).

the parasympathetic division of the autonomic nervous system. In the sympathetic division, most postganglionic neurones are noradrenergic – but there are two kinds that are acetylcholinergic:

(1) Those supplying the eccrine sweat glands.
(2) Those providing a vasodilator pathway to the arterioles of skeletal muscle.

Muscarinic acetylcholine receptors are probably located over the entire surface of effector cells. They are also found on cells that do not receive an acetylcholinergic innervation, for example, the ventricular myocardium and the endothelial cells of blood vessels (see the footnote to Table 2.7).

Normal sequence of events during acetylcholinergic transmission to autonomic effector cells

See Figure 2.10.

(1) Arrival of action potential in the terminal branches of the postganglionic neurone.

(2) Release of acetylcholine into the junctional cleft (width 20–1000 nm).

(3) Diffusion of acetylcholine down a concentration gradient towards the effector cell.

(4) Association of acetylcholine with muscarinic acetylcholine receptors on the effector cell.

(5) Induction of postjunctional events. The muscarinic acetylcholine receptors contain seven transmembrane domains and transduce occupation by the agonist into activation of a G-protein.

   (a) In exocrine gland, smooth muscle and vascular endothelium cells where acetylcholine has an excitatory action (Table 2.7), the activated G-protein activates phospholipase C to catalyse the formation of the second messengers IP_3 and DAG. The former agent acts to release Ca^{2+} from stores in the endoplasmic reticulum (see Figure 3.7) while the latter agent activates protein kinase C (see p. 13) and may thereby increase the Ca^{2+} sensitivity of the intracellular contractile or secretory machinery. The activator Ca^{2+} released by IP_3 may itself activate the intracellular machinery. Additionally, it may amplify the second messenger signal by increasing the membrane permeability to Cl^-, resulting in depolarization (excitatory postjunctional potential). The depolarization results in the opening of L-type voltage-sensitive Ca^{2+} channels, leading to the influx of Ca^{2+}, and (in those cells that exhibit action potentials) an increase in action potential frequency.

   (b) In effector cells where acetylcholine has an inhibitory action, the activated G-protein evokes a selective increase in membrane permeability to K^+-ions, resulting in hyperpolarization (inhibitory postjunctional potential) and (in those cells that exhibit action potentials) a decrease in action potential frequency.

   Note that since many autonomic effector cells exhibit spontaneous electrical activity, the interaction of acetylcholine with the muscarinic acetylcholine receptor tends not to initiate but rather to modify on-going electrical activity.

(6) Dissociation of the acetylcholine/acetylcholine receptor complex.

(7) Hydrolysis of acetylcholine by neural acetylcholinesterase and diffusion of acetylcholine away from the site of action.

(8) Transport of choline back into the nerve terminal.

(9) Resynthesis of acetylcholine.

(10) Storage of acetylcholine in vesicles.

Effects of agonists at muscarinic acetylcholine receptors

Acetylcholine, methacholine (Figure 2.22), *pilocarpine* and muscarine (see Figure 1.4) activate muscarinic acetylcholine receptors and cause changes (depolarization and/or IP_3 production; hyperpolarization) in effector cell activity analogous to the changes evoked by acetylcholine released from acetylcholinergic nerve terminals. Hence the agonists at muscarinic acetylcholine receptors can give rise to the excitatory and inhibitory effects listed in Table 2.7. Since many of the agonists at

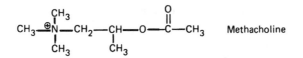

Figure 2.22 The structure of methacholine, an agonist at muscarinic acetylcholine receptors. Compare it with the structure of acetylcholine (see Figure 1.4)

muscarinic acetylcholine receptors are less susceptible than acetylcholine to hydrolysis by acetylcholinesterase, the cellular changes evoked by them are longer lasting that those evoked by stimulation of acetylcholinergic nerves.

The effects of agonists at muscarinic acetylcholine receptors are called (rather imprecisely) parasympathomimetic effects. Hence agonists at muscarinic acetylcholine receptors can also be called directly acting parasympathomimetic drugs. Contrast these agents with other drugs that can cause the same effects but by different mechanisms – the indirectly acting parasympathomimetic drugs. Examples include the agonists at the nicotinic acetylcholine receptors of ganglia (see p. 62) and anticholinesterase drugs (see p. 73).

Acetylcholine and muscarine are not used clinically.

Pilocarpine eye-drops cause miosis, contraction of the ciliary muscle and increase the drainage of aqueous humour. They are useful in reducing intra-ocular pressure in acute attacks of closed-angle glaucoma (long-term relief from attacks requires surgery) and in long-term control of open-angle glaucoma.

Effects of competitive antagonists at muscarinic acetylcholine receptors

Atropine, **hyoscine** [scopolamine], *cyclopentolate, tropicamide*
Quaternary ammonium derivatives – *ipratropium*
Antimuscarinic drugs used in parkinsonism – *benzhexol*
Tricyclic antidepressant drugs – **imipramine**
Antipsychotic drugs – *thioridazine*
Antidysrhythmic drugs – *quinidine*

These agents are all competitive antagonists of acetylcholine at muscarinic acetylcholine receptors. Injection of these agents results in the effects shown in Table 2.8.

Measurements of the relative potencies of antagonists at muscarinic acetylcholine receptors and molecular biology techniques suggest that such receptors can exist in the form of four distinct subtypes, designated M_1, M_2, M_3 and M_4 acetylcholine receptors. *Pirenzepine* is a competitive antagonist exhibiting selectivity for the M_1 acetylcholine receptor. By blocking M_1 acetylcholine receptors on gastric parietal cells, *pirenzepine* can inhibit neurogenic gastric acid and pepsin secretion without exhibiting many of the other effects of **atropine**.

Atropine is the type substance of the non-selective antagonists at muscarinic acetylcholine receptors. It has two actions that cannot be

Table 2.8 Some effects of competitive antagonists at muscarinic acetylcholine receptors

Eye	
Ciliary smooth muscle	Relaxed (cycloplegia)
Circular smooth muscle of iris	Relaxed (mydriasis)
Lacrimal and salivary glands	Reduced secretion
Heart	
SA node	Tachycardia
AV node	Reduced refractory period
Respiratory tract	
Airway smooth muscle	Relaxed
Bronchial glands	Reduced secretion
Gut, stomach to rectum	
Propulsive smooth musculature	Reduced motility
Alimentary and pancreatic exocrine glands	Reduced secretion
Bladder	Difficulty in micturition
Skin	
Eccrine sweat glands	Reduced secretion

Note:
(1) In vivo, blockade of acetylcholinergic autonomic neuroeffector transmission by **atropine** is more readily produced in some organs than in others. The order of susceptibility to blockade is: sweat, bronchial and salivary glands > heart and muscles of eye > smooth muscle of bladder and gastrointestinal tract > gastric glands. The reason for this difference in susceptibility is unclear.
(2) It is easier to prevent the effects of exogenous (injected) acetylcholine than endogenous (released from nerve terminals) acetylcholine. (The concentration of acetylcholine in a narrow cleft during neuroeffector transmission can be large enough to surmount the effects of relatively large doses of atropine-like drugs.)

explained in terms of blockade of acetylcholinergic transmission in the periphery:

(1) It causes histamine release, by virtue of its basicity (Table 4.12), which results in dilatation of cutaneous vessels.
(2) It stimulates the CNS.

In therapeutic doses **atropine** stimulates the medullary vagal centre to evoke a transient bradycardia. This precedes the tachycardia due to occupation of SA nodal muscarinic acetylcholine receptors by **atropine**. In toxic doses it causes restlessness, excitement, hallucinations, delirium and convulsions. Therapeutic uses are:

(1) Anaesthetic pre-medication for effects on bronchial secretions and heart: **hyoscine** (sedative) is often preferred to **atropine** (CNS stimulant).
(2) Routine mydriasis (diagnostic retinoscopy) carries a risk of precipitating glaucoma, particularly in the elderly, so choose a short-acting mydriatic agent -- *tropicamide*.
(3) Accurate diagnostic refraction in children who are unable voluntarily to relax the ciliary muscle requires cycloplegia – *cyclopentolate*.
(4) Iritis and iridocyclitis are inflammatory conditions in which the iris tends to adhere to the anterior surface of the lens. A mydriatic agent with a long action is preferred – **atropine**.

(5) Protection against undesired effects of anticholinesterase drugs during anticholinesterase drug therapy and poisoning (see p. 75).

(6) Parkinson's disease (see p. 228). Highly lipid-soluble antagonists at muscarinic acetylcholine receptors (e.g. *benzhexol*) are able to penetrate the CNS. They are used to control tremor and excessive salivation associated with Parkinson's disease.

(7) Muscarinic (rapid-type mushroom) poisoning results from ingestion of toadstools that contain appreciable amounts of muscarine (e.g. the red-staining inocybe, *Inocybe patouillardii*) – **atropine** is a specific antidote

(8) Travel sickness – **hyoscine** is useful (see p. 241).

(9) Bronchoconstriction of chronic bronchitis has an element mediated by acetylcholine release. The quaternary N-containing compound *ipratropium* is useful in controlling the bronchoconstriction. Under administration by inhalation, it shows distributional selectivity.

(10) Gastric and duodenal (peptic) ulceration — *pirenzepine* usefully reduces gastric acid and pepsin secretion and thereby promotes healing (see p. 463). The use of *pirenzepine* in the treatment of gastric and duodenal ulceration is less frequent than that of other forms of therapy (eradication of *Helicobacter pylori* infection, blockade of histamine H_2 receptors, inhibition of the gastric proton pump; see p. 464).

Summary

(1) Muscarinic acetylcholine receptors are found on smooth muscle cells, cardiac muscle cells, exocrine gland cells and cells of the vascular endothelium.

(2) Muscarinic acetylcholine receptors differ from nicotinic acetylcholine receptors in the relative affinities of both agonists and antagonists.

(3) There is evidence to suggest the existence of several subtypes of muscarinic acetylcholine receptor.

(4) By activating the muscarinic acetylcholine receptor, agonists (e.g. *pilocarpine*) can evoke changes in the activity of a wide variety of effector cells.

(5) By occupying the muscarinic acetylcholine receptor without causing its activation, antagonists (e.g. **atropine**) can evoke changes in the activity of a wide variety of effector cells.

Cholinesterases and their inhibitors

Acetylcholinesterase

Acetylcholinesterase (E.C. 3.1.1.7) is found in and near the endings of all acetylcholinergic axons and in erythrocytes. It is the activity of acetylcholinesterase that is primarily responsible for transmitter inactivation during acetylcholinergic transmission (Figure 2.10).

Acetylcholinesterase exhibits relatively high substrate specificity – it hydrolyses certain of the esters of choline (Table 2.9). Substrate attachment occurs both at the anionic and esteratic sites of the active centre of acetylcholinesterase (Figure 2.23).

Cholinesterase

Cholinesterase (pseudocholinesterase, butyrylcholinesterase, E.C. 3.1.1.8) is found in blood serum, in the liver and in certain effector cells.

The substrate specificity of cholinesterase is low (cf. acetylcholinesterase). It not only hydrolyses certain choline esters (compare and contrast with acetylcholinesterase, Table 2.9) but it also hydrolyses esters unrelated to choline (e.g. the ester kind of local anaesthetic agent, see p. 105).

Table 2.9 Hydrolysis of choline esters by acetylcholinesterase and cholinesterase

Substrate	Rate of hydrolysis by acetylcholinesterase	Rate of hydrolysis by cholinesterase
Acetylcholine	+++	++
Methacholine	+	0
Suxamethonium	0	+

+++ = very rapid hydrolysis; + = slow hydrolysis; 0 = no hydrolysis.

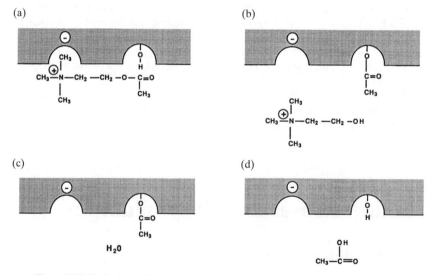

Figure 2.23 Hydrolysis of acetylcholine by acetylcholinesterase: (a) attachment of acetylcholine to anionic and esteratic sites; (b) acetylation of esteratic site with liberation of choline; (c) and (d) hydrolytic reactivation of esteratic site with liberation of acetic acid

Roughly 1 in every 3000 individuals is a homozygote with an abnormal gene pair that directs the synthesis of an atypical form of cholinesterase. The atypical enzyme hydrolyses **suxamethonium** exceedingly slowly, so that a homozygote producing the atypical enzyme stays paralysed for some hours when given this drug (see p. 55). Heterozygotes may hydrolyse **suxamethonium** slower than normal individuals but rapidly enough to present no clinical problem.

The atypical form of cholinesterase is relatively resistant to inhibition by cinchocaine [dibucaine]. Measurement of the dibucaine number (percentage inhibition of serum cholinesterase activity produced by a standard concentration of dibucaine) gives an indication of whether the subject possesses abnormal genes for synthesizing cholinesterase. A dibucaine number close to 80 indicates the absence of atypical cholinesterase. A dibucaine number significantly smaller than 80 indicates the presence of atypical enzyme.

Inhibitors of cholinesterases

Competitive inhibitors

Neostigmine, *physostigmine* (eserine), *pyridostigmine, edrophonium, carbaryl*

The inhibition of acetylcholinesterase produced by these agents can be overcome by increasing the substrate (e.g. acetylcholine) concentration and the inhibited enzyme can readily be reactivated by subjecting it to dialysis – the inhibition is reversible. With the exceptions of *carbaryl* and *physostigmine*, all agents in this group have molecular structures that contain a quaternized N-atom, and hence are fully ionized over a wide pH range. The positive charge on the quaternized N atom facilitates attachment of these agents to the anionic site of the active centre of acetylcholinesterase (Figure 2.23).

Since *physostigmine* is a tertiary amine its inhibition of acetylcholinesterase is pH dependent. Attachment of *physostigmine* to the anionic site of acetylcholinesterase only occurs when the N atom of the amine group is positively charged.

Edrophonium is unique among the competitive inhibitors of acetylcholinesterase in that it is not an ester. *Edrophonium* cannot therefore combine with the esteratic site of acetylcholinesterase. This may explain the very brief duration of action of *edrophonium* in vivo.

Acetylcholinesterase and cholinesterase are equally sensitive to the actions of the competitive inhibitors.

Active site-directed irreversible inhibitors

Malaoxon from *malathion*, military nerve gases (e.g. sarin)

The inhibition of acetylcholinesterase produced by these agents cannot be overcome by increasing the substrate (e.g. acetylcholine) concentration and the inhibited enzyme cannot be reactivated by dialysis – the inhibition is irreversible.

STAFFS UNIVERSITY LIBRARY

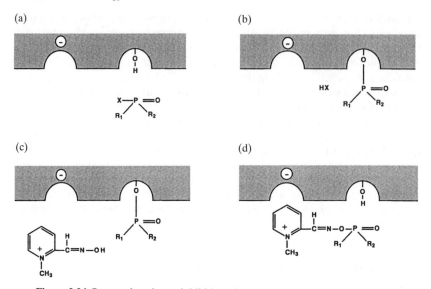

Figure 2.24 Organophosphorus inhibition of acetylcholinesterase: (a) and (b) phosphorylation of esteratic site with liberation of acid (HX); (c) and (d) reactivation of esteratic site by pralidoxime

The irreversible inhibitors of acetylcholinesterase are organophosphorus esters and all can bind firmly to (phosphorylate) the esteratic site of acetylcholinesterase (Figure 2.24).

The irreversible inhibitors have greater affinities for cholinesterase than for acetylcholinesterase.

Consequences of cholinesterase inhibition

Inhibition of acetylcholinesterase delays the biotransformation of acetylcholine. The resulting accumulation of endogenous acetylcholine at muscarinic acetylcholine receptors evokes parasympathomimetic effects (see p. 67 and Table 2.1), including excessive sweating, salivation and bronchial secretion, miosis, bradycardia and diarrhoea. These effects can be minimized by the administration of an antagonist at muscarinic acetylcholine receptors – **atropine**.

Inhibition of acetylcholinesterase can cause fasciculation of skeletal muscle and convulsions. However, when acetylcholinesterase is inhibited by approximately 80%, the accumulation of acetylcholine at the skeletal neuromuscular junction evokes depolarizing blockade of neuromuscular transmission (see p. 55 and Figure 2.14). At this point death may ensue from respiratory paralysis – effectively due to acetylcholine poisoning.

Uses of inhibitors of cholinesterases

Competitive inhibitors of acetylcholinesterase are used in the diagnosis and treatment of myasthenia gravis. This disease is believed to have an autoimmune basis. The sufferer produces antibodies to his/her nicotinic acetyl-choline receptors in skeletal muscle. The reduced number of functional receptors leads to impairment of acetylcholinergic transmission at the skele-tal neuromuscular junction, producing weakness and ready fatiguability of skeletal muscle. *Edrophonium* is a diagnostic agent – a positive result is indicated by a brief increase in muscular power following its injection.

Neostigmine and *pyridostigmine* are used in the symptomatic treatment of myasthenia usually in conjunction with **atropine**, which minimizes the effects of acetylcholine at muscarinic acetylcholine receptors. Overdosage with **neostigmine** or *pyridostigmine* can itself precipitate muscle weakness due to excessive accumulation of acetylcholine causing depolarizing block-ade of neuromuscular transmission – a <u>cholinergic crisis</u>. *Edrophonium* can be used to distinguish between a cholinergic crisis and the effects of undertreatment or increased disease severity. An injection of *edropho-nium* briefly exacerbates a cholinergic crisis but briefly increases muscle power in the case of underdosage with an inhibitor of acetylcholinesterase.

Neostigmine is used to accelerate the offset of the neuromuscular block-ade evoked by **tubocurarine** or *vecuronium* (Table 2.3). The injection of **neostigmine** is preceded by an injection of **atropine** in order to minimize the effects of acetylcholine at muscarinic acetylcholine receptors.

Physostigmine is useful for reducing intra-ocular pressure in closed-angle glaucoma. Its use in the eye carries a risk of systemic toxicity, since it is well absorbed from the conjunctival sac.

Malathion and *carbaryl* are used as insecticides in the treatment of pediculosis (see p. 288). A number of different organophosphorus inhibitors of cholinesterase are used as agricultural insecticides or military nerve gases.

Reactivation of cholinesterases inhibited by organophosphorus compounds

The inhibition of esterases evoked by organophosphorus compounds is irreversible in the sense that the phosphorylated esteratic site cannot spontaneously hydrolyse. If, and only if, the phosphorylation is recent, the enzyme can be reactivated by agents that are more nucleophilic than water (e.g. **pralidoxime**) (Figure 2.24). **Pralidoxime** administered some time after phosphorylation of the enzyme has occurred is ineffective because even more stable chemical bonds develop between the inhibitor and the ester-atic site of the enzyme.

Industrial, agricultural or military poisoning with organophosphorus anticholinesterase agents is treated by injection of both **atropine** and **prali-doxime**.

Summary

(1) Enzymes that hydrolyse acetylcholine include acetylcholinesterase and cholinesterase.
(2) Acetylcholinesterase is associated with acetylcholinergic nerve termi-nals and erythrocytes and exhibits high substrate specificity.

(3) Cholinesterase is found in the liver, blood serum and certain effector cells; its substrate specificity is relatively low.
(4) A genetically determined atypical form of cholinesterase hydrolyses **suxamethonium** very slowly.
(5) Competitive, reversible inhibitors of acetylcholinesterase (e.g. **neostigmine**) slow the hydrolysis of acetylcholine and cause its accumulation within the synaptic or junctional cleft. This results in more intense and prolonged activation of both muscarinic and nicotinic acetylcholine receptors.
(6) Active site-directed irreversible inhibitors of cholinesterase (e.g. sarin) also cause intense activation of acetylcholine receptors. They phosphorylate the active site of cholinesterase. Provided that such phosphorylation is recent, the enzyme can be reactivated by **pralidoxime**.

Noradrenergic neuroeffector transmission as a target of drug action

Revise

- The anatomy and physiology of the sympathetic nervous system (see pp. 34 and 40).
- The effects of stimulating sympathetic neurones (Table 2.1).

Noradrenergic neurones synthesize, store and release noradrenaline as their transmitter. They include:

(1) Most postganglionic sympathetic neurones (except those neurones supplying the eccrine sweat glands and those providing a vasodilator pathway to the arterioles of skeletal muscle – although anatomically sympathetic, these neurones are acetylcholinergic).
(2) Some neurones lying entirely within the CNS.

Anatomy of sympathetic neuroeffector junctions

The anatomy of sympathetic neuroeffector junctions is comparable with that of parasympathetic neuroeffector junctions (see p. 40). Those effector cells that receive a noradrenergic innervation (smooth muscle, cardiac muscle and exocrine gland cells) are supplied by postganglionic sympathetic neurones. The receptor sites for noradrenaline (α- and β-adrenoceptors, see p. 91) are located over the entire surface of the effector cells. They can also be found on cells that do not receive noradrenergic innervation (Table 2.14).

Drugs with noradrenergic prejunctional sites of action

Noradrenergic transmission

The process of noradrenergic neuroeffector transmission (Figure 2.25) is basically similar at all sites in the body. Drugs that act on noradrenergic axons and their terminals (drugs that interfere with stages A, B, C, D and H in Figure 2.25) modify noradrenergic transmission similarly at all sites.

Synthesis of noradrenaline

The biosynthesis of noradrenaline may arbitrarily be regarded as the first stage in the process of noradrenergic transmission. The starting material

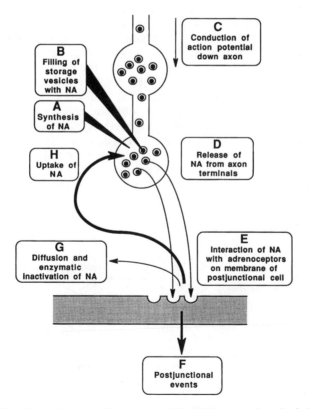

Figure 2.25 Noradrenergic neuroeffector transmission (NA = noradrenaline). The relative thicknesses of the lines representing removal of NA from the receptors indicates the relative physiological importance of the two processes

is dietary L-phenylalanine. This amino acid is actively absorbed from the gut and oxidized in the liver by phenylalanine hydroxylase to form L-tyrosine, which circulates in the bloodstream. Like other neutral amino acids entering mammalian cells, it is co-transported across the cytoplasmic membrane of noradrenergic neurones with Na^+. The membrane Na^+/K^+-ATPase then actively pumps the Na^+ outwards.

Within the cytoplasm of the noradrenergic neurone (Figure 2.26) L-tyrosine is hydroxylated to form L-dihydroxyphenylalanine (L-dopa, **levodopa**). This reaction is catalysed by tyrosine hydroxylase and is the rate-limiting step in the biosynthesis of noradrenaline. The activity of tyrosine hydroxylase is governed by the cytoplasmic concentration of noradrenaline, a large noradrenaline concentration inhibiting enzyme activity. This is an example of <u>feedback</u> (product) <u>inhibition</u>.

Tyrosine hydroxylase exhibits some substrate specificity but is susceptible to inhibition by *metirosine* (α-methyltyrosine). This inhibits tyrosine hydroxylase and reduces catecholamine synthesis. It is useful in limiting the catecholamine output of a rare tumour of the adrenal medullary chromaffin cells (phaeochromocytoma), both preoperatively or as a long-term therapy in inoperable cases.

Aromatic L-amino acid decarboxylase is a cytoplasmic enzyme of low substrate specificity that converts L-dopa to dopamine. Levodopa is useful to replace a functional deficiency of dopamine in the treatment of Parkinson's disease (see p. 229). Aromatic L-amino acid decarboxylase can be inhibited by *benserazide* and by *carbidopa*. These agents are hydrophilic analogues of L-dopa and so they do not enter the brain (see p. 342). They can therefore produce an inhibition selectively restricted to peripherally located enzyme. This property makes the utilization of **levodopa** more efficient in central than peripheral dopaminergic and noradrenergic neurones. Hence, the unwanted peripheral effect of cardiac tachy-dysrhythmias, due to excessive catecholamine production, and the dose of **levodopa** needed for the treatment of Parkinson's disease are reduced.

Dopamine, synthesized within the neuronal cytoplasm, is actively transported into the transmitter storage vesicles of the axon terminals. There,

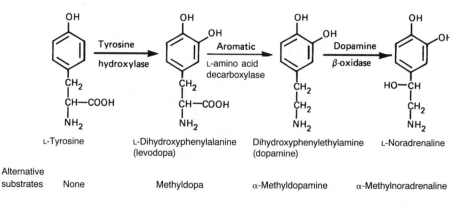

Figure 2.26 Synthesis of noradrenaline

it is oxidized by dopamine β-hydroxylase (an enzyme of low substrate specificity) to form noradrenaline.

Storage of noradrenaline in vesicles

Endogenous noradrenaline is stored in membrane-limited vesicles, which are formed in the neuronal cell body and transported to the varicosities of the axon terminal by axoplasmic flow. Within the vesicles, noradrenaline is weakly complexed with ATP and a soluble protein called chromogranin. The retention of noradrenaline inside vesicles results from its affinity for the vesicular contents and from the continued operation of the amine uptake process in the vesicle membrane (a process requiring energy from the breakdown of ATP by Mg^{2+}-dependent ATPase).

Drugs that interfere with the vesicular retention of noradrenaline

Reserpine and *tetrabenazine* inhibit the amine uptake process in the vesicle membrane and thereby allow the leakage of noradrenaline into the cytoplasm where it is largely metabolized by neuronal monoamine oxidase (MAO, see p. 85). Furthermore, since vesicular dopamine uptake is inhibited, noradrenaline synthesis is impaired. For these two reasons the storage vesicles become depleted of noradrenaline (chromaffin cells of the adrenal medulla and noradrenergic, dopaminergic and 5-hydroxytryptaminergic neurones within the CNS are also susceptible to this action of reserpine, see p. 231).

Noradrenaline depletion induced by reserpine or *tetrabenazine* is accelerated by action potential activity in the neurone. Noradrenergic neuroeffector transmission fails when the noradrenaline content is reduced to approximately 25% of normal. When large doses of reserpine are used, recovery of neurone function depends upon the synthesis of new vesicles and their transport to the axon terminals (approximately 10 days).

Pretreatment with reserpine:

(1) Abolishes the effects of sympathetic noradrenergic neurone activity.
(2) Abolishes the effects of agents that cause the release of noradrenaline from axon terminals – the <u>indirectly acting sympathomimetic agents</u> (see p. 82).
(3) Does not reduce responses of effector cells to exogenous noradrenaline or to other agonists acting on adrenoceptors (see p. 91).
(4) Has similar effects on noradrenergic, dopaminergic and 5-hydroxytryptaminergic neurotransmission in the CNS (see p. 221).

Reserpine was formerly useful in the treatment of severe hypertension. Part of the hypotensive action of reserpine results from the impairment of monoaminergic transmission in BP control centres of the CNS. It is now rarely used because it can induce severe (suicidal) depression.

Tetrabenazine is of use in Huntington's chorea (see p. 230) and related disorders of movement, presumably because its action depletes the transmitter stores of central dopaminergic neurones. The usefulness of *tetra-*

benazine, like reserpine, is limited by the development of severe depression.

Drugs that compete with noradrenaline for vesicular storage

Certain drugs, on gaining access to the neuronal cytoplasm, can compete with dopamine or noradrenaline for uptake into the vesicles. They may then stoichiometrically displace noradrenaline from its storage site. Drugs in this group include α-methyldopamine formed from *methyldopa* and certain indirectly acting sympathomimetic agents (tyramine, amphetamine).

As a consequence of noradrenaline displacement:

(1) Less noradrenaline is available for release during neuroeffector transmission.
(2) The displacing drug may be released in the place of noradrenaline during neuroeffector transmission (false transmission).
(3) The response of the effector cell to the displacing drug may result from the pharmacological effects of displaced noradrenaline (see indirectly acting sympathomimetic agents, p. 82).

Methyldopa (cf. triethylcholine acting on acetylcholinergic transmission, p. 50) is a substrate for aromatic L-amino acid decarboxylase and hence can be converted to α-methyldopamine. α-Methyldopamine is not a substrate for neuronal MAO (because it carries the α-methyl substituent, see p. 85) so it competes very successfully with dopamine for transport into the storage vesicles. Vesicular dopamine β-hydroxylase then oxidizes α-methyldopamine to yield α-methylnoradrenaline. This substance functions as a false transmitter since it can be stored in the vesicles and is subsequently released into the junctional cleft on arrival of the nerve action potential. α-Methylnoradrenaline is approximately equipotent with noradrenaline in evoking a response from effector cells in the periphery by agonist action at postjunctional α_1-adrenoceptors (see p. 91) but is more potent than noradrenaline at prejunctional α_2-adrenoceptors. It reduces neuroeffector transmission by reducing the amount of neurotransmitter released.

Pretreatment with *methyldopa*:

(1) Reduces the effects of noradrenergic neurone activity, and of dopaminergic neurone activity in the CNS.
(2) Reduces the effects of agents that cause the release of noradrenaline from axon terminals – the indirectly acting sympathomimetic agents (see p. 82).
(3) Does not reduce the responses of effector cells to exogenous noradrenaline or to other agonists acting on adrenoceptors (see p. 91).

Methyldopa is useful in the treatment of moderate to severe hypertension in patients in whom antagonists at β-adrenoceptors are contraindicated (see p. 102) and in pregnancy (see p. 412). Its main site of action in reducing cardiac output and peripheral resistance seems to be the central noradrenergic neurones involved in the control of BP. Unwanted effects include drowsiness, depression and retention of salt and water by the kidney (see p. 197).

Neuronal action potential conduction

Action potential conduction in noradrenergic neurones is comparable with that in other neurones.

Noradrenergic neurone blocking agents

The noradrenergic neurone blocking agents (e.g. *guanethidine*) selectively impair transmission at noradrenergic neuroeffector junctions. These agents show weak local anaesthetic activity on non-noradrenergic neurones, but are selectively accumulated by noradrenergic neurones by the same mechanism that transports noradrenaline into the cell – the neuronal uptake pump (see p. 87). Thus the noradrenergic neurone blocking agents are accumulated within noradrenergic neurones to a concentration sufficiently large to exert a local anaesthetic effect. Noradrenaline release is abolished mainly by the prevention of nerve action potential conduction in terminal neuronal branches. In addition, these drugs cause depletion of stored noradrenaline and may interfere with exocytosis. Large doses of *guanethidine* may cause structural damage in noradrenergic nerve terminals, so that the axon partly and temporarily dies back towards the cell body.

The noradrenergic neurone blocking agents:

(1) Prevent the effects of noradrenergic neurone activity.
(2) Prevent the effects of agents that cause the release of noradrenaline from axon terminals – the indirectly acting sympathomimetic agents (see p. 82).
(3) Do not reduce the effects of exogenous noradrenaline or other agonists at adrenoceptors (see p. 91). Indeed, such an agent is potentiated if it is a substrate for the neuronal noradrenaline uptake process.

The selectivity of the noradrenergic neurone blocking agents and their ability to modify the actions of indirectly acting sympathomimetic agents and of some agonists acting on adrenoceptors all depend on their being substrates for the neuronal noradrenaline uptake process. The actions of noradrenergic neurone blocking agents are impaired by other drugs that either compete for uptake into the neurone (tyramine) or block the uptake process (*cocaine*, **imipramine**, see p. 88).

Guanethidine eye-drops (formulated with *adrenaline*, see p. 96) can reduce intraocular pressure in chronic, open-angle glaucoma. The noradrenergic neurone blocking agents were sometimes useful in the treatment of severe hypertension that was resistant to other drugs. The wide range of unwanted effects included postural and exercise hypotension, retention of salt and water by the kidney (see p. 197), diarrhoea and failure of ejaculation.

Release of noradrenaline from axon terminals

The release of noradrenaline from noradrenergic axons is comparable with the release of acetylcholine from acetylcholinergic axons (see p. 49).

In the absence of action potential traffic in noradrenergic nerves, the random migration of storage vesicles to the cell surface occasionally results in exocytosis. Although the amount of noradrenaline released is small, it can still influence the membrane of the postjunctional cell if the cleft is narrow. For example, spontaneous postjunctional potentials are seen in some noradrenergically innervated smooth muscles (cf. the miniature epp seen at the motor end-plate of skeletal muscle, Figure 2.12).

Reserpine, by depleting the vesicles of stored noradrenaline (see p. 79), prevents both the spontaneous and action potential-evoked release of noradrenaline (see below).

When an action potential invades the varicosities, membrane permeability changes occur. Na^+, Cl^- and Ca^{2+} enter the axon terminals and K^+ emerges. N-type voltage-sensitive Ca^{2+} channels are activated (see p. 127). The influx of Ca^{2+} triggers many storage vesicles to release noradrenaline, ATP, chromogranin and dopamine β-hydroxylase into the extracellular space (exocytosis) and this noradrenaline diffuses down its concentration gradient to stimulate adrenoceptors on the effector cell surface. The empty vesicles are probably retained within the cell and subsequently refilled with transmitter.

Since transmitter release by this mechanism requires the nerve action potential, it is prevented by noradrenergic neurone blocking agents.

Since transmitter release by this mechanism requires the influx of Ca^{2+}, release is reduced if the extracellular environment is deficient in this ion or contains a large concentration of Mg^{2+}.

After treatment of tissues with *methyldopa*, neuronal action potentials release less noradrenaline but this is accompanied by the release of α-methylnoradrenaline (false transmission, see p. 80) from the terminals of noradrenergic axons.

Indirectly acting sympathomimetic agents

The effects of activation of noradrenergic neurones are called (rather imprecisely) sympathomimetic effects. Hence an agonist at adrenoceptors could also be called a directly acting sympathomimetic agent. An indirectly acting sympathomimetic agent does not itself activate adrenoceptors. It evokes sympathomimetic effects either (nicotine, tyramine) by promoting the release of neuronal noradrenaline or (*cocaine*) by preventing the inactivation of noradrenaline.

Agonists at the nicotinic acetylcholine receptors of ganglia

Acetylcholine and nicotine cause action potentials to be generated in noradrenergic neurones and so evoke release of neural noradrenaline (Figure 2.19), thereby indirectly inducing sympathomimetic effects.

Tyramine-like indirectly acting sympathomimetic agents

Certain chemical modifications of the noradrenaline molecule (loss of catechol-OH groups; loss of the β-OH group; methylation of the α-C atom) yield agents that are sympathomimetic despite being unable

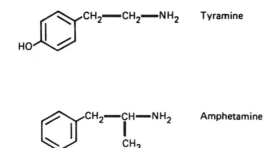

Figure 2.27 The structures of some indirectly acting sympathomimetic drugs

themselves to activate adrenoceptors. Examples include tyramine and amphetamine (Figure 2.27). However, these drugs do act as substrates for the noradrenaline uptake process in the neuronal membrane (see p. 88) and gain access to the neuronal cytoplasm by that route. In addition, amphetamine is sufficiently lipid soluble to enter the neurone by diffusion across the neuronal membrane. From the cytoplasm they are then transported into the transmitter storage vesicles where they stoichiometrically (molecule for molecule) displace noradrenaline. A large proportion of the displaced noradrenaline escapes from the neurone and subsequently activates postjunctional adrenoceptors because the MAO associated with the mitochondria (see p. 85), which would normally break down excess cytoplasmic noradrenaline, is occupied by a competing molecule. Tyramine is a substrate and amphetamine an inhibitor of MAO.

Noradrenaline release evoked by tyramine-like agents does not require the discharge of neuronal action potentials.

The properties of the tyramine-like group of indirectly acting sympathomimetic agents are compared with those of noradrenaline and adrenaline, the physiological agonists acting on adrenoceptors, in Table 2.10.

Inhibitors of the neuronal uptake of noradrenaline

Cocaine and **imipramine** inhibit the neuronal uptake of noradrenaline (see p. 88). Endogenous noradrenaline (spontaneously released or released by neuronal action potentials) therefore accumulates in the junctional cleft and activates adrenoceptors. *Cocaine* and **imipramine** are sufficiently lipid soluble to be able to penetrate into the CNS. Their central effects are, in part, consequences of inhibition of neuronal uptake of noradrenaline there.

Summary

(1) Most postganglionic sympathetic neurones are noradrenergic, as are some CNS neurones.
(2) The synthesis of dopamine, noradrenaline and adrenaline can be modified by drugs acting as substrates (e.g. **levodopa**, *methyldopa*) or inhibitors of the synthetic enzymes.

Table 2.10 Comparison of the properties of physiological agonists acting on adrenoceptors and indirectly acting on sympathomimetic agents

Physiological agonists acting on adrenoceptors, noradrenaline, adrenaline	Indirectly acting sympathomimetic agents, e.g. tyramine, amphetamine	Explanation for different property of indirectly acting drug
Chemically unstable	Chemically more stable	Drug molecule lacks catechol –OH groups
Pharmacological effects are brief	Pharmacological effects are more prolonged	Drug molecule relatively resistant to biotransformation
Poorly absorbed from gut	Better absorption from gut	Drug molecule lacks catechol –OH groups and is less polar
Poor penetration of CNS and thus CNS effects unremarkable	Better penetration of CNS and thus CNS effects more prominent	Drug molecule lacks catechol –OH groups and is less polar
Postganglionic sympathetic denervation potentiates	Postganglionic sympathetic denervation prevents action	Drug must enter neurone to be active; neurones degenerate
Cocaine and **imipramine** potentiate	*Cocaine* and **imipramine** prevent action	Drug must enter neurone to be active; entry into neurone prevented
Summates with noradrenaline	Potentiates noradrenaline	Drug competes with noradrenaline for neuronal uptake
Reserpine does not prevent action	Reserpine prevents action	Drug cannot displace neural noradrenaline; transmitter stores are depleted
Phenelzine does not modify action	**Phenelzine** potentiates	MAO inhibition delays biotransformation of drug or of noradrenaline released by drug
Repeated equal doses have equal effects	Tachyphylaxis occurs	Neuronal noradrenaline stores become depleted by repeated drug challenge

(3) A non-physiological substrate leads to the synthesis, storage and release of a false transmitter.
(4) Drugs are available that disrupt the vesicular storage of noradrenaline – their effects are widespread.
(5) Drugs are available that prevent the propagation of action potentials through noradrenergic nerve terminals – their effects are widespread.
(6) A drug that activates adrenoceptors <u>indirectly</u> does so, not by combining with them itself but by increasing the local concentration of the physiological agonists, either by causing their release or reducing their inactivation.
(7) Tyramine-like indirectly acting sympathomimetic agents displace noradrenaline from the neuronal storage granules so that it leaves the nerve endings and produces noradrenergic effects.

Drugs that modify the inactivation of noradrenaline

Enzymatic degradation is not an important mechanism for the inactivation of noradrenaline released during neuroeffector transmission. The noradrenaline in the junctional cleft is largely inactivated by neuronal uptake (see p. 87).

Metabolic inactivation of noradrenaline

Sympathomimetic amines circulating in the bloodstream (amines from the diet, drugs absorbed from their site of administration, adrenaline released from the adrenal medulla) are inactivated by enzymatic destruction to a variable extent. Metabolic inactivation assumes greatest importance if the circulating amines are present in large amounts and are not substrates for neuronal uptake.

Circulating sympathomimetic amines may be metabolized by catechol-O-methyl transferase (COMT), by MAO, or by both enzymes (Figure 2.28).

Catechol-O-methyl transferase is found in the liver and certain effector cells but not in noradrenergic neurones. This enzyme can utilize any catechol as substrate. The O-methylated product may undergo conjugation (see p. 354) to form a sulphate or glucuronide, or may be oxidized by MAO (see below) to inactive products.

MAO is found in the intestine, in the liver and in mitochondria in the cytoplasm of noradrenergic neurones. MAO oxidatively deaminates its substrate. It can utilize many aryl- and alkyl-amines (noradrenaline, *adrenaline*, tyramine, 5-HT) as substrates but not those with a large N-substituent (*isoprenaline*, see p. 94) or those with an α-methyl substituent (amphetamine, α-methyldopamine). The product is the corresponding carboxylic acid (in the periphery, Figure 2.28) or glycol (in the CNS), which are inactive.

The major product of biotransformation of both noradrenaline and adrenaline released in the periphery is 3-methoxy-4-hydroxymandelic acid (vanillylmandelic acid, VMA). The urinary excretion rate of VMA is increased in phaeochromocytoma and can be measured as a diagnostic test.

Drugs that interfere with the biotransformation of noradrenaline

All catechols can act as competitive inhibitors of catechol-O-methyl transferase, an interaction that is not therapeutically exploited.

Inhibitors of MAO are of three major kinds:

(1) Competitive and rapidly reversible – *moclobemide*.
(2) Competitive but slowly dissociating – *tranylcypromine*.
(3) Irreversible – **phenelzine** (the hydrazine group), *selegiline*.

STAFFS UNIVERSITY LIBRARY

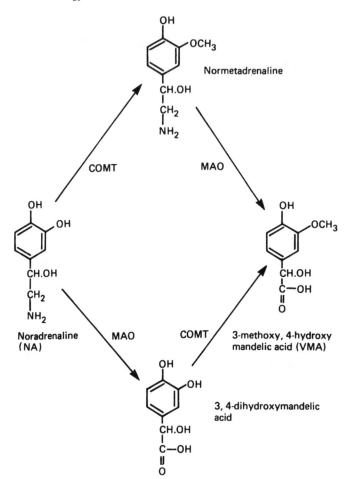

Figure 2.28 Metabolism of noradrenaline (COMT = catechol-*O*-methyl transferase, MAO = monoamine oxidase)

Phenelzine first forms a reversible complex with the active centre of the enzyme (its action is thus <u>site directed</u>). It is oxidized (it is a substrate) to form a reactive intermediate that makes a covalent addition compound with the flavin co-factor of the enzyme, thus irreversibly inhibiting enzyme activity. The enzyme can be thought of as committing suicide by oxidizing this substrate. The drug can thus be referred to as a <u>suicide substrate</u> and the mechanism of action as <u>suicide inhibition</u>.

By inhibiting MAO in the intestine, liver and noradrenergic neurones, **phenelzine**, *tranylcypromine* and *moclobemide* potentiate dietary tyramine. Significant amounts of tyramine are found in cheese, meat extracts (e.g. Bovril), yeast extracts (e.g. Marmite), pickled herrings, broad bean pods and some alcoholic drinks (those made using long extraction of red grape skins). Some sympathomimetic agents that are administered therapeutically (*adrenaline*, **levodopa**, indirectly acting sympathomimetic agents that are ingredients of proprietary cold remedies) are also potentiated and these, as well as tyramine in foodstuffs, can cause dangerous hypertensive crises.

MAO inhibition can potentiate sympathomimetic drugs by:

(1) Delaying the biotransformation of the drug itself (e.g. *adrenaline*, tyramine).
(2) Delaying the biotransformation of any noradrenaline released by the drug (e.g. tyramine).

The hydrazine group of inhibitors of MAO (e.g. **phenelzine**) lack selectivity for they can also inhibit the mixed function oxidase (MFO) enzymes (see p. 353) of the liver. They can therefore delay the biotransformation of (and thus potentiate) many drugs that are not substrates for MAO (e.g. amphetamine, *pethidine*, **morphine**).

Tranylcypromine is a close structural and functional analogue of amphetamine; hence it has CNS-stimulant properties, in addition to being an inhibitor of MAO, that further limit its usefulness.

Inhibitors of MAO have a place in the treatment of depression but their usefulness is limited because of their multiplicity of interactions with dietary constituents and other drugs.

MAO is actually composed of several isoenzymes, the most abundant of which are called MAO-A and MAO-B. Both are found in most peripheral noradrenergic neurones but the liver and gut mucosa contain mainly MAO-A. Parts of the brain contain mainly MAO-B – particularly the dopaminergic structures in the striatum. It is inhibition of MAO-A that is responsible for the augmented hypertensive response to sympathomimetic agents.

Moclobemide is a selective inhibitor of MAO-A that is claimed to be effective in depression yet to cause less potentiation of tyramine.

Selegiline is a suicide substrate selective for MAO-B and therefore an irreversible inhibitor. Potentiation of tyramine is not a problem during *selegiline* treatment because MAO-A is not inhibited. *Selegiline* is useful as an adjunct to **levodopa** in the treatment of Parkinson's disease (cf. *carbidopa*, see p. 78), as it makes the utilization of **levodopa** more efficient in dopaminergic than noradrenergic neurones.

Neuronal uptake of noradrenaline

Uptake into the cytoplasm of noradrenergic neurones is the major mechanism for inactivating noradrenaline released during neuroeffector transmission or noradrenaline injected as a small i/v dose. Blockade of uptake therefore potentiates noradrenaline released by nerve impulses or administered exogenously.

The uptake process is located in the axonal membrane and:

(1) Operates against a concentration gradient.
(2) Requires an energy supply (to generate the ATP that is substrate for the membrane Na^+/K^+-ATPase that pumps Na^+ from the cytoplasm).

(3) Requires Na$^+$ (the transporter associates with noradrenaline and Na$^+$ together and is inwardly directed by the Na$^+$ concentration gradient).
(4) Is saturable (it has a small capacity but a high affinity).
(5) Is moderately substrate specific.

Substrates for the neuronal noradrenaline uptake process

These include:

(1) The physiological directly acting sympathomimetic agents – noradrenaline and *adrenaline* (note that the synthetic drugs, *phenylephrine*, *isoprenaline* and **salbutamol** are not substrates).
(2) Certain indirectly acting sympathomimetic agents – tyramine, amphetamine.
(3) The noradrenergic neurone blocking agents – *guanethidine*.

Drug interactions among the substrates for neuronal noradrenaline uptake

(1) The tyramine-like indirectly acting sympathomimetic agents and the noradrenergic neurone blocking agents potentiate noradrenaline and *adrenaline* by competing for neuronal uptake.
(2) The tyramine-like indirectly acting sympathomimetic agents and the noradrenergic neurone blocking agents are mutually antagonistic, since they compete for the uptake process (and thus for access to their sites of action).

Non-transported inhibitors of neuronal noradrenaline uptake

Cocaine inhibits the noradrenaline uptake process at concentrations less than those required to produce local anaesthesia. *Cocaine* thus potentiates endogenous noradrenaline released either spontaneously or in response to an action potential from the axon terminal. This is the mechanisms of the mydriasis evoked by *cocaine* eye-drops. No other local anaesthetic drug has this property.

The antidepressant actions of the tricyclic agents **imipramine** and **amitriptyline** may be attributed to their blockade of monoamine uptake in the CNS (see p. 233).

Drug interactions with non-transported inhibitors of noradrenaline uptake

By blocking neuronal uptake, *cocaine* and tricyclic antidepressant drugs:

(1) Potentiate noradrenaline and *adrenaline* (by delaying their inactivation).
(2) Antagonize the tyramine-like indirectly acting sympathomimetic agents and the noradrenergic neurone blocking agents (by preventing their access to their sites of action).

Fate of noradrenaline transported into the neuronal cytoplasm

A small proportion of the noradrenaline entering the cytoplasm by way of the neuronal uptake process is metabolized by mitochondrial MAO. The majority is transported into the storage vesicles for subsequent transmitter use (cf. uptake of choline and its use in acetylcholine synthesis, see p. 51).

Figure 2.29 summarizes the mechanisms of noradrenaline uptake and release from noradrenergic neurones.

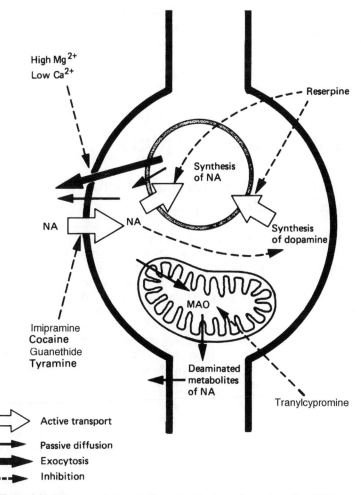

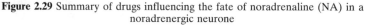

Figure 2.29 Summary of drugs influencing the fate of noradrenaline (NA) in a noradrenergic neurone

Extraneuronal uptake of noradrenaline

Uptake of catecholamines (*isoprenaline* > *adrenaline* > noradrenaline), by a large-capacity, small-affinity, active transport process, occurs at the effector cell membrane. This is their route of access to catechol-*O*-methyl transferase. Inhibitors of extraneuronal uptake are not exploited therapeutically.

Summary

(1) Inhibition of MAO type A potentiates substrates of the enzyme (e.g. tyramine).
(2) Noradrenaline is inactivated more by noradrenergic neuronal reuptake than by biodegradation.
(3) Inhibition of neuronal uptake (e.g. **imipramine**) potentiates substrates acting upon adrenoceptors (noradrenaline, adrenaline), but antagonizes substrates acting within the neurone (e.g. tyramine, *guanethidine*).

Agonists at adrenoceptors

The interaction of noradrenaline with postjunctional adrenoceptors

The noradrenaline/adrenoceptor interaction is comparable with the acetylcholine/muscarinic acetylcholine receptor interaction (see p. 68).

Neurotransmitter noradrenaline that has been released into the junctional cleft diffuses down its concentration gradient and forms reversible complexes with receptors (adrenoceptors) on the surface of the membrane of the effector cell. The size of the response is determined by the occupancy of the adrenoceptors (see pp. 15, 18). The nature of the response is determined by the effector cascade to which the adrenoceptors are coupled (see p. 11) and its physiological role in the effector cells on which the adrenoceptors are located. The signal transduction process for adrenoceptors initiates the activation of a G-protein.

(1) In smooth muscle cells where noradrenaline has an excitatory action (Tables 2.12 and 2.14), the activated G-protein activates phospholipase C with all the consequences described when acetylcholine acting at muscarinic acetylcholine receptors elicits excitatory postjunctional events (see p. 68 and Figure 3.7).

In the heart the G-protein activates adenylyl cyclase to produce cAMP. This promotes the opening of L-type Ca^{2+} channels in the cell membrane and hence increases the force of cardiac contraction (contrast with the inhibitory effects of cAMP observed in smooth muscles – see (2) below).

(2) In effector cells where noradrenaline has an inhibitory action, the activated G-protein may evoke a selective increase in membrane permeability to K^+, resulting in hyperpolarization (inhibitory postjunctional potential) and (in those cells that exhibit action potentials) a decrease in action potential frequency. Alternatively, the G-protein may stimulate the production of cAMP, which reduces the concentration of free Ca^{2+} by inhibiting the cellular influx of Ca^{2+}, enhancing the uptake of Ca^{2+} into intracellular stores or promoting the extrusion of Ca^{2+} from the cell.

Since many autonomic effector cells exhibit spontaneous electrical activity, the interaction of noradrenaline with adrenoceptors tends less to initiate but rather more to modify on-going electrical activity.

There are two major kinds of adrenoceptor, which can be distinguished by characteristic relative orders of potencies for both agonists and antagonists: the α-adrenoceptor (Table 2.11) and the β-adrenoceptor (Table 2.13). Each of these receptors exists in the form of several subtypes.

Agonists at the α-adrenoceptor

The effects mediated by α-adrenoceptors are listed in Table 2.12.

The physiological role of prejunctional α_2-adrenoceptors is illustrated in Figure 2.30 and is believed to be associated with transmitter conservation. Activation of α_2-adrenoceptors results in a reduction in the amount of noradrenaline released at any given frequency of neuronal activity. This mechanism operates when the noradrenergic nerve terminal is exposed to large concentrations of noradrenaline.

Agonists at the β-adrenoceptor

The effects mediated by β-adrenoceptors are listed in Table 2.14.

All types of β-adrenoceptor seem to be coupled to a stimulatory G-protein that activates adenylyl cyclase. Thus, in many effectors, the

---

Table 2.11 The α-adrenoceptor: relative orders of potency

Non-selective agonists
Noradrenaline	=	*Adrenaline*	>>	*Isoprenaline*

Agonists selective for subtypes of the α-adrenoceptor
α_1 *Phenylephrine*
α_2 α-Methylnoradrenaline

Non-selective antagonists
Phentolamine	>>	**Propranolol**
Phenoxybenzamine		

Antagonists selective for subtypes of the α-adrenoceptor
α_1 *Prazosin*

Note: Compounds to the left of the >> symbol are potent but not equally so; those to the right are of such low potency that they may be regarded as inactive at the α-adrenoceptor.

STAFFS UNIVERSITY LIBRARY

Table 2.12 Some effects of agonists mediated by α_1- and α_2-adrenoceptors

α_1-Adrenoceptors	
Eye	
Radial smooth muscle of iris	Contracted
Smooth muscle of eyelids	Contracted
Gut, stomach to rectum	
Propulsive smooth musculature	Inhibited
Urinary system smooth muscle	
Bladder neck and trigone	Contracted
Genital apparatus	
Smooth muscle of seminal vesicles and vas deferens	Contracted
Blood vascular system	
Smooth muscle of arteries, arterioles and veins	Constricted
α_2-Adrenoceptors	
Noradrenergic neurone terminals*	Inhibition of noradrenaline release

*Agonist action at α_2-adrenoceptors is coupled by an inhibitory G-protein to adenylyl cyclase, cAMP production is reduced and this reduces neuronal Ca^{2+} entry through N-type voltage-sensitive Ca^{2+} channels in response to an action potential and so reduces noradrenaline release.

Table 2.13 The β-adrenoceptor: relative orders of potency

Non-selective agonists				
Isoprenaline	>	*Adrenaline*	>	Noradrenaline
Agonists selective for subtypes of the β-adrenoceptor				
β_1 *Dobutamine*				
β_2 **Salbutamol**				
Non-selective antagonists				
Propranolol		>>		**Phentolamine**
				Phenoxybenzamine
Antagonists selective for subtypes of the β-adrenoceptor				
β_1 **Atenolol**				

Note: Compounds to the left of the >> symbol are potent but not equally so; those to the right are of such low potency that they may be regarded as inactive at the β-adrenoceptor.

activation of β-adrenoceptors is accompanied by an increase in cellular content of cAMP. The role of adenylyl cyclase in lipolysis and glycogenolysis is illustrated in Figure 2.31.

The effects of agonists at adrenoceptors

Adrenaline, dopamine, dobutamine, isoprenaline, noradrenaline, *phenylephrine,* **salbutamol***, salmeterol*

These drugs activate one or both kinds of adrenoceptor and cause changes in effector cell activity analogous to the changes evoked by

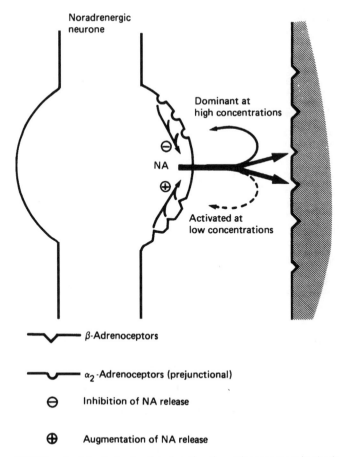

Noradrenergic
neurone

Dominant at
high concentrations

NA

Activated at
low concentrations

β-Adrenoceptors

α_2-Adrenoceptors (prejunctional)

$\ominus$ Inhibition of NA release

$\oplus$ Augmentation of NA release

Figure 2.30 The physiological role of prejunctional α_2-adrenoceptors in the heart

noradrenaline released from noradrenergic nerve terminals (depolarization and/or IP$_3$ production; hyperpolarization and/or cAMP production). Hence agonists at adrenoceptors can give rise to the excitatory and inhibitory effects listed in Tables 2.12 and 2.14. Since many agonists at adrenoceptors are less susceptible than noradrenaline to the disposal mechanisms of uptake and biotransformation, the cellular changes evoked by them are longer lasting than those evoked by stimulation of noradrenergic nerves.

Structure/activity relationships and selectivity of agonists at adrenoceptors

Agonists that activate adrenoceptors are structural analogues of *adrenaline*. This agent is a potent agonist at both α- and β-adrenoceptors. Slight changes in the structure of the *adrenaline* molecule can yield compounds that selectively activate either α- or β-adrenoceptors. Figure 2.32 shows a classification of agonists at adrenoceptors according to their α/β selectivity.

Table 2.14 Some effects of agonists that are mediated by β₁- and β₂-adrenoceptors

β₁-Adrenoceptors

Heart	
SA node	Increased firing rate
AV node	Reduced refractory period
Conducting tissue	Reduced refractory period and increased automaticity
Ventricular myocardium	Increased contractile force
Gut, stomach to rectum	
Propulsive smooth musculature	Inhibited
Kidney	
Juxtaglomerular cells	Renin release
Adipocytes*†	Lipolysis

β₂-Adrenoceptors

Respiratory tract	
Airway smooth muscle	Relaxed
Genital apparatus smooth muscle	
Uterus	Relaxed
Blood vascular system smooth muscle‡	
Arterioles	Dilated
Liver cells*	Glycogenolysis
Skeletal muscle cells*	Tremor, glycogenolysis, uptake of K^+

*β-Adrenoceptors can be found on cells that do not receive a noradrenergic innervation (cf. muscarinic acetylcholine receptors, Table 2.7).
†In infants β₃-adrenoceptors lie on brown (thermogenic) adipose tissue (agonist potencies *isoprenaline* ≈ noradrenaline > *adrenaline*; **propranolol** is of low potency as an antagonist). These receptors regress with age; lipolysis in adults is mediated by both β₁- and β₂-adrenoceptors.
‡These vessels receive noradrenergic innervation but the noradrenaline released activates only α-adrenoceptors causing vasoconstriction (Table 2.12). β-Adrenoceptors here are activated by circulating agonists (e.g. adrenaline from the adrenal medulla) – the resulting reduction in BP is largely due to dilatation of arterioles in skeletal muscle because of the large proportion of body mass that skeletal muscles constitute.

Notes:

(1) An alternative name for 1,2-dihydroxybenzene is catechol, therefore 3,4-dihydroxyphenylethylamines are catecholamines.

(2) The β-carbon atom of phenylethanolamines is asymmetric; the biosynthesis of the physiological compounds noradrenaline and adrenaline yields the L-isomer (in which much the greater biological activity resides).

(3) The physiological compounds, noradrenaline and adrenaline, have relatively low selectivity and therefore elicit effects mediated by both α- and β-adrenoceptors. The synthetic agonist agent *isoprenaline* elicits only the effects mediated by β-adrenoceptors (Table 2.14).

(4) In general, increasing the size of the alkyl substituent on the nitrogen atom of the 3,4-dihydroxyphenylethanolamine molecule increases

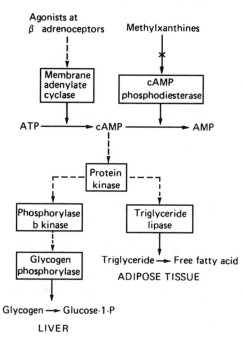

Figure 2.31 The second messenger function of cyclic nucleotide in mediating glycogenolysis and lipolysis. Note: in liver, protein kinase also phosphorylates and inhibits glycogen synthetase. Broken arrow represents activation

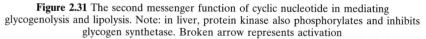

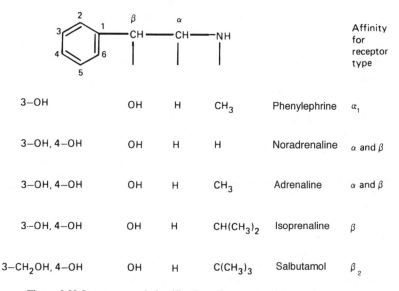

	β	α			Affinity for receptor type
3–OH	OH	H	CH$_3$	Phenylephrine	α$_1$
3–OH, 4–OH	OH	H	H	Noradrenaline	α and β
3–OH, 4–OH	OH	H	CH$_3$	Adrenaline	α and β
3--OH, 4–OH	OH	H	CH(CH$_3$)$_2$	Isoprenaline	β
3–CH$_2$OH, 4–OH	OH	H	C(CH$_3$)$_3$	Salbutamol	β$_2$

Figure 2.32 Structures and classification of some agonists at adrenoceptors

selectivity first for β- rather than α-adrenoceptors and then for $β_2$-rather than $β_1$-adrenoceptors.

(5) Provided that excessive drug concentrations are avoided, the synthetic agonist drug *phenylephrine* elicits only the effects mediated by $α_1$-adrenoceptors (Table 2.12) and the synthetic agonist drug **salbutamol** elicits only the effects mediated by $β_2$-adrenoceptors (Table 2.14).

Dopamine has complex peripheral actions on noradrenergic mechanisms. It is a precursor in the synthesis of noradrenaline (see p. 78). Furthermore, when exogenously administered, it is an agonist at both $β_1$- and $α_1$-adrenoceptors. *Dopamine* is also an agonist at renal vascular dopamine receptors, mediating vasodilatation, and it is an indirectly acting sympathomimetic agent.

Dobutamine is an analogue of *isoprenaline* that is an agonist at both $β_1$- and $α_1$-adrenoceptors. It has little chronotropic effect (contrast *isoprenaline*) because the $α_1$-adrenoceptor-mediated vasoconstriction induces an increase in mean arterial BP and therefore a baroreceptor-mediated reflex restraint on the heart rate.

Salmeterol is an analogue of **salbutamol** that has a very long alkyl substituent on the nitrogen atom. This confers a long duration of binding close to the $β_2$-adrenoceptor and a long duration of action.

Therapeutic uses

Eye-drops containing *phenylephrine* produce mydriasis, which is useful as an aid in diagnostic retinoscopy. *Adrenaline* eye-drops are effective in reducing intraocular pressure (probably both by reducing the production by ultrafiltration and by increasing the drainage of aqueous humour) in primary open-angle glaucoma.

Adrenaline is included in the formulation of some local anaesthetic agents for injection (see p. 109). By causing vasoconstriction at the injection site it prolongs the local anaesthesia.

Adrenaline is given i/m or i/v in the control of anaphylactic shock (see p. 425) and i/m in other severe forms of anaphylaxis. It usefully evokes vasoconstriction, bronchodilatation and a reduction in the protein permeability of the endothelium of postcapillary venules.

Salbutamol is useful for reducing airways resistance in bronchial asthma (see p. 487). It can relax bronchial smooth muscle at doses that have little or no cardiac stimulant activity. There is therefore less risk of tachycardia, ectopic beats and dangerous dysrhythmias than with the non-selective agent, *isoprenaline*. Most of the agonists selective at $β_2$-adrenoceptors that are used as bronchodilator drugs are neither substrates for uptake (see p. 88) nor for enzymatic degradation by MAO or catechol-*O*-methyl transferase (see p. 85). Their resistance to catechol-*O*-methyl transferase endows them with bronchodilator activity that outlasts that of *isoprenaline*. Selectivity in asthma is achieved by a combination of this pharmacodynamic selectivity for $β_2$-adrenoceptors, and dispositional selectivity from the inhaled route of administration. **Salbutamol** is also useful as a relaxant of uterine smooth muscle when attempting to suppress premature labour.

Salmeterol is useful as a bronchodilator in bronchial asthma, the action of which persists for 12 h.

Dopamine and *dobutamine* are useful, by i/v infusion, to increase the force of contraction of the failing heart (see p. 472).

Summary

(1) Agonists that are non-selective between the kinds of adrenoceptor exert a wide range of effects. The possession of a mixture of effects in appropriate proportions occasionally confers therapeutic usefulness (e.g. *adrenaline, dopamine, dobutamine*); more often it confers a wide range of unwanted effects.

(2) More selective agonists show a narrower range of effects, a few of which are therapeutically useful; *phenylephrine* (an agonist at α_1-adrenoceptors) for mydriasis and **salbutamol** (an agonist at β_2-adrenoceptors) for relaxation of bronchial or uterine smooth muscle.

Antagonists at adrenoceptors

These drugs resemble noradrenaline structurally and are therefore able to combine with adrenoceptors. However, because they have little or no intrinsic efficacy, they are unable to activate adrenoceptors, and most do not evoke an active biological response from the effector cell.

Antagonists at the α-adrenoceptor

By combining with the α-adrenoceptor, these antagonists reduce the access of agonists. They thereby reduce those effects of noradrenergic nerve activity or sympathomimetic drug (both directly and indirectly acting) action that are mediated by α-adrenoceptors (Table 2.12).

Non-selective

Phentolamine, phenoxybenzamine, chlorpromazine
These antagonists, while very selective for α- as opposed to β-adrenoceptors, have equal potency at the α_1- and α_2-adrenoceptor subtypes.

Phentolamine and **chlorpromazine** are competitive (surmountable and reversible) antagonists (see p. 23) at α-adrenoceptors.

In contrast, **phenoxybenzamine** is a non-equilibrium (insurmountable and irreversible) antagonist (see p. 24) at α-adrenoceptors. **Phenoxybenzamine** is a β-haloalkylamine (specifically a β-chloroethylamine). In neutral or alkaline solution it forms the highly reactive ethyleniminium ion. This ion either alkylates reactive groups of the cell membrane (e.g.

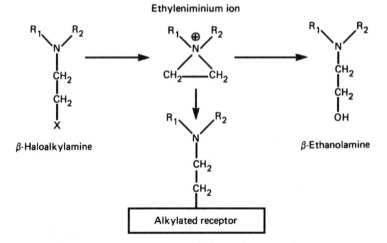

Figure 2.33 Mechanism of alkylation by **phenoxybenzamine**

the α-adrenoceptor) or spontaneously condenses with water to form an inactive alcohol (Figure 2.33).

A small concentration or short exposure time restricts **phenoxybenzamine** to alkylating α-adrenoceptors only. A larger concentration or longer exposure time leads to the alkylation of more α-adrenoceptors but also of other kinds of receptor – H_1 histamine receptors, 5-HT_2 receptors and muscarinic acetylcholine receptors.

Selective

Prazosin is a competitive antagonist that is very selective for α- as opposed to β-adrenoceptors and also has a much greater affinity for α_1- than α_2-adrenoceptors.

Therapeutic uses

Phentolamine is occasionally a useful aid in the diagnosis of phaeochromocytoma. The diagnosis is supported when an i/v injection of **phentolamine** produces a dramatic but brief reduction in BP to near or below normal by antagonizing the catecholamines that are circulating in excessive concentrations.

Phenoxybenzamine protects vascular smooth muscle from large circulating concentrations of catecholamines produced by phaeochromocytoma and is useful in providing this protection during surgical removal of such tumours or as symptomatic treatment in inoperable cases. In both circumstances it should be combined with an antagonist at β-adrenoceptors (see p. 101). Its irreversible action affords prolonged protection.

Neither **phentolamine** nor **phenoxybenzamine** has proved useful in the treatment of essential hypertension, despite the fact that each produces a marked decrease in peripheral resistance. This is because the resultant

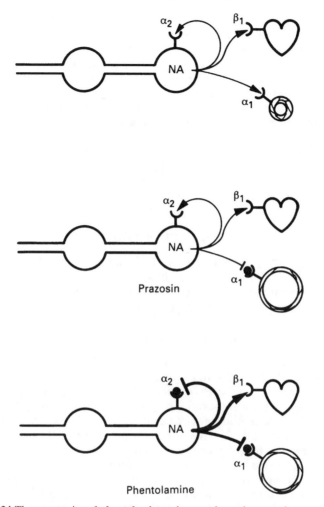

Figure 2.34 The propensity of **phentolamine**, when used as a hypotensive agent, to cause tachycardia is not shared by *prazosin*

reduction in BP is accompanied by an unacceptable degree of reflex tachycardia.

Prazosin, however, produces much less tachycardia than **phentolamine** for the same reduction in peripheral resistance and as a result has proved more useful in treating hypertension. This difference arises because of the existence of prejunctional α_2-adrenoceptors with structural requirements slightly different from the α_1-adrenoceptors on effector cells (see p. 91).

Phentolamine generates an excessive amount of reflex tachycardia because the normal feedback inhibition of noradrenaline release from cardiac noradrenergic nerves by released noradrenaline is abolished, due to occupation of prejunctional α_2-adrenoceptors (Figure 2.34). However, *prazosin* does not occupy the prejunctional α_2-adrenoceptors and the size of the reflex tachycardia can still be limited by the normal feedback inhibition via prejunctional α_2-adrenoceptors.

Prazosin, because it is able to inhibit contraction of the smooth muscle of the trigone, urethra and perhaps prostate gland, has been exploited to reduce the symptoms of benign prostatic hypertrophy – obstruction of urine flow through the bladder neck.

Other antagonists at α-adrenoceptors have useful properties unrelated to α-adrenoceptor blockade. **Chlorpromazine** (a phenothiazine) is an antipsychotic drug, which is valuable in the treatment of schizophrenia and can suppress vomiting. These actions of **chlorpromazine** on the CNS result from its interaction with dopamine receptors (see p. 237). The antagonism at α-adrenoceptors evoked by **chlorpromazine** is responsible for some unwanted effects (e.g. hypotension).

Antagonists at the β-adrenoceptor

By combining with β-adrenoceptors, these antagonists reduce the access of agonists. They thereby reduce those effects of noradrenergic nerve activity or sympathomimetic drug (both directly and indirectly acting) action that are mediated by β-adrenoceptors (Table 2.14).

Non-selective between β_1- and β_2-adrenoceptors

Propranolol, while very selective for β- as opposed to α-adrenoceptors, has equal potency at the β_1- and β_2-adrenoceptor subtypes. **Propranolol** is a competitive antagonist at β-adrenoceptors. In a concentration greater than that required for blockade of β-adrenoceptors, **propranolol** can directly stabilize the membranes of excitable cells (see p. 119), prolonging the action potential and effective refractory period of cardiac muscle. With *sotalol* this latter action is more prominent.

Labetalol has a structure that confers affinity for both β- and α-adrenoceptors but it is three times more potent as a competitive antagonist at β- than α-adrenoceptors. It exhibits no selectivity between the β_1- and β_2-adrenoceptor subtypes but it is selective for α_1-adrenoceptors, reducing the arteriolar response to noradrenaline without affecting the neuronal negative feedback mechanisms mediated by α_2-adrenoceptors (see p. 99).

Selective for β_1-adrenoceptors

Atenolol is a competitive antagonist that is very selective for β- as opposed to α-adrenoceptors and also has a greater affinity for β_1- than β_2-adrenoceptors. That is, it can antagonize noradrenaline on the heart at doses that have little or no effect on the relaxant action of noradrenaline on respiratory tract smooth muscle. **Atenolol** does not directly stabilize the membranes of excitable cells.

Other properties of antagonists at β-adrenoceptors

Oxprenolol exhibits some intrinsic efficacy at β-adrenoceptors, that is it is a partial agonist. In situations where there is little noradrenergic tone to an organ (e.g. the heart in a healthy person at rest) the agonist action can be seen. Where there is significant noradrenergic tone to an organ (e.g. the heart in a person undergoing vigorous exercise) the antagonist action predominates.

Atenolol and *sotalol* are relatively water soluble compared to the other antagonists. Hence, they penetrate less into the CNS.

Some differences in properties among the antagonists at β-adrenoceptors are summarized in Table 2.15.

Therapeutic uses

Antagonists at β-adrenoceptors reduce the heart rate by occupying cardiac pacemaker β-adrenoceptors. This prolongs diastole and reduces myocardial oxygen demand, thereby increasing the exercise tolerance of patients with angina pectoris (see p. 483).

Antagonists at β-adrenoceptors are useful to reduce the BP of hypertensive patients (see p. 475). *Labetalol* is useful in both chronic hypertension and hypertensive emergencies (see p. 477).

Antagonists at β-adrenoceptors are effective in the correction of certain cardiac dysrhythmias, especially those due to **digoxin** toxicity or thyrotoxicosis, that are associated with either increased local or circulating concentrations of catecholamines or increased sensitivity to their tendency to produce dysrhythmias. *Sotalol* is useful against a broader range of dysrhythmias.

Antagonists at β-adrenoceptors are useful in protecting cardiac β-adrenoceptors from large concentrations of circulating catecholamines prior to, or during, the surgical removal of a phaeochromocytoma.

Some of the symptoms of thyrotoxicosis (tachycardia, palpitations, tremor) can be controlled by antagonists at β-adrenoceptors. The similar symptoms of anxiety are also amenable, but here an action within the CNS may also contribute.

Antagonists at β-adrenoceptors are useful prophylactically in migraine.

Eye-drops containing an antagonist at β-adrenoceptors provide useful

Table 2.15 Differences between antagonists at β-adrenoceptors

Selectivity for subtypes of adrenoceptors	
Labetalol	($\beta \approx \alpha$)
Atenolol, *metoprolol*	($\beta_1 > \beta_2 \gg \alpha$)
Propranolol, *oxprenolol, sotalol*	($\beta_1 = \beta_2 \gg \alpha$)
Intrinsic efficacy	
Oxprenolol	(partial agonist)
Propranolol, atenolol, *labetalol, metoprolol, sotalol*	(competitive antagonist)
Antidysrhythmic activity	
Sotalol	(β-blockade and Class III antidysrhythmic action)
Propranolol, atenolol, *labetalol, metoprolol, oxprenolol*	(β-blockade only)
Polarity (physicochemical)	
Atenolol, *sotalol*	(water-soluble)
Propranolol, *oxprenolol, metoprolol, labetalol*	(lipid-soluble)

control of intraocular pressure in chronic open-angle glaucoma, by reducing the rate of secretion of aqueous humour. The drug can be absorbed from the conjunctival sac so that unwanted systemic effects can occur.

Unwanted effects

Unwanted effects of antagonists at β-adrenoceptors include excessive bradycardia and the precipitation of cardiac failure in patients with a small cardiac reserve. Many patients experience easy fatiguability, stemming from a reduced ability to increase the cardiac output, and coldness of the extremities, stemming either from the same source or from antagonism of a vasodilator response to a small concentration of circulating adrenaline; these problems may be less marked with a partial agonist at β-adrenoceptors.

There is aggravation of bronchoconstriction in asthmatic patients. The risk is less with **atenolol** than with the non-selective antagonists at β-adrenoceptors, and is less with eye-drop than with oral routes of administration, but it is nevertheless still significant.

Sleep disturbance and unpleasant dreams are experienced with the more lipid-soluble agents (e.g. **propranolol**).

Unwanted effects of *labetalol* also include those mediated at α-adrenoceptors (e.g. postural hypotension, failure of ejaculation).

Summary

(1) Antagonists that are non-selective between the kinds of adrenoceptor exert a wide range of effects. The possession of a mixture of effects in appropriate proportions occasionally confers therapeutic usefulness (e.g. *labetalol*); more often it confers a wide range of unwanted effects.

(2) More selective antagonists show a narrower range of effects, a few of which are therapeutically useful; e.g. *prazosin* (an antagonist at α_1-adrenoceptors) for relaxation of vascular and bladder neck smooth muscle.

(3) The greatest usefulness is shown by **atenolol** (an antagonist at β_1-adrenoceptors) for cardiac overactivity in angina pectoris, and hypertension. Similar drugs are also useful in glaucoma, thyrotoxicosis, anxiety and migraine.

The adrenal medulla

The chromaffin cells that comprise the adrenal medulla arise embryologically from the same cells as those giving rise to postganglionic noradrenergic neurones. However, the embryonic adrenal medullary cells do not develop long axons or exhibit threshold electrical characteristics.

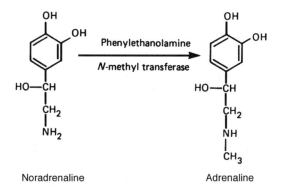

Figure 2.35 The synthesis of adrenaline by the adrenal medulla

Instead they develop a great capacity for the storage and release of catecholamines.

The medullary chromaffin cells synthesize noradrenaline (Figure 2.26) but also possess an additional enzyme for conversion of noradrenaline to adrenaline (Figure 2.35).

Adrenal medullary chromaffin cells bear nicotinic acetylcholine receptors (see p. 60) and are innervated by preganglionic acetylcholinergic sympathetic neurones. Receptor activation causes a small non-propagated depolarization (analogous to an epsp, see p. 61 and Figure 2.18), Ca^{2+} influx and the subsequent Ca^{2+}-dependent release of adrenaline by exocytosis into the bloodstream.

The released adrenaline can activate α- and β-adrenoceptors at all sites in the body. The effects of circulating adrenaline are thus all those of stimulating sympathetic noradrenergic neurones (Table 2.1), together with:

(1) arteriolar dilatation (skeletal muscle);
(2) reduced protein permeability (endothelium of postcapillary venules);
(3) lipolysis (adipose tissue);
(4) glycogenolysis (liver);
(5) glycogenolysis (skeletal muscle);
(6) tremor (skeletal muscle);
(7) restlessness and anxiety (CNS).

Drug action on the adrenal medulla

Secretion of adrenaline is stimulated by agonists at nicotinic acetylcholine receptors (see p. 61) and inhibited by antagonists at nicotinic acetylcholine receptors (see p. 64) of ganglia.

The chromaffin cells are susceptible to the amine-depleting actions of reserpine and *guanethidine* (see p. 81).

3

Drug action on peripheral tissues – drugs acting on signalling mechanisms other than those directly related to receptors for neurotransmitters and hormones

Aims

The drugs described in this section exert their effects on peripheral tissues but their targets of action do not involve structural relationships with the peripheral neurotransmitters acetylcholine or noradrenaline or with hormones.

For each drug you should seek to know:

- Its mechanism of action and the direct and indirect consequences that stem from that fundamental process.
- The rationale behind its principal therapeutic applications.
- Its principal adverse effects.

Local anaesthesia

Revise

- The basis of the resting membrane potential and of the generation and propagation of action potentials.

Local anaesthesia is the result of drug-induced reversible blockade of impulse generation and propagation in a restricted number of neurones. Sensation and motor control of effectors are impaired only in that part of the body innervated by the locally anaesthetized neurones.

Active form of the local anaesthetic drug molecule

Local anaesthetic drugs are weak bases (pK_a = 8–9), which are combined with a strong acid (HCl) to provide a soluble salt for clinical use. They consist of a substituted amino group (hydrophilic) connected by an intermediate chain (usually a carbon chain) to an aromatic residue (lipophilic) (Figure 3.1). The linkage between the intermediate and aromatic groups may be an amide (**lignocaine**, *prilocaine, bupivacaine*) or an ester (*amethocaine* [tetracaine], *benzocaine*).

At a tissue pH of 7.4, local anaesthetic drugs exist in both ionized and unionized (base) forms, the proportion of each being dependent on the pK_a of the drug. Only the unionized (lipid-soluble) form of the drug is able to cross membranous barriers (nerve sheath, cell membrane) before its site of action inside the pore of the Na^+ channel is reached. Once inside the cell, the cationic form, which comprises about 75–95% (depending on the pK_a) of the drug in solution at pH 7.4, binds to its receptor site within the Na^+ channel.

Local anaesthetic drugs: site and mechanism of action

Local anaesthetic drugs exert their effects by blocking voltage-sensitive Na^+ channels.

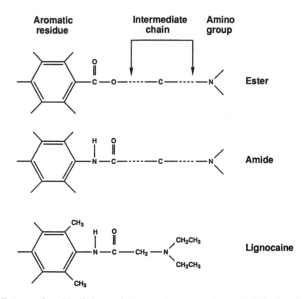

Figure 3.1 Ester and amide linkages between the aromatic part of the local anaesthetic molecule and the intermediate chain leading to the terminal amine. The structure of **lignocaine**, an amide-type local anaesthetic agent

Neuronal impulse generation and propagation depends on the movement of ions through pores in the neuronal cell membrane. These pores constitute the innermost region of specialized protein structures known as <u>ion channels</u>. The opening and closing (<u>gating</u>) of those Na^+, K^+ and Ca^{2+} channels that are important in neuronal signalling is voltage- and time-sensitive. This means that their gating is a function of both the prevailing magnitude of membrane potential and the time for which that potential has been maintained.

The pore-forming regions of voltage-sensitive Na^+, K^+ and Ca^{2+} channels are remarkably similar (Figure 3.2). In the case of Na^+ and Ca^{2+} channels, they consist of a single α-subunit that is the product of a single gene. The α-subunit is a single protein that consists of four almost identical repeating domains (I–IV), each of which contains six membrane-spanning α-helical regions (S1–S6). Polypeptide loops link the membrane-spanning regions and the repeating domains. The four P-loops, which link α-helices S5 and S6 in each domain, are believed to be oriented inwards to form the lining of a Na^+- or Ca^{2+}-permeable pore.

Voltage-sensitive K^+-channels are formed similarly but from four separate proteins (α-subunits), which can be the products of up to four different genes (Figure 3.2).

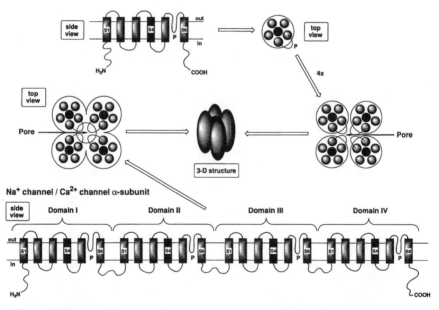

Figure 3.2 Structural features of the pore-forming region (α-subunit) of voltage-sensitive Na^+, Ca^{2+} and K^+ channels. Lower panel: the protein which forms the α-subunit of voltage-sensitive Na^+ and Ca^{2+} channels is a single gene product. It consists of four similar domains, each of which contains six membrane-spanning α-helices (rectangles S1–S6). S4 is the voltage sensor. Upper panel: voltage-sensitive K^+ channels are formed from four gene products, each comprising six membrane-spanning α-helical segments. The single proteins (Na^+ or Ca^{2+} channel) or tetramers of four proteins (K^+ channel) assemble as shown to form functional channels. For each channel, the four polypeptide chains linking S5 to S6 (P-loops) help to form the pore

The channel itself exists in three basic configurations (open, closed, inactivated). In its open state, the pore of the channel provides a water-filled passage between the extra- and intracellular compartments. The channel pore contains a selectivity filter that determines which ions may flow through the open channel down their concentration gradient. When the channel is in the closed state, there is no movement of ions across the membrane. The gating between these two states is controlled by the voltage-sensor (S4, Figure 3.2) regions, which contain a high density of positively charged amino acids. At typical resting membrane potentials, voltage-sensitive channels are predominantly closed. However, in response to membrane depolarization during a nerve impulse, movement of charges in the S4 regions modifies the configuration of the protein and allows the channel to open. From the open state, many kinds of voltage-sensitive ion channel rapidly enter a non-conducting, inactivated state (even if the depolarization is maintained). Inactivation of the channel is thought to result from the movement of an intracellular component of the channel, which acts as a gate by physically blocking the channel. In the case of the Na^+ channel the gate is formed by the intracellular loop linking domains III and IV. To return to the closed state from which opening is possible, the membrane potential must return to its resting (or even to a hyperpolarized) level for several milliseconds.

When a neurone is stimulated by an action potential a small depolarization occurs, due to the opening of some Na^+ channels. This initiates the opening of further channels and further depolarization. If a critical threshold potential is reached, many Na^+ channels progressively rapidly open and this may be recorded as the upstroke of the action potential. With this further rapid depolarization towards the Na^+ equilibrium potential (transmembrane potential at which the effects of any electrical potential gradient are balanced by the effects of the concentration gradient so that no net Na^+ flux occurs), the driving force for Na^+ ions through the channel decreases, the channel becomes inactivated and repolarization commences. The process of repolarization is assisted by the efflux of K^+ through the voltage-sensitive K^+ channels that open shortly after the upstroke of the action potential. Following repolarization a further action potential can be initiated but only after a short recovery period. This refractory period is the time taken for the Na^+ channels to recover from inactivation.

The active (cationic) form of a local anaesthetic drug blocks voltage-sensitive Na^+ channels by binding to an intracellular receptor site located inside the channel pore. Many local anaesthetic agents demonstrate the phenomenon of use-dependence, which means that the degree of anaesthesia increases with the frequency of action potentials. These drugs bind to those channel states (open and inactivated) that are favoured by depolarization, having gained access to their receptor while the channel was open. Thus the frequency with which the membrane is depolarized (and therefore the relative proportion of time the channel spends in these states) is an important determinant of the degree of local anaesthesia. (See also use-dependency of blockers of L-type voltage-sensitive Ca^{2+} channels, p. 128).

Most local anaesthetic drugs are relatively non-specific, in that they block voltage-sensitive Na^+ channels in the cell membranes of all kinds of

STAFFS UNIVERSITY LIBRARY

excitable cells. At large concentrations the membranes even of non-excitable cells such as erythrocytes may be stabilized.

Effects on the neuronal action potential

The action potential normally propagates because it acts as a suprathreshold stimulus for the opening of voltage-sensitive Na^+ channels in adjacent inactive regions of the neuronal membrane (linked by local circuit currents). For this reason, and also because the blockade of Na^+ channels is concentration dependent, local anaesthetic drugs can exert graded effects on the action potential and its propagation.

A small concentration of a local anaesthetic drug increases the stimulus strength required to elicit an action potential (the safety factor for conduction decreases). The rate of rise, amplitude and conduction velocity of that action potential are all reduced.

If sufficient local anaesthetic drug is applied, the action potential becomes so reduced in amplitude that it ceases to act as a suprathreshold stimulus for adjacent inactive regions of the neuronal membrane and conduction ceases. Action potentials can then no longer be initiated or recorded, irrespective of stimulus strength.

The blockade of Na^+ channels in a small part of an axon does not guarantee local anaesthesia. The local circuit currents responsible for action potential propagation can effectively jump over a small section of anaesthetized neurone. To prevent this, approximately 5 mm of a non-myelinated axon or three successive nodes in a myelinated neurone must be stabilized.

Differential blockade in mixed bundles of nerve fibres

Several factors can influence neuronal susceptibility to local anaesthesia. Neurones of small diameter are more readily blocked than those of large diameter. This may result from their larger surface area/volume ratio and therefore their poorer ability to conduct a membrane potential change passively through an anaesthetized area. In myelinated neurones, the Na^+ channels are concentrated in the nodal region, and the internodal distance (0.3–1.5 mm) varies with neurone diameter.

Since blockade of Na^+ channels by local anaesthetic drugs is often use-dependent, fibres with a high firing rate are blocked more readily than those conducting at a lesser frequency. Thus, when a local anaesthetic drug is applied to a nerve bundle, the sensation of pain, which is carried by small diameter fibres of a high firing rate (myelinated A_δ and non-myelinated C fibres), is usually lost before the sensations of cold, warmth, touch or pressure (A_β fibres); motor fibres (large diameter fibres of low firing rate at rest) are blocked last.

Recovery from local anaesthesia

A local anaesthetic drug diffuses away from its site of administration down its concentration gradient, and is carried away by bulk flow of the interstitial fluid to enter the venous ends of the local capillaries. Most local anaesthetic drugs (e.g. **lignocaine**) dilate blood vessels by anaesthesia of the peri-arterial sympathetic vasoconstrictor neurones, and by increasing local blood flow promote their systemic absorption and limit their duration of local anaesthesia. Some (e.g. *prilocaine*) do not. On reaching the systemic circulation, esters are more rapidly destroyed (plasma and liver esterases including cholinesterase) than are amides (liver microsomes).

Systemic effects of local anaesthetic drugs

Local anaesthetic drugs readily pass into the CNS where neurones are sensitive to plasma concentrations incapable of affecting peripheral nervous system activity. All nitrogenous local anaesthetic drugs cause stimulation of the CNS, resulting in restlessness, tremor, convulsions and respiratory stimulation. These effects may result from a selective depressant action of voltage-sensitive Na^+ channels in inhibitory neurones. Central stimulation is followed by depression; death following overdosage usually results from respiratory failure. Depressant effects (drowsiness, slurred speech) are prominent with **lignocaine**.

Local anaesthetic drugs also affect the cardiovascular system, resulting mainly in myocardial depression and vasodilatation. The antidysrhythmic action of **lignocaine** is useful clinically (see p. 118). Vasodilator effects are due to a direct effect on vascular smooth muscle. Combined myocardial depression and peripheral vasodilatation may result in life-threatening hypotension.

Because of their systemic adverse effects, the doses of local anaesthetic agents must be limited. The formulation of the agent and patient factors (e.g. age, medical and drug status) affect the maximal safe dose.

Formulations of local anaesthetic drugs

Local anaesthetic drugs are available in a variety of formulations and presentations; eye-drops (beware masking the process of corneal abrasion caused by foreign bodies), lozenges, gels, tinctures and ointments (beware contact dermatitis, see p. 426) and solutions for injection. The latter usually contain the hydrochloride salt buffered to pH 2.0–6.0.

Solutions for injection may also contain a catecholamine vasoconstrictor drug (usually *adrenaline*, sometimes noradrenaline). This prolongs the local anaesthesia to a variable degree by reducing the rate of systemic absorption. Formulations containing a catecholamine should not be used if the injection is intended for a digit or appendage. Patients receiving tricyclic antidepressant drugs (see p. 233), which potentiate catecholamines (see p. 88), may be at risk from cardiac dysrhythmias (especially by adrenaline) and hypertension (especially by noradrenaline). For such patients, local anaesthetic drug formulations containing felypressin, an analogue of ADH, may need to be considered.

Other components of a local anaesthetic drug formulation for injection may include an antioxidant (to stabilize the vasoconstrictor if adrenaline), a buffering agent (to maintain pH), and sodium chloride (to achieve isotonicity with interstitial fluids).

Method of administration

Topical or surface anaesthesia

The drug is applied directly to mucous membranes, or the skin. To be effective for topical anaesthesia, a drug must: (a) be relatively lipid soluble in its non-ionized form; (b) exist in appreciable amounts as its non-ionized form at pH 7.4 (that is, have a pK_a of 8.5 or less, see p. 330)

Lignocaine, like most local anaesthetic drugs, penetrates mucosal surfaces readily. Only limited penetration of skin occurs. Enhanced transdermal absorption of local anaesthetic agents can be achieved by combining **lignocaine** and *prilocaine* in equal quantities. They form an oily eutectic mixture that can be emulsified into a cream for skin application. This, applied under an occlusive dressing, can provide surface anaesthesia for venepuncture. There is a risk of systemic adverse effects, increasing with the concentration employed and the area to which it is applied.

Infiltration anaesthesia

The drug is injected s/c or submucosally to anaesthetize fine sensory nerve branches. This is suitable for small areas only, as the risk of systemic adverse effects increases with the area infiltrated. Solutions containing vasoconstrictor agents should not be used on fingers and toes because of the risk of ischaemia.

Intravenous regional anaesthesia

The local anaesthetic drug is injected into the emptied veins of a limb, the circulation through which has been arrested by means of an inflated sphygmomanometer cuff. The whole limb becomes anaesthetized and surgery or reduction of a bone fracture can take place. Release of the cuff must be controlled to avoid too large a dose of local anaesthetic agent entering the systemic circulation too quickly.

Nerve block anaesthesia

The local anaesthetic drug is injected alongside a nerve trunk, so less drug is needed compared with infiltration anaesthesia. The transmission of both afferent and efferent impulses is prevented, which results in loss of sensation and muscle paralysis in the area supplied by the nerve trunk. The larger the nerve trunk bathed in drug, the greater is the region anaesthetized. A special form of nerve block anaesthesia is termed epidural (or extradural) block. Here a relatively large concentration of the local anaesthetic drug is injected into the fatty material (Figure 3.3) outside the dura mater. The drug may have to diffuse into the subarachnoid space or outside the spinal canal before its effects can be mediated. However, it cannot penetrate to the brain because the epidural space terminates at the foramen magnum.

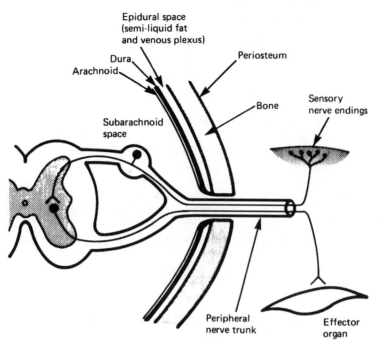

Figure 3.3 Sites for the production of local anaesthesia

Spinal (or intrathecal) anaesthesia

The drug is injected to the subarachnoid space (Figure 3.3), usually in the lower spine where there is no danger of damage to the spinal cord. The dispersion of the injected fluid and hence the locus and extent of local anaesthesia depends on the:

(1) Site of the injection.
(2) Volume and speed of the injection.
(3) Postinjection position of the patient.
(4) Specific gravity (SG) of the injected solution.

The SG of the cerebrospinal fluid (CSF) varies (1.003–1.009). A hypobaric solution (SG less than 1.003) tends to rise through the CSF, while a hyperbaric solution (SG greater than 1.009) tends to sink through the CSF. An isobaric solution tends to remain at the level of the injection site.

Spinal anaesthesia produces analgesia (loss of pain sensation) and muscle relaxation without the patient losing consciousness. However, the level of anaesthesia within the spinal cord cannot be precisely controlled. Unwanted effects may include reduced cardiac output, hypotension and neurological complications.

Properties of individual local anaesthetic drugs

Lignocaine is widely used for all kinds of local anaesthesia. **Lignocaine** i/v is effective in the control of cardiac dysrhythmias (see p. 118).

Prilocaine is suitable for all kinds of local anaesthesia. If large amounts enter the circulation, methaemoglobin is formed. This can be reversed using the reducing agent, methylene blue.

Bupivacaine has a slow onset of action. However, its long duration of action (up to 8 h) makes it particularly suitable for nerve block, epidural and spinal anaesthesia. It is not indicated for i/v regional anaesthesia because of cardiotoxicity.

Amethocaine is an ester that is well and rapidly absorbed across mucous membranes. It provides useful topical anaesthesia of the skin, buccal mucous membranes and eye. Its toxicity and tendency to produce hyper-sensitivity reactions preclude its systemic use.

Benzocaine is an ester that is almost insoluble in water. It is not signif-icantly ionized at physiological pH values and reaches the Na^+ channel from the lipid membrane. Its actions can be reversed by increasing the hydrostatic pressure and thus its mechanism of channel blockade is similar to that of the general anaesthetic agents (increased surface pressure in the phospholipid bilayer), which can also prevent action potential propaga-tion. It provides useful topical anaesthesia of mucous membranes of the mouth and the perianal area.

Other agents causing local anaesthesia

Cocaine has limited use in topical anaesthesia of the eye, nose and throat. In concentrations less than those required to produce local anaesthesia, *cocaine* inhibits the uptake of noradrenaline and dopamine into noradren-ergic and dopaminergic neurones (see p. 88 for the consequences of the uptake-inhibiting properties of *cocaine*). This produces a powerful stimu-lant action on the cerebral cortex, which is the basis for *cocaine* abuse and addiction. Euphoria, indifference to pain and fatigue, appetite suppression (anorexia) and an elevation of body temperature (pyrexia) are all produced. Tolerance develops to the stimulant effects but not to the CNS depression that follows.

The noradrenergic neurone blocking agents (e.g. *guanethidine*) selec-tively anaesthetize the fine terminals of noradrenergic neurones (see p. 81).

Other agents affecting sodium channels

Tetrodotoxin (produced by the puffer fish) and saxitoxin (from marine flagellates) both block voltage-sensitive Na^+ channels. Their action is exerted on the extracellular face of the channel pore and does not exhibit use-dependence. Both tetrodotoxin and saxitoxin are useful research tools in the study of the Na^+ channel. They selectively prevent action-potential production involving voltage-sensitive Na^+ channels but they do not influ-ence the action potentials of smooth muscle cells since these are associated with the influx of Ca^{2+}. Hence tetrodotoxin can be used in vitro function-ally to denervate smooth muscle leaving its contractility unaffected; this can be used to determine whether the action of a drug on a smooth muscle-containing tissue occurs directly on the smooth muscle cell itself or involves nerve action potentials and the release of neurotransmitter.

Various lipid-soluble substances, for example veratridine, batrachotoxin and the insecticides, DDT and pyrethroids (see p. 285), produce the opening of voltage-sensitive Na⁺ channels. This initially leads to cell hyper-excitability and spontaneous discharges, although eventually cells become permanently depolarized and inexcitable. Such agents affect the heart causing dysrhythmia and may cause spontaneous discharges in nerve and muscle cells leading to twitching and convulsions.

Summary

(1) Local anaesthetic agents are weak bases containing hydrophobic (aromatic) and hydrophilic (amine) moieties, which can exist in an unionized lipid-soluble form and an ionized water-soluble form.
(2) In their unionized form they readily penetrate lipid barriers within tissues, nerve sheaths, neuronal cell membranes and the blood–brain barrier.
(3) In their cationic (charged) form, local anaesthetic agents inhibit action potentials by blocking voltage-sensitive Na⁺ channels.
(4) Local anaesthetic agents act by binding to a site inside the Na⁺ channel, blocking Na⁺ entry during the upstroke of the action potential and so stabilizing the neuronal membrane.
(5) The degree of local anaesthesia usually increases with action potential frequency (use-dependence).
(6) The various techniques in local anaesthesia exploit knowledge of the anatomy of innervation and differing routes of administration – surface, infiltration, i/v regional, nerve block, epidural and spinal.
(7) Duration of action depends on chemical structure, physicochemical properties, the volume and concentration used, the local vascularity, and the presence of a vasoconstrictor agent.
(8) Unwanted systemic effects result mainly from action on the CNS and cardiovascular system.

Cardiac antidysrhythmic drugs

General features

Any disorder of cardiac rhythm is termed a dysrhythmia. This can result from disorders of impulse generation, impulse conduction or a combination of these.

Ionic basis of normal cardiac action potentials

In the normal heart the site (focus) for the generation of the heart beat is the SA node. From here electrical impulses are conducted through the atrial muscle to the AV node and thus, via the bundle of His and the Purkinje fibres, to the ventricular muscle cells. The contractile cells of the atria and ventricles show a characteristic form of action potential associated with the movement of Na^+, Ca^{2+} and K^+ through specific ion channels. The opening and closing of these channels (their gating) is variously influenced by membrane potential, intracellular ionic concentrations and ligands, such as noradrenaline, acetylcholine and adenosine. Gating processes are also usually time dependent.

The cardiac action potential is conventionally divided for descriptive purposes into five phases (Figure 3.4). These broadly correlate with the opening and/or closing of different ion channel types as follows.

Phase 0: rapid depolarization

The main upstroke of the cardiac action potential involves influx of Na^+ through voltage-sensitive Na^+ channels. These are identical to those in neurones (Figure 3.2) and can be inhibited by tetrodotoxin. The activation of this channel is rapid and is triggered when the pacemaker potential (phase 4) reaches approximately –60 mV.

In nodal tissues, the upstroke of the action potential is carried by Ca^{2+}.

Phase 1: the peak or notch

Rapid inactivation of the Na^+ channels produces a short-lived repolarization of the membrane potential. This generates the notch, which is especially prominent in ventricular cells.

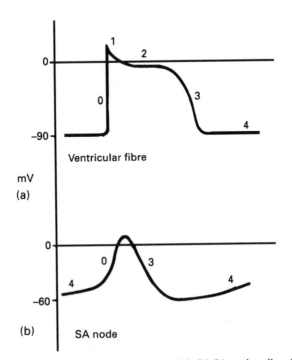

Figure 3.4 (a) Ventricular muscle cell action potential; (b) SA node cell action potential

Phase 2: the plateau
The depolarization generated during phase 0 initiates the relatively slow activation of L-type voltage-sensitive Ca^{2+} channels (see p. 127). The influx of Ca^{2+} through these maintains the depolarized state of the cardiac muscle cell and gives rise to the plateau phase, which is very prominent in the ventricle.

Entry of Ca^{2+} during this phase is of critical importance in generating cardiac force. Additionally, the maintained depolarization causes voltage-sensitive Na^+ channels to remain inactivated and inwardly rectifying K^+ channels to remain closed. Under normal conditions, this ensures that the refractory period of cardiac cells will be relatively long and that synchronous contractions driven by the SA node will occur.

Noradrenaline and adrenaline, agonists at β_1-adrenoceptors, activate an excitatory G-protein (G_s). This stimulates adenylyl cyclase and thus increases the production of cAMP. The resulting phosphorylation of L-type Ca^{2+} channels enhances Ca^{2+} influx and generates the increased force of contraction (positive inotropic effect) characteristic of such agonists.

Opposite effects (negative inotropic effects) are induced by the interaction of acetylcholine with muscarinic acetylcholine receptors. This activates an inhibitory G-protein (G_i), which inhibits adenylyl cyclase and consequently reduces the phosphorylation of L-type Ca^{2+} channels.

Phase 3: repolarization
The repolarization phase terminates the action potential. It results from the combined activation of voltage-sensitive delayed rectifier K^+ channels and the time-dependent inactivation of L-type Ca^{2+} channels. As the membrane potential becomes more negative, inwardly rectifying K^+ channels are also activated, enhancing the rate of repolarization.

Phase 4: pacemaking
In nodal cells, a slow depolarization during diastole, the <u>pacemaker potential</u>, is a prominent feature. The basic depolarization is generated by the flow of Na^+ inwards and of K^+ outwards through a cation channel, which becomes activated during phase 3. The flow of Na^+ and K^+ down their respective concentration gradients exerts a net depolarizing effect (reversal potential = -20 mV).

When the pacemaker potential has depolarized the cell to approximately -60 mV, voltage-sensitive Ca^{2+} channels (in nodal cells) are activated and an action potential is initiated. The slope of the pacemaker potential can be modulated by activity of the autonomic nervous system. Agonists at β_1-adrenoceptors activate L-type Ca^{2+} channels, the current through which summates with the pacemaking cation current to increase the slope of the pacemaker potential. The voltage at which many additional Ca^{2+} channels become activated is reached more rapidly and heart rate increases (a positive chronotropic effect). Agonists at muscarinic acetylcholine receptors reduce the opening of L-type Ca^{2+} channels (via inhibition of adenylyl cyclase, see above) and simultaneously they activate a special inwardly rectifying K^+ current. These effects combine to reduce the slope of the pacemaker potential and reduce the heart rate (a negative chronotropic effect).

Kinds of dysrhythmia

Disorders of impulse generation

The most common problem is the development of an ectopic focus, a group of cardiac cells that generate pacemaker activity additional to the SA node. Ectopic foci may be induced by mild damage to the cardiac muscle (neighbouring myocardial infarction), drugs (general anaesthetic agents, see p. 259) or metabolic disturbances (hyperthyroidism, see p. 177). Such cells are not usually abnormally depolarized and their Na^+ channels undergo normal cycles of activation and inactivation (contrast severely damaged cells in which Na^+ channels exist for a greater time in the inactivated state). These dysrhythmias may be subdivided by the location of the focus into supraventricular (with the ectopic focus in the atria or AV node) and ventricular dysrhythmias.

Supraventricular dysrhythmias

The main problem for the patient arises from the increased ventricular rate, resulting in a reduced stroke volume and increased workload for the heart.

(1) Atrial flutter. This is characterized by a regular and very fast atrial rate (150–350/min). The AV nodal cells with their long refractory period cannot conduct impulses at this high rate; nevertheless, the ventricular rate becomes abnormally high, although regular. The cause is a single ectopic focus in the atrial muscle and the ECG shows several P waves for each QRS complex (in a 2 : 1, 3 : 1 or 4 : 1 ratio).
(2) Atrial fibrillation. The atrial action potential rate is in the range 200–600/min and the dysrhythmia is due to the presence of multiple atrial ectopic foci. There are no normal P waves and the ventricular rate is high and irregular, although much lower than the atrial rate.
(3) Supraventricular paroxysmal tachycardia. Sporadic episodes of increased heart rate occur due to the intermittent appearance of an atrial ectopic focus. Normal sinus rhythm can often be restored by inducing acetylcholine release via reflex vagal stimulation (pressure applied to the eyeballs or to one carotid sinus).

Ventricular dysrhythmias

(1) Ventricular fibrillation. This is caused by the development of ventricular ectopic foci, leading to rapid uncoordinated ventricular contractions and a consequent severe reduction in cardiac output. Since this is rapidly fatal, pharmacological intervention has a limited role, and DC electric shock (cardioversion) is indicated.
(2) Ventricular paroxysmal tachycardia. This dysrhythmia is characterized by sporadic episodes of increased heart rate due to the intermittent appearance of a ventricular ectopic focus. It is distinguished from the atrial kind by an ECG record on which the QRS complexes outnumber the P waves.

Disorders of impulse conduction

Heart block

The most common sites of heart block occur in the AV node and the bundle of His. Different degrees of heart block are recognized. In general, drug treatment is of limited value for heart block, although agonists at β-adrenoceptors may be useful in the short term. In the long term, the use of an artificial pacemaker is indicated.

Re-entry dysrhythmias

Since the whole heart muscle behaves like a complex syncytium, it might at first seem surprising that reverberatory circuits of excitation do not occur more frequently. This is avoided by the long refractory period (during which voltage-sensitive Na^+ and Ca^{2+} channels are inactivated) and the rapid conduction velocity that are characteristic of healthy cardiac muscle cells. However, if part of the heart muscle becomes severely damaged, as a consequence of myocardial infarction, or if its excitability is affected by drugs (agonists at β-adrenoceptors, **digoxin**, *quinidine*), abnormal conduction pathways may arise. In damaged regions of the heart, the cardiac muscle cells tend to depolarize. Such an effect tends to inactivate several kinds of cardiac ion channel with important consequences for antidysrhythmic drug action (see below).

One possible situation is illustrated in Figure 3.5. In the normal heart, shown in Figure 3.5a, the conduction wave passes down into the two bundle branches and is then conducted away on either side. The waves of excitation moving from the bundle branches towards the central portion

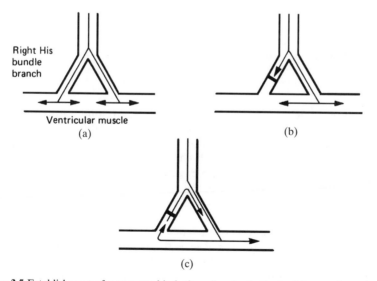

Right His bundle branch

Ventricular muscle

(a)

(b)

(c)

Figure 3.5 Establishment of a re-entry kind of cardiac dysrhythmia: (a) normal conduction; (b) unidirectional block in right His bundle branch; (c) retrograde transmission through right His bundle branch

of ventricular muscle extinguish each other. If, however, one of the bundle branches is damaged, anterograde conduction may be blocked because the voltage-sensitive Na^+ and Ca^{2+} channels of the affected bundle remain inactivated (Figure 3.5b). However, a short time later, the wave of conduction from an undamaged bundle may be able to excite the damaged branch retrogradely (Figure 3.5c) because the time-dependent inactivation of Na^+ and Ca^{2+} channels no longer exists. Therefore the excitation wave may reappear (prematurely) in the normal branch, thus completing a re-entry circuit. Such pathways could occur anywhere in the cardiac muscle when damaged and normal muscle exist side by side.

A rare form of re-entry dysrhythmia occurs in the Wolff–Parkinson–White syndrome. Here an anatomically abnormal bundle of cardiac muscle joins the atria to the ventricles, bypassing the AV node. Thus the ventricles may be excited prematurely via this short-circuit in addition to the normal pathway via the AV node to the bundle of His. Following excitation via the latter pathway, the ventricular impulse may re-enter the atria through the bypass to set up a circus of excitation.

Some mild dysrhythmias (e.g. occasional extrasystoles) require little treatment beyond reassurance of the patient. Others (e.g. supraventricular paroxysmal tachycardia) may revert to normal rhythm spontaneously or can be induced to revert by reflex vagal stimulation. DC electroshock effectively induces the reversion of several kinds of tachycardia.

Antidysrhythmic drugs

Two basic mechanisms underlie the action of these agents. Some (classes I and IV) directly block the ion channels that carry the excitatory cations, Na^+ and Ca^{2+}. This effect can also be achieved indirectly by:

(1) Antagonism at β_1-adrenoceptors (class II).
(2) Opening of K^+ channels (adenosine, class IV).
(3) Blockade of K^+ channels (class III).

Class I: inhibitors of Na^+ influx

This group includes **lignocaine** and **phenytoin**, *quinidine* and *procainamide*. These drugs produce use-dependent inhibition of the influx of Na^+ through the rapidly activating and inactivating Na^+ channels (cf. local anaesthetic agents, p. 107) which open during phase 0 of the cardiac action potential. Since action potentials in the SA node cells involve relatively little Na^+ influx compared with those in atrial or ventricular cells, these drugs are more effective in suppressing ectopic rather than normal pacemaker activity.

Lignocaine and **phenytoin** are particularly effective in the suppression of the ventricular dysrhythmias observed after myocardial infarction. This occurs because the block is use-dependent, that is, the higher the frequency of the ectopic focus, the greater the inhibition. Furthermore, if the damaged cells become depolarized, the Na^+ channels are inactivated, and binding of **lignocaine** and **phenytoin** is enhanced. **Lignocaine** and

phenytoin also reduce the action-potential duration and shorten the effective refractory period, which may improve conduction in damaged cells in the bundle of His, reducing the likelihood of re-entry dysrhythmias.

Lignocaine has a rapid onset of action and a short $t_{1/2}$ (approximately 1 h), which means that it must be given by i/v infusion. It is useful in emergency treatment during surgery. It is also an antagonist at muscarinic acetylcholine receptors and may therefore evoke mild tachycardia by removing the effect of vagal tone on the SA node. Adverse effects may be attributed to actions on the CNS and include confusion, fits, sweating and drowsiness.

Phenytoin is particularly effective in blocking ventricular dysrhythmias attributable to **digoxin** toxicity. Its general antidysrhythmic effectiveness is less than that of **lignocaine**. Unwanted effects include hypotension.

Quinidine and *procainamide* have actions that are broadly similar and they also produce use-dependent blockade of voltage-sensitive Na^+ channels. They are effective in blocking ectopic pacemaker activity both in atria and ventricles. In addition, they prolong the action potential and lengthen the effective refractory period, an action that probably results from K^+ channel blockade. This may prevent the occurrence of re-entry dysrhythmias caused by retrograde transmission of the kind illustrated in Figure 3.5c.

Quinidine and *procainamide* each has a small therapeutic index and depresses the force of myocardial contraction at concentrations close to those required for the suppression of dysrhythmias. They may therefore precipitate cardiac failure in patients with small cardiac reserve. Their negative inotropic effects extend to skeletal muscle (aggravation of myasthenia gravis) and vascular smooth muscle (hypotension).

Quinidine is also an antagonist at muscarinic acetylcholine receptors (see p. 69). By removing the effect of vagal tone at the SA node it induces a mild tachycardia. This action at the AV node may precipitate a hazardous 'paradoxical' tachycardia in patients with atrial flutter or fibrillation. Cardiotoxic doses of *quinidine* directly depolarize Purkinje fibres and increase their automaticity (an effect opposite to that seen at therapeutic concentrations). Toxic doses may therefore induce hazardous ventricular dysrhythmias.

Class II: antagonists at β$_1$-adrenoceptors

Sympathetic stimulation produces a general increase in the excitability of cardiac muscle by phosphorylation of L-type Ca^{2+} channels. Antagonists at β-adrenoceptors (**propranolol, atenolol**) reduce the incidence of dysrhythmias by reducing automaticity, increasing the effective refractory period and decreasing conduction velocity. They reduce ventricular rate in atrial flutter and fibrillation by slowing AV conduction.

The use of **propranolol** and **atenolol** is limited to the treatment of dysrhythmias induced by catecholamines (phaeochromocytoma and thyrotoxicosis) and to those attributed to **digoxin** toxicity. In concentrations close to those required for suppression of dysrhythmias, antagonists at β-adrenoceptors may also depress the force of cardiac contraction and precipitate cardiac failure. The use of these drugs is particularly hazardous

STAFFS UNIVERSITY LIBRARY

in patients with ventricular failure or small cardiac reserve who may depend on sympathetic drive to obtain an adequate cardiac output.

The use of a selective antagonist at β_1-adrenoceptors (e.g. **atenolol**) may minimize the incidence of bronchospasm and cold extremities that follow from the additional blockade of β_2-adrenoceptors by the less selective **propranolol**.

Class III: drugs that prolong both the action potential and refractory period

Delayed rectifier K^+ channels play a crucial role in terminating the cardiac action potential. Their blockade delays repolarization, lengthens the plateau (phase 2) and increases the time during which voltage-sensitive Na^+ and Ca^{2+} channels remain inactivated. This prolongs the refractory period of cardiac cells and reduces the chance that ectopic foci will arise.

Amiodarone is a blocker of the delayed rectifier K^+ channels, but it is not selective. However, it does delay repolarization, with a consequent lengthening of the effective refractory period. It is useful in the treatment of supraventricular tachycardias, particularly in the Wolff–Parkinson–White syndrome.

Amiodarone must be administered in several doses daily for 2 weeks before therapeutic plasma concentrations are achieved. Its molecule contains iodine and this may cause thyroid dysfunction during its long-term use. The large plasma concentrations of *amiodarone* encourage its deposition as microcrystals in the cornea, skin and other tissues. These act as reservoirs of the drug, so that its effects may persist for some time (weeks) after dosing is stopped.

Class IV: inhibitors of Ca^{2+} influx

This can either be achieved by direct block of L-type Ca^{2+} channels or indirectly by hyperpolarizing the membrane via the opening of K^+ channels.

Verapamil directly blocks the influx of Ca^{2+} through the slowly inactivating, voltage-sensitive L-type Ca^{2+} channels. It predominantly affects pacemaker cells in which the upstroke of the action potential is carried by Ca^{2+}. **Verapamil** is therefore effective in blocking AV conduction and thus slows the ventricular rate in supraventricular tachycardias. The effect of **verapamil** is most marked when the frequency of action potentials is high – a phenomenon known as use-dependency. It is effective when the Ca^{2+} channels are either activated or inactivated. **Verapamil** is effective in some types of re-entry tachycardia in which the AV node is involved (in nodal tissue, the action-potential upstroke is carried by Ca^{2+}). However, in the Wolff–Parkinson–White syndrome, in which the AV shunt pathway is formed from ordinary cardiac muscle, verapamil is ineffective because voltage-sensitive Na^+ channels play an important excitatory role. **Verapamil** can even increase the frequency of conduction in the accessory tissue and is therefore contraindicated in the Wolff–Parkinson–White syndrome. **Verapamil** inhibits the contribution that L-type Ca^{2+} channels make to phase 2 of the cardiac action potential. It thus exerts a negative inotropic action, and should therefore only be used with great care in patients receiving antagonists at β-adrenoceptors.

Adenosine indirectly inhibits Ca^{2+}-influx. It activates adenosine receptors (also known as P_1-purinoceptors) that are G-protein coupled to the ATP-sensitive K^+ channel. The resulting hyperpolarization holds the membrane potential too negative for the activation of L-type Ca^{2+} channels involved in phases 3 and 4 of the cardiac action potential.

Adenosine is administered by rapid i/v injection and its effects last less than 1 min. It can be used in all forms of supraventricular tachycardia and, because of its short duration of action, even after administration of an antagonist at β-adrenoceptors.

Other antidysrhythmic drugs

Digoxin, by reducing conduction through the AV node, can reduce the rate at which the ventricles beat in response to atrial tachycardia, flutter or fibrillation (see below).

Summary

(1) The cardiac action potential comprises five phases:

Phase 0 (depolarization) – the opening of voltage-sensitive Na^+ channels (or L-type Ca^{2+} channels in nodes).

Phase 1 (peak) – the start of the time-dependent inactivation of voltage-sensitive Na^+ channels (or L-type Ca^{2+} channels in nodes).

Phase 2 (plateau) – activation of L-type Ca^{2+} channels, enhanced by agonists at $β_1$-adrenoceptors and inhibited by agonists at muscarinic acetylcholine receptors.

Phase 3 (repolarization) – the resultant of (a) time-dependent inactivation of L-type Ca^{2+} channels together with (b) activation of delayed and inwardly rectifying K^+ channels. K^+-channel activation is enhanced by agonists at muscarinic acetylcholine receptors and by agonists at $β_1$-adrenoceptors resulting in the shortening of the duration of the action potential.

Phase 4 (pacemaker) – activation of a mixed (Na^+/K^+) cation channel. The resulting slow diastolic depolarization can be augmented by agonists at $β_1$-adrenoceptors (opening of L-type Ca^{2+} channels) and diminished by agonists at muscarinic acetylcholine receptors (opening of K^+ channels).

(2) Dysrhythmias are deviations from normal cardiac rhythm. They are caused by: ectopic foci – pacemakers additional to the SA node. These generate flutters, fibrillations and tachycardias, of which those in the ventricle are life-threatening.

(3) Impulse conduction disorders – serious damage to cardiac muscle tends to depolarize it, inactivating voltage-sensitive ion channels. The resulting increase in refractory period modifies impulse conduction from the SA node. Heart block in the AV node and bundle of His and re-entry dysrhythmias are recognized.

(4) Antidysrhythmic drugs reduce excitability by direct or indirect inhibition or voltage sensitive Na^+ or Ca^{2+} channels. Four main classes are recognized:

Class I (inhibitors of Na^+ channels) – **lignocaine, phenytoin,** *quinidine* and *procainamide* each produce direct use-dependent inhibition of voltage-sensitive Na^+ channels.

Class II (antagonists at β_1-adrenoceptors) – **propranolol** and **atenolol** inhibit the actions of agonists at β-adrenoceptors and of noradrenergic nerve activity on L-type Ca^{2+} channels.

Class III (inhibitors of K^+ channels) – *amiodarone* inhibits delayed rectifier K^+ channels. This delays repolarization and increases the time over which voltage-sensitive Na^+ and Ca^{2+} channels remain inactivated.

Class IV (inhibitors of Ca^{2+} channels) – verapamil produces direct, use-dependent inhibition of L-type Ca^{2+} channels. Adenosine opens the ATP-sensitive K^+ channel and the resulting hyperpolarization prevents L-type Ca^{2+} channels from opening.

Cardiac glycosides

Digoxin is a sugar-containing compound (glycoside) extracted from the leaves of the foxglove, *Digitalis lanata*. The pharmacodynamic activity of **digoxin** resides in the sugar-free (aglycone) part of the molecule. This consists of a steroid nucleus (folded in a different way from the steroid hormones) and lactone ring. Three digitoxose (sugar) residues are also attached to the steroid nucleus and these influence the pharmacokinetic properties of **digoxin** (see Figure 7.28). Other glycosides, which differ only in their pharmacokinetic properties, are available but are little used.

Direct actions on cardiac cells

The most important therapeutic action of **digoxin** is in increasing the force of contraction in the failing heart (a positive inotropic effect). This results from inhibition of a Na^+/K^+ transporter located in the cell membrane of myocardial cells.

Membrane effects

Na^+/K^+-ATPase is an energy-dependent transporter that hydrolyses one molecule of ATP and uses the released energy to remove three Na^+ from the cell interior in exchange for a gain of two K^+ from the extracellular fluid. Each transporter unit probably forms a pore through which Na^+ and K^+ can pass. The transporter comprises a tetramer of two α- and two β-subunits, each of which is a separate gene product. The α-subunit is a complex protein with three Na$^+$ binding sites and the locus of the ATP hydrolysis on its inward-facing aspect, and two K$^+$ binding sites facing extracellularly.

Digoxin binds to the extracellular face of the transporter α-subunit. This reduces the affinity of the transporter for K$^+$, and effectively inhibits the exchange of three Na$^+$ for two K$^+$. Since the transporter is normally electrogenic (the loss of three Na$^+$ for every two K$^+$ gained helps to maintain the negative membrane potential), a depolarization ensues together with an increase in intracellular Na$^+$ concentration (Figure 3.6).

Myocardial cells also contain a Na$^+$/Ca^{2+} exchanger (an antiporter), by which the outward movement of one Ca^{2+} is coupled obligatorily with the inward transport of three Na$^+$. The increase in intracellular Na$^+$ concentration resulting from inhibition of the Na$^+$/K$^+$-ATPase by **digoxin** reduces

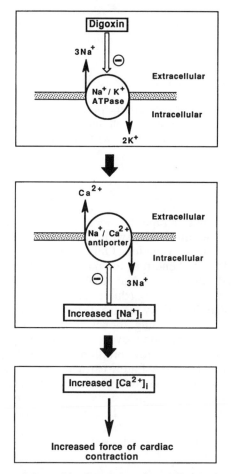

Figure 3.6 Summary of the positive inotropic action of digoxin. Inhibition of Na$^+$/K$^+$-ATPase results in an excessive intracellular Na$^+$ concentration. This inhibits Ca^{2+} extrusion by the Na$^+$/Ca^{2+} antiporter, resulting in an increased intracellular Ca^{2+} concentration, thereby increasing the force of contraction

the efficiency of the Na^+/Ca^{2+} exchanger, leading to an increase in intra-cellular Ca^{2+} concentration (Figure 3.6). This ensures that myocardial Ca^{2+} stores remain full and results in an increase in myocardial force with every heart beat (Figure 3.6). Tension development and relaxation occur faster and with relatively little increase in O_2 demand. This effect is best seen in patients with both heart failure and atrial fibrillation.

The depolarization that results from inhibition of the Na^+/K^+-ATPase has two consequences:

(1) In some cells action-potential propagation (and generation) is inhib-ited, resulting in transmission block, especially in the AV node (useful in atrial fibrillation, see above).
(2) In other cells, especially in the bundle of His, automaticity is increased and ventricular dysrhythmias are produced (see below). K^+ depletion (e.g. associated with diuretic therapy and secondary hyperaldostero-nism) reduces the availability of K^+ at the K^+-binding sites of the Na^+/K^+-ATPase. This further limits $3Na^+/2K^+$ exchange and may lead to the development of fatal ventricular dysrhythmias.

Indirect actions on cardiac cells

Digoxin augments vagal nerve activity partly by central vagal stimulation and also by increased myocardial cell sensitivity to acetylcholine. These actions slow the heart and summate with the direct AV nodal blocking actions.

Toxicity

Digoxin has a very small therapeutic index. The normal functioning of the Na^+/K^+-ATPase and its interaction with the Na^+/Ca^{2+} exchanger are criti-cal features of myocardial function. Only small deviations can be toler-ated and exploited to the benefit of the patient. All toxic actions probably result from marked inhibition of Na^+/K^+-ATPase.

Nausea, anorexia and vomiting (due to stimulation of the CTZ) are all early features of **digoxin** toxicity, as are disturbances of colour vision and impaired vision acuity (including snowy vision, flickering or flashes of light, coloured spots surrounded by coronas, dimming of vision, glare sensitivity), which may be due to inhibition of the Na^+/K^+-ATPase neces-sary for normal cone function. Later, cardiac dysrhythmias are common and almost any pathological dysrhythmia can be imitated by **digoxin** toxic-ity. Ectopic beats are common early signs and ventricular tachycardia and fibrillation terminate the sequence. The increased automaticity respons-ible for this arises in the Purkinje fibres, where a large intracellular Ca^{2+} concentration causes membrane-potential oscillations.

Treatment

In addition to terminating **digoxin** administration, increasing the plasma K^+ concentration stimulates the membrane Na^+/K^+-ATPase and hence aids

Ca^{2+} extrusion via the Na^+/Ca^{2+} exchanger. The antidysrhythmic drugs **phenytoin** (see p. 119) and **propranolol** are also useful. Digoxin-specific antibody fragments are also available for use in life-threatening situations.

Summary

(1) **Digoxin** inhibits Na^+/K^+-ATPase. This decreases Na^+/Ca^{2+} exchange and effectively increases intracellular Ca^{2+} concentration. The force of myocardial contraction increases.
(2) **Digoxin** reduces impulse transmission in the AV node, which inhibits supraventricular tachycardias.
(3) Toxic effects, especially cardiac dysrhythmias, are exacerbated by hypokalaemia, which can occur during diuretic therapy.

Blockers of calcium channels

These drugs are also known as inhibitors of calcium influx (or, less satisfactorily, as calcium antagonists).

Role of calcium within the cell

In many effector cells (e.g. muscle, neuronal, secretory) an increase in free intracellular Ca^{2+} concentration activates Ca^{2+}-sensitive protein kinases, phosphatases and ATPases. These enzymes then initiate a variety of biochemical cascades that culminate in the cellular response (e.g. contraction, release of neurotransmitter, secretion). The activator Ca^{2+} may be derived from:

(1) Intracellular stores, from which it is released by IP_3 (or by methylxanthines).
(2) The ECF, through voltage-sensitive Ca^{2+} channels (see below) in the cell membrane. Ca^{2+} entering the cell can also stimulate the release of Ca^{2+} from stores (Ca^{2+}-induced Ca^{2+} release).

In all muscles Ca^{2+} is a critical element of excitation–contraction coupling. Contraction of skeletal muscle depends largely on Ca^{2+} release from intracellular stores. In cardiac and smooth muscle the influx of extracellular Ca^{2+} (Figure 3.7a) contributes to the contraction to a degree determined both by the cell and by the excitatory stimulus.

The dissipation of the Ca^{2+} signal (Figure 3.7b), once excitation wanes, is by:

(1) Active sequestration of Ca^{2+} into intracellular storage sites (prominent in skeletal muscle and other tissues that use an intracellular source of activator Ca^{2+}).

STAFFS UNIVERSITY LIBRARY

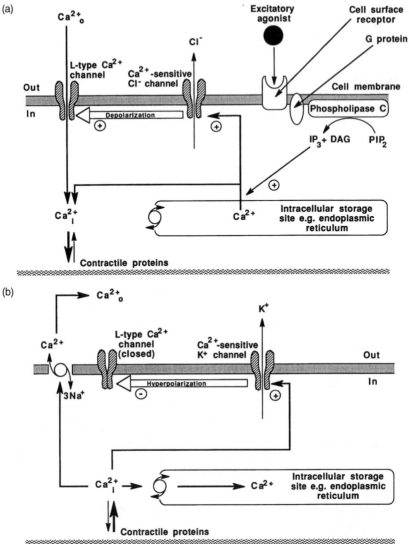

Figure 3.7 Typical cascade of events following the interaction of an excitatory agonist with a cell surface receptor, using smooth muscle as a model. (a) Initiation of contraction. The agonist–receptor interaction often activates a G protein-coupled cascade leading to the formation and release of IP_3. Interaction of IP_3 with a specific receptor on the endoplasmic reticulum releases Ca^{2+} from storage sites. This is a self-amplifying process (Ca^{2+}-induced Ca^{2+} release) and one which also activates Ca^{2+}-sensitive Cl^- channels, allowing Cl^- efflux. The resulting membrane depolarization activates voltage-sensitive channels such as the L-type Ca^{2+} channel. The intracellular Ca^{2+} pool is thus further augmented and Ca^{2+}-sensitive enzymes, such as myosin light chain kinase, are activated (PIP_2 = phosphatidyl inositol (4,5) bisphosphate). (b) Termination of excitation. The excitation-driven increase in intracellular free Ca^{2+} concentration activates Ca^{2+}-sensitive K^+ channels. The resulting K^+ efflux hyperpolarizes the membrane, closing L-type Ca^{2+} channels. The intracellular Ca^{2+} concentration decreases further by resequestration into stores and exchange of Ca^{2+} for Na^+ at the Na^+/Ca^{2+} antiporter. Basal conditions are re-established by the continuous action of Na^+/K^+-ATPase (not shown)

Table 3.1 Properties of voltage-sensitive Ca^{2+} channels

	L	T	N
Nifedipine, verapamil, *diltiazem*-sensitive	Yes	No	No
ω-Conotoxin-sensitive	No	No	Yes
Duration of activation	Long	Transient	Intermediate
Channel conductance (Ca^{2+} flux per unit time)	Large	Small	Intermediate
Location	Cardiac, skeletal and smooth muscles, brain and endocrine cells	Widespread in excitable cells	Neurones

(2) Extrusion from the cell (prominent in tissues that use an extracellular source of activator Ca^{2+}) via transport systems such as the 3Na$^+$/Ca^{2+} antiporter.

Types of Ca^{2+} channel

Several types of voltage-sensitive Ca^{2+} channel are now recognized and some of the key properties of the three major types are summarized in Table 3.1. L-channels (long-lasting) are activated for a relatively long time on marked membrane depolarization. The α-subunits of such channels closely resemble those of voltage-sensitive Na$^+$ channels (Figure 3.2). T-channels (transient) require little depolarization to become transiently activated.

Blockade of L-type Ca^{2+} channels

Blockade of Ca^{2+} entry from the ECF can inhibit cellular excitation. This occurs when Ca^{2+} entry forms a significant portion of the membrane excitation process as in:

(1) Certain smooth muscle cells.
(2) Cells of the SA node and AV node in the heart.
(3) Other myocardial cells that are depolarized and where voltage-sensitive Na$^+$ channels have become inactivated.

Blockers of L-type Ca^{2+} channels

Three kinds of blocker of L-type Ca^{2+} channels can be distinguished, typified by **nifedipine**, **verapamil** and *diltiazem*, largely on the basis of ligand binding and electrophysiological studies. Detailed observations have shown that they interact with three distinct (but allosterically linked) sites on the α-subunit of the channel.

These drugs are <u>calcium antagonists</u> by virtue of their ability to reduce the access of Ca^{2+} to its site of action within the cell.

Nifedipine is the prototype dihydropyridine blocker of Ca^{2+} entry. It binds with a site on the extracellular surface of the α-subunit of the L-channel, a process that is greatly enhanced the more depolarized the cell and if the channel is in an inactivated state. In general, vascular smooth muscle cells have a less negative resting membrane potential than cardiac muscle cells. Hence, in the former, a greater proportion of the L-type channels may normally be in the inactivated state. This could explain why **nifedipine** is more potent in relaxing vascular smooth muscle than in depressing the activity of cardiac tissue. The interaction between **nifedipine** and the L-type channel shows little dependency on the frequency with which the channel opens (lack of use-dependency).

Nifedipine has little action on the cardiac SA or AV nodes. The myocardium is mildly affected but prominent peripheral vasodilatation occurs. **Nifedipine** is therefore useful in the management of essential hypertension (see p. 476) and angina pectoris (see p. 483). Unwanted effects are largely the predictable consequences of vasodilatation – headache, flushing, dizziness, tachycardia, palpitations, and salt and water retention by the kidney leading to peripheral oedema (see p. 197).

Verapamil is the prototype phenylalkylamine blocker of Ca^{2+} entry. Its site of action on the α-subunit faces the cell interior and can only be accessed by **verapamil** when the channel is open. Hence the interaction of **verapamil** with the L-channel shows marked use-dependency (potency increases the more the channel opens). This feature may confer some selectivity for the heart.

Verapamil inhibits Ca^{2+} entry in cardiac, vascular and gastrointestinal tissues.

In the myocardium **verapamil** interferes with Ca^{2+} entry occurring during the plateau of the cardiac action potential and thereby reduces the contractility. Elsewhere in the heart it interferes with the Ca^{2+} entry that is important for excitation; this is exploited in the treatment of paroxysmal supraventricular tachycardia (see p. 120). It is also responsible for the very prolonged AV node transmission times that can result from overdosage or combination of **verapamil** with an antagonist at β-adrenoceptors.

In arteriolar smooth muscle **verapamil** produces vasodilatation. This is exploited in the management of essential hypertension and angina pectoris. It should not be used in congestive heart failure where further reduction in cardiac contractility cannot be tolerated.

In gastrointestinal propulsive smooth musculature, contraction is weakened. This underlies the constipation that occurs as a side-effect of **verapamil**. Other unwanted effects resemble those of **nifedipine**.

Diltiazem is the prototype benzothiazepine blocker of Ca^{2+} entry. It interacts in a use-dependent manner with a third site on the L-channel α-subunit. In profile, *diltiazem* is more like **verapamil** than **nifedipine** and it is capable of inhibiting cardiac tachycardias and producing bradycardia. Its main use is the treatment of angina pectoris.

Summary

(1) Blockers of Ca^{2+} channels inhibit the opening of voltage-sensitive L-type Ca^{2+} channels.
(2) Three kinds of agent are recognized, typified by **nifedipine**, **verapamil** and *diltiazem*.
(3) **Nifedipine** acts on the outer face of the channel; its actions are not use-dependent. **Verapamil** and *diltiazem* interact with inward-facing components of the channel; their actions are use-dependent.
(4) **Nifedipine** is relatively selective for smooth muscle. It is useful in the treatment of hypertension and angina pectoris.
(5) **Verapamil** is relatively selective for the heart. It is useful in the treatment of supraventricular dysrhythmias.
(6) Unwanted effects include ankle oedema (**nifedipine**) and constipation (**verapamil**). Co-administration of **verapamil** with an antagonist at β-adrenoceptors can precipitate heart failure.

Openers (activators) of potassium channels

Nicorandil is a simple pyridine derivative containing a nitrate ester moiety. It increases cell membrane permeability to K^+, predominantly in vascular smooth muscle.

Mechanism of action

Several subtypes of K^+ channel exist and one of these, designated K_{ATP}, is sensitive to the intracellular concentration of ATP. The K_{ATP} channel opens as the intracellular concentration of ATP decreases and vice versa. *Nicorandil* can open K_{ATP} channels even when the intracellular concentration of ATP is relatively large, but the exact mechanism by which this action is exerted is not understood. The opening of K_{ATP} channels hyperpolarizes the cell membrane, leading to the closure of voltage-sensitive ion channels, especially the L-type Ca^{2+} channel, and relaxation (Figure 3.7b).

While the opening of K_{ATP} may represent the principal action of nicorandil in relaxing smooth muscle, the nitrate moiety in the drug molecule also causes the activation of guanylyl cyclase (see p. 133). Hence part of the relaxant effect may reflect the intracellular accumulation of cGMP and activation of cGMP-dependent protein kinase.

Although all sorts of smooth muscle are relaxed in vitro, relaxation of vascular smooth muscle is the predominant effect of *nicorandil* in vivo. There is generalized vasodilatation. Skin flushing may occur and a throbbing headache may be experienced on initial dosing. *Nicorandil* is useful clinically in the treatment of angina pectoris.

Methylxanthines

Theophylline and *aminophylline* are the commonly prescribed methyl-xanthines, *aminophylline* being a more water-soluble complex of *theophylline* with ethylenediamine. Coffee, tea, cocoa, chocolate and cola usually contain methylxanthines (caffeine, theobromine, theophylline), although the methylxanthines can be removed (decaffeinated beverages).

Actions

Airways smooth muscle

Providing that plasma concentrations can be limited to the range 10–20 mg/L, *theophylline* and *aminophylline* evoke bronchodilatation with little effect on other smooth muscle-containing organs or on the heart. These agents are thus useful in the treatment of bronchial asthma (see p. 487).

The contribution of relaxation of airways smooth muscle to the therapeutic effect of the methylxanthines in bronchial asthma may depend on the treatment situation. When *aminophylline* is administered by i/v infusion during the treatment of acute, severe asthma, the rapidity of the therapeutic response indicates that relaxation of airways smooth muscle plays a more important role than resolution of inflammation. However, in the oral prophylaxis of asthma using sustained-release formulations of *theophylline*, it is possible that anti-inflammatory actions of the drug (see below) assume greater importance.

Vascular smooth muscle

Methylxanthines dilate most blood vessels and thereby reduce peripheral resistance, although they may constrict cerebral vessels. Dilatation of veins results in reduced central venous pressure and cardiac pre-load.

Other smooth muscles

In large concentrations, *theophylline* is capable of causing the relaxation of all kinds of smooth muscle.

Cells involved with inflammation in the lung

Mast cells, platelets, eosinophils and macrophages are all involved with the process of inflammation in the lung. *Theophylline* can inhibit both the release of mediators of tissue anaphylaxis from mast cells and eosinophil accumulation within the lung. Such actions may allow *theophylline* to exert some anti-inflammatory activity in the asthmatic lung.

Kidney

Methylxanthines are diuretic agents, although the maximal effect is small. Diuresis results mainly from inhibition of Na^+ reabsorption, with some contribution from an increased GFR. This increase is the consequence of the cardiac stimulant and vasodilator actions of the methylxanthines.

The heart

Theophylline and other methylxanthines stimulate the heart, producing an increase in force of contraction and heart rate.

Milrinone produces a positive inotropic effect in congestive heart failure when administered i/v, with less of the other actions characteristic of methylxanthines. Its selectivity for the heart may result from the selective inhibition of a phosphodiesterase enzyme in the heart that differs from the isoenzymes in many other tissues.

Large concentrations of these drugs may induce dysrhythmias.

The central nervous system

The methylxanthines stimulate the CNS (see p. 249). They increase alertness and reduce fatigue. Insomnia, restlessness, delirium and seizures are part of the acute toxic syndrome associated with overdosage.

Mechanism of action

Several mechanisms have been proposed for the pharmacodynamic actions of methylxanthines.

Inhibition of cyclic nucleotide phosphodiesterases

Inhibition of cyclic nucleotide phosphodiesterases can increase intracellular cAMP and cGMP concentrations (see Figure 2.31 and Figure 3.9b).

Theophylline inhibits cyclic nucleotide phosphodiesterases. However, significant increases in the tissue cAMP content are observed only at concentrations close to, or in excess of, those causing maximal relaxation of smooth muscle. This does not necessarily rule out inhibition of phosphodiesterase as a mechanism for the smooth muscle-relaxant action of *theophylline*, because the changes in cAMP turnover crucial for relaxation may occur in a minor compartment not detectable by the assay of whole-tissue cAMP content.

Antagonism of adenosine

Antagonism of adenosine (and related nucleotides) occurs at cell surface adenosine receptors. During the process of neurochemical transmission, adenosine (a co-transmitter) is often released simultaneously with the main neurotransmitter substance. The neurally released adenosine may participate in a negative feedback process. By activating adenosine receptors on the presynaptic or prejunctional nerve terminal, adenosine inhibits the release of the main neurotransmitter. The methylxanthines act as antagonists at neuronal adenosine receptors and thereby augment neurotransmitter release. Such antagonism at adenosine receptors may underlie the ability of the methylxanthines to stimulate the CNS (see p. 249) and to cause gastric irritation.

In the asthmatic lung adenosine may activate adenosine receptors. Accordingly, antagonism of adenosine could partly explain the anti-asthma efficacy of *theophylline*.

Alteration of the Ca^{2+} handling of effector cells

Large concentrations of caffeine and *theophylline* are agonists at the so-called ryanodine receptor located on intracellular Ca^{2+} stores in smooth muscle. This action results in Ca^{2+} release and does not depend on the intracellular accumulation of cAMP. When store refilling is compromised (e.g. when the extracellular concentration of Ca^{2+} is small), methylxanthines can be used experimentally as tools to prevent the actions of spasmogenic agents that are dependent on a functional Ca^{2+} store and to study the properties of these stores.

Summary

Theophylline and other methylxanthines:

(1) Relax smooth muscle; they are used orally to treat bronchial asthma.
(2) Increase the rate and force of cardiac contraction.
(3) Stimulate the CNS, increasing alertness.
(4) Inhibit cyclic nucleotide phosphodiesterases, an action that probably underlies many of their cellular effects.
(5) Are antagonists at adenosine receptors.

Nitrates

Glyceryl trinitrate (Figure 3.8) and *isosorbide mononitrate* are organic esters of nitric acid and are sufficiently lipid soluble to penetrate cell membranes. The molecules can be regarded as carriers of the nitrite ion (NO_2^-) that is the precursor of the active species nitric oxide (see below and Figure 3.9a).

Mechanism of action

Within the smooth muscle cells, organic nitrates are reduced by sulphydryl groups to release nitric oxide (NO) via a nitrite intermediate. The pool of sulphydryl groups available for this step can become exhausted resulting

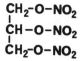

$$CH_2-O-NO_2$$
$$CH-O-NO_2$$
$$CH_2-O-NO_2$$

Figure 3.8 Structure of **glyceryl trinitrate**

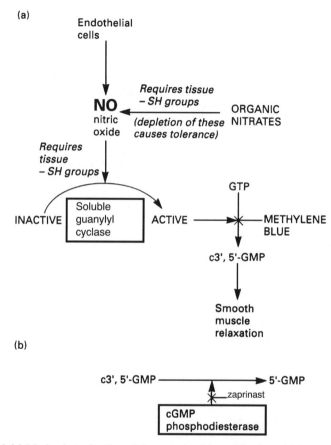

(a)

Endothelial
cells

NO
nitric
oxide

*Requires tissue
– SH groups
(depletion of these
causes tolerance)*

ORGANIC
NITRATES

*Requires
tissue
– SH groups*

INACTIVE | Soluble
guanylyl
cyclase | ACTIVE ────→ METHYLENE
BLUE

GTP

c3', 5'-GMP

Smooth
muscle
relaxation

(b)

c3', 5'-GMP ──────────────→ 5'-GMP

zaprinast

cGMP
phosphodiesterase

Figure 3.9 (a) Mechanism of action of the organic nitrates. These synthetic agents mimic
the action of the body's endogenous vasodilator, nitric oxide, which is liberated from the
vascular endothelium; (b) breakdown of cyclic 3'5'-GMP

in tolerance to the relaxant actions of the organic nitrate. (Dithiothreitol,
a source of sulphydryl groups, has been used experimentally to reverse the
tolerance.) Nitric oxide activates soluble guanylyl cyclase, a process that
also requires –SH groups, although the pool of these seems different from
that involved in the formation of NO. The resulting increase in cGMP
concentration produces smooth muscle relaxation by activating a cGMP-
dependent protein kinase. This initiates a series of biochemical changes
that effectively reduces intracellular free Ca^{2+} concentration (Figure 3.9a).

The actions of organic nitrates can be inhibited experimentally by methylene blue, an inhibitor of soluble guanylyl cyclase, and potentiated by inhibitors of phosphodiesterase that slow the breakdown of cGMP (Figure 3.9b).

Actions

Smooth muscle

Blood vessels

There is generalized relaxation of vascular smooth muscle leading to vasodilatation. The effect on veins and venules is greater than that on the arteriolar tree, resulting in skin flushing. The filling pressure at the heart (pre-load) is reduced to a greater extent than total peripheral resistance (after-load).

Unwanted effects that follow from the vasodilatation include skin warmth and sweating, throbbing headache (stretching of cranial vessels) and fainting. Therapeutic exploitation of the reduced pre-load occurs in angina of effort (see p. 482) and in congestive heart failure (see p. 471).

Other smooth muscle

Organic nitrates are capable of relaxing all kinds of smooth muscle, including that of the bronchi, biliary tract, gut and genitourinary tract.

The heart

Tachycardia arises reflexly from nitrate-induced vasodilatation (see above). However, the load on the heart (principally pre-load) is also reduced so that the cardiac work required per unit of cardiac output is reduced.

Pharmacokinetics

Glyceryl trinitrate is rapidly inactivated by hepatic reductase enzymes. Sublingual administration (tablets, aerosol spray) is effective and initially avoids the hepatic circulation (first-pass effect). Onset of action is rapid, within 1 min, but the duration of action is short, normally 15–30 min. Percutaneous administration (self-adhesive skin patches) is useful in the prophylaxis of attacks of angina occurring at night and at rest.

Isosorbide mononitrate is more stable and therefore suitable for oral administration.

Summary

Organic nitrates:

(1) Act as donors of nitric oxide.
(2) Relax all kinds of smooth muscle in vitro by activating guanylyl cyclase and increasing intracellular cGMP concentrations.

(3) Dilate veins and so reduce cardiac pre-load in vivo and are useful in the treatment of angina and congestive heart failure.
(4) Are absorbed rapidly across mucous membranes. Presystemic metabolism, development of tolerance and headache are practical problems in their use.

Diuretic agents

Diuretic agents increase the urine output of fluid and ions from the kidney. They do this by interfering with one or more of the tubular reabsorptive processes located between the glomerular capsule and junction of the collecting ducts with the ureter. To understand the actions of the diuretic agents it is necessary to understand the normal reabsorptive processes that take place after filtration at the glomerular capsule. These processes reduce the filtrate from about 125 mL/min to a volume of urine of about 1 mL/min, as well as drastically changing the ionic composition. The regions involved in these processes and the functions performed in each are as follows.

Proximal convoluted tubule

(1) Reabsorption of a substantial portion of the filtered Na^+, accompanied by Cl^- and water to maintain electrochemical and osmotic balance.
(2) Reabsorption of approximately 50% of the filtered K^+ accompanied by Cl^- and water.
(3) Reabsorption of filtered HCO_3^-. This involves the production of HCO_3^- and H^+ within the tubular epithelial cells under the influence of cytoplasmic carbonic anhydrase, the transfer of the HCO_3^- to the peritubular vessels and the exchange of the H^+ with Na^+ in the filtrate. This Na^+ is transferred to the peritubular fluid, the H^+ interacts with HCO_3^- in the filtrate, catalysed by carbonic anhydrase on the brush border membrane, producing water and CO_2 (which may diffuse into the epithelial cells and be used in the production of more HCO_3^-). HCO_3^- reabsorption can take place throughout the nephron but the major site appears to be the proximal tubule.

Descending limb of the loop of Henle

The tubular membranes are relatively impermeable to anything other than water, which is removed by osmotic forces.

Ascending limb of the loop of Henle

Reabsorption of Na^+, K^+ and Cl^- by a co-transport mechanism. The tubule cell membranes are relatively impermeable to water. Thus the rate of absorption of the ions exceeds that of water, leaving a tubule fluid that is hypotonic as it enters the distal tubule. Ca^{2+} and Mg^{2+} are also reabsorbed in this region.

Distal convoluted tubule

Reabsorption of Na^+, accompanied by Cl^-, and further reabsorption of Ca^{2+}.

Collecting duct

(1) Active reabsorption of Na^+ in connection with secretion of K^+. This 'exchange' is increased by aldosterone (see p. 181) and by increased delivery of Na^+ to the collecting duct.
(2) Reabsorption of water unaccompanied by ions, a process that is regulated by ADH released from the posterior pituitary gland (see p. 193). ADH increases the permeability of the tubule cells and normally results in a tubule fluid that is hypertonic relative to the general ECF when it leaves the collecting duct. Changes in plasma tonicity influence the release of ADH such that more, or less, water is reabsorbed to restore the tonicity to normal.

Compounds reducing or blocking these reabsorptive processes for solutes result in the production of an increased volume of urine with increased concentration of one or more ions.

Benzothiadiazides and related diuretic agents

This large group of diuretic agents includes the benzothiadiazides (thiazides), having a basic structure in common (**bendrofluazide** [bendro-flumethiazide]), and related compounds (*chlorthalidone*) that do not have the basic structure of the thiazides but produce essentially the same effects. All members of the group appear to have the same mechanism of action. They produce the same maximum effect on urine production and have the same potential for unwanted effects. The drugs are concentrated in the kidney partly by glomerular filtration and partly by active secretion into the proximal tubule by the organic acid secretory mechanism located there. These diuretic agents differ from each other mainly in their onset and duration of action. The latter appears to depend on lipid solubility and on the degree of plasma protein binding, the longer-acting compounds being more extensively bound.

The major action of the drugs is in reducing the reabsorption of Na^+ (and Cl^-) in the distal tubule. The mechanism is not clear but may involve a decreased permeability to Na^+ (and Cl^-) at the luminal membrane. The increased delivery of Na^+ to the collecting ducts results in increased K^+ secretion in association with increased Na^+ reabsorption at this site. Some members of the group are able to inhibit carbonic anhydrase and potentially increase HCO_3^- loss in the urine, but this does not explain their main diuretic activity. The net effect is an increased urine volume with an increased loss of Na^+ and Cl^- and possible accompanying K^+ and HCO_3^-

loss. The thiazides exhibit moderate efficacy and can produce excretion of 5–10% of the filtered Na^+ (cf. 1% excreted in the absence of diuretic agent administration).

Other renal effects are a reduction in uric acid secretion (due in part to competition for proximal secretory processes), enhanced excretion of Mg^{2+}, a decreased excretion of Ca^{2+} (due to increased reabsorption in the distal tubule) and a decreased GFR possibly due to a direct action on the renal blood vessels.

The increased K^+ secretion may result in hypokalaemia and cause problems, particularly in patients receiving **digoxin** (see p. 124). This disadvantage may be reduced by the use of K^+ supplements (effervescent potassium tablets), or of K^+-sparing diuretic agents (see below). In susceptible patients the hyperuricaemia may induce gout.

Adverse effects that are not of renal origin include the induction of hyperglycaemia (due mainly to a reduction in insulin secretion, although resistance to insulin or increased breakdown of glycogen may contribute) and aggravation of pre-existing diabetes mellitus.

In patients with diabetes insipidus (due either to lack of ADH or lack of responsiveness of the kidney to ADH), the thiazides produce a reduction in the urine volume. The Na^+-depleting effect appears to be essential for this action. It is suggested that the loss of Na^+ causes a reduction in ECF volume and GFR and an increased reabsorption of Na^+ and water in the proximal tubule. A reduced Na^+ and water load is delivered to the distal tubule and a smaller volume of less dilute urine is produced.

The thiazide and related diuretic agents also produce a sustained antihypertensive effect, which may be due, initially, to the diuretic action but subsequently is independent of this effect. It may be obtained with lower doses and is probably due to a direct relaxation of arteriolar smooth muscle through the opening of membrane K^+ channels. *Diazoxide*, a thiazide analogue useful in the treatment of chronic hypoglycaemia (see p. 192), causes profound relaxation of arterioles whilst causing salt and water retention and antagonizing **bendrofluazide**, thus lending support to the suggestion that the antihypertensive effect of the thiazides is distinct from their diuretic action. *Indapamide*, a *chlorthalidone* analogue, is claimed to lower the BP with less metabolic disturbance, and is being promoted solely for use in the treatment of hypertension.

High ceiling or loop diuretic agents

Like the thiazides, **frusemide** [furosemide] and *bumetanide* are absorbed after oral administration, are protein bound in the plasma and enter the kidney partly by filtration and partly by active secretion into the proximal tubule by the organic acid secretory mechanism. Unlike that of the thiazides, their diuretic action is rapid in onset, short in duration and dose related. As the group name suggests, the response is more marked than with other diuretic agents.

Their major action is to reduce the $Na^+/K^+/2Cl^-$ co-transport from the lumen to the cell in the ascending limb of the loop of Henle, although there may be minor actions on Na^+ reabsorption in the proximal tubule.

Na^+/K^+-ATPase is involved in the movement of Na^+ from the tubule lumen to the peritubular fluid but although loop diuretic agents can be shown to inhibit the enzyme in vivo it is not clear if inhibition plays any role in their diuretic effect. K^+ secretion (associated with Na^+ reabsorption) is increased because of the greater Na^+ load delivered to the collecting duct. There is thus an increased urine volume with loss of Na^+ (15–30% of the filtered Na^+ may be lost), Cl^- and K^+. The Cl^- loss may induce alkalosis and the K^+ loss provoke **digoxin** intoxication. In contrast to the thiazides, loop diuretic agents cause the loss of both Ca^{2+} and Mg^{2+}. They also increase renal blood flow, an action that may be mediated via PGE_2 and $PGF_{2\alpha}$. Uric acid secretion may be reduced, resulting in gout in susceptible patients. The very rapid, marked reduction in ECF volume has resulted in cardiovascular collapse and may cause urinary retention in patients with an enlarged prostate gland.

In acute left ventricular failure/pulmonary oedema (see p. 472), **frusemide** rapidly reduces ECF volume by its diuretic action but further reduces ventricular filling pressure by a dilator action on veins, which may be direct or mediated, at least in part, by PGs.

The loop diuretics are also capable of producing a sustained reduction in BP. *Piretanide* has marked vasodilator action and is promoted solely for use in the treatment of hypertension.

Potassium-sparing diuretic agents

Amiloride and triamterene

The major action of **amiloride** and *triamterene* is to reduce K^+ secretion in the collecting duct by a primary effect on Na^+ reabsorption (which normally provides a potential to aid K^+ secretion). The mechanism of action of these drugs is not clear but does not involve antagonism of aldosterone (see below). **Amiloride** binds to a receptor on the luminal membrane, blocking the Na^+ channels and limiting the entry of Na^+ to the tubular cells. As a result, K^+ secretion and the Na^+/H^+ exchange are reduced. *Triamterene* may have a similar action. This gives a mild diuresis with loss of Na^+ (up to 5% of that filtered) and a reduced loss of K^+. Diuretic agents of this kind are generally used in combination with thiazide diuretic agents to reduce the loss of K^+ normally associated with the use of this group. The main problem associated with the use of these compounds is the danger of hyperkalaemia.

Antagonist of aldosterone

Spironolactone, and its major metabolite canrenone, inhibit the Na^+ reabsorption and associated K^+ secretion in the distal nephron promoted by aldosterone by competing with it for intracellular receptors. The magnitude of the effect depends on the involvement of aldosterone in the reabsorption. **Spironolactone** is useful in combination with the thiazides to reduce the K^+ loss normally associated with their diuretic effect. Again the main adverse effect is the likelihood of increased plasma K^+ concentrations but disturbances of endocrine function (gynaecomastia) may also occur, presumably due to the ability of **spironolactone** to interact with steroid receptors.

Other diuretic agents of more limited use

Inhibitors of carbonic anhydrase

Acetazolamide produces a reversible inhibition of carbonic anhydrase and therefore reduces the formation of H^+ and HCO_3^- within the epithelial cells of the tubule; this reduces the reabsorption of HCO_3^-. The loss of HCO_3^- may result in metabolic acidosis as the plasma buffer concentration decreases; this limits the diuresis as sufficient H^+ is generated from metabolism to exchange with Na^+ in the tubule and thus re-establish HCO_3^- reabsorption from the tubule fluid.

Adverse effects include paraesthesiae (tingling and similar sensations), hypokalaemia, anorexia, drowsiness and depression. These problems, and the self-limiting nature of the diuresis, restrict the use of these agents.

Acetazolamide is useful in the treatment of open-angle glaucoma (inhibition of carbonic anhydrase reduces both the formation of HCO_3^- and the secretion of aqueous humour causing intraocular pressure to decline) and epilepsy (see p. 519).

Osmotic diuretic agents

Osmotic diuretic agents (*mannitol*) are compounds that are filtered at the glomerulus and are not significantly reabsorbed from the tubules. The presence in the filtrate of the osmotically active solute limits the reabsorption of water and therefore increases urine output and increases the tonicity of the ECF. Osmotic diuretic agents, by this mechanism, are able to reduce the volume and pressure of both CSF and intraocular fluid (in acute closed-angle glaucoma).

Summary

(1) Diuretics increase ion and fluid output from the kidney by inhibiting tubular reabsorption processes.
(2) Benzothiadiazides and related compounds (e.g. **bendrofluazide**):
    (a) have moderate efficacy as diuretics;
    (b) reduce Na^+ and Cl^- reabsorption in the distal tubule;
    (c) increase K^+ loss (in association with Na^+ reabsorption) in the collecting ducts;
    (d) reduce uric acid excretion;
    (e) produce a sustained antihypertensive effect independent of the diuresis;
    (f) reduce the urine output in diabetes insipidus;
    (g) are useful in oedema and hypertension and may cause K^+ depletion, hyperuricaemia and hyperglycaemia.

(3) High ceiling (loop) diuretic agents (e.g. **frusemide**):
  (a) have high efficacy as diuretics;
  (b) inhibit the $Na^+/K^+/2Cl^-$ co-transporter in the ascending limb of the loop of Henle;
  (c) increase K^+ loss (in association with Na^+ reabsorption) in the collecting ducts;
  (d) reduce uric acid excretion;
  (e) reduce BP by a vasodilator action;
  (f) are useful in oedema;
  (g) may cause K^+ depletion, hyperuricaemia and hypovolaemia.
(4) The potassium-sparing diuretic agents:
  (a) act in the collecting ducts to reduce K^+ secretion;
  (b) **amiloride** and *triamterene* act by reducing Na^+ reabsorption there;
  (c) **spironolactone** is an antagonist at intracellular aldosterone receptors;
  (d) may produce unwanted hyperkalaemia.

Anticoagulant, antiplatelet and fibrinolytic compounds

These are used:

(1) To prevent the clotting of blood in extravascular situations (blood samples, heart–lung machines, kidney dialysis equipment).
(2) In an attempt to prevent the formation or enlargement of thrombi (intravascular clots) in the venous circulation and on prosthetic heart valves (anticoagulant drugs) or in the arterial circulation (antiplatelet drugs).
(3) To break down pre-existing thrombi (fibrinolytic drugs).

Normally, clotting of blood in vivo only occurs as part of a physiological protective process (haemostasis) that, along with vasoconstriction, aids arrest of blood loss from damaged blood vessels. Coagulation is the part of the clotting process that can occur in plasma; it is the conversion of a soluble protein (fibrinogen) to strands of insoluble fibrin. The clotting process comprises a complex cascade of enzyme-mediated events, with amplifying or positive feedback stages, that lead up to coagulation, plus the aggregation of platelets (thrombocytes).

Pathologically clots can form (thrombosis) within the lumen of components of the cardiovascular system – veins, the chambers of the heart and arteries. In veins the thrombus is composed principally of fibrin while platelets form the major component in arteries. Inappropriate coagulation is the indication for anticoagulant therapy, as is thrombosis for thrombolytic therapy.

Fibrin formation

Blood coagulation can be considered to be initiated when tissue damage releases a tissue factor or thromboplastin, which in turn activates the coagulation factor VII. This extrinsic pathway, so called because it starts outside the blood, combines with the intrinsic pathway, a process that occurs entirely within the blood and so can occur in vitro. The intrinsic pathway starts with the contact of a coagulation factor with a negatively charged surface; the factor is converted to its active form which results in a cascade of coagulation factors (including IX) being successively converted to their active forms.

These two pathways converge to activate coagulation factor X (Figure 3.10). The inactive precursor prothrombin, normally present in plasma, is subsequently converted to the enzyme thrombin. Thrombin catalyses the conversion of the soluble protein fibrinogen (also normally present in plasma) to the insoluble fibrin, activates fibrin stabilizing factor (coagulation factor XIII) which causes the formation of covalent bonds between the monomers of fibrin, thus stabilizing it, and acts on platelets to promote aggregation.

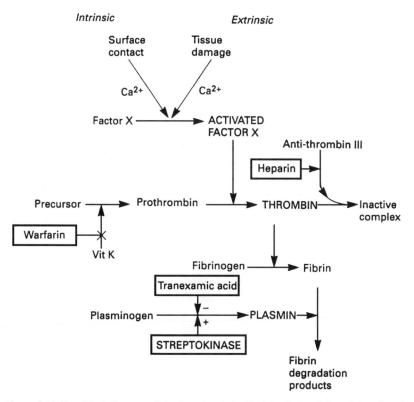

Figure 3.10 Simplified diagram of the key events in the blood coagulation (above) and dissolution of clot (below) processes. Words in CAPITALS represent active proteases. Boxes enclose the names of drugs acting at the sites indicated

The coagulation factors are proteases or enzyme co-factors, and activation is achieved by limited proteolysis.

Normally coagulation is limited to a site of injury, as healthy vascular endothelial cells generate several anticoagulant substances and these cells express a receptor that binds thrombin.

Platelet aggregation

Damage to the vascular endothelium causes platelets to adhere, which results in their activation. Activation involves a shape change and the release of many substances, such as adenosine diphosphate (ADP), 5-hydroxytryptamine (see p. 203), fibrinogen, platelet-activating factor and thromboxane A_2 (see p. 207), the latter synthesized from arachidonic acid. These substances are pro-aggregatory, causing platelets to form links with fibrinogen. Fibrin becomes associated with negatively charged phospholipids on the surface of activated platelets to form a blood clot.

Normally platelet aggregation is limited to a site of injury as healthy vascular endothelial cells release the anti-aggregatory substances prostacyclin (see p. 207), synthesized from arachidonic acid, and nitric oxide (see p. 132).

Several of the pro-aggregatory substances, such as 5-hydroxytryptamine and thromboxane A_2, are vasoconstrictor, aiding the haemostatic process, while the anti-aggregatory substances, prostacyclin and nitric oxide, are vasodilator.

Thrombus formation

Thrombi (unwanted intravascular clots) occur most commonly in the deep veins of the calf following surgery and bed rest when blood flow is sluggish and there may be changes in the blood (elevated platelet count, increased stickiness of platelets and increased concentration of fibrinogen). Thrombus formation starts with the aggregation of platelets at the vessel endothelium, the activation of coagulation resulting in the formation of fibrin and the entanglement of passing red cells. The resulting mass of platelets, fibrin and red cells is the thrombus.

In arterial thrombus formation, which typically occurs in a fast-flowing circulation, platelet aggregation plays a more important role than does coagulation. For this reason compounds with anticoagulant activity are less successful than those inhibiting platelet function in the prevention of arterial thrombosis.

Part of the thrombus may detach (an embolus) and be carried in the blood to another organ. There it may retard or obstruct blood flow, resulting in ischaemia (lack of blood) and death of the tissue beyond.

Atherosclerosis is a disease of arteries in which the vascular endothelium is initially damaged and leads over many years to fatty deposition (plaques). These plaques have a tendency to promote thrombus formation, especially in the coronary and cerebral arteries, which can result in acute myocardial and cerebral infarction respectively.

Drug interference with coagulation or thrombus formation

There are several means by which compounds can affect coagulation.

Removal of calcium ions

In practice this method is restricted to in vitro application. Removal of Ca^{2+} inhibits several stages of the process. Ca^{2+} can be removed by precipitation (as the insoluble fluoride, sulphate, oxalate) or by chelation (with sodium edetate). Blood for transfusion may be prevented from clotting by the use of citrate, which forms a soluble complex with Ca^{2+}. Citrate has the advantage that it is metabolized in the Krebs' cycle.

Heparin

Heparin occurs naturally in the body at a number of sites including the liver, lungs and mast cells. Heparin is a family of sulphated mucopolysaccharides of varying MW (4–30 kDa), built up of repeating units of glucosamine and glucuronic acid, and glucosamine and iduronic acid. The anionic sulphate and carboxylic acid groups result in a highly acid molecule with a large net negative charge, and these negative groups are essential for activity. The activity of **heparin** as an anticoagulant requires the presence in plasma of a naturally occurring inhibitor of serine proteases, plasma antithrombin III. This co-factor inhibits the activity of thrombin (and activated coagulation factors IX and X) by forming inactive complexes (Figure 3.10). **Heparin** greatly increases the rate at which these inactive complexes are formed by binding to antithrombin III and causing a conformational change that aids its access to the active site of thrombin. High MW (unfractionated) **heparin** shows greater activity because it contains more of the necessary binding sites, but the low MW **heparins** (e.g. *dalteparin*) are claimed to show selective activity at different points in the cascade (especially activated coagulation factor X) and to be free of effects on platelet behaviour (see below). They also have a longer duration of action. The anticoagulant effects of **heparin** are exerted both in vivo and in vitro. Despite the presence of heparin in the body and the mechanism of its anticoagulant activity, there is no evidence that it plays any role in the physiological control of blood clotting.

Platelet aggregation may be decreased by **heparin**, because of the decrease in thrombin activity. Paradoxically some 25–30% of patients experience a mild reduction in the number of circulating platelets (thrombocytopenia) because of aggregation and destruction, and a smaller number experience a severe reduction, which may be due to the formation of antiplatelet antibodies against the **heparin**/antithrombin III complex. By releasing or activating lipoprotein lipase (clearing factor) from tissues, **heparin** increases the removal of lipids from the plasma.

As a fully ionized molecule **heparin** is not absorbed after oral administration and it is therefore given by i/v injection or infusion or s/c injection. It should not be given by i/m injection because of possible haematoma formation at the site of injection. **Heparin** may be used in vivo, in extracorporeal circulations and to preserve fluidity of blood samples.

The main problem associated with the use of **heparin** is haemorrhage, especially if the patient has a hidden potential source of bleeding (e.g. peptic ulcer). Transient alopecia (hair loss) may occur several months after use. **Heparin** is of non-human animal origin and thus hypersensitivity and anaphylactic reactions may occur but these are not frequent.

Antagonists of heparin

Excessive anticoagulant activity or minor haemorrhage is controlled by ceasing administration of **heparin**. For major haemorrhage resulting from **heparin**, use of an antagonist is required. **Protamine sulphate** is a simple, low MW protein that is strongly basic and combines with the negatively charged heparin forming a stable complex with no anticoagulant properties. It is given by slow i/v injection, usually 1 mg to 100 units of **heparin**, but the dose required decreases with the time after **heparin** administration. **Protamine sulphate** has some anticoagulant properties (inhibits thrombin/fibrinogen interaction), so care must be taken not to exceed the amount required to neutralize **heparin**.

The injection of **protamine sulphate** may cause bradycardia, dyspnoea, flushing and a feeling of warmth by releasing histamine (see p. 198), but it is usually not antigenic.

Warfarin

Vitamin K is normally synthesized in the gastrointestinal tract by bacteria, and is essential for the formation in the liver of prothrombin and coagulation factors VII, IX and X. During the carboxylation of precursors of these factors, vitamin K is oxidized to its inactive epoxide and then reduced back to its active form for reuse. **Warfarin**, which has a similar chemical structure to vitamin K, is a competitive inhibitor of vitamin K reductase. Hence it prevents the reduction of vitamin K to its active form, inhibiting further formation of prothrombin and coagulation factors VII, IX and X (Figure 3.10). There is a delay of a few days before the onset of the anticoagulant effect as the preformed factors prothrombin and VII, IX and X must first be depleted. The varying plasma $t_{1/2}$ of these factors (prothrombin 60 h, factor VII 6 h) complicates control. The action is exerted only in vivo and is influenced by the vitamin K intake and the fat content of the diet, which affects absorption of vitamin K. Concurrent use of broad-spectrum antibiotic agents that alter gut bacterial flora, and thus vitamin K production, may affect the action of the oral anticoagulant agents, particularly if there is a concurrent deficiency of vitamin K in the diet.

Warfarin, a racemic mixture of dextro *R*- and laevo *S*-isomers, is completely absorbed after oral administration, is almost totally protein bound in the plasma and is metabolized by non-specific MFO in the liver. The peak anticoagulant effect is exerted from 36 to 72 h, the *S*-isomer being four times more potent than the *R*-isomer. The duration of this effect after withdrawing the drug is 4–5 days.

It is necessary carefully to monitor **warfarin** use, to strike a balance between underdosing, leaving excessive coagulation unaffected, and overdosing, leading to haemorrhage. Therapy is monitored by its effect on prothrombin time, the time for citrated plasma to clot on addition of calcium and tissue factor. The results are expressed as the International Normalized Ratio – the ratio of the measured prothrombin time relative to a standard.

Adverse effects other than haemorrhage or interaction with other drugs (see below) rarely occur. **Warfarin** crosses the placenta and should be avoided in pregnancy (see p. 436).

Drug interactions

Warfarin is subject to several clinically important pharmacokinetic interactions by the mechanisms of induction of MFO (see p. 442), competition for plasma protein binding sites (see p. 441) and inhibition of metabolism (see p. 443). *Sulphinpyrazone* selectively inhibits the metabolism of the more active *S*-isomer and so potentiates **warfarin**.

Aspirin, at high dosage, causes a reduction in prothrombin concentration in the blood and may add to the effects of the oral anticoagulant agents. Gastric haemorrhage commonly produced by **aspirin** may cause greater problems in the presence of **warfarin**.

Drugs affecting platelet function (by influencing thromboxane A_2 and prostacyclin formation) may also interact with **warfarin**.

Antagonists of *warfarin*

Minor haemorrhages and excessively reduced prothrombin concentration respond to withdrawal of the drug. Some situations may need more rapid action, whole blood (containing the missing coagulation factors) or vitamin K_1 (**phytomenadione** [phytonadione]) may be given.

Drugs affecting platelet function

Epoprostenol

Epoprostenol (prostacyclin, PGI_2) is available for use in extracorporeal circulations (e.g. renal dialysis) to inhibit aggregation of platelets, with or without **heparin**. It cannot be used in other situations because of its extremely short $t_{1/2}$ (30 s to 3 min) and marked vasodilator action exerted at IP receptors (see p. 207), leading to hypotension, headache and flushing.

Dipyridamole

By inhibiting the enzyme phosphodiesterase, *dipyridamole* reduces the metabolism of cAMP and results in its elevated concentration within the platelet. This decreases release of pro-aggregatory substances and may reduce thrombus formation. For best effect it is used in combination with **aspirin** or **warfarin**.

Aspirin

Drugs that inhibit cyclo-oxygenase reduce the synthesis of the products of the arachidonic acid pathway (see p. 204). **Aspirin** inhibits cyclo-oxygenase irreversibly by acetylating the active centre of the enzyme. Other inhibitors (e.g. salicylic acid, the propionic acid derivatives *ibuprofen* and *naproxen*) act competitively. With a low dose of **aspirin** it is possible to inhibit thromboxane A$_2$ formation without inhibiting that of prostacyclin (because of the inability of the non-nucleated platelet to synthesize more cyclo-oxygenase, and possibly greater sensitivity of the platelet enzyme to inhibition) and thus reduce thrombus formation. The daily dose used appears to be critical and is well below that used for analgesia or anti-inflammatory activity. Too large a daily dose reduces the formation of prostacyclin by vascular endothelial cells, in addition to that of thromboxane by platelets. Given for a month after myocardial infarction, low-dose **aspirin** has been shown to reduce mortality. Encouraging results have also been obtained in other kinds of patient considered to be at risk of thrombus formation.

Dissolution of thrombus

In the normal clotting process in vivo the clot is finally broken down to soluble fibrin degradation products (Figure 3.10) by the action of plasmin (fibrinolysin). This is formed from an inactive precursor plasminogen (fibrinolysinogen) by a coagulation factor XII-dependent activator formed during the clotting process. Activators of this mechanism may be used in an attempt to break down pre-existing thrombi and so are useful in acute myocardial infarction. **Streptokinase** (from haemolytic streptococci) and urinary-type plasminogen activator (*urokinase* from urine) are both able to activate this mechanism and show most success in dissolving fresh clots. **Streptokinase** may cause allergic reactions and anaphylaxis. Additionally, tissue-type plasminogen activator (*alteplase*, produced by recombinant DNA techniques) can be used and is not antigenic.

One danger associated with such attempts to dissolve clots is that fibrinogen and other coagulation factors may be used up in maintaining the clot with the resultant risk of haemorrhage. Should this occur an inhibitor of plasminogen activation, *tranexamic acid*, or an inhibitor of plasmin, *aprotinin*, may be used. Another danger associated with attempts at dissolution is formation of emboli as portions of the thrombus break away, move through the circulation and lodge in small vessels, blocking them.

Summary

(1) Anticoagulants are used to prevent clotting in extravascular situations and prevent formation of thrombi in the venous circulation.
(2) **Heparin**: is a family of sulphated mucopolysaccharides of varying MW; has a high net negative charge that is essential for activity; increases the rate of formation of inactive complexes between

antithrombin III and thrombin and factors IX and X; is active both in vivo and in vitro; requires parenteral (s/c, i/v) administration because it is not absorbed from the gastrointestinal tract; has an immediate onset of action; produces few unwanted effects, other than haemorrhage; can be antagonized by neutralization with **protamine**.

(3) **Warfarin**: has a similar chemical structure to vitamin K; inhibits vitamin K reductase, preventing the activation of vitamin K essential for the formation of prothrombin and factors VII, IX and X; has a delayed onset of action as preformed factors must be depleted; is active in vivo only; requires careful monitoring to avoid haemorrhage; has clinically significant interactions with a wide range of drugs; can be antagonized slowly by vitamin K_1 and rapidly by blood transfusion.

(4) Antiplatelet drugs are used to prevent formation or enlargement of thrombi in the arterial circulation. *Epoprostenol*: inhibits platelet aggregation; has a very short $t_{1/2}$ and is limited to use in extracorporeal circulation; causes marked vasodilatation. *Dipyridamole*: increases platelet cAMP concentration by inhibiting phosphodiesterase; decreases platelet aggregation and possibly thrombus formation. **Aspirin**: irreversibly inhibits cyclo-oxygenase; in a low dose reduces thromboxane A_2 formation without influencing prostacyclin formation.

(5) Thrombolytic agents are used to break down pre-existing thrombi. **Streptokinase**, *urokinase* and *alteplase* all activate the conversion of plasminogen to plasmin; *tranexamic acid* and *aprotinin*, which inhibit fibrinolysis, may be used in haemorrhage resulting from thrombolytic drugs.

Lipid-lowering drugs

Hyperlipidaemia, excess cholesterol and triglyceride circulating in combination with low density lipoproteins (LDL), is associated with the development of atherosclerosis.

Lipids are transported in the bloodstream between sites of absorption, synthesis (liver), storage (adipose tissue) and utilization (other tissues) in association with lipoproteins of four density (as determined by ultracentrifugation) bands (Figure 3.11).

(1) After absorption from the intestine, lipids are transported in the blood within chylomicrons. These are the lipid transporting lipoproteins of lowest density. They are broken down at the interface of adipose tissue and capillaries, liberating their lipid (95% triglyceride : 5% cholesterol) content. Most of the lipid is absorbed into the tissue but the remnants of the chylomicrons (80% triglyceride : 20% cholesterol) are transported to and metabolized by the liver.

(2) The very low density lipoproteins (VLDL) represent a carrier for lipid (70% triglyceride : 30% cholesterol) synthesized in the liver, transporting such lipid to the adipose tissue.

STAFFS UNIVERSITY LIBRARY

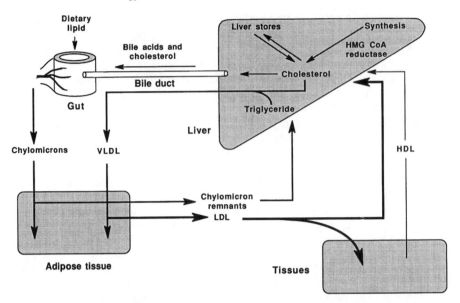

Figure 3.11 The carriage of lipids, triglyceride and cholesterol in the blood. VLDL = very low density lipoprotein; LDL = low density lipoprotein; HDL = high density lipoprotein. The thicker of the lines tracing the various processes for lipid transport in the blood reflects the higher risk factor for atherosclerosis

(3) The LDL represent a carrier for lipid (10% triglyceride : 90% cholesterol) mobilized from the adipose tissue. They transport such lipid to other tissues (e.g. vascular endothelium and macrophages in the wall of the blood vessel) and the liver.

(4) The high density lipoproteins (HDL) represent a carrier for excess lipid (25% triglyceride : 75% cholesterol) back from the tissues to the liver.

The risk factors for atherosclerosis are thus excessive serum concentrations of cholesterol, LDL-cholesterol or LDL-triglyceride and a reduced serum concentration of HDL-cholesterol.

Hyperlipidaemia is difficult to define quantitatively and the pathology is often obscure. Lipid concentrations fluctuate widely within an individual. However, it is generally thought that plasma cholesterol concentrations above 6.5 mmole/L require treatment.

Dietary modification, along with the reduction of other risk factors, e.g. lowering of BP and cessation of smoking, is always the first treatment.

Severe hypercholesterolaemia may be alleviated by *cholestyramine*, an anion exchange resin that promotes cholesterol excretion. It does this by binding bile acids within the gut lumen, preventing their normal reabsorption and reutilization. The liver responds by using more cholesterol, derived from circulating LDL-cholesterol, to synthesize bile acids for excretion. Fat-soluble vitamins may be lost from the body. *Cholestyramine* reduces absorption of other drugs – this interaction can be avoided by instructing the patient to swallow the *cholestyramine* several hours before or after swallowing other drugs.

Bezafibrate alters the pattern of hepatic lipid metabolism and the beneficial effects may arise from stimulation of lipoprotein lipase and hence a reduction in the circulating concentration of triglycerides. *Bezafibrate* also evokes reduced production of LDL-cholesterol, reduced production of cholesterol and increased production of HDL-cholesterol.

Simvastatin is a competitive inhibitor of 3-hydroxy-3-methylglutaryl coenzyme A (HMG CoA) reductase, a hepatic enzyme that catalyses the rate-limiting step involved in the synthesis of cholesterol. It is effective against hypercholesterolaemia.

Summary

(1) Lifestyle change is the preferred method of decreasing cardiovascular risk.
(2) Drugs that affect the hepatic handling of lipid act by reducing the synthesis of lipids or increasing their metabolism or excretion.

4

Endocrine pharmacology

Aims

- To provide a framework of physiology of the important endocrine systems.
- To explain the site and mechanism of action of endogenous hormones, their structural analogues and other compounds that interact with endocrine systems.
- To produce a scientific basis for the therapeutic use of compounds that interact with endocrine systems.

Introduction

In the mammalian body chemical messengers are often employed to transmit information from a cell to itself (autocrine), within the tissue (paracrine) and to distant organs (endocrine). The second (peripheral) and fifth (CNS) sections deal with the theme of drugs that interact with one class of chemical messengers – the neurotransmitters. The theme of this section is interaction with chemical messengers other than neurotransmitters (Table 4.1).

Hierarchy of endocrine hormones

Several endocrine systems consist of a hierarchy of endocrine glands and hormones, in which the secretion of one hormone influences the secretion of a second hormone, that in turn affects the production of a third

Table 4.1 Classification of chemical messengers

	Cell of origin	Transport medium
Neurotransmitter (paracrine)	Nerve	Interstitial fluid
Local hormone (auto- or paracrine)	Non-nerve	Interstitial fluid
Neurohumour (endocrine)	Nerve	Blood
Hormone (endocrine)	Non-nerve	Blood

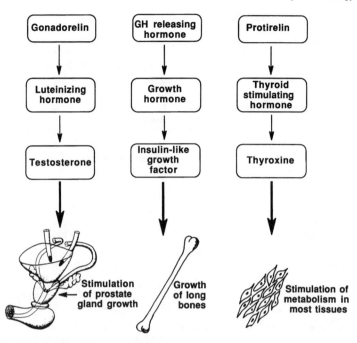

Figure 4.1 A typical hierarchy of hormones (a thin arrow represents promotion of synthesis/release; a thick arrow represents action upon)

hormone. This third hormone may act on a peripheral target tissue. An example is shown in Figure 4.1.

Usually homeostasis is maintained by a negative feedback whereby a change in the plasma concentration of the peripherally produced hormone alters the secretion of the centrally produced hormone in the opposite direction. A similar but simpler link occurs between plasma glucose concentration and insulin secretion. Consequently, pharmacological manipulation at one point in an endocrine system tends to influence the whole system because of this hierarchy and feedback.

Mechanisms of hormone action

Hormones act by regulating pre-existing processes. The actions of hormones can be divided into those that are cell plasma membrane mediated (see cell surface receptor coupled by a G-protein to an effector enzyme or kinase-linked receptor in Figure 1.8) and those that are cell nucleus mediated (Table 4.2).

Most reproductive and non-reproductive steroid hormones have a similar molecular mechanism of action. Tissue selectivity is achieved by the presence of one of a family of specific soluble protein receptors, which are occasionally found in the cytoplasm (may be an artefact) but are mainly in the nucleus of the target cell (e.g. oestrogen specific in the uterus, androgen specific in the prostate). Steroid hormones pass from the

Table 4.2 Mechanisms of hormone action

Membrane-mediated	Nucleus-mediated
Hormone action mediated extracellularly	Hormone action mediated intracellularly (Figure 4.2)
Mechanism of action	
Interaction with a cell membrane receptor	Interaction with a soluble intracellular receptor
Change in intracellular activities of second messengers (Ca^{2+}, cAMP, protein kinase)	Binding of receptor complex to hormone response element of gene
	Change in transcription
Increase in cellular metabolic activities	Synthesis of mRNA, proteins and enzymes
Examples: hormone – target	
Insulin – liver	Glucocorticosteroids – liver
Adrenaline – adipose cells	Oestrogens – uterus
Protirelin – anterior pituitary	Androgens – prostate
Thyroxine – most tissues	Thyroxine – most tissues
Onset of action	
Rapid (min)	Slow (h), often with a delay
Offset of action	
Rapid	Persistent due to slow turnover of enzymes/proteins
Correlation between plasma concentration of hormone and time-course of action	
Good	Poor as action slow and delayed

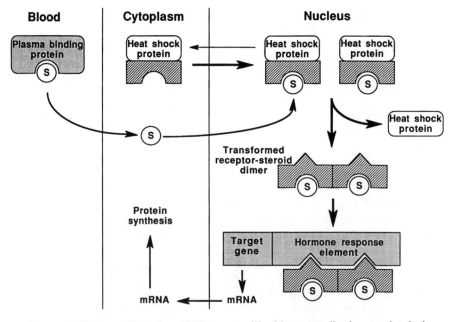

Figure 4.2 The interaction of steroid hormones (S) with target cells; the cross-hatched element represents the steroid hormone receptor

blood into the cell, combine with the receptor which promotes the dissociation of a heat shock protein and allows receptors to dimerize. The complex then binds to the DNA to act as a transcription factor (Figure 4.2).

The time-course of onset and offset of a drug modifying an endocrine system is influenced by whether the actions are membrane mediated or nuclear mediated. For example, *soluble insulin* given i/v has a very rapid onset and offset of action, due in part to the membrane-mediated nature of the action of insulin and in part to its rapid metabolism. Therefore, many formulations of insulin have been developed to produce a slower onset and more prolonged duration of action (see p. 188). Conversely, the benefits of glucocorticosteroids given in the relief of chronic asthma take several hours rather than a few minutes to appear, due to the genomically mediated action of these drugs.

Therapeutic uses of drugs affecting endocrine systems

Most therapeutic uses can be divided into four categories:

Replacement therapy

Where there is hyposecretion of an endogenous hormone, this can be replaced by the administration of the hormone or a structural analogue.

> *Examples:*
> Insulin for diabetes mellitus
> *Thyroxine sodium* for hypothyroidism

Many hormones, unlike neurotransmitters, are proteins or polypeptides and, therefore, it is more difficult to produce structural analogues and such analogues are unlikely to be orally active.

Alternatively, residual endogenous hormone secretion can be stimulated by drugs either directly at the site of endocrine deficiency or by an action higher in the endocrine hierarchy.

> *Examples:*
> **Tolbutamide** to stimulate insulin secretion
> *Gonadorelin* to treat female infertility

The dosage used is such that the endocrine system is functioning within the normal physiological range and, therefore, unwanted effects are usually few. Treatment is particularly easy when a constant action is required (e.g. treatment of hypothyroidism).

However, when a varying magnitude of effect is required (e.g. diabetes mellitus, see p. 189) replacement therapy may present more problems.

Decrease of hormone action

Endocrine diseases due to hypersecretion of a hormone or excess response of a peripheral target tissue to a hormone can be treated by surgical (e.g.

Cushing's disease of adrenal origin) or radiological (e.g. hyperthyroidism, see p. 178) removal of the source of the hormone. Alternatively drug treatment may be used:

(1) By antagonism of the hormone at its receptor.

> *Examples:*
> **Clomiphene** antagonism of 17β-oestradiol in anovulatory infertility
> **Cyproterone** antagonism of testosterone in prostate cancer
> **Spironolactone** antagonism of aldosterone in hypertension

(2) By functional opposition at the tissues affected by the hormone.

> *Examples:*
> **Propranolol** opposition of thyroid hormones – the sensitivity of β-adrenoceptors or their effector mechanisms is increased in thyrotoxicosis
> Progestogen opposition of oestrogens – hyperplastic endometrium produced by oestrogens is converted to a secretory endometrium

(3) By reduction of hormone production and/or secretion.

> *Examples:*
> **Carbimazole** reduction of thyroid hormone formation in thyrotoxicosis
> *Aminoglutethimide* reduction of extraovarian formation of oestrogens in postmenopausal breast cancer
> **Captopril** prevention of conversion of angiotensin I to angiotensin II in hypertension
> Combined oestrogen and progestogen inhibition of gonadotrophin secretion and prevention of ovulation in contraception

Functional tests of endocrine systems

An endogenous hormone, structural analogue or inhibitor of synthesis is given to determine the site of under or excess secretion of a hormone.

> *Examples:*
> Hypothalamic–pituitary–adrenal system (see p. 184)
> Hypothalamic–pituitary–thyroid system (see p. 179)

Drugs affecting endocrine systems for non-endocrine diseases

The commonest uses of some of the drugs fall in this category:

> *Examples:*
> Glucocorticosteroids (**prednisolone**) for inflammatory reactions and immune responses in suppression of rheumatoid arthritis and asthma
> Antagonists at mineralocorticosteroid receptors (**spironolactone**) for hypertension

As the dosage required for agonists is greater than in the replacement dose situation, so the unwanted effects tend to be greater.

Summary

Steroid hormones act primarily by alteration of gene transcription, initiated by a soluble nuclear receptor. Other hormones usually modulate intracellular second messenger systems via receptors located in the cell membrane.

Hypothalamopituitary axis

The pituitary gland is situated at the base of the brain and is connected by the pituitary stalk to the hypothalamus (Figure 4.3). The posterior pituitary gland secretes the neurohumours antidiuretic hormone (ADH, vasopressin, see p. 193) and oxytocin (see p. 194) from the endings of nerves. These nerves have their cell bodies in the hypothalamus. The anterior pituitary gland comprises non-innervated endocrine glands cells of five kinds that synthesize, store and secrete the proteinaceous pituitary trophic hormones:

(1) Follicle-stimulating hormone (FSH) and luteinizing hormone (LH).
(2) Prolactin (PRL).
(3) Thyroid-stimulating hormone (thyrotrophin, TSH, see p. 176).

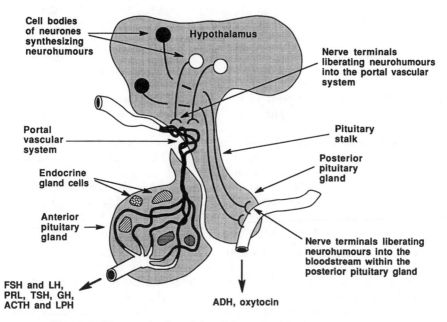

Figure 4.3 The organization of the pituitary gland for hormone secretion

(4) Adrenocorticotrophic hormone (corticotrophin, ACTH, see p. 180) and β-lipotrophin (see p. 225).
(5) Growth hormone (GH). Biosynthetic human *somatropin* is expensive but effective in the treatment of children of short stature due to a deficiency of GH secretion.

The secretion of pituitary trophins is controlled by neurohumours synthesized in neurones in the hypothalamus. The neurohumours are released into the blood of capillaries, which unite to form the sole blood supply of the anterior pituitary gland (a portal system).

Hypothalamopituitary neurohumours

These are substances that promote or inhibit the synthesis and secretion of an anterior pituitary hormone. They are also called hypothalamic releasing or release inhibiting hormones. Generally there is one neurohumour for each anterior pituitary hormone but supraphysiological doses of the neurohumours may affect the secretion of other anterior pituitary hormones.

(1) There is only one neurohumour controlling FSH and LH secretion, FSH/LH releasing hormone or *gonadorelin*, which is a decapeptide (made up of 10 amino acids). The mechanism of differential release of FSH and LH is poorly understood. In both men and women gonadotrophin (see p. 158) secretion is episodic.
   Gonadorelin or analogues given in short i/v pulses stimulate ovarian and testicular development and can be used to treat infertility. Sustained activity at the receptor causes down-regulation and inhibition of gonadal activity, an observation that has lead to the introduction of potent agonist analogues (*goserelin*) for the treatment of hormone-dependent breast and prostate cancer.
(2) Prolactin secretion is inhibited by prolactin release inhibiting hormone, the major component of which is dopamine, acting upon dopamine receptors in the pituitary gland.
(3) TSH secretion is promoted by TSH releasing hormone, which is a tripeptide, *protirelin*. This is not entirely specific as it can also cause release of prolactin.
(4) Corticotrophin releasing hormone, which controls ACTH (see p. 180), β-lipotrophin and β-endorphin (see p. 225) secretion, is a large molecule and consists of 41 amino acids.
(5) Somatostatin or GH release inhibiting hormone is a tetradecapeptide (made up of 14 amino acids) that inhibits GH secretion, whereas the GH releasing factors are larger polypeptides of between 37 and 44 amino acids. Somatostatin also inhibits release of prolactin and TSH.

These neurohumours are not exclusively localized in the hypothalamus and may possess other actions, both centrally and peripherally. For example, somatostatin is found in the pancreas and may inhibit secretion of both insulin and glucagon (see p. 191), and *octreotide*, a long-acting analogue of somatostatin, can relieve the symptoms of tumours that secrete gut hormones as well as inhibiting GH release in acromegaly. The plasma $t_{1/2}$ of each naturally occurring neurohumour is very short (less than 5 min), therefore clinical applications are mainly limited to diagnostic procedures that require tests of pituitary gland integrity.

Feedback mechanisms

Feedback in the control of anterior pituitary hormone secretions involves the central (hypothalamus and/or anterior pituitary gland) monitoring of the plasma concentration of a peripherally produced hormone and the consequent alteration of anterior pituitary hormone secretions to maintain a predetermined concentration. Feedbacks may be overridden by higher physiological processes, for example, stress increases ACTH and hence adrenal glucocorticosteroid secretion so that normal physiological plasma concentrations are exceeded. A unique transient positive feedback operates to promote gonadotrophin secretion above the set point in pubertal and adult females and is usually seen where high plasma concentrations of oestrogen follow low priming concentrations – as occur preceding ovulation.

Adverse and useful effects of drugs mediated by neurohumours

Various drugs that disturb hypothalamic neurotransmitter processes also produce disturbances in anterior pituitary secretion (barbiturates, phenothiazines and **morphine** inhibit gonadotrophin secretion, leading to decreased libido and infertility).

Phenytoin increases GH secretion, so producing hyperplasia of the gums. *Bromocriptine* suppresses GH release in acromegalic patients (and so is useful in preventing excessive growth in stature), whereas in normal subjects GH release is paradoxically increased.

A high serum prolactin concentration can result from the use of drugs that decrease dopamine storage, release and action. **Chlorpromazine** reduces the neuronal drive from higher centres to the hypothalamic dopaminergic nerve endings. *Metoclopramide* (and perhaps **chlorpromazine**) antagonize prolactin release inhibiting hormone at its pituitary gland (dopamine) receptor. The high serum prolactin concentration causes gynaecomastia (increased breast size), galactorrhoea (inappropriate breast secretion), impotence and infertility.

An agonist at dopamine receptors, *bromocriptine*, is useful therapeutically to decrease prolactin secretion and is also the drug of choice to suppress lactation. In addition, it promotes fertility in both sexes where increased prolactin plasma concentrations, possibly as a result of a pituitary adenoma, are associated with disturbances of gonadal activity and/or impotence. Oestrogens promote the synthesis and subsequently the secretion of prolactin. This accounts for the increased plasma concentrations of prolactin seen late in pregnancy and after combined oral contraceptive preparations and *stilboestrol* for prostatic carcinoma.

STAFFS UNIVERSITY LIBRARY

The feedback mechanisms are also exploited for therapeutic purposes. Combined oral contraceptive preparations inhibit gonadotrophin release and therefore ovulation does not occur. Oestrogens and progestogens are administered to men to reduce LH, and hence secretion of androgen, in an attempt to influence androgen-dependent prostatic cancer. **Clomiphene** (an antagonist at oestrogen receptors) prevents the negative feedback action of oestrogens, so generating a surge of gonadotrophin secretion and ovulation. Therefore it is useful in infertility associated with high plasma oestrogen concentration (Stein–Leventhal syndrome characterized by polycystic ovaries, infertility and oligomenorrhoea (decreased menstrual blood loss)).

Summary

(1) The anterior pituitary endocrine system can be supplemented by drugs acting directly upon target organ receptors (e.g *somatropin* in short stature) or inhibited or stimulated indirectly via feedback systems located in the hypothalamus or anterior pituitary gland (e.g. **clomiphene** in infertility).
(2) Synthetic peptide hypothalamic neurohumours are used to promote (e.g. *gonadorelin* in infertility) or inhibit (e.g. *octreotide* in acromegaly) pituitary trophin secretion.
(3) Autonomous pituitary prolactin secretion is inhibited by dopamine.

Gonadotrophins

A gonadotrophin is a substance producing growth and development of the gonads. The gonadotrophins, except prolactin, are high MW (25–70 kDa) glycoproteins. Prolactin is a protein (MW approximately 25 kDa). FSH, LH, *chorionic gonadotrophin* (and TSH too) consist of a common α-chain and different β-chains. The β-chain provides specificity of action. *Human menopausal gonadotrophins* is a mixture of gonadotrophins, mainly FSH, extracted from the urine of postmenopausal women. *Chorionic gonadotrophin* is similarly obtained from pregnant women. Pure pituitary trophins are now produced by recombinant DNA technology.

Gonadotrophic action in the female

It is the cyclical changes in the pituitary gonadotrophin secretions that produce corresponding ovarian changes, and hence the changes characteristic of the human menstrual cycle.

At birth each human ovary contains approximately 200 000 oocytes, each enclosed in follicular cells to form primordial follicles. Oocytes have

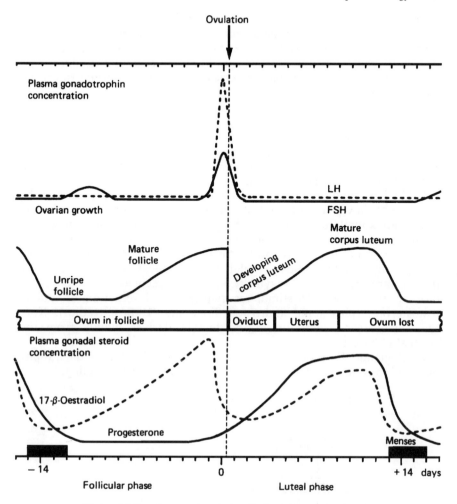

Figure 4.4 Events occurring during the human menstrual cycle

partially undergone first meiotic division. FSH (cooperating with a small concentration of LH), during the follicular phase of the menstrual cycle, promotes the growth of many follicles. It also promotes 17-β-oestradiol secretion by the thecal cells of these follicles (Figure 4.4), which leads to a surge of LH secretion (positive feedback, see p. 157).

The LH induces final maturation of the oocyte in the dominant follicle and completion of first meiotic division. Ovulation and conversion of the follicle to a corpus luteum occurs approximately 10 h later. This corpus luteum secretes 17-β-oestradiol and progesterone under the influence of LH.

If the oocyte is fertilized the resulting blastocyst implants onto the endometrium of the uterus approximately 7 days after ovulation. The trophoblast soon secretes human chorionic gonadotrophin (HCG), which maintains the steroid-synthesizing activity of the corpus luteum. Immuno-assay of HCG may be used for the diagnosis of pregnancy. In a menstrual cycle in which the ovum is not fertilized, the corpus luteum regresses, due to lack of gonadotrophins and steroid hormone secretion declines. This withdrawal of steroid hormones produces loss of endometrium (menstruation).

Steroid synthesis

Steroid synthesis to the progesterone stage is common for the adrenal cortex, testis and ovary (Figure 4.5).

FSH, LH (and ACTH) increase steroid synthesis, probably by increasing conversion of cholesterol to pregnenolone. FSH and LH selectively stimulate synthesis in the gonads. This selective synthesis of testosterone and 17-β-oestradiol derives from the presence of receptors and enzymes in the gonads and the relative absence of enzymes capable of forming corticosteroids. Similarly, only thecal cells of the ovary possess large amounts of enzymes converting precursors to 17-β-oestra-diol. In the testis, LH stimulates synthesis and secretion of mainly testosterone (plus some androstenedione and 17-β-oestradiol). Note that testosterone secretion in the female derives mainly from the adrenal cortices.

Prostaglandin $F_{2\alpha}$ reduces progesterone synthesis by causing the atrophy of the corpus luteum. This may be the basis of menstrual cycling.

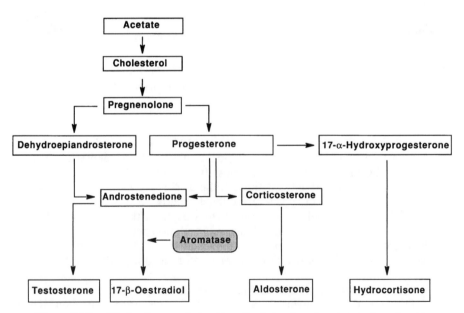

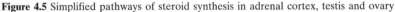

Figure 4.5 Simplified pathways of steroid synthesis in adrenal cortex, testis and ovary

Gonadotrophic action in the male

In the pubertal male, gametogenesis is mainly controlled by FSH and steroid hormone synthesis by LH. In the adult, spermatogenesis is mainly dependent upon LH-stimulated androgen. Sites of sperm production are the seminiferous tubules of the testes. Between the tubules are Leydig cells, which are the major site of testosterone synthesis and secretion.

Before puberty, the seminiferous tubules are lined by diploid spermatogonia. FSH stimulates continued cell divisions so that there are increased numbers of diploid spermatogonia and spermatocytes (Figure 4.6). Also, FSH induces the Sertoli cells to secrete an androgen binding protein, which maintains a high androgen concentration in the tubule lumen. Meiosis is stimulated by FSH and testosterone. Spermatozoa pass to the epididymides where final maturation occurs and it can be 1–3 weeks before sperm appear in the ejaculate. The total duration of spermatogenesis and sperm transport into the ejaculate in man is 12–15 weeks. Gametogenesis is therefore a continuous process in the male, in contrast to a cyclical process in female.

Gonadotrophic activity

Gonadotrophins can be subdivided and defined by the actions they produce (Table 4.3). *Chorionic gonadotrophin* has mainly LH-like actions.

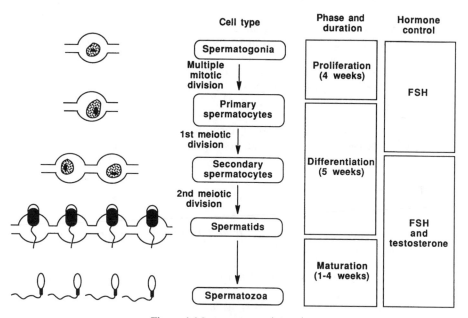

Figure 4.6 Spermatogenesis in man

Table 4.3 Classification of gonadotrophic activity

FSH-like activity	LH-like activity
In the female	
Oocyte growth	Maturation of ova
Follicular growth	Ovulation
Mainly 17-β-oestradiol secretion	Structural integrity of corpus luteum
	17-β-oestradiol and progesterone secretion
In the male	
Spermatogenesis	Testosterone secretion

Therapeutic use

One cause of female infertility is irregular and insufficient endogenous gonadotrophin secretion and therefore absence of ovulation. Replacement therapy with FSH as *human menopausal gonadotrophins* or *urofollitrophin*, followed by *chorionic gonadotrophin* mimicking the physiological sequence can lead to ovulation and pregnancy if the ovaries are capable of responding. Ovarian stimulation is easier to manage if endogenous gonadotrophin secretion is inhibited by a gonadorelin agonist. Excessive response leads to ovarian enlargement and haemorrhage, multiple ovulations and multiple pregnancy. This can be avoided by monitoring the number of follicles developing in response to *human menopausal gonadotrophins* (using ultrasound imaging). If this is excessive, then *chorionic gonadotrophin* is not given. Multiple ovulations are deliberately induced for subsequent collection of ova for in vitro fertilization of the ovum in the treatment of infertility.

Exogenous gonadotrophins have proved of little value in the treatment of male infertility that is due to reduced secretion of endogenous gonadotrophins. In part this may be due to the long time (10–13 weeks) between the first cell division of spermatogonia and final maturation.

Replacement therapy for steroid hormone deficiencies usually involves the use of steroid hormones rather than pituitary trophins.

Summary

(1) Gonadotrophins, of pituitary, urinary or biosynthetic origin, with FSH-like activity (e.g. *human menopausal gonadotrophins*) produce ovarian follicular growth, maturation and steroid hormone secretion, and with LH-like activity (e.g. *chorionic gonadotrophin*) precipitate ovulation. This activity can be used to treat female infertility.

(2) Gonadotrophins also support spermatogenesis in men, but male infertility is usually unrelated to deficiency of gonadotrophins.

Oestrogens, progestogens and androgens

An oestrogen, progestogen or androgen is a compound that produces a similar range of effects to those produced by 17-β-oestradiol, progesterone or testosterone respectively. Most such compounds show selectivity of action as they show high affinity at one kind of receptor and low affinities at the other kinds. However, some compounds possess properties of the other kinds of steroid hormone at higher doses. Such lesser selectivity arises either because the compound itself or a metabolite is less selective (e.g. an androgen could possess progestogenic activity due to an inherent property of the compound or due to the production of a metabolite possessing progestogenic activity). Some non-endocrine drugs combine with steroid hormone receptors and this accounts for some of their adverse effects. **Spironolactone** and **digoxin** can produce gynaecomastia by acting as agonists at the oestrogen receptor. **Cimetidine**, an antagonist at H_2 histamine receptors, also displaces testosterone from its receptor so that the effects of endogenous oestrogens can be expressed (removal of functional opposition).

All naturally occurring steroid hormones have a short plasma $t_{1/2}$ (less than 4 h) and are inactive orally due to high first-pass metabolism. Simple structural alterations of the steroid hormone molecule produce dramatic

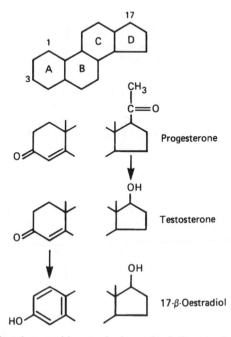

Figure 4.7 The steroid nucleus, position numbering and substituents of some physiological steroids

changes in biological activity (Figure 4.7). Modification of the basic structure by conjugation, esterification or alkylation (at positions 1 or 17) extends the $t_{1/2}$ into the therapeutically useful range. The esters exhibit significant first-pass metabolism but a sustained effect (days) occurs after parenteral administration by slow de-esterification. Steric hindrance by alkylation at position 17 (by an ethinyl group $-C{\equiv}CH$) greatly reduces first-pass metabolism, so these derivatives are orally active with a $t_{1/2}$ of approximately 1 day.

Steroid hormones are extensively bound to albumin or specific binding globulins. Free steroid hormones are metabolized by the liver and conjugated to form the sulphate and glucuronide. Excretion of the metabolite is mainly in the urine but some is excreted in the bile. Once in the gut, bacteria act upon some of the conjugates to release free steroid hormone, which is then reabsorbed – a process referred to as enterohepatic circulation (see Figure 7.9). The remainder is excreted in the faeces.

Oestrogens

The major secretory product of the ovarian follicles is 17-β-oestradiol, which is rapidly metabolized to less potent oestrogens – oestriol and oestrone. Figure 4.4 shows the steroid hormone secretion pattern during the menstrual cycle.

Preparations

Steroidal

Oestradiol is available as trans- and sub-dermal preparations, to avoid the low systemic bioavailability resulting from the extensive metabolism during its first pass through the liver (see p. 337) that occurs on oral administration.

Ethinyloestradiol is active orally because its 17-ethinyl group sterically hinders first-pass metabolism by mixed function oxidase (MFO). Mestranol is the 3-methyl ether of ethinyloestradiol and is an active prodrug converted by the liver and the gut wall to the more potent ethinyloestradiol.

Non-steroidal

These are orally and topically active preparations: *stilboestrol* [diethylstilbestrol] and dienoestrol. This group of oestrogens is suspected of carcinogenic activity, therefore their use is restricted to topical applications or postmenopausal breast cancer or prostate cancer.

All are agonists at oestrogen receptors producing the effects in Table 4.4.

Therapeutic use

Oestrogens are used for either their direct actions or indirect hypothalamus/pituitary gland negative feedback actions. Oestrogen therapy alone is

Table 4.4 Some effects of oestrogens

System affected	Consequence
Female reproductive organs	
Fallopian tubes, uterus, vagina	Growth and development
Mammary glands	Growth and development of ducts
Uterine endometrium	Proliferation (irregular menstruation)
Cervical epithelium	Thin and copious mucus (good sperm penetration)
CNS	
FSH and LH secretion	Positive and negative feedback
Prolactin secretion	Increases
Libido	Indispensable in non-primate mammals; role in people not clear
Chemosensitive trigger zone	Nausea and vomiting
Metabolic actions	
Coagulation factors	Predisposition to thromboembolic phenomena
Hormone binding globulins	Increases plasma concentration
Carbohydrate metabolism	Weak diabetogenic action
Fluid mobilization	Salt and water retention
High density lipoproteins increased	Protection against atherosclerosis
Other actions	
Long bones	Growth early; reduces bone reabsorption
Epiphyses	Closure
Axillary and pubic hair	Growth in female pattern
Oestrogen-dependent cancers	Growth after low doses
Carcinogenesis	Endometrial carcinoma may be induced in postmenopausal women by chronic treatment

not recommended due to the high incidence of side-effects, for example thromboembolic phenomena or uterine endometrial hyperplasia, which in postmenopausal women is associated with progression to carcinoma. Progestogens are usually administered concurrently, in the form of combined oral contraceptive preparations, to obtain the desired effect (see p. 169).

Replacement therapy

These effects occur with small doses and result from direct actions on target tissue receptors.

(1) *Primary ovarian failure.* Oestrogens initiate pubertal changes, which are maintained with combination therapy.
(2) *Relief of menopausal symptoms* (natural or premature), which include vasomotor instability, anxiety, depression and atrophy of secondary sexual organs. Oestrogens do not relieve osteoporosis but may prevent its development. Oestrogen should only be used alone as replacement therapy if the patient has had a hysterectomy. The incidence of atherosclerosis is decreased.
(3) Atrophic vaginitis or vulvitis is the only indication for topical (pessary or cream) application to produce a local effect.

Neoplastic disease

Large doses of oestrogens may palliate certain neoplastic diseases. This results from a combination of direct actions on receptors in target tissues and non-receptor-mediated effects.

> *Examples:*
> Androgen-dependent carcinoma of the prostate
> Advanced breast cancer (see p. 325).

Antagonists at oestrogen receptors

These compete with 17-β-oestradiol for the soluble receptors (Figure 4.2). **Clomiphene** and **tamoxifen** are non-steroidal orally active compounds that antagonize oestrogens at all their specific target organ receptors. However, the drug–oestrogen receptor complex is not inert – the drugs are partial agonists with very long $t_{1/2}$.

Therapeutic use

Induction of ovulation

Antagonists at oestrogen receptors can induce ovulation in an infertile patient with an intact hypothalamus–pituitary–ovarian axis and increased plasma oestrogen concentration, for example, Stein–Leventhal syndrome (see p. 158), or in amenorrhoea on discontinuing contraceptive preparations. In combination with *chorionic gonadotrophin* they produce multiple ovulations for ovum collection for in vitro fertilization. A short period of administration induces ovulation and initiates menstrual cycles by preventing the inhibitory (negative feedback) action of oestrogen at the hypothalamus, allowing gonadotrophin secretion and therefore follicular development.

Advanced breast cancer

Thirty per cent of breast tumours respond by regression to hormone manipulations, that is, empirical treatment that may involve the removal of the hormone-producing gland, ovary or adrenal (premenopause), or the administration of large doses of androgens, oestrogens or antagonists at oestrogen receptors. Breast tumours containing detectable oestrogen receptors respond more favourably. **Tamoxifen** has replaced all other endocrine manipulations as the treatment of choice. Regression can only be obtained during continuous therapy, which is relatively free of adverse effects.

Progestogens

Physiologically the major progestogen is progesterone, which is secreted by the corpus luteum of the ovary as well as by the placenta during

Table 4.5 Some effects of progestogens

System affected	Consequence
Female reproductive organs	
Fallopian tubes, uterus, vagina	Growth and development
Mammary glands	Growth and development of the lobular-alveolar system
Uterine endometrium	Increased secretion. Withdrawal leads to tissue necrosis and menstruation
Cervical epithelium	Viscous and scanty mucus (poor sperm penetration)
CNS	
FSH and LH secretion	Negative feedback
Libido	Synergistic with oestrogens in lower mammals
Consciousness	Sedative (large doses)
Body temperature	Thermogenic
Pregnancy	
Uterus, placenta, fetus	Necessary for normal course of pregnancy
Metabolic actions	
Fluid mobilization	Salt and water loss (aldosterone antagonism)
High density lipoprotein concentration	Adversely reduced

pregnancy. Most progestational effects (Table 4.5) are only seen after previous priming of the target organs with oestrogens, which induces the synthesis of progestogen receptors.

Preparations

Progesterone derivatives

Medroxyprogesterone acetate is an ester and only weakly active after oral administration, due to high first-pass metabolism; it is given by deep i/m injection.

19-Nortestosterone derivatives

Norethisterone is one of a group of steroids having an ethinyl substitution at the 17-α-position, which makes them orally active and extends the $t_{1/2}$. Ethynodiol is a prodrug that is converted to norethisterone. Levonorgestrel is the commonest progestogen in combined oral contraceptive preparations. Desogestrel is an orally active, potent and selective derivative of levonorgestrel, used only as the progestogen component in combined oral contraceptive preparations.

These compounds are all agonists at progestogen receptors and produce the same effects as progesterone (Table 4.5). In addition, members of this group may possess androgenic, oestrogenic or oestrogen antagonistic activity because of either intrinsic efficacy of the parent molecule or metabolism to active compounds. Relative to the peripheral progestational effects, they more strongly inhibit gonadotrophin secretion than the progesterone derivatives.

Testosterone derivatives

Danazol is a mixed androgen and progestogen that inhibits pituitary gonadotrophin secretion but shows less peripheral progestogenic and androgenic effects.

Therapeutic use

Progestogens are usually used in combination with oestrogens. However, the following list indicates where a progestogen has been found useful alone.

Contraception

(1) Continuous oral administration of 19-nortestosterone derivatives in doses smaller than those contained in combined oral contraceptive preparations has a contraceptive effect. The action is a combination of the effects (Table 4.5) upon the CNS, pituitary, ovary, Fallopian tube, endometrium and cervical mucus. Ovulation is suppressed in approximately 50% of women and menstrual irregularities are common. Ectopic pregnancy is not prevented.

(2) Three-monthly i/m depot injections of the esters *medroxyprogesterone acetate* or *norethisterone enanthate*, or implants containing levonorgestrel lasting up to 5 years, have a contraceptive effect. Gonadotrophin secretion is suppressed so ovulation does not occur. Menstruation is irregular and amenorrhoea may occur after 12 months. Continued patient compliance is not required therefore it is useful when pregnancy is contraindicated, for example, following rubella vaccination.

Both approaches are useful during lactation and in women who suffer from oestrogen-related unwanted effects of the combined oral contraceptive preparations.

Endometriosis

Endometriosis is the growth of endometrial tissue in inappropriate (ectopic) positions, such as·in the peritoneal cavity. Continuous long-term use of progestogens is aimed at producing regression of the tissue mass by the withdrawal of endogenous oestrogen support.

Neoplastic disease

Large doses of progestogens produce remission in inoperable endometrial carcinoma and breast cancer, which is maintained for approximately 15 months.

Antagonist at progestogen receptors

Mifepristone is an antagonist at progestogen receptors. As progesterone is necessary for the maintenance of pregnancy, **mifepristone** can be useful for the termination of early pregnancy.

Oestrogen plus progestogen

Oral combined therapy (one oestrogen (**ethinyloestradiol** or mestranol) plus one progestogen (a 19-nortestosterone derivative)) is used at smaller doses than single drug therapy, as the constituents are synergistic.

The synthetic steroidal oestrogens are combined with the orally active progestogens. The combination is usually administered as a 21-day course, followed by a 7-day tablet-free interval during which withdrawal bleeding from the endometrium occurs (not true menstruation). Practically any cycle length can be produced by continuing administration of these drugs. The oestrogen plus progestogen exert a negative feedback action at the hypothalamus-anterior pituitary, resulting in decreased FSH and LH secretion and preventing the mid-cycle surge of secretion of these gonadotrophins. Consequently, ovulation is prevented and endogenous 17-β-oestradiol and progesterone secretion markedly reduced. However, the peripheral action of the steroid hormones is replaced by that of the synthetic analogues. The pattern of administration of these synthetic compounds is in a different sequence from that of the endogenous hormones so disrupting the finely tuned processes necessary for ovulation, fertilization and pregnancy. Reduction of the daily dose of oestrogen to less than 20 μg is likely to lead to breakthrough bleeding and smaller contraceptive efficacy due to failure to inhibit gonadotrophin secretion and suppress the endogenous cycle.

Drug interactions

Drugs that increase the MFO activity of the liver (see p. 442; e.g. **rifampicin** [rifampin], **phenytoin**, barbiturates) decrease the plasma concentrations of the steroid analogues and hence the effectiveness of the contraceptive preparation – recognized by breakthrough bleeding or later by pregnancy. Oral antibiotic agents that reduce the gut content of bacteria may also produce these effects by decreasing the enterohepatic circulation of the steroid analogues (Figure 7.9).

Therapeutic uses

Replacement therapy

In the treatment of menopausal symptoms and primary ovarian failure where there is deficient endogenous hormone secretion, the combination provides better cycle control than oestrogens alone and avoids continuous therapy. Oestradiol as an ester or conjugate is the preferred oral steroid.

Menstrual irregularities

In the treatment of dysmenorrhoea (painful menses) and dysfunctional uterine bleeding (abnormal menstrual pattern), the therapeutic aim is to impose regular drug-induced cycles by inhibiting the endogenous ovarian hormonal rhythm.

STAFFS UNIVERSITY LIBRARY

Contraception

Combined oral contraceptive preparations produce almost complete suppression of gonadal activity and therefore no ovulation. Other progestational effects contribute to the contraceptive action (see p. 168). Triphasic and biphasic formulations seek to mimic the pattern of hormone secretion during the menstrual cycle. Adverse effects can be alleviated by changing the dose and kind of oestrogen/progestogen content.

Postcoital contraception

The contraceptive action can occur up to 72 h after intercourse. Possible mechanisms are interference with sperm migration, increases in tubal transport of the ovum or prevention of implantation by asynchronous development of the endometrium. The incidence of acute unwanted effects is increased compared to that seen with conventional oral contraception, as a larger dose is necessary for effectiveness postcoitally.

Unwanted effects

Unwanted effects that show tolerance

Some unwanted effects tend to disappear after the first month of administration.

(1) Oestrogenic – nausea, vomiting, headache, weight gain, enlarged and tender breasts, decreased libido.
(2) Progestogenic – increased appetite, weight gain, decreased libido, depression, cramps, acne.

Less transient unwanted effects

Most of these effects arise because the dose of the administered steroids is greater than the replacement dose, and are similar to the changes that can occur in early pregnancy. The overall risk is less than that of pregnancy.

(1) Thromboembolic disorders. The mortality due to deep vein thrombosis is increased two times and that due to cerebral thrombosis is increased four times. These mortality increases are greater above 35 years of age and with longer medication and higher dose of the oestrogenic and possibly progestogenic component. Combined oral contraceptive preparations contain 50 µg or less of **ethinyloestradiol** or mestranol to reduce the incidence of thromboembolic disorders.
(2) Arterial diseases. Cerebrovascular and ischaemic heart disease is associated with the progestogenic component, which increases cholesterol and reduces high density lipoprotein concentrations in the serum. Their incidence is increased by two to six times, while that of hypertension is reversibly increased by approximately three times. The risk of dying from a vascular disease is greater with age, cigarette smoking, obesity and family history of hypertension. Desogestrel may

have smaller adverse effects on circulating lipid concentrations than the other 19-nortestosterone derivatives.

(3) Genitourinary tract infections. The incidence is increased by approximately 1.5 times, probably by increasing vaginal pH.

(4) Glucose tolerance is decreased but the incidence of diabetes mellitus is not increased.

(5) Thyroid function tests are impaired.

(6) Amenorrhoea may follow cessation of use; however, fertility is not significantly different from that in non-users 18 months after ceasing treatment.

(7) There is no association between usage and cancer, except cancer of the cervix, which is increased. This may be due to changes in pregnancy rate and sexual practices and not to the drugs.

Advantageous effects

Beneficial health effects can be demonstrated for dysmenorrhoea, menorrhagia, iron-deficiency anaemia, pelvic inflammatory disease, uterine fibroids, endometrial and ovarian cancer as well as benign breast disease.

Contraindications

Breast feeding, diabetes mellitus and migraine (not absolute), cardiovascular disease including hypertension and thromboembolism, liver disease, pregnancy, young oligomenorrhoeic girls, abnormal vaginal bleeding, hormone-dependent cancer, elective surgery and immobilization.

Androgens

Androgens are substances that cause masculinization (Table 4.6). Testosterone is the most important androgen and is secreted by the Leydig cells of the testis, and to a smaller extent, by the adrenal cortex of both sexes. Testosterone is converted to the more potent derivative 5-α-dihydrotestosterone in some target tissues of the body.

Preparations

Testosterone

Testosterone esters are given by i/m injection in oil. They are hydrolysed to the active drug testosterone. The dosage interval can be manipulated by administering a mixture of *testosterone esters* that are hydrolysed at different rates.

Mesterolone

Alkylation in position 1 results in oral activity and the lack of 17-α-alkylation in a low incidence of hepatotoxicity. *Mesterolone* is a weak androgen that has primarily peripheral actions.

Table 4.6 Some effects of androgens

System affected	Consequence
Reproductive organs	
Internal and external genitalia	Sexual differentiation in the fetus
	Growth and development
Spermatogenesis	Low concentrations stimulate
	High concentrations inhibit via negative
	feedback on gonadotrophin secretion
CNS	
LH secretion	Negative feedback
FSH secretion	Negative feedback in combination with
	the testicular factor inhibin
Fetal hypothalamus	Imprinting of male behavioural and acyclic
	control of gonadotrophin secretory patterns
Libido and aggression	Augmented in both sexes
Metabolic actions	
General	Marked net anabolic action (nitrogen retention)
Fluid mobilization	Salt and water retention
Other actions	
Long bone	Growth
Epiphyses	Closure
Muscle	Growth
Hair	Growth in male pattern. Paradoxically responsible
	for male pattern baldness
Skin	Thickening. Increased secretion from sebaceous
	glands (acne)
Vocal cords	Growth
Blood	Increased erythropoiesis
Liver	17-α-alkylated derivatives cause cholestatic jaundice

Anabolic steroids

Nandrolone is alkylated at the 17-α-position, which reduces the rate of metabolism. This results in oral activity but also some hepatotoxicity (cholestatic jaundice). Androgens have useful anabolic actions and nandrolone shows some separation between the anabolic and androgenic actions but its ratio of anabolic to androgenic potency is only two to three times that of testosterone, which militates against its use, particularly in women and children. Abuse of these drugs is common among athletes.

Therapeutic use

Replacement therapy

Androgens initiate or maintain the growth of the male secondary sexual characteristics, for example, after castration or gonadal failure with delayed puberty. *Mesterolone* is useful as it acts peripherally and does not decrease gonadotrophin secretion. Premature fusion of the epiphyses may occur in boys.

Treatment of infertility

Male infertility of endocrine cause is usually resistant to treatment. Spermatogenesis requires gonadotrophins plus androgens, while the latter usually suppress gonadotrophin secretion by negative feedback. In hypopituitarism fertility can be restored with *chorionic gonadotrophin* and FSH (as *urofollitrophin*), which stimulate both androgen production and spermatogenesis.

Advanced breast cancer

Androgens are sometimes used after recurrence of metastatic breast cancer. The action may be exerted via the negative feedback at the pituitary or directly upon the tissue. The adverse effects are virilization (growth of facial hair), hoarseness of voice and an increase in libido.

Stimulation of erythropoiesis

Large doses of the anabolic steroids are administered for at least 2 months in aplastic and refractory anaemias. The effectiveness is variable and unclear.

Antagonists at androgen receptors

Cyproterone competes with testosterone for the androgen receptor (see p. 151) and antagonizes androgens at all their specific target organs. It is also a very potent progestogen, so activating the negative feedback upon gonadotrophin secretion. **Finasteride** decreases androgen action by inhibiting the enzyme that converts testosterone to 5-α-dihydrotestosterone.

Therapeutic use

Cyproterone decreases sexual drive in sexual offenders but does not alter the direction of the desire. Severe hirsutism in women, due to excess adrenal androgen secretion, can be treated with **cyproterone**. Severe acne in women may be treated with an oral preparation of **ethinyloestradiol** and **cyproterone**. Prostate cancer also responds to this antagonist at androgen receptors. **Finasteride** is useful in benign prostatic disease.

Antispermatogenic effects of drugs

A number of drugs and chemicals modify spermatogenesis, although none are currently suitable for use as male contraceptive agents. Such compounds either inhibit spermatogenesis or modify the sperm such that fertilization does not ensue. There are two major mechanisms of drug action as follows.

STAFFS UNIVERSITY LIBRARY

Direct action on sperm cells

Many alkylating agents and antimetabolites when used in cancer chemotherapy (see p. 322) inhibit spermatogenesis at specific stages leading to infertility. The time from commencement of drug administration to sterility is dependent on the stage of spermatogenesis affected. For example, *busulphan* selectively kills spermatogonia. The stages from spermatocytes onward continue at the normal rate and therefore sterility does not occur for upwards of 14 weeks. Irreversible ablation of spermatogenesis often occurs after **cyclophosphamide** and *procarbazine*. The ovary is also affected. Infertility is a particular problem after the successful treatment of young people for Hodgkin's disease or children for acute lymphoblastic leukaemia. The effects of these drugs are related to widespread inhibition of cell proliferation. The mechanism producing reversible infertility during treatment of inflammatory bowel disease with *sulphasalazine* is unknown.

Indirect action via suppression of secretion of gonadotrophins

As the gonadotrophins are necessary for spermatogenesis, any drug that suppresses their secretion sufficiently and for a prolonged period eventually produces sterility. Therefore oestrogens, progestogens and androgens can all produce sterility via their negative feedback actions at the hypothalamus or anterior pituitary gland. The time to the onset of sterility is usually at least 14 weeks. Most endocrine drugs do not affect the stem cells within the seminiferous tubules, so that fertility usually returns after cessation of drug treatment. This may take several months.

Summary

(1)   Steroid hormones have a short biological $t_{1/2}$. Therapeutic effects are achieved by formulation (e.g. oestradiol skin patches) or chemical modification. Esterification (e.g. *medroxyprogesterone acetate*) effectively forms a biological depot. Alkylation (e.g. levonorgestrel) confers protection from metabolism and oral activity.

(2)   Oestrogens maintain the secondary sexual characteristics of women after the menopause or in ovarian failure.

(3)   **Ethinyloestradiol** is the most widely used oestrogen. *Stilboestrol* is a potent non-steroidal oestrogen reserved for topical use, or the treatment of breast or prostate cancer. Oestrogens are not usually used alone.

(4)   Progestogens only act after their receptor has been synthesized by oestrogen stimulation. They contribute towards the development of secondary sexual characteristics.

(5)   Levonorgestrel is the most widely used oral progestogen. *Medroxyprogesterone acetate* must be injected. Unwanted effects arise from cross-reaction with other steroid hormone receptors by the parent molecule or its metabolites. Their most widespread use is

as a component of combined oral contraceptive preparations, or alone as oral or parenteral progestogen-only contraceptives.

(6) Combinations of oestrogen and progestogen (e.g. for contraception) are more efficacious and possess fewer unwanted effects than either used alone. The contraceptive action of the combined oral therapy is primarily established via negative feedback, reducing gonadotrophin secretion so that ovulation cannot take place.

(7) Relatively common and often transient unwanted effects of the combined oral contraceptive preparations include nausea, weight gain, breast tenderness, mood changes and acne. Rare life-threatening adverse effects are thromboembolic disorders (oestrogenic), cerebral haemorrhage and ischaemic heart disease (progestogenic). Beneficial effects can also be demonstrated (e.g. reduction in the incidences of anaemia and ovarian cancer).

(8) The efficacy of the contraceptive steroids is reduced by drugs that promote their clearance by either increasing metabolism by the MFOs or promoting faecal excretion by reducing enterohepatic circulation.

(9) *Mesterolone* is a weak orally active androgen; male secondary sexual characteristics are usually maintained with injections of *testosterone esters*. Anabolic steroids (e.g. nandrolone) are weak androgens widely abused in sport.

(10) Non-steroidal competitive antagonists at steroid hormone receptors include **tamoxifen**, an antagonist at oestrogen receptors used for breast cancer, **mifepristone**, an antagonist at progestogen receptors used for termination of pregnancy and **cyproterone**, an antagonist at androgen receptors used in acne.

The thyroid gland and drugs used in thyroid abnormalities

The function of the thyroid gland is the synthesis, storage and release of the thyroid hormones L-thyroxine (T_4) and L-tri-iodothyronine (T_3).

Synthesis and release

Dietary iodine is converted to I^- and absorbed from the alimentary canal. The thyroid concentrates I^- 20–200 times with respect to the plasma concentration by active transport (the I^- pump) involving a cAMP-dependent Na^+/I^- co-transport system, from the blood to the thyroid follicular cells and, ultimately, by diffusion, to the colloid-containing lumen of the follicle. At the apical surface of the follicular cell the I^- is converted to an active iodinating species by the action of a haem-containing thyroid peroxidase that requires H_2O_2. The iodinating species appears not to be iodine itself but an intermediary, which (probably as free radicals) reacts with tyrosine residues within the thyroglobulin (a complex glycoprotein present in the luminal colloid of the thyroid follicle) to yield mono-iodotyrosine (MIT) and di-iodotyrosine (DIT). These compounds have respectively one or two molecules of iodine attached to the benzene ring of tyrosine. Two molecules of DIT undergo condensation, with the elimination of alanine, to form T_4. Some T_3 is similarly formed from the condensation of MIT and DIT. The condensation reactions are oxidative and utilize thyroid peroxidase as a catalyst. In normal circumstances more T_4 than T_3 is produced but when iodine is deficient the ratio may be reduced. At this stage MIT, DIT, T_3 and T_4 are in peptide linkage to the thyroglobulin. Release involves the proteolytic breakdown of the peptide bonds between iodinated compounds and thyroglobulin. T_4 and T_3 pass out of the thyroid cells into the circulation. MIT and DIT are de-iodinated by microsomal iodotyrosine de-iodinase to I^- and tyrosine, which are reused in synthesis. Ninety-nine per cent of the plasma thyroid hormones are protein bound, particularly to an α-globulin called thyroxine binding globulin. Ninety per cent of the circulating hormone is T_4, the remainder is T_3. T_4 is slowly eliminated from the body ($t_{1/2}$ 6–7 days), whereas the $t_{1/2}$ of T_3 is 2 days. Both compounds are conjugated in the liver with glucuronic and sulphuric acids. There is an enterohepatic circulation of the hormones.

In peripheral tissues, T_4 is converted to T_3, which is approximately four times as active as T_4. The rate of this conversion in each tissue is therefore a determinant of its biological response to thyroid hormone.

Control of synthesis and release

This involves the hypothalamus and anterior pituitary gland (see p. 155). TSH stimulates all stages of synthesis (but especially I^- uptake) and release of the thyroid hormones. Most of the actions of TSH are dependent upon cAMP as an intracellular second messenger. A negative feedback system exists such that increased concentration of free thyroid hormone in the blood reduces the output of TSH from the anterior pituitary gland.

Effects of thyroid hormone

In general, thyroid hormones increase the O_2 consumption of most metabolically active tissues (exceptions: brain, testes, uterus, spleen and anterior pituitary gland). They stimulate lipid catabolism, protein synthesis and intestinal carbohydrate absorption. These actions are believed to be exerted through interaction with both membrane and nuclear receptors (see p. 152). The effect on body systems can best be illustrated by comparison between the hypothyroid and hyperthyroid states (Table 4.7).

Use of thyroid hormone

Thyroxine sodium and *liothyronine sodium* are only used as replacement therapy to treat hypothyroid states (adult myxoedema, childhood

Table 4.7 Comparison of hypothyroid and hyperthyroid states

Effect	Hypothyroid state	Hyperthyroid state
Body weight	Gain	Loss
Oxygen consumption	Decreased	Increased
Heat production	Decreased	Increased
Basal metabolic rate	Decreased	Increased
CNS	Impaired mentality Poor memory and concentration Drowsiness	Excitability, restlessness apprehension, insomnia
Somatic motor nervous system	Decreased activity	Increased activity
Sympathetic nervous system	Decreased activity	Increased activity
Cardiovascular system	Bradycardia, reduced cardiac output and BP	Tachycardia, increased cardiac output and BP
Gastrointestinal tract	Activity diminished, constipation	Activity increased, diarrhoea
Sensitivity to catecholamines	Decreased	Increased

cretinism). *Thyroxine sodium* is normally the drug of choice for maintenance therapy but *liothyronine sodium* may be preferred when a rapid onset of action (hypothyroid coma) or shorter duration of action (hypothyroidism with ischaemic heart disease) is required.

Thyroid hormones may enhance the effects of the oral anticoagulant agents, although the mechanism of the interaction is not clear. The hormones can be shown to inhibit the metabolism of anticoagulant agents, and to displace them from protein binding sites, but this is probably not the case with therapeutic plasma concentrations and other mechanisms are likely to be involved.

Thyrotoxicosis

In hyperthyroidism (thyrotoxicosis) there is an excess of circulating thyroid hormones. This may be due to:

(1) A diffusely enlarged gland producing excess hormone – this is Graves' disease, which is associated with auto-antibodies directed against TSH receptors on the thyroid follicular cells. Unlike TSH, the synthesis of these thyroid-stimulating antibodies is not subject to feedback control by thyroid hormones.
(2) A multinodular goitre.
(3) Stimulation of the thyroid by excess TSH from a tumour of the pituitary thyrotroph cells (not subject to feedback control).
(4) An autonomously functioning nodule (toxic adenoma).

Drugs used in thyrotoxicosis

Thioamide derivatives

Carbimazole and *propylthiouracil* prevent both the iodination of the tyrosine residues and also the condensation reaction between the mono- and di-iodotyrosines; this latter occurs at a concentration smaller than that needed to inhibit the iodination. As both stages of the synthesis involve tyrosine peroxidase and a reactive oxidation derivative of iodine, it seems likely that the thioamide compounds interfere with the action of the peroxidase enzyme or interact with the intermediate itself. *Propylthiouracil* also prevents the peripheral metabolism of T_4 to the more active T_3. The drugs are well absorbed from the intestine and widely distributed in tissues. Response to treatment takes several weeks, with the euthyroid state produced in 1–2 months. To avoid relapse treatment should be prolonged (1.5–2 years), even then relapse is common; it occurs in up to 50%, and in many within 3 months of stopping treatment. Thioamides may also be used before thyroid surgery and to hasten euthy- roidism after radiation therapy. Unwanted effects include skin rashes, lymphadenopathy and fever (3–5% of patients treated) and agranulocy- tosis (0.5%). If the dosage is too high and a hypothyroid state is produced, enlargement of the gland (goitre) may result, with TSH being released from the anterior pituitary gland in response to the low circulating concen- trations of thyroid hormones and stimulating the gland causing hyperpla- sia. *Propylthiouracil* is useful when rashes develop to **carbimazole** as there is not usually cross-sensitivity. When used during pregnancy or lactation, there is a danger of neonatal goitre and hypothyroidism as the drugs can enter the fetus from the placenta and the newborn from the milk.

Monovalent ions

The daily intake of iodide (I^-), in amounts considerably above the normal requirement of 100–200 µg, is able to control hyperthyroidism. The mecha- nism of action is unclear but I^- promotes involution of the hypertrophied tissue with an increased colloid storage and a decreased release of thyroid hormones. A possible explanation for this action (autoregulation) is that I^- reduces the stimulation by TSH on cAMP synthesis in thyroid cells. The effects are rapid in onset (10–15 days for maximal effect) but not sustained. I^- is useful before surgery to prepare the gland for subtotal thyroidectomy, but only after prior treatment with antithyroid drugs, and together with other antithyroid drugs and supportive measures in thyro- toxic crisis. It is prescribed as *iodine aqueous solution*. Unwanted effects include hypersensitivity reactions and painful salivary glands.

Radioactive iodide

Radioactive I^- (given as sodium iodide) is treated exactly as unlabelled iodide by the body and is rapidly and efficiently trapped by the thyroid gland, incorporated into the iodoamino acids and deposited into the colloid of the follicles. ^{131}I ($t_{1/2}$ 8 days; emits β-particles and γ-rays) is the radioac- tive isotope of iodine normally used in the treatment of hyperthyroidism.

The dose needed is large compared with that used in diagnostic tests. The radioactive iodine is deposited in the colloid of the follicles from where the destructive β-particles originate. The average depth of penetration of the particles is 0.5 mm, which means that radiation damage occurs to the parenchymal cells lining the follicles of the thyroid gland with little or no damage to surrounding tissue. The response is slow (this is overcome by administering antithyroid drugs after dosing) and there is a high incidence of myxoedema (up to 50% of cases in 8 years after dosing) due to the difficulty in estimating the effective dose. There is a late increase in the incidence of thyroid cancer. Radioactive isotopes are also used in the testing of thyroid function (see below).

Antagonists at β-adrenoceptors

Propranolol (see p. 100) and other antagonists at β-adrenoceptors reduce many of the signs and symptoms of thyrotoxicosis, including nervousness, atrial fibrillation and increased myocardial contractility and cardiac output. There is no effect on basal metabolic rate or I^- utilization. **Propranolol** is valuable before thyroidectomy, after irradiation and in thyrotoxic crisis (in conjunction with antithyroid drugs and supportive measures). As sole treatment for thyrotoxicosis the success rate differs little from the spontaneous remission rate, and the patient remains biochemically hyperthyroid throughout the treatment.

Testing of the hypothalamic-pituitary-thyroid system

TRH stimulation test

Protirelin (TRH) is used as a diagnostic aid because of its ability to stimulate the anterior pituitary gland and increase the output of TSH (see p. 156). A patient with normal thyroid function responds to an i/v injection of *protirelin* with an increased output of TSH (and consequential increased plasma concentrations of T_3 and T_4). In thyrotoxicosis this increased output is prevented by the negative feedback exerted by the increased concentrations of thyroid hormones. TSH concentrations may also fail to increase in hypothyroidism due to pituitary failure.

Radioactive iodide uptake test

The percentage of an administered dose of radioactive sodium iodide (^{131}I) absorbed by the thyroid at set time intervals is determined. The pattern of uptake distinguishes thyroiditis from the common causes of hyperthyroidism.

Summary

(1) Drug use in hypothyroidism: *thyroxine sodium* (T_4) is normally used for maintenance therapy; *liothyronine sodium* (T_3) is used when a rapid onset and short duration of response is required.

STAFFS UNIVERSITY LIBRARY

(2) Drug use in hyperthyroidism: thioamides (e.g. **carbimazole**) reduce synthesis of thyroid hormones by preventing iodination and condensation of tyrosine residues; cause rashes and pruritus and, rarely, agranulocytosis.
(3) Iodine, in high doses: produces a rapid, but not sustained, reduction in release of thyroid hormones; is used prior to surgery and in thyrotoxic crisis.
(4) Radioactive iodine (^{131}I) as sodium iodide: deposits in the colloid and emits β-particles that damage follicular cells; frequently produces hypothyroidism.
(5) Antagonists at β-adrenoceptors: reduce many signs and symptoms whilst leaving the patient biochemically hyperthyroid; are used prior to surgery, after irradiation and in thyrotoxic crisis.

The adrenal cortex and the corticosteroids

The function of the adrenal cortex is the synthesis and release of the adrenal corticosteroids hydrocortisone [cortisol], corticosterone and aldosterone (minor amounts of 11-deoxycorticosterone and androgens are also produced).

Synthesis is from cholesterol (Figure 4.5).

Control of synthesis and release

The rate of release of adrenocortical hormones is virtually identical to the rate of synthesis as the hormones are not stored. The role of the hypothalamus and anterior pituitary gland in the synthesis and release of adrenocortical hormones is discussed on page 156. ACTH stimulates the production of hydrocortisone by increasing activity of the enzyme, cholesterol esterase, that regulates the conversion of cholesterol to pregnenolone. ACTH release is under hypothalamic control mediated by corticotrophin releasing hormone, which is secreted into the hypophyseal portal venous circulation.

A negative feedback system operates, with increased plasma concentration of free hydrocortisone reducing release of corticotrophin releasing hormone and ACTH. A circadian rhythm exists in hydrocortisone production, output being maximal shortly after awakening. In the plasma, hydrocortisone is largely protein bound to a high-affinity α_2-globulin (transcortin). Metabolism occurs in the liver, giving water-soluble metabolites with little or no activity that are excreted by the kidney. Approximately 0.5% of hydrocortisone is excreted unchanged in the urine. This is of clinical significance as urinary free hydrocortisone reflects plasma free hydrocortisone and can be used to assess adrenal cortical hyperactivity.

Aldosterone synthesis and release is under the control of the renin-angiotensin mechanism (see p. 195). Renin is released from the juxtaglomerular apparatus in the kidney in response to a reduction in blood volume, renal perfusion pressure or Na^+ concentration in the distal tubule. Both the action of the released angiotensin II in the constriction of the glomerular efferent arteriole and aldosterone in the promotion of Na^+ retention offset the stimulus for further renin release.

Effects of the adrenal corticosteroids

The adrenal cortex functions as an organ of homeostasis, enabling the body to maintain a constant internal environment in response to changing environmental demands. The adrenal corticosteroids exert a number of actions on all aspects of metabolism, resulting in effects classed as mineralocorticoid and glucocorticoid.

Mineralocorticoid effects are:

- electrolyte balance – increased Na^+ retention and K^+ loss by the kidney.

Glucocorticoid effects are:

- peripheral amino acid mobilization;
- decreased glucose uptake and increased gluconeogenesis;
- mobilization of fatty acids from adipose tissue.

These effects are believed to be exerted by interaction of the steroids with specific steroid hormone receptors (see p. 15).

Suprahysiological doses of steroids with glucocorticoid activity reduce immune and inflammatory responses. The effect on the immune response is in part the result of decreased release of interleukin 2 (IL-2) by T-cells in response to antigenic stimuli. The anti-inflammatory action reduces manifestations of the inflammatory response, both macroscopic (warmth, redness, swelling, pain) and microscopic (leucocyte accumulation and activation of mononuclear cells), regardless of the cause. This involves the stimulation of synthesis and release by leucocytes of a protein, lipocortin, that inhibits phospholipase A_2 activity. This inhibition reduces the synthesis of the products of the arachidonic acid pathway, prostaglandins (PGs) and leukotrienes (LTs), that are involved in the causation of inflammatory responses (see p. 212). There is also a decreased production or release of other mediators, including histamine, IL-1 and other cytokines. Associated with these functions is a reduction in lymphoid tissue mass. These actions on immune and inflammatory responses are classed as glucocorticoid.

Aldosterone exerts exclusively mineralocorticoid effects, hydrocortisone exerts mainly glucocorticoid activity but large doses also influence electrolyte balance.

The use of ACTH

Preparations

ACTH is a 39-amino acid polypeptide chain in which the first 24 amino acids are common to all species and are essential for the physiological activity. The remaining 15 amino acids are species specific, not essential for activity and confer specific antigenicity.

Tetracosactrin is a synthetic analogue consisting of the adrenocorticotrophic component of ACTH, that is, the first 24 amino acids. It has a short plasma $t_{1/2}$, but a formulation with zinc gives a depot preparation and a longer duration of action.

Uses

Tetracosactrin is used diagnostically to determine whether adrenal insufficiency is due to pituitary or adrenal gland failure. This test assesses adrenal cortex reserve. Blood for assay of hydrocortisone is collected at standard times in relation to an injection of a standard dose of a short-acting preparation. In the normal individual a significant increment and peak value is seen. In adrenal insufficiency both increment and peak value are smaller.

The main problem with the use of polypeptides is the necessity for parenteral administration to avoid proteolytic destruction of the polypeptide structure. Hypersensitivity reactions occur only infrequently with *tetracosactrin*.

The use of adrenal corticosteroids

Corticosteroids are useful for replacement therapy or in non-endocrinological diseases for their other (particularly anti-inflammatory) actions.

Preparations

Modification of the structures of the adrenal corticosteroid hormones has produced analogues that have the following properties:

(1) Mainly glucocorticoid activity but with some significant mineralocorticoid activity, **prednisolone**.
(2) Glucocorticoid activity with no significant mineralocorticoid activity, *beclomethasone, betamethasone, dexamethasone, fluocinolone*.
(3) Mineralocorticoid activity with no significant glucocorticoid activity, **fludrocortisone**.

It has not yet proved possible to produce compounds showing anti-inflammatory activity without the other glucocorticoid actions.

Alteration in structure also changes plasma $t_{1/2}$ by influencing protein binding and metabolism. Hydrocortisone has a very short $t_{1/2}$ of approximately 2 h, synthetic glucocorticosteroids can be classified as intermediate acting (biological $t_{1/2}$ 12–36 h, e.g. **prednisolone**) or longer acting (biological $t_{1/2}$ 36–72 h, e.g. *dexamethasone*).

Replacement therapy

There is little risk of side-effects when adrenal corticosteroids are used for replacement therapy, as plasma concentrations are in the physiological range. The kind of analogue (mineralocorticosteroid or glucocorticosteroid) that is appropriate depends on the condition treated. Acute adrenal failure usually requires only a glucocorticosteroid (*hydrocortisone sodium succinate* given i/v), together with measures to correct fluid and electrolyte imbalance. Chronic adrenal insufficiency requires both glucocorticosteroid (*hydrocortisone*) and mineralocorticosteroid (**fludrocortisone**) replacement. In anterior pituitary gland failure a glucocorticosteroid alone is sufficient, as ACTH does not regulate aldosterone secretion. In congenital adrenal hyperplasia, abnormalities in the synthetic pathway for steroid hormones lead to deficient glucocorticosteroid secretion, increased ACTH secretion and androgen production as the precursors are diverted from the non-functioning to the functioning pathways. Potent and longer-acting compounds (*dexamethasone*) are preferred in this instance, as they have to replace deficient steroid hormones and suppress ACTH secretion in order to reduce androgen production. Mineralocorticosteroid replacement may be necessary depending on the nature of the defect in the synthetic pathway.

Treatment of non-endocrinological disorders

The corticosteroids are used for their effects on immune and inflammatory responses. Analogues with high glucocorticoid and low mineralocorticoid activity (e.g. **prednisolone**) are used.

Among conditions treated with glucocorticosteroids are those in which tissue inflammation and autoimmunity play a part (asthma, see p. 487, allergic rhinitis and conjunctivitis, eczema, systemic lupus erythematosus). Topical application of glucocorticosteroids can be useful in reducing inflammation in skin (see p. 545) and eye diseases. However, care should be taken to avoid their use in infective situations such as herpes simplex. Glucocorticosteroids can be used for their ability to cause involution of lymphoid tissue in achieving temporary remission in leukaemia (see p. 325) and prevent transplant rejection. In all these situations glucocorticosteroids themselves are not curative.

Treatment with glucocorticosteroids presents two main risks:

(1) Abrupt withdrawal after prolonged high dosage may result in life-threatening acute adrenal insufficiency due to suppression of ACTH secretion and atrophy of the gland. When treatment is discontinued the dose should be reduced gradually over several weeks or months. However a glucocorticosteroid given for periods less than 7 days, as in acute severe asthma, can be withdrawn rapidly with little danger. Alternate-day therapy and the use of minimal effective doses can be used to prevent suppression of the hypothalamopituitary-adrenal axis. High doses, especially those larger than 7.5 mg daily, can cause hypothalamopituitary-adrenal axis suppression. Attempts to reduce the dose often results in disease relapse.

(2) Prolonged treatment in supraphysiological doses always carries risks, which must be weighed against benefits in serious disabling illness. Many of these unwanted effects are clearly extensions of the physiological actions and include hyperglycaemia, salt and water retention, increased susceptibility to infection, muscle wasting, osteoporosis and

a state resembling Cushing's syndrome. Disruption of the local gastric defence against the acid environment may predispose to peptic ulceration. Other adverse reactions include cataract, euphoria, psychosis and increased intraocular pressure. This latter is genetically determined in patients with a predisposition to open-angle glaucoma and occurs more readily to topical treatment.

Non-systemic application or administration of glucocorticosteroids does not necessarily protect against these two risks – liberal application of the older, more potent compounds in the treatment of various skin problems was associated with suppression of the hypothalamopituitary-adrenal axis (sparing application of less potent compounds is now employed). More recently, asthma therapy with inhaled glucocorticosteroids has been implicated in the development of cataracts. In both these situations there is sufficient absorption from the site of application to produce a significant systemic drug concentration.

Interference with synthesis or action of the adrenal corticosteroids

Metyrapone decreases the synthesis of hydrocortisone, corticosterone and, to a lesser extent, aldosterone by inhibiting the enzyme (11β-hydroxylase) that catalyses the final step in their production. It can be used to test pituitary gland function and in the treatment of ectopic ACTH secretion and malignant adrenal tumours to reduce the output of these steroids.

Aminoglutethimide, which inhibits conversion of cholesterol to pregnenolone, can also be used to treat such tumours. The ability of *aminoglutethimide* to inhibit the conversion of androgens to oestrogens in peripheral tissues leads to its use in the treatment of breast cancer in postmenopausal women. Concurrent glucocorticosteroid replacement therapy (e.g. *dexamethasone*) is required.

Spironolactone acts as an antagonist of aldosterone and is a potassium-sparing diuretic (see p. 138).

Dynamic testing of the hypothalamic-pituitary-adrenal system

Dexamethasone suppression tests

These are used to diagnose and establish the cause of Cushing's syndrome. *Dexamethasone* suppresses the secretion of corticotrophin releasing hormone (and thus of ACTH and of hydrocortisone, which is assayed) by acting on the hypothalamus. A low dose of *dexamethasone* decreases the concentration of hydrocortisone in plasma in most normal patients; a maintained high concentration of hydrocortisone in plasma is suggestive of Cushing's syndrome. A high dose of *dexamethasone* then produces suppression in Cushing's syndrome of pituitary origin

(Cushing's disease), but not when it is due to an adrenal neoplasm or an ectopic source of ACTH.

Insulin tolerance test

Hypoglycaemia induced by insulin usually stimulates the secretion of corticotrophin releasing hormone (and thus ACTH and hydrocortisone, which is assayed) by acting on the hypothalamus. Failure of the concentration of hydrocortisone in plasma to increase indicates Cushing's syndrome or anterior pituitary or adrenocortical insufficiency.

Tetracosactrin tests

These are used to aid the diagnosis and establish the cause of adrenocortical insufficiency. *Tetracosactrin* stimulates the secretion of hydrocortisone (which is assayed) by acting on the adrenal cortex. *Tetracosactrin* injection produces a marked increase in the concentration of hydrocortisone in plasma in normal patients; failure to increase denotes adrenocortical insufficiency. Injection of a depot formulation produces an increase in the concentration of hydrocortisone in plasma that is delayed but usually normal in size in adrenal insufficiency of pituitary origin (or following long-term glucocorticosteroid treatment). A small response indicates primary adrenocortical insufficiency (Addison's disease).

Metyrapone test

Metyrapone blocks the synthesis of hydrocortisone and so causes a reduction in the concentration of hydrocortisone in plasma. This reduction stimulates the secretion of corticotrophin releasing hormone (and thus of ACTH, which stimulates the adrenal cortex to liberate precursors of adrenocorticosteroids and their metabolites, which are assayed). A large response indicates Cushing's syndrome of pituitary origin. A small one occurs in Cushing's syndrome due to ectopic ACTH, or in anterior pituitary or adrenocortical insufficiency.

Summary

(1) Adrenal corticosteroids, natural and synthetic, are used in replacement therapy or in non-endocrinological diseases.
(2) Replacement therapy: may require a glucocorticosteroid (*hydrocortisone, dexamethasone*) alone, or in combination with a mineralocorticosteroid (*fludrocortisone*); has little risk of unwanted effects.
(3) Treatment of non-endocrinological diseases: utilizes the effects on immune and inflammatory responses; is not curative; involves compounds with mixed (**prednisolone**) or glucocorticoid (*betamethasone*) activity; involves high risk of serious unwanted effects, from the high plasma concentrations; may suppress the pituitary-adrenal axis and result in adrenal failure if high-dose prolonged therapy is discontinued abruptly.

Drugs in diabetes mellitus

Insulin

Occurrence

Insulin is a hormone secreted by the β-cells of the islets of Langerhans in the pancreas. Islet cells comprise 1–3% of pancreatic cell mass and number 100 000–2 500 000. Islets also contain α-cells that secrete glucagon, δ-cells that secrete somatostatin and PP cells that secrete pancreatic polypeptide.

Biosynthesis

Insulin is synthesized in the rough endoplasmic reticulum as prepro-insulin, a large precursor molecule. This is almost immediately split to form pro-insulin, which is stored in the Golgi apparatus in small granules. The connecting or C peptide is also stored in these granules. The insulin molecule consists of two chains of amino acids: A with 21 amino acids and B with 30 amino acids (Figure 4.8). The insulins of different species are remarkably similar, with human and porcine insulins differing only at the

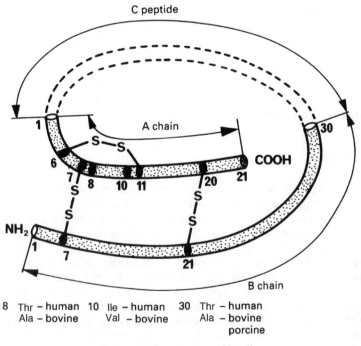

8	Thr – human	10	Ile – human	30	Thr – human
	Ala – bovine		Val – bovine		Ala – bovine
					porcine

Figure 4.8 The structure of insulin

B30 position and human and beef insulins differing at the A8, A9 and B30 positions. The granules of insulin and C peptide are transported via the microtubular system to the cell surface where they are extruded by reverse pinocytosis.

Release

A number of different agents, including glucose, amino acids and gut hormones, act as insulin secretagogues. Glucagon stimulates the release of insulin, somatostatin inhibits it. Neural regulation mechanisms also exist, with sympatho-adrenal activity inhibiting and parasympathetic activity stimulating insulin release. Insulin is secreted in anticipation of ingestion of food in the cephalic phase of insulin secretion, which is thought to be mediated by the vagus nerve. After ingestion of food two further stages of release occur. The first is rapid and is due to release of preformed insulin from granules, the second involves the release of newly formed insulin. Insulin is secreted into the portal vein and is extensively metabolized in the liver and kidneys and has a short $t_{1/2}$ (4–5 min). This may therefore be prolonged in patients lacking substantial amounts of renal tissue.

Mechanism of action

Insulin binds to a specific receptor situated in the cytoplasmic membranes of fat, muscle, liver and brain cells. The receptor is intimately linked with the enzyme tyrosine kinase on its cytoplasmic side. Insulin binding causes a change in the conformation of the receptor–enzyme complex that activates the enzyme to phosphorylate itself. The phosphorylated tyrosine kinase in turn activates other enzymes that modify cellular synthetic processes. Thus insulin facilitates entry of glucose into muscle and adipose tissue while inhibiting glycogenolysis and gluconeogenesis in the liver. In general it promotes anabolic and inhibits catabolic processes.

The insulin receptor concentration is regulated in the long term by prevailing insulin concentrations and can be reduced in hyperinsulinaemic states, as occurs in obesity.

Diabetes mellitus

Diabetes mellitus is a clinical syndrome, characterized by hyperglycaemia due to an absolute or relative deficiency of insulin. On the basis of aetiology, two major categories have been described:

(1) Insulin-dependent diabetes mellitus (IDDM).
(2) Non-insulin-dependent diabetes mellitus (NIDDM).

Table 4.8 compares the typical features of these two categories.

Treatment

Insulin treatment has remained the mainstay of treatment of IDDM patients over the last 60 years, while patients with NIDDM may be treated

STAFFS UNIVERSITY LIBRARY

Table 4.8 Comparison of insulin-dependent and non-insulin-dependent diabetes mellitus

Typical features	Insulin-dependent diabetes mellitus	Non-insulin-dependent diabetes mellitus
Age at onset	Younger, from 2 years	Older, from 25 years
Prevalence	0.2%	1%
Plasma insulin concentration	Very low or absent	Normal or reduced (delayed secretion to glucose stimulus)
β-Cell function	Very low or absent	Normal or reduced
Ketosis	Yes (if treatment delayed)	No
Treatment	Insulin	Diet ± oral hypoglycaemic agents
Others	Insulin responsive	Tendency to insulin resistance

with dietary control alone or in combination with oral hypoglycaemic agents or insulin. The role of insulin therapy in NIDDM is not clear and studies are in progress to assess this.

Insulin formulations

Insulin formulations can be classified in terms of duration of action (Table 4.9), source or purity. For clinical use, insulin has been formulated for short, intermediate or long duration of action. *Soluble insulin* consists of insulin in simple solution that is rapidly absorbed when injected. Insulin zinc suspensions can be prepared, as insulin is relatively insoluble in a zinc acetate buffer. *Amorphous insulin zinc suspension* has small particles and is absorbed more slowly than *soluble insulin*. *Crystalline insulin zinc suspension*, with larger particle size, is absorbed more slowly still and has a prolonged duration of action lasting up to 24 h. *Insulin zinc suspension* is a mixture of 30% amorphous and 70% crystalline insulin zinc suspensions.

Isophane insulin (a suspension of insulin with protamine) is another formulation from which insulin is released slowly. *Biphasic isophane insulin* is available containing both soluble and isophane insulins.

Purity and source of insulin

The duration of action of an insulin formulation can also vary with the purity and source of insulin. The highly purified insulins have a much

Table 4.9 Formulation and duration of action of insulins

Insulin	Time of onset (h)	Duration of effect
Soluble insulin	1/2–1	Short (4–6 h)
Isophane insulin	2	Intermediate (12 h)
Insulin zinc suspension (amorphous)	1–2	Intermediate
Insulin zinc suspension (mixed)	2–7	Intermediate
Insulin zinc suspension (crystalline)	4–7	Long (24–30 h)

shorter duration of action than the older insulins, which had a high content of antigenic contaminants (pro-insulin, pancreatic polypeptide, somatostatin). Similarly, human insulins have a more rapid onset and shorter duration of action than porcine or bovine insulins. These differences may be explained in part by the reduced formation of antibodies to the insulin.

Human insulin is produced by enzymatic modification of animal insulins or by using recombinant DNA techniques to induce *Escherichia coli* to synthesize human sequence insulin. Some patients have reported changes in the symptoms that warn of impending hypoglycaemia after transfer to human insulin. This may be explained by the smaller antibody binding to human insulin, which leads to rapid onset of action with rapid reduction in blood glucose concentration. In such instances, the release of the counter-regulatory hormones (e.g. catecholamines) that produce the warning symptoms may not be sufficiently rapid. Controversy exists as to whether human insulins can cause sudden death by this mechanism. The vast majority of patients treated with human insulin experience no problems and those who do can be changed back to treatment with animal insulins.

Administration of insulin

Insulin is commonly administered as a s/c injection using a disposable plastic syringe. However, increasing numbers of patients are now using pen devices instead of syringes. These devices resemble a fountain pen and contain cartridges of insulin. Visually handicapped patients may be helped by syringes that draw up a fixed dose or ones that give an audible click at each mark on the syringe, enabling them to do a click count and vary the dose. Insulin may be delivered intraperitoneally in patients on continuous peritoneal dialysis. This method of insulin delivery is more physiological; insulin is absorbed into the portal circulation rather than the systemic circulation (as occurs with s/c injection) and patients often find that control is easier. Continuous s/c infusion of insulin by syringe pump is possible but a significant number of patients using such pumps develop ketoacidosis, electrolyte disturbances and infections.

Insulin regimens

In non-diabetic individuals, insulin is secreted at two rates, a basal rate in the fasting state and an accelerated rate in response to a meal. The aim of insulin replacement therapy is to mimic this as closely as possible. It is possible to achieve this using computerized glucose sensor/insulin delivery systems. However, these are used in research but are not yet suitable for routine use. A twice-daily injection of a combination of short- and intermediate-acting insulins is commonly used. The intermediate-acting component mimics the basal insulin secretion, while the short-acting component mimics the response to a meal. A near physiological pattern can also be achieved by using a single long-acting injection with short-acting insulin before each meal. The latter regimen is preferred by many younger patients, as it permits a greater flexibility in lifestyle.

In elderly patients and those whose compliance is suboptimal, a single daily injection of long-acting insulin may be adequate to reduce or suppress symptoms.

Oral hypoglycaemic agents

The mainstay of treatment of NIDDM is weight reduction, diet and exercise. All NIDDM patients should have an adequate trial of these methods before drug treatment is considered. An appreciable proportion of NIDDM patients fail to achieve adequate control by these methods and oral hypoglycaemic agents are then indicated.

Sulphonylureas

These drugs require the presence of functioning β-cells in the pancreas for their action. They act in part by stimulating the release of insulin in response to a glucose load. They bind to a sulphonylurea receptor on the β-cell, an action that results in the closure of membrane ATP-sensitive K^+-channels. The resultant depolarization and Ca^{2+} influx through voltage-sensitive Ca^{2+} channels triggers insulin release. The sulphonylureas also enhance the effect of insulin on the liver and promote peripheral glucose utilization by increasing the number of insulin receptors. The net result is an improvement in glucose tolerance. Sulphonylurea drugs are indicated in patients at or near ideal body weight, when diet and weight reduction alone are insufficient to produce satisfactory control of blood glucose. They are best avoided in overweight patients because sulphonylureas encourage weight gain. Data on the safety of sulphonylurea drugs in pregnancy are not sufficient and they are best avoided in females in the reproductive years.

The pharmacokinetic profiles of some sulphonylurea drugs are shown in Table 4.10. These properties must be considered when selecting a drug for an individual patient. In the presence of impaired renal function, or if such impairment is likely as in the elderly, drugs with a long $t_{1/2}$ (*chlorpropamide*) and drugs excreted mainly by renal mechanisms (*glibenclamide*) are best avoided. Drugs excreted by hepatic pathways (**tolbutamide**, *gliclazide*) are less likely to cause dose-related hypoglycaemia in these patients.

The principal adverse effect is hypoglycaemia. (Fatal hypoglycaemic episodes have occurred in elderly patients taking *chlorpropamide* or *glibenclamide*.) All patients must be advised of this danger, and carry sugar or sweets to take when a warning is felt. Other unwanted effects (gastrointestinal irritation, nausea, skin rashes, rarely blood dyscrasias and

Table 4.10 Sulphonylurea oral hypoglycaemic agents

Drug	$t_{1/2}$ (h)	Dosage frequency per day
Tolbutamide	4	2
Chlorpropamide	35–40	1
Glibenclamide	12	1–2

inappropriate diuretic hormone secretion) may occur. Some patients taking *chlorpropamide* may experience flushing with ingestion of alcohol due to a disulfiram-like interference with metabolism (see p. 263).

Biguanides

The action of the biguanide, *metformin*, requires the presence of functioning pancreatic tissue. It acts by increasing peripheral glucose utilization. As it does not stimulate endogenous insulin secretion it does not cause hypoglycaemia. *Metformin* is used mainly in the management of obese NIDDM patients. Lactic acidosis may occur in patients with impaired renal function and cardiac failure. *Metformin* is therefore best avoided in elderly patients in whom both renal impairment and cardiac failure are common.

Inhibitor of alpha glucosidase

The inhibitor of alpha glucosidase, *acarbose*, binds to the polysaccharide hydrolytic enzymes (alpha glucosidases) in the microvilli of the small intestine, reversibly inhibiting their activity in a dose-dependent fashion. Thus, the release of glucose from complex carbohydrates is slowed by up to 80%. As this drug does not stimulate endogenous insulin secretion, it is not associated with hypoglycaemia. In common with *metformin*, *acarbose* is not associated with weight gain and can be used in obese patients with diet alone, in combination with sulphonylureas or with biguanides. The principle unwanted effects of this drug include flatulence, diarrhoea, abdominal distension and discomfort.

Diabetogenic hormones and drugs

(1) Glucagon, a polypeptide secreted by the α-cells of the islets of Langerhans, is a very potent hormone that increases blood glucose concentration and increases free fatty acid release from adipocytes.
(2) GH promotes growth in the immature animal by laying down protein, but in the adult is diabetogenic.
(3) Glucocorticosteroids have many actions that are opposite to those of insulin and when given at unphysiologically high doses are diabetogenic.
(4) Adrenaline inhibits insulin release (via α-adrenoceptors) and promotes glycogenolysis (via β-adrenoceptors).

Other diabetogenic agents are summarized in Table 4.11.

Table 4.11 Pharmacological agents that can produce or unmask diabetes

Agent	Mechanism of action
Antagonists at β-adrenoceptors	Inhibit insulin secretion
Thiazide diuretic agents, *diazoxide*, **phenytoin**	Inhibit insulin secretion
Combined oral contraceptive steroids	Gluconeogenesis, lipolysis (or tissue resistance to insulin)

Hypoglycaemia

Normal fasting blood glucose concentrations average 3.3–5.6 mmole/L; smaller than 2.6 mmole/L is termed hypoglycaemia. The signs and symptoms of hypoglycaemia fall into two groups:

(1) Those due to adrenaline release. These include hunger, pallor, sweating, apprehension and tachycardia. The adrenaline response is sometimes sufficient to increase blood glucose concentration by mobilization of liver glycogen (mediated by β-adrenoceptors, see above).
(2) those due to neuroglycopenia – lack of glucose fuel for cerebral cells. If the adrenaline response is insufficient then the signs and symptoms due to neuroglycopenia occur and include mental confusion, incoherent speech, retrograde amnesia and coma.

The main causes of hypoglycaemia are insulin administration and sulphonylurea drugs. Precipitating factors may be the omission of a meal or unaccustomed exercise.

Treatment

Glucose

When the patient recognizes the symptoms of hypoglycaemia, sugar should be swallowed. If consciousness is lost glucose should be given i/v.

Glucagon

Glucagon is given by injection and increases the output of glucose from the liver. The response is proportional to the glycogen reserve of the liver.

Diazoxide

Diazoxide is related to the thiazide diuretic agents (see p. 137). It is given orally and reserved for treating the chronic hypoglycaemia of excess insulin secretion (tumour – insulinoma). It may cause an increase in circulating catecholamine concentration, which indirectly alters glucose concentration or it may directly block insulin release from the β-cells.

Summary

(1) Diabetes mellitus is a chronic metabolic problem, characterized by hyperglycaemia, due to absolute or relative deficiency of insulin. There are two forms, insulin-dependent diabetes mellitus (IDDM) and non-insulin-dependent diabetes mellitus (NIDDM).
(2) Treatment of IDDM is with parenteral insulin which may be:
    (a) porcine or bovine (extracted from animal pancreas) or 'human' (prepared by enzymic modification of animal insulin or DNA recombinant technology);

(b) short (*soluble insulin*), intermediate (*insulin zinc suspension*) or long (*crystalline insulin zinc suspension*) acting.

Hypoglycaemia is the main adverse effect of insulin.

(3) Treatment of NIDDM involves diet, use of oral hypoglycaemic drugs (sulphonylureas, biguanides) and *acarbose*.

(4) Sulphonylureas (e.g. **tolbutamide**):
(a) require the presence of functioning β-cells;
(b) induce closure of membrane ATP-sensitive K^+ channels;
(c) stimulate the release of insulin;
(d) produce hypoglycaemia as the main adverse effect.

(5) Biguanides (e.g. *metformin*):
(a) require the presence of functioning β-cells;
(b) increase peripheral glucose utilization;
(c) do not induce hypoglycaemia, but may produce lactic acidosis.

(6) *Acarbose*:
(a) inhibits alpha glucosidase;
(b) reduces the release of glucose from complex carbohydrates during digestion;
(c) does not induce hypoglycaemia, but may cause gastro-intestinal disturbances.

(7) Hypoglycaemia, from administration of insulin or sulphonylurea drugs, is treated with glucose (oral, i/v) or *glucagon*, which increases plasma glucose concentrations.

Posterior pituitary hormones

Vasopressin

Synthesis, release and actions

Antidiuretic hormone (ADH, vasopressin) is a cyclic nonapeptide (made up of nine amino acids) synthesized in the hypothalamus. Bound to neurophysin, it is transported to the posterior pituitary gland within the axons running between the two areas. The release of ADH into the circulation from the nerve terminals is Ca^{2+}-dependent and occurs in response to an increase in plasma osmotic pressure (including that due to diuretic agents) or haemorrhage. Release is also stimulated by nicotine and **morphine** and perhaps by *chlorpropamide* (alternatively this may sensitize the kidney to ADH) and is inhibited by ethanol.

The main physiological action of ADH is to increase the water permeability of the kidney tubule membranes leading to reabsorption of water, unaccompanied ·by ions, from the collecting ducts of the kidney tubules to reduce the osmotic pressure of the plasma. In most circumstances this results in the production of a small volume of

STAFFS UNIVERSITY LIBRARY

concentrated urine. The mechanism involves agonist action of ADH at a membrane V_2 vasopressin receptor, which produces activation of adenylate cyclase, generation of cAMP and an increase in the number of water channels.

Diabetes insipidus is characterized by the passage of large volumes of dilute urine (polyuria), with consequential thirst and water drinking (polydipsia). It results from either an absence of ADH release (pituitary diabetes insipidus) or a lack of responsiveness of the kidney tubule membranes to ADH (nephrogenic diabetes insipidus). **Lithium carbonate** may greatly reduce the sensitivity of the tubule to vasopressin leading to such an adverse effect.

At much higher concentration, vasopressin causes constriction of blood vessels, especially capillaries and venules, by agonist action at the V_1 vasopressin receptor, which promotes phosphatidylinositol breakdown and calcium mobilization.

Uses of vasopressin and its analogues

As an antidiuretic agent

Diabetes insipidus of pituitary gland origin is treated with the analogue of synthetic vasopressin (arginine vasopressin), *desmopressin*. This is longer acting than vasopressin and is also free of vasoconstrictor effects (it is a selective agonist at V_2 vasopressin receptors).

To prevent splitting of the peptide bonds in the stomach the compounds are administered by i/m, i/v, s/c or intranasal routes.

As a vasoconstrictor agent

Oesophageal varices   Vasopressin or terlipressin is given by i/v infusion or injection in the control of the bleeding from oesophageal varicose veins that occurs in portal hypertension due to hepatic scarring, usually due to cirrhosis.

Local anaesthesia   Felypressin, an analogue that is a selective agonist at V_1 vasopressin receptors and has little or no antidiuretic action, is useful mixed with *prilocaine* to prolong the duration of local anaesthesia (see p. 109).

Oxytocin

Oxytocin, another hypothalamic nonapeptide, acts as an agonist at oxytocin (OT) receptors selectively to increase the frequency and duration of bursts of action potentials of uterine smooth muscle, leading to contraction, and of the myoepithelial cells of the mammary glands, leading to milk ejection. High sensitivity of the two tissues to oxytocin is only seen in the appropriate hormonal environment, namely in late pregnancy (uterine action) or postpartum (mammary action). This may reflect an increase in the numbers of OT receptors.

Uses of oxytocin

Beginning of labour

Oxytocin is used to augment labour or, along with rupture of the amniotic membranes, to induce labour at or near term by direct stimulation of phasic uterine contractions. Excessive response of the uterus to *oxytocin* consists of a maintained spasm, which can result in fetal hypoxia, due to restriction of placental blood flow, or rupture of the uterus, particularly if the patient has had a previous caesarean section. This narrow therapeutic range, together with the short $t_{1/2}$ due to rapid metabolism, makes it necessary to administer *oxytocin* by i/v infusion (see p. 373) with dose rate titrated to uterine response. *Oxytocin* can interact with V_2 vasopressin receptors in the kidney (see p. 194) and so at high infusion dose rates *oxytocin* can produce water retention. PGE_2 (*dinoprostone*) may alternatively be used and have the advantage of softening the cervix.

End of labour

The maintained spasm of the uterus produced by *oxytocin* is the basis of the use of the drug after delivery, by single bolus i/v or i/m administration, for the prophylaxis of postpartum haemorrhage. More commonly the alkaloid *ergometrine* (with or without *oxytocin*) is used. This agonist at α-adrenoceptors selectively contracts uterine smooth muscle, although some vasoconstriction producing an increase in BP may be observed. *Ergometrine* has a longer duration of action than *oxytocin*.

Summary

(1) Vasopressin and analogues are agonists at the V_2 vasopressin receptors on renal tubules to increase water reabsorption.
(2) Higher concentrations are agonists at the V_1 vasopressin receptors on vascular smooth muscle to cause contraction.
(3) *Oxytocin* produces phasic smooth muscle contractions in low concentrations and tonic contractions at higher concentrations.
(4) *Oxytocin* and PG analogues are useful in the management of labour.
(5) Postpartum uterine bleeding can be controlled by the spasmogens *oxytocin* and *ergometrine*.

Angiotensin

Occurrence, biosynthesis and metabolism

Angiotensin (angiotensin II) is an octapeptide (made up of eight amino acids) formed by the action of the kidney enzyme, renin, on an inactive

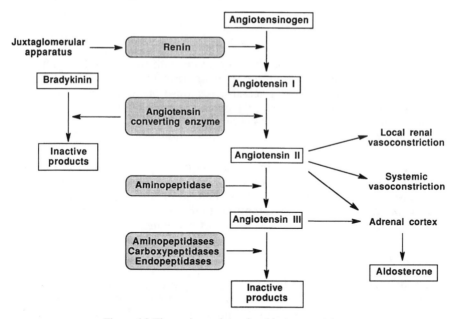

Figure 4.9 The renin–angiotensin–aldosterone system

plasma α_2-globulin, angiotensinogen (Figure 4.9). A relatively inert inter-mediate, the decapeptide angiotensin I is formed initially. This is subse-quently converted to angiotensin II by angiotensin converting enzyme (ACE). This enzyme, which is bound to endothelial cells and located mainly in the lungs, is identical to one of the two enzymes responsible for the breakdown of bradykinin.

Angiotensin II is rapidly destroyed (plasma $t_{1/2}$ = 1–2 min) by angiotensi-nases (mainly aminopeptidases) to yield angiotensin III, a heptapeptide (made up of seven amino acids), and various inactive peptides.

Actions of angiotensin

Angiotensin II is the most potent pressor agent known (the equi-effective molar dose ratio, angiotensin : noradrenaline is 1 : 40), causing arteriolar constriction and an increase in diastolic and systolic BP. This effect is mainly exerted directly on the vessels by agonist action at angiotensin receptors (coupled by a G-protein to phospholipase C), but facilitation of noradrenaline release from noradrenergic nerves may contribute.

Angiotensin II also causes contraction of the smooth muscle of the intestine, bronchioles and uterus. It stimulates the adrenal medulla (to release catecholamines) and stimulates parasympathetic and sympathetic ganglia (to elicit nerve impulses that release acetylcholine and noradren-aline respectively).

By acting on specific receptors in the adrenal cortex, angiotensin II and III increase the synthesis and release of aldosterone. This in turn increases the Na^+ re-absorption and linked K^+ excretion in the distal nephron (see pp. 138, 181).

Role in physiology and pathophysiology

Renin is released from juxtaglomerular cells in the afferent arteriole of the kidney by stimuli of reduced distension of its wall (reduced blood volume or pressure) or reduced delivery of Na^+ to the distal part of the nephron. The release is greater in magnitude if the β_1-adrenoceptors on the juxtaglomerular cells are concurrently occupied by an agonist agent (see p. 94). The stimuli tending to reduce renin secretion are the expansion of ECF volume by aldosterone action, the constriction of the efferent arteriole by angiotensin II action, a negative feedback effect by angiotensin II and an increase in BP due to general vasoconstriction evoked by angiotensin II.

The renin-angiotensin system is important in the maintenance of cardiovascular homeostasis and the control of electrolyte balance (see p. 181). It may also play a modulatory role in the control of small blood vessel tone by virtue of a facilitation of noradrenergic neuroeffector transmission. A large concentration of circulating renin and hence of angiotensin is a common finding in malignant (but not benign) hypertension (see p. 474).

Any drug that reduces BP, without disrupting the renin–angiotensin–aldosterone detection and response system, is liable to activate the system and cause as an (usually unwanted) effect salt and water retention by the kidney, ECF volume expansion and gravitationally directed oedema.

Pharmacological and therapeutic exploitation

Inhibitors of ACE (**captopril** and *enalapril*) produce a small reduction in arterial BP in normal people, suggesting that the renin-angiotensin system contributes to the regulation of BP even in health. Inhibitors of ACE are useful in the treatment of hypertension (see pp. 383, 476) when antagonists at β-adrenoceptors and thiazide diuretic agents have failed or are contraindicated. These agents produce a much greater reduction in BP in hypertensive patients than in normal subjects.

Inhibitors of ACE are also valuable in the management of heart failure (see p. 471) when this condition is not adequately controlled by a loop diuretic agent. Addition of the inhibitor of ACE to diuretic therapy is likely to cause a profound reduction in BP, hence treatment with the inhibitor of ACE should be started at a very low dose.

Unwanted effects of the inhibitors of ACE include persistent dry cough, which may be attributable to the drug causing the accumulation of bradykinin in the bronchial mucosa.

A non-peptide antagonist at angiotensin receptors (*losartan*) has been developed and is being evaluated in the treatment of hypertension.

Summary

(1) Angiotensin I is formed by the enzyme renin, which is released from the juxtaglomerular apparatus in the kidney.
(2) Renin release is stimulated by reduced distension of the wall of the afferent glomerular arteriole or reduced delivery of Na^+ to the distal part of the nephron. It is augmented by the activation of β-adreno-ceptors on the juxtaglomerular cells.
(3) Angiotensin I is converted to angiotensin II by angiotensin converting enzyme (ACE) found in the lungs.
(4) Angiotensin II causes smooth muscle contraction, the release of catecholamines from noradrenergic neurones and the adrenal medulla and the secretion of aldosterone from the adrenal cortex.
(5) Inhibitors of ACE (e.g. **captopril**, *enalapril*) reduce arterial BP in normal subjects and (more so) in those suffering from essential hypertension.
(6) Inhibitors of ACE are useful in the control of congestive cardiac failure that is resistant to therapy with loop diuretics.

Local hormones

Histamine

Occurrence, biosynthesis and metabolism

Histamine (2-(4-imidazolyl) ethylamine) is formed from the amino acid L-histidine by the action of histidine decarboxylase. Histamine is present in many mammalian tissues, with especially high concentrations in lung, skin and intestine. Most is stored in the granules of tissue mast cells (basophils in blood) bound electrostatically to the carboxyl groups of protein to form a heparin/protein complex (Figure 4.10).

The electrostatic forces binding histamine to the carboxyl groups are relatively weak, nevertheless the bound form of histamine is inactive. This arrangement is significant for the mechanism of histamine release described below. Some histamine is located not in mast cells but in neurones in the CNS and in cells of the epidermis, gastric mucosa and growing or regenerating tissues where there is a rapid turnover of histamine. More than 90% of an exogenous histamine load is metabolized either by deamination (enzyme: diamine oxidase or 'histaminase'; product: imidazolylacetic acid) or by a combination of N-methylation and deamination (enzymes: imidazole-N-methyltransferase and MAO; product: methylimidazolylacetic acid).

Release of histamine

The antigen/antibody reaction of anaphylaxis releases histamine from tissue stores (mast cells), as do trauma and certain compounds including

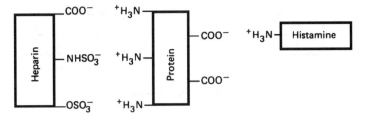

Figure 4.10 The granular storage of histamine in mast cells

Table 4.12 Agents that release histamine from mast cells

Kind of activator	Examples
Tissue damage	Mechanical, chemical, heat
Complex macromolecules	Snake and wasp venoms Bacterial toxins
High MW polymers	*Dextran*
Detergents and surface active agents	Bile salts
Basic drugs	**Atropine, morphine, tubocurarine** Antagonists at H_1 histamine receptors

basic drugs such as antagonists at H_1 histamine receptors due to their structural similarity to histamine (Table 4.12).

The underlying principle of histamine release is that the heparin/protein complex acts as a weak cation-exchange resin. Exposure of the granules to a cation-containing medium results in an instantaneous exchange of histamine with the cation. Basic drugs and polypeptides with many basic groups displace the similarly basic histamine from its binding sites. Detergents, proteolytic enzymes and the antigen/antibody reaction of anaphylaxis cause cell disruption, with expulsion of granules into the extracellular cation-containing medium (degranulation), where instantaneous amine release by cation exchange occurs. Since the predominant extracellular cation is Na^+, the mechanism can be represented as in Figure 4.11.

Anaphylaxis develops by the following stages:

(1) Exposure of a person or an animal to a foreign macromolecule (antigen) results in the formation of specific antibodies by B-lymphocytes.
(2) Circulating antibodies are taken up and firmly bound on the surface of tissue cells.
(3) Re-exposure to antigen results in its combination with tissue-bound antibody and tissue damage.
(4) Histamine (and other cell constituents) are released 'explosively': other mediators implicated in anaphylaxis include plasma kinins, 5-hydroxytryptamine (5-HT), PGs and LTs.

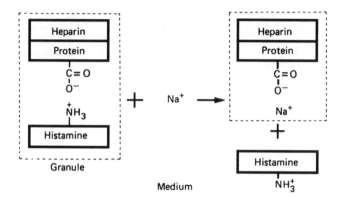

Figure 4.11 The cation exchange mechanism of mast cell degranulation

Suppression of release

Sodium cromoglycate [cromolyn sodium] selectively suppresses the release of chemical mediators (histamine, LTs) arising from antigen/antibody reactions or degranulating agents. The precise mode of action is unknown but it may stabilize the mast cell membrane so that steps between antigen/antibody union and the release of chemical mediators are prevented.

It does not affect the course of the response to mediators already released if given after the antigen/antibody interaction and has no direct anti-inflammatory activity.

Sodium cromoglycate is a very effective drug in allergic rhinitis and allergic conjunctivitis, and moderately effective in food allergies in children and asthma. It is poorly absorbed from the gut and is administered either by inhalation as an aerosol, into the nose and respiratory tract, or is applied topically, for example, to the conjunctiva in cases of allergic conjunctivitis.

Actions of histamine

The actions of histamine are mediated by cell surface receptors that are of two kinds, H_1 and H_2 histamine receptors. On the cardiovascular system histamine dilates small arteries and venules. Thus the BP declines but the heart rate increases due to reflex baroreceptor nerve stimulation (and an agonist action at H_2 histamine receptors in the heart). Cerebral blood vessels are especially sensitive to the dilator action of histamine. Histamine increases the permeability of the endothelial lining of postcapillary venules to plasma protein. It also produces increased cerebrospinal fluid pressure and histamine headaches.

In the skin, Lewis's triple response consists of:

(1) A red mark due to capillary dilatation at the injury site.
(2) A pink flare that is diffuse and surrounds the injury site due to arteriolar dilatation from an axon reflex triggered by sensory nerve stimulation.

(3) A wheal (a raised oedematous area close to the injury site) due to the increased permeability of the microcirculation to plasma protein.

Histamine also stimulates sensory neurones to give itching and sometimes pain. The response arises from injurious stimuli releasing endogenous histamine. It can be mimicked by a small quantity of histamine injected intradermally.

Histamine directly stimulates the smooth muscle of intestine and bronchioles. It is a powerful stimulant of gastric secretion (mainly direct but also facilitates the secretagogue action of the vagus nerve), with both parietal and peptic gland cells being affected. In high doses, histamine stimulates the adrenal medulla and autonomic ganglia causing release of catecholamines.

Role in physiology and pathophysiology

Histamine plays a role in the normal regulation of gastric secretion, in the body's protective mechanism at an injury site (triple response, acute inflammation) and as a mediator in allergic and anaphylactic conditions.

Pharmacological and therapeutic exploitation

Histamine itself has no therapeutic value. Compounds that are antagonists at histamine receptors or prevent the release of histamine are used therapeutically.

Antagonists at histamine receptors

These selectively and competitively antagonize histamine whether it is injected or endogenously released. The antagonists can be divided into two groups, as can histamine receptors (Table 4.13).

Antagonists at H_1 histamine receptors

Competitive antagonists at H_1 histamine receptors are stable lipid-soluble amines having in common the ethylamine chain of histamine. The group

Table 4.13 Histamine receptors

H_1 histamine receptors	H_2 histamine receptors
Effects mediated	
Contraction of smooth muscle of:	
intestine	Stimulation of gastric secretion
bronchioles	Stimulation of the heart
Most of depressor effects on BP	Inhibition of antigenic release
Increased capillary permeability	of histamine from basophils
Stimulation of sensory neurones	
Selective competitive antagonist	
Chlorpheniramine	**Cimetidine**

Table 4.14 Other actions at some H₁ receptor antagonists

	Sedation	Anti-emesis	Antagonism at muscarinic acetylcholine receptors
Promethazine	++++	+++	++
Chlorpheniramine	++	0	0
Terfenadine	0	0	0

++++ = strong; + = weak; 0 = no activity.

includes older (**chlorpheniramine**, *promethazine*) and newer drugs (*terfenadine*). Most drugs from both groups are absorbed rapidly after oral administration. All are metabolized by liver MFO enzymes and most have a duration of action of 4–6 h, but some (e.g. *promethazine, terfenadine*) act for up to 12 h.

The antagonists at H₁ histamine receptors block the action of histamine by reversible competitive antagonism at the H₁ histamine receptor site (Table 4.13). However most members of this group also have actions that are not related to antagonism at H₁ histamine receptors. Some of these other important actions are outlined in Table 4.14.

The main usefulness of antagonists at H₁ histamine receptors is the relief of the effects that are mediated by histamine in allergic (seasonal rhinitis or 'hay fever', insect bites and stings) and anaphylactic reactions. They are largely ineffective in asthma, arthritic inflammation and systemic anaphylaxis where other local hormones are involved. Their other actions (Table 4.14) make them useful in the alleviation of motion sickness and as mild hypnotic agents (*promethazine*). Unwanted effects are frequent but tend to be mild. They include sedation, anorexia, nausea and vomiting, dizziness, blurred vision and dry mouth. Most of these effects are thought to be due to action in the CNS, some can be explained by antagonism at muscarinic acetylcholine receptors. The sedation, which is additive to the effects of alcohol, may be such that the ability of users to drive or operate machinery is impaired. *Terfenadine* causes less sedation than the other antagonists at H₁ histamine receptors and does not cause psychomotor disturbances because blood–brain barrier penetration is slight. Rarely cardiac dysrhythmias are associated with *terfenadine* use in situations where the plasma concentration is increased through high dosage, impaired liver function or inhibition of metabolism by **erythromycin** or imidazole antifungal agents.

Antagonists at H₂ histamine receptors

Competitive antagonists at H₂ histamine receptors include **cimetidine** and *ranitidine*. Unlike the antagonists at H₁ histamine receptors, these are imidazole derivatives. They inhibit cardiac stimulation evoked by histamine and gastric acid secretion evoked by histamine, gastrin, physiological stimuli and agonists at muscarinic acetylcholine receptors. The latter three stimuli have histamine release as a final common pathway. **Cimetidine** and *ranitidine* are inhibitors of gastric secretion for use in the treatment of gastric and duodenal ulcer (see p. 463) and reflux oesophagitis (heart-burn).

Cimetidine (but not *ranitidine*) binds to androgen receptors occasion-ally causing gynaecomastia (see p. 163), and may potentiate such drugs as **phenytoin** and **warfarin** due to inhibition of cytochrome P_{450}.

5-Hydroxytryptamine

Occurrence, biosynthesis and metabolism

5-Hydroxytryptamine (serotonin) is present in many mammalian tissues with highest concentrations in the enterochromaffin cells of the gastroin-testinal tract. In rodent mast cells, 5-hydroxytryptamine is complexed with heparin and protein. Elsewhere, 5-hydroxytryptamine is stored in associ-ation with ATP in intracellular storage particles within intestinal chromaf-fin cells, platelets and the specific 5-hydroxytryptamine-containing (5-hydroxytryptaminergic) neurones of the brain (see p. 221).

The amino acid L-tryptophan is hydroxylated by tryptophan-5-hydroxy-lase to 5-hydroxytryptophan, which is then decarboxylated to 5-hydroxy-tryptamine by aromatic L-amino acid decarboxylase.

The degradation of 5-hydroxytryptamine occurs mainly in the liver where it is converted to 5-hydroxyindole acetaldehyde by MAO. This aldehyde is rapidly converted to the excretory product 5-hydroxyindole acetic acid by aldehyde dehydrogenase.

Actions of 5-hydroxytryptamine

5-Hydroxytryptamine has complex cardiovascular actions. In general it acts directly to constrict arteries, resulting in increased peripheral resis-tance.

5-Hydroxytryptamine stimulates intestinal and bronchial smooth muscle, the adrenal medulla and ganglia of the autonomic nervous system. It is a potent stimulant of sensory nerve endings and gives pain when applied to an exposed blister base. It is pro-aggregatory on platelets.

Recent nomenclature identifies at least four families of receptors for 5-hydroxytryptamine and these have been designated 5-HT_1, 5-HT_2, 5-HT_3 and 5-HT_4. Most peripheral 5-hydroxytryptamine receptors (in platelets and smooth muscle) appear to be of the 5-HT_2 kind. 5-HT_4 receptors in the atria mediate increases in contractile force. 5-HT_1, 5-HT_2 and 5-HT_3 kinds of 5-hydroxytryptamine receptor have been identified in the brain. Although the functional implications for kinds of 5-hydroxytryptamine receptor in the brain remain unclear, there is some evidence to suggest therapeutic roles for drugs acting at 5-HT_1 receptors in depression, anxiety and migraine, at 5-HT_2 receptors in psychoses and at 5-HT_3 receptors in emesis.

Role in physiology and pathophysiology

The selective localization of 5-hydroxytryptamine in platelets and its vasoconstrictor properties suggest a role in haemostasis. 5-Hydroxytryptamine may be involved in the genesis of atrial fibrillation and associated thromboembolic stroke. A tumour of enterochromaffin or related cells (carcinoid) may develop in the gastrointestinal or respiratory tracts, that secretes excessive quantities of 5-hydroxytryptamine (in addition to polypeptides and PGs). In the CNS 5-hydroxytryptamine has a neurotransmitter role (see p. 221).

Pharmacological and therapeutic exploitation

There are no selective antagonists at 5-HT$_1$ or 5-HT$_4$ receptors that are available for clinical use. Antagonists at 5-HT$_3$ receptors usefully control nausea and vomiting (see p. 241).

Antagonists at 5-HT$_2$ receptors

Pizotifen is an antagonist at 5-HT$_2$ and H$_1$ histamine receptors. It is an orally active, effective prophylactic agent in migraine (see p. 501). Its mechanism of action may involve inhibition of the local inflammatory response evoked by 5-hydroxytryptamine. *Pizotifen* also controls the increased intestinal motility but not the flushing (may be due to kinins or PGs) associated with carcinoid tumour. In addition, it possesses antagonist activity at muscarinic acetylcholine receptors and is sedative. These unwanted effects are frequent, as are increased appetite and weight gain.

Lysergic acid diethylamide (LSD) is an antagonist at 5-HT$_2$ and α-adrenoceptors but, like other ergot alkaloids, has partial agonist properties at central dopamine and 5-HT$_1$ receptors. These agonist actions may be relevant to its hallucinogenic properties (see p. 257).

Phenoxybenzamine and **phentolamine** are potent but not specific antagonists at 5-HT$_2$ receptors (see p. 98).

Eicosanoids

The term eicosanoid is used to describe a vast array of substances that includes the PGs (including prostacyclin), thromboxanes and the LTs, since they are all derived from the same eicosanoic (eicosa = 20 carbon; enoic = containing double bonds) acid precursors.

Eicosanoid biosynthesis

The substrates for eicosanoid biosynthesis are generated mainly by the action of phospholipase A$_2$ on the phospholipid fraction of the cell (Figure 4.12). Some of the anti-inflammatory actions of glucocorticosteroids can be explained by their ability to induce the production of a group of proteins called lipocortins that are inhibitors of phospholipase A$_2$ activity.

Released PG precursor (principally arachidonic acid) is acted upon by an enzyme (cyclo-oxygenase, COX), either constitutively expressed (COX1) or induced by inflammatory stimuli (COX2), resulting in the formation of PG endoperoxides. Non-steroidal anti-inflammatory drugs (NSAIDs, e.g. **aspirin**, *ibuprofen*) act by inhibiting cyclo-oxygenase (see p. 213).

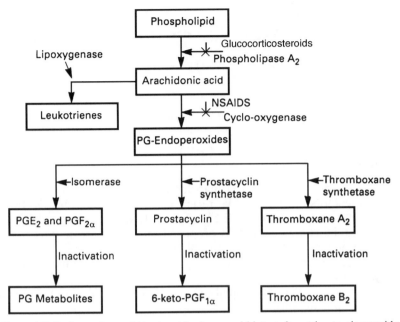

Figure 4.12 Pathways in arachidonic acid release and biotransformation to eicosanoids

The endoperoxides are then converted to one or other of the relatively stable PGs. A number of other derivatives is also formed from the endoperoxides, including prostacyclin (PGI$_2$) and thromboxane A$_2$ (TxA$_2$). These three groups of products are termed prostanoids.

Arachidonic acid also acts as precursor for another group of biologically active substances, the LTs and certain hydroperoxide derivatives. The enzyme responsible for this conversion is 5-lipoxygenase (Figure 4.12).

Prostaglandins

The term PG is the generic name for a family of closely related cyclic, oxygenated, 20-carbon unsaturated fatty acids. The hypothetical basic 20-carbon skeleton of the PGs has been given the name <u>prostanoic acid</u>. On the basis of their structures, the PGs have been separated into nine groups, named A–I. All have in common a double bond at the 13,14 position and an OH-group at C$_{15}$ (except PGG). In naming them the number of unsaturated carbon bonds is denoted by a subscript numeral and the subscript α or β denotes the orientation of an OH-group in position 9 below or above the molecular plane (Figure 4.13).

The PGs are synthesized and released by virtually every tissue in the body. Since there is no evidence for storage of PGs (except in the seminal fluid), the rate of release reflects that of biosynthesis. A wide variety of stimuli (allergies, inflammatory conditions, trauma) is capable of releasing PGs. Several of the PGs are very rapidly metabolized in the kidneys, lungs and liver.

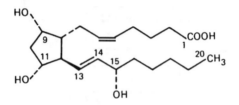

Figure 4.13 Prostaglandin $F_{2\alpha}$

Actions of prostaglandins

PGs have many and varied pharmacological actions that are mediated by several receptors. There are five receptors more or less selective for the natural prostanoids PGD_2, PGE_2, $PGF_{2\alpha}$, PGI_2 and TxA_2 named DP, EP, FP, IP and TP respectively. It is proposed that there are subtypes of the EP receptor and that PGE_2 exerts differing action at these. Table 4.15 summarizes the effects of the E and F PGs and the receptors mediating these effects.

The actions of PGs are usually exerted close to their site of release (local hormone action).

Role in physiology and pathophysiology

The PGs are believed to be involved in many physiological processes. In female reproductive physiology they have been implicated in uterine and Fallopian tube contractility, labour (at term) and maintaining the patency of the fetal ductus arteriosus. There is good evidence that PGs play a role in gastric mucus secretion and modulation of renal blood flow.

Excessive production of PGs has been implicated in many pathological processes, in particular the acute inflammatory response (see p. 212), fever (see p. 252) and various female reproductive disorders (spasmodic dysmenorrhoea, habitual abortion and premature labour).

Pharmacological and therapeutic exploitation

Clinical application is based on either mimicking physiological effects by exogenous PGs or, in pathological situations, preventing their synthesis.

Table 4.15 Some effects of PGs typified by PGE_2 and $PGF_{2\alpha}$, and the prostanoid receptors that mediate them

	PGE_2 (prostanoid receptor)	$PGF_{2\alpha}$ (prostanoid receptor)
Blood vessels	Dilated (EP, DP)	Constricted (TP)
Capillary permeability	Increased (EP, DP)	Little effect
Gastric secretion	Decreased (EP)	Little effect
Bronchiolar smooth muscle	Relaxed (EP)	Contracted (FP, TP)
Uterine smooth muscle	Contracted* (FP)	Contracted (FP)
Sensory nerve fibres	Sensitized*	?

*Generalization – the responses produced are often complex.

The uterine smooth muscle stimulating properties of PGs and their analogues form the basis of most of their clinical usage. Both the PGE_1 analogue, *gemeprost*, and PGE_2, *dinoprostone*, are useful for second trimester pregnancy termination. Unwanted effects are frequent but mild, and include nausea, vomiting, diarrhoea, flushing, shivering, headache and dizziness and, when given i/v, local tissue irritation and erythema, due to actions at other EP and FP receptors. Local application to the uterus helps to reduce these adverse effects.

PGE_2 (*dinoprostone*) is also useful for the induction of labour. A combination of *dinoprostone* and *oxytocin* has been used successfully for induction of labour, with a reduction in the incidence of adverse effects due to the PG (a result of the smaller dose now required). A $PGF_{2\alpha}$-analogue, *carboprost*, is useful to control severe postpartum haemorrhage.

PGE_1 (*alprostadil*) is used to maintain patency of the ductus arteriosus in neonates with congenital heart defects, and, by direct intracavernous injection, to manage impotence.

Misoprostol, a synthetic analogue of PGE_1, is relatively selective for the EP receptors that mediate decreased gastric acid secretion (and possibly increased gastric mucus secretion) and is useful to promote healing of gastric and duodenal ulcers, including ulcers induced by NSAIDs in patients from whom the drugs cannot be withdrawn.

Thromboxane A_2 and prostacyclin

Occurrence, biosynthesis and metabolism

Thromboxane A_2 (TxA$_2$, synthesized predominantly by platelets) and prostacyclin (PGI$_2$, synthesized predominantly by heart, vascular endothelium and stomach) are derived from PG endoperoxides and have short half-lives of 30 s and 3 min respectively.

Actions of thromboxane A_2 and prostacyclin

Thromboxane A_2 and prostacyclin have directly opposing pharmacological actions in many systems, as shown in Table 4.16.

Role in physiology and pathophysiology

Generation of prostacyclin by the endothelial cells lining blood vessels is probably the biochemical mechanism underlying their unique ability to

Table 4.16 Main actions of prostacyclin and thromboxane A_2, and the prostanoid receptors that mediate them

Prostacyclin (prostanoid receptor)	Thromboxane A_2 (prostanoid receptor)
Vasodilatation (IP)	Vasoconstriction (TP)
Inhibition of platelet aggregation (IP)	Platelet aggregation (TP)
Bronchodilatation (EP)	Bronchoconstriction (TP)
Cytoprotective (vascular endothelium)	Cytolysis

STAFFS UNIVERSITY LIBRARY

resist platelet adhesion. A balance between the formation of anti-aggregatory vasodilator substances (prostacyclin) and pro-aggregatory vasoconstrictor substances (thromboxane A_2) could contribute to the maintenance of the integrity of vascular endothelium. Loss of this balance may explain the mechanism of formation of intra-arterial thrombi in certain pathophysiological conditions.

Pharmacological and therapeutic exploitation

Synthetic prostacyclin (*epoprostenol*) can be used during surgical procedures and renal dialysis involving extracorporeal circulation of the blood to prevent platelet aggregation. There are no drugs available for clinical use that selectively modify the synthesis, actions or metabolism of prostacyclin or thromboxane A_2 (but see p. 146).

Leukotrienes

Occurrence, biosynthesis and metabolism

Six groups of LTs have currently been identified and designated LTA–LTF. They are synthesized from arachidonic acid by 5-lipoxygenase in a variety of tissues, in particular lung tissue and white blood cells.

Actions of leukotrienes

The LTs possess a wide variety of pharmacological actions but LTB_4 is a particularly potent chemotactic and chemokinetic agent on polymorphonuclear leucocytes. All LTs contract to varying degrees smooth muscle from the gut, bronchioles and various vascular beds, cause oedema formation and potentiate other inflammatory mediators.

Role in physiology and pathophysiology

The LTs are believed to be intimately involved in various inflammatory and allergic disorders, notably bronchial asthma, with LTC_4 and LTD_4 being the principal LTs generated during tissue anaphylaxis.

Exploitation

Compounds that selectively modify the synthesis, actions or metabolism of LTs are not clinically available. Antagonists at LT receptors have been developed but are not yet being prescribed clinically.

Kinins

Occurrence, biosynthesis and metabolism

The kinins are bradykinin (a nonapeptide), kallidin (lysyl-bradykinin, a decapeptide) and related vasodilator peptides. Bradykinin and kallidin are formed from the same circulating α_2 globulin precursors, known as kininogens and kallidinogens, by the action of specific proteolytic enzymes, kallidinogenases (synonym kallikreins). Kallidinogenases are found in many organs and in urine, saliva, lymph, pancreatic secretions, blood, sweat and tears. Plasma kallidinogenase exists in the form of an inactive precursor (prekallidinogenase) but when plasma equilibrium is disturbed (e.g. by change in pH, temperature or contact with water insoluble materials), various activators (including Factor XII, the Hageman factor of blood clotting) convert it to its active form, with subsequent formation of kinins. *Aprotinin* is a non-specific inhibitor of kallidinogenase. Its medical application (to limit blood loss during and after surgery) rests on its ability to inhibit both plasmin and kallidinogenase.

Kinins are rapidly destroyed in blood ($t_{1/2}$ less than 1 min) by kininases, which remove one (carboxypeptidase-N) or two (kininase II or ACE, see p. 196) amino acids from both bradykinin and kallidin.

Actions of kinins

The actions of bradykinin, which are mediated through interaction with at least two receptors, are typical of the vasodilator kinins.

Bradykinin has potent action on the cardiovascular system, both as a relaxant of vascular smooth muscle (causing a reduction in systemic BP) and as a promoter of increased capillary permeability.

Bradykinin contracts the smooth muscle of the intestine and bronchioles, stimulates the release of transmitters via actions at the adrenal medulla and sympathetic ganglia and stimulates sensory nerve endings, as demonstrated by the pain when applied to an exposed blister base.

Role in physiology and pathophysiology

Kinins have been implicated in many physiological functions, including functional and reactive hyperaemia, regulation of tissue blood flow, BP control and neonatal circulatory changes. They may be involved in various pathological states (allergy, inflammation, pancreatitis, shock) and the *pizotifen*-resistant flushing and bronchoconstriction seen with carcinoid tumour.

Pharmacological and therapeutic exploitation

No selective antagonist of bradykinin is available for clinical use.

Cytokines

Occurrence, biosynthesis and metabolism

Cytokines are a heterogeneous group of proteins, distinct from immunoglobulins, released by cells of the immune system and elsewhere (e.g. endothelium). Alternative terms reflect the cell source (lymphokines from lymphocytes, monokines from monocytes). Some individual cytokines have, or used to have, a descriptive name, sometimes several, based on the biological activity of interest (e.g. tumour necrosis factor, TNF). The large number of descriptive names and related acronyms is now being reduced by the systematic allocation of interleukin (IL) numbers, as the nature of each cytokine is established by its physicochemical, rather than its biological properties. However, some cytokines retain familiar non-systematic names (e.g. TNF; interferons, IFN).

Cytokines contain between 100 and 200 amino acids. They can be variably glycosylated and can form oligomers, hence conflicting reports on their molecular size. Production, controlled primarily at the level of transcription, is increased, usually in response to signals from the cell surface.

Internalization of cytokine/receptor complexes, enzymatic degradation, endogenous inhibitors, dilution in body fluids and excretion (e.g. urine) contribute to a short $t_{1/2}$ for most cytokines.

Actions of cytokines

Cytokines bind to specific surface receptors. Most of their biological effects are localized near their site of release and confined to cells of the immune system. In general terms, these actions are concerned with:

(1) Modulation of leucocyte margination and emigration (see p. 211).
(2) Coordination of responses (including antibody formation and phagocytosis) from different kinds of leucocytes to infection and inflammatory stimuli.
(3) Production and maturation of blood cells (haematopoiesis).

A few cytokines also appear to act as hormones affecting cells outside the immune system. For example, the monokine, interleukin-1 (IL-1), produces effects on the brain (fever), liver (synthesis of acute-phase proteins) and skeletal muscle (proteolysis).

Role in physiology and pathophysiology

The immunomodulatory, cytotoxic, haematopoietic and other effects of cytokines are important in the maintenance of health, the defence against infection and the development of inflammation.

Pharmacological and therapeutic exploitation

Interferons (IFN) have complex effects on immunity and cell function. Interferon alpha has some antitumour effect in certain lymphomas and solid tumours. Interferon gamma-1b can be used as an adjunct to antibiotic treatment in patients with chronic granulomatous disease. Adverse reactions include influenza-like symptoms, depression and lethargy.

There are no drugs available for clinical use that selectively antagonize cytokines. Some cytokine effects (e.g. fever) are mediated indirectly by PGs and are blocked by NSAIDs (see p. 253).

Summary

Local hormones:

(1) Are produced and/or released near their site of action.
(2) Help to regulate many physiological functions.
(3) In abnormal amounts, contribute to the pathophysiology of many diseases.
(4) Can have their activity modified by drugs, resulting in desirable and/or undesirable effects.

Inflammation

Inflammation is an active defensive response from the body to injury of any kind. The inflammatory stimuli include chemical or physical trauma, infestation with helminths, infection with protozoa, fungi, bacteria, rickettsia or viruses and antigen/antibody interaction. In acute inflammation, a succession of changes takes place over a short period (minutes to days), which ends either by return of tissue to normal or by conversion to chronic inflammation. Chronic inflammation may last months or years and is characterized by periods of regression and repair, which may be punctuated by further acute inflammatory changes.

The inflammatory response

General characteristics

In the skin an inflammatory stimulus results in the area becoming warm and red due to increased blood flow, swollen due to leakage of plasma protein, followed by salt and water, into the interstitial space as a result of increased protein permeability of microcirculatory vessel walls, and painful due to stimulation of sensory pain fibres. This is similar to Lewis's triple response (see p. 200). Loss of function may consequently occur. Similar inflammatory processes occur at all other sites.

Emigration of leucocytes and phagocytosis

In the early stages of inflammation, polymorphonuclear leucocytes (polymorphs) adhere to the endothelium of vessels (mainly venules), then emigrate through the vessel wall into the interstitial space. At an inflamed site, polymorphs come within the chemotactic (chemical attractive) orbit of living or dead bacteria, or tissue or plasma factors (cytokines, eicosanoids, kinins). Polymorphs move up the concentration gradient of the chemotactic stimulus and, if not killed in the process, ingest the invading organisms or tissue debris (phagocytosis).

Repair and regeneration

When an inflammatory lesion subsides, vasodilatation diminishes and oedema disappears due to exuded fluid being reabsorbed into lymphatic vessels. Macrophages (monocytes and histiocytes) ingest dead polymorphs, microbes and tissue debris. When loss or destruction of tissues has occurred, new capillaries and fibroblasts grow into previously inflamed tissues. Collagen is laid down (fibrosis) and the tissue becomes less vascular (granulation). Epithelium gradually extends over this granulation tissue. Blood vessels, nerves and lymphatic vessels grow into the repair tissue, more collagen is formed and fibres already laid down by fibroblasts shorten, drawing the edges of the wound together and forming a scar (cicatrix).

Chemical mediators

The pattern of the response to various inflammatory stimuli is similar. This similarity indicates that certain chemicals commonly mediate the response.

The following criteria should be satisfied by a putative endogenous chemical mediator of inflammation.

(1) It should be demonstrably present during the inflammatory reaction. The following have been demonstrated:
   (a) Histamine released from mast cells and 5-hydroxytryptamine from platelets.
   (b) K^+ released from all damaged cells and H^+ from hypoxic cells.
   (c) Bradykinin and kallidin formed from kallidinogen.
   (d) Eicosanoids formed from fatty acids (e.g. arachidonic acid).
   (e) Numerous enzymes, including fibrinolysin, hyaluronidase and collagenase, activated due to breakdown of lysosomes.
   (f) Cytokines synthesized and released by cells of the immune system and elsewhere (e.g. endothelium).
(2) It should produce effects that mimic one or more features of inflammation. The relevant effects of some putative chemical mediators are given in Table 4.17.
(3) Selective antagonists, that inhibit one or more of the effects of the postulated mediator, should inhibit similar components of the inflam-

Table 4.17 Some effects of putative mediators of acute inflammation in people

Putative mediator	Oedema	Increased blood flow	Pain	Cell damage
Histamine	+	+	+	
Kinins	+	+	+	
Eicosanoids*	+	+	+	
Cytokines	+	+	+	
K^+			+	+
H^+			+	+

*Effects vary depending on the individual eicosanoid involved. PGs enhance the effect of other painful stimuli rather than initiating pain themselves.

matory reaction. Of the putative mediators, only specific antagonists for histamine are clinically available. Antagonists at H_1 histamine receptors inhibit the acute inflammatory response, but only during the first 30–60 min, when histamine is detectable in the exudate.

(4) Depletion of tissues of the postulated mediator, or inhibition of its means of production and release, should suppress appropriate components of the inflammatory reaction. **Aspirin**-like drugs inhibit cyclo-oxygenase in vitro and suppress the secondary phase of inflammation associated with the presence of PGs in the exudate.

Thus many of the features of inflammation can be explained by a combination of histamine with one or more of the other compounds observed to be present. Histamine is thought to be significant only during the first 30–60 min of the response. Eicosanoids, kinins and cytokines are strong candidates for mediating the inflammatory response beyond this time.

Anti-inflammatory drugs

Defence reactions to trauma and infection are initially desirable but may become unacceptable or unhelpful to the patient. Inflammatory reactions to extrinsic (pollen – allergic rhinitis/conjunctivitis) or intrinsic (host tissue – rheumatoid arthritis) allergens may always be inappropriate. In both of these situations, the symptoms associated with acute inflammation can be suppressed by anti-inflammatory drugs.

The non-steroidal anti-inflammatory drugs

This group includes **aspirin**, propionic acid derivatives (*ibuprofen* and *naproxen*) and *indomethacin*. All relieve pain, reduce swelling and increase mobility in inflammatory diseases (acute rheumatic fever, osteoarthritis, rheumatoid arthritis). They do not alter the course of the underlying disease (chronic inflammation, fibrosis).

Anti-inflammatory effects

Their anti-inflammatory action is due to suppression of PG formation by inhibiting cyclo-oxygenase. Inhibition of cyclo-oxygenase may also explain the analgesic and antipyretic activity of the anti-inflammatory drugs (see p. 253). Although there appears to be a central component (see p. 253), the analgesic action of **aspirin** is a substantially peripheral effect. By preventing PG synthesis (and release) in inflammation, **aspirin** prevents the sensitization of the pain receptors to mechanical stimulation or to chemical mediators. This would also explain why **aspirin** is less effective as an analgesic in non-inflamed tissues.

The relative activities of NSAIDs as anti-inflammatory, analgesic or antipyretic agents may depend on the susceptibility of different tissue cyclo-oxygenases to inhibition by these drugs. Thus in clinical concentrations **aspirin** and *indomethacin* inhibit cyclo-oxygenase in peripheral and central nervous tissues and each displays anti-inflammatory activity (a peripheral action) and antipyretic activity (a central action).

Unwanted effects

Major toxic effects of NSAIDs are uncommon but minor toxic effects are very common and shared by all the group.

Mucosal irritation due to the acidic nature of most NSAIDs and inhibition of production of a mucosal protective PGE lead to gastric erosion, epigastric discomfort and minor bleeding. With large doses, major gastric bleeding or insidious chronic blood loss leading to iron-deficiency anaemia (see p. 530) is sometimes seen.

NSAIDs also produce allergic disorders or may precipitate asthma in susceptible individuals by inhibition of production of a bronchodilatory PG or diversion of free fatty acid precursors (arachidonic acid) towards LT production.

NSAIDs promote salt and water retention by the kidney by inhibiting the production of a PG regulating blood flow in the renal blood vessels. They may also produce renal damage manifest as increased urinary excretion of epithelial cells and leucocytes. Aspirin and salicylates antagonize the uricosuric drugs (probenecid, sulphinpyrazone) used to decrease renal tubular reabsorption of uric acid in gout.

Most NSAIDs are organic acids with affinity for plasma albumin binding sites. This may result in the displacement of other drugs from plasma albumin, with a consequent undesired increase in the free plasma concentration, leading to increased effect (see p. 441).

Adverse effects expressed primarily in the CNS are important features (see p. 253).

Aspirin inhibits the formation of prothrombin, an effect that may result in haemorrhage and is reversible by injection of vitamin K.

Indomethacin is effective in rheumatoid arthritis and gout but is a poorly tolerated drug. It is usually reserved for cases that are unresponsive to other drugs and then used only in short courses to reduce the risks.

Glucocorticosteroids

This group includes **prednisolone**, *beclomethasone, betamethasone, dexamethasone* and *hydrocortisone*. All suppress initial and secondary characteristics of the inflammatory response, including emigration of polymorphs, phagocytosis and the process of repair and regeneration. They are used to suppress inflammation in a wide variety of disease processes, including systemic lupus erythematosus, asthma (see p. 487), cranial arteritis, polyarteritis nodosa and some cases of rheumatoid arthritis (though chronic use is to be avoided, see p. 538). As with the NSAIDs, their actions are palliative and the underlying cause of the lesion remains. Long-term therapy holds many hazards (see p. 183).

They stimulate the production of lipocortin, which inhibits phospholipase A_2 activity thus decreasing the availability of substrate for eicosanoid synthesis. They also stabilize lysosomal membranes, thereby preventing the liberation of enzymes including phospholipase A_2.

Antirheumatic drugs

These drugs, unlike NSAIDs and glucocorticosteroids, do influence the underlying disease process but are drugs with low therapeutic indices. Their beneficial effects are not immediate and it may take several months for a full response to be achieved.

Chloroquine

Chloroquine may be indicated in those patients whose rheumatoid arthritis does not respond to the NSAIDs. The anti-inflammatory effect of *chloroquine* is brought about in part by inhibition of phospholipase A_2. Prolonged use of a dose larger than that effective in malaria is necessary (see p. 281), consequently the risk of irreversible retinopathy is greater.

Penicillamine

Penicillamine is a reserve drug for severe rheumatoid arthritis that has not responded to other treatments. The mechanism may involve reduction of IgM concentration. Toxic effects are common and may be serious (see p. 537).

Organic gold compounds

Gold by i/m injection of *sodium aurothiomalate* [gold sodium thiomalate] or by mouth as *auranofin*, has long-lasting anti-inflammatory effects. This compound is chiefly employed against the early stages of rheumatoid arthritis. Its mode of action is unknown, current hypotheses attribute it to inhibition of mononuclear cell phagocytosis and suppressed immune responsiveness. As with *penicillamine*, toxic effects are common and may be serious (see p. 537).

Despite this wide range of drugs, the ideal anti-inflammatory and antirheumatic agent has yet to be discovered. The toxicity of these compounds (see p. 537) in effective doses often leaves NSAIDs as the mainstay of patient management.

Immunosuppressive drugs

Cytotoxic agents

Alkylating agents (see p. 323), antimetabolites (see p. 322) and drugs affecting DNA (see p. 322) are used to suppress rejection by recipients of transplanted organs and tissues, as too are glucocorticosteroids (see p. 183). They are also used to treat a variety of autoimmune and collagen diseases, including systemic lupus erythematosus, severe progressive rheumatoid arthritis, polyarteritis nodosa, polymyositis and scleroderma. Cytotoxic immunosuppressive drugs (*azathioprine*, **methotrexate**, **cyclophosphamide**, *chlorambucil*) are non-specific in their action, but are most effective on dividing cells such as lymphocytes proliferating and differentiating in response to allo-antigens.

Patients receiving these drugs are prone to atypical infections. Frequent and regular determinations of complete blood cell counts are essential during the use of immunosuppressive drugs for the regulation of drug dosage and determination of the degree of bone marrow suppression.

Cyclosporin

Cyclosporin [cyclosporine], a lipid-soluble cyclic undecapeptide (made up of 11 amino acids) isolated from a soil fungus, is a potent immunosuppressant, which is virtually non-myelotoxic, in marked contrast with other currently used means of immunosuppression (see above). Consequently, it has become an important drug in the field of organ and tissue transplantation, for prevention of graft rejection following bone marrow, kidney, liver, pancreas, heart and heart–lung transplantation, and for prophylaxis of graft-versus-host disease. It may also be used in atopic dermatitis and severe psoriasis when conventional therapy is ineffective or inappropriate.

Cyclosporin selectively and reversibly suppresses activation of helper T lymphocytes (T_H) by blocking gene transcription of interleukin 2 (IL-2), a lymphocyte growth factor. **Cyclosporin** can inhibit both cell-mediated and humoral immune responses but at therapeutic concentrations, synthesis by T_{H1} cells of lymphokines that promote cell-mediated rejection (IL-2, IFN-γ, TNF-β) is inhibited more than that by T_{H2} cells of those that promote B-cell and suppressor T-cell growth and differentiation (IL-4, IL-5, IL-10).

Cyclosporin is nephrotoxic. A dose-dependent increase in serum creatinine and urea concentrations may necessitate a dose reduction in transplant patients or discontinuation in non-transplantation patients.

Summary

Inflammation:

(1) Is a common active defence response to various kinds of injury.
(2) Is mediated by several different sorts of endogenous chemical.
(3) Is often controlled by NSAIDs or glucocorticosteroids, inhibiting PG production.
(4) In specific severe conditions, may be treated with drugs that have a low therapeutic ratio and marked toxicity.

5

Drug action on the central nervous system

Aims

- To describe those chemicals that have a neurotransmitter role in the CNS.
- To describe how defects and imbalances in neurotransmitters can explain CNS disorders.
- To describe the range of mechanisms by which drugs can interfere with neurotransmission.
- To describe how defects and imbalances in neurotransmitters can be restored by drugs, thereby leading to a rational treatment of CNS disorders.
- To anticipate how an understanding of neurotransmitters and of mechanisms of drug action can further lead to more selective treatment of brain disorders.

Introduction

The CNS has many functions and each involves an altered brain chemistry. Every thought, decision, perception and mood change is chemically mediated. In their simplest form the principles of drug action on the CNS are the same as those described for the peripheral nervous system. Drugs affect both peripheral and central neuronal functions by interfering with neurochemical transmission. Remember:

(1) Neurotransmitters can be excitatory or inhibitory;
(2) Drugs act by mimicking or antagonizing neurotransmitters.
(3) Mimics may act directly (agonists at receptors) or indirectly (e.g. releasing agents, inhibitors of uptake, inhibitors of enzymes).
(4) Antagonists may act directly (competitive and non-equilibrium antagonists at receptors) or indirectly (e.g. preventing release, depleting neurotransmitter stores).

However, in the CNS the situation is infinitely more complex for several reasons, including the following:

(1) The very large number of neurones in the brain.
(2) Each neurone may be in synaptic contact with thousands of other neurones.
(3) In addition to the two major neurotransmitters of the periphery, there may be around 40 other neurotransmitters in the CNS and, as in the periphery, most are excitatory or inhibitory dependent on location.
(4) Some neurotransmitters can interact with several different kinds of receptor (as in the periphery), but it is likely that receptors exist in the brain that have no peripheral equivalent.
(5) Drug interaction with presynaptic receptors that modulate the release of neurotransmitters is a more frequently used mechanism of drug action in the brain than in the periphery.
(6) At some synapses transmission is effected by the release of more than one neurotransmitter from the same neurone, but the full significance of this co-transmission has still to be determined.

To illustrate this complexity, consider the neurotransmission that governs the functioning of a particular brain area. The system is analogous to that in the autonomic nervous system where function is the result of a balance between inhibitory and excitatory inputs (Figure 5.1). Four sites at which chemical transmission occurs are shown involving four different neuro-transmitters: A, B, C and D, the later two being released by presynaptic inhibitory neurones.

Assuming absolute selectivity of drug action, the overall phenomenon of excitation can be caused by mimics of neurotransmitters A and D, or antagonists of B and C. Conversely, the phenomenon of inhibition can be caused by mimics of B or C, or antagonists of A and D.

Accepting that this example is a massive oversimplification, and that most drugs interfere with more than one neurotransmitter (e.g. **chlorpromazine** see p. 237), some idea of the complexity emerges. Nevertheless, because there is a range of chemical neurotransmitters in the brain, which may be associated with certain brain areas (and therefore brain functions), and because some drugs have some selectivity of action, some degree of selective alteration of brain activity is possible. Good examples are found in the pharmacology of strychnine (see p. 224), **levodopa** (see p. 229) and **morphine** (see p. 242).

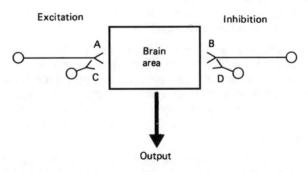

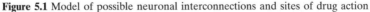

Figure 5.1 Model of possible neuronal interconnections and sites of drug action

Chemical transmission in the central nervous system

Criteria for identification of a neurotransmitter

(1) It must be present at the synapse.
(2) It should be stored in the presynaptic terminal.
(3) Processes for its synthesis should be present in the presynaptic neurone.
(4) It should be released on nerve stimulation.
(5) Postsynaptic application of the putative neurotransmitter should mimic stimulation.
(6) Processes for its inactivation should be present at the synapse.

Note that the above criteria are not yet met fully by some of the more recent additions to the list of neurotransmitters.

Many techniques are required to determine whether these criteria are satisfied, including:

(1) Micro-electrodes for recording from, or applying electrical stimuli to, neurones.
(2) Micropipettes for application of putative neurotransmitters and dialysis probes for removal of ECF for analysis.
(3) Biochemical and isotopic techniques for detection of neurotransmitters or their precursors and metabolites.
(4) Ligand binding, immunological and molecular (e.g. in situ hybridization) techniques to map the distribution of a receptor and its subtypes in the CNS.
(5) Histochemical fluorescence techniques for localization of putative monoamine neurotransmitters.
(6) Immunological techniques for the localization of enzymes involved in neurotransmitter synthesis and breakdown, or for identification of putative peptide neurotransmitters.
(7) Lesion-making and neuroanatomical tracing.

Substances acting as neurotransmitters

Progress in our understanding of putative neurotransmitters has generally depended on the availability of drugs that interfere with them.

Whilst some CNS neurotransmitters also carry out similar functions in the periphery, others, such as the amino acids, which are by far the most abundant CNS neurotransmitters, have only a small role as peripheral neurotransmitters.

Monoamines

Dopamine, noradrenaline and 5-hydroxytryptamine all have important neurotransmitter functions in the CNS. Three ascending monoamine tracts have been identified in mammalian brain. Their cell bodies are located in specific areas of the midbrain and their axons transmit impulses to many brain areas (Figures 5.2, 5.3).

The ascending nigrostriatal dopaminergic tract (Figure 5.2) plays an important role in the maintenance of gait and posture. Degeneration of the nigral neurones forming this tract leads to Parkinson's disease, a neurological disorder named after the physician James Parkinson who first described it in 1817 (see p. 228).

The ascending noradrenaline and dopamine tracts to the limbic system are shown in Figure 5.2. The limbic system is a complex neuronal loop that connects the hippocampus, fornix bundle, mammillary body, thalamus, cingulate gyrus and amygdala. The limbic system plays an important role in the regulation of mood. Disorders of mood and behaviour are likely to have as their basis altered function of neurotransmitters in the limbic system. Many drugs that affect mood and behaviour can be shown to interact with either noradrenaline or dopamine. Empirically this has led to the monoamine theory of nervous and mental disease, which suggests that clinical depression is related to a functional monoamine deficiency, whilst mania and other behavioural excitations are related to a functional monoamine excess. At present it is not possible to define a separate role for any one of the monoamines in any one mental disorder. However, the theory receives support when the effects of drugs on the CNS are compared with their known mechanism of action. Drugs that cause excite-

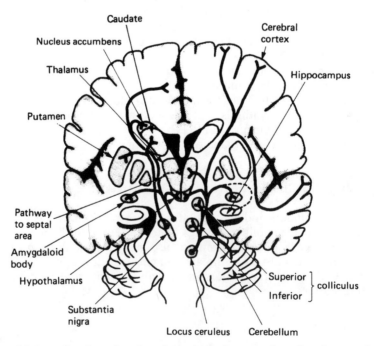

Figure 5.2 Ascending dopaminergic and noradrenergic tracts; dopaminergic tracts shown on the left half of diagram, noradrenergic tracts on the right

ment are known to increase functional monoamine activity (*cocaine* inhibits uptake of monoamines into nerve terminals (see p. 88), and therefore delays inactivation; amphetamine releases stored monoamines from nerve terminals (see p. 82)). Antidepressant drugs, like **imipramine**, are inhibitors of monoamine uptake. On the other hand, some drugs that cause sedation are known to decrease functional monoamine activity. Reserpine depletes neuronal stores (see p. 79) and **chlorpromazine** is an antagonist at monoamine receptors (see p. 237). Many drugs useful in treating disorders of mood are only effective on chronic treatment and acute pharmacological effects may not be relevant.

In the CNS α-adrenoceptors (α_1- and α_2-subtypes) and β-adrenoceptors are present. Chronic treatment with tricyclic antidepressant drugs causes β-adrenoceptors to become less responsive and α_1-adrenoceptors to become more responsive. Since antidepressant activity is slow to develop, these changes may be more relevant to the therapeutic activity than inhibition of monoamine uptake.

Dopamine receptors have been subdivided, dependent on whether they are linked with adenylyl cyclase (D_1) or not (D_2).

The ascending 5-hydroxytryptamine tracts, which also innervate the limbic areas, are shown in Figure 5.3. The monoamine theory of nervous and mental disease includes the functions of 5-hydroxytryptamine. Alterations in 5-hydroxytryptamine functions are linked to changes in sensitivity to painful stimuli, altered sexual behaviour, sleep patterns,

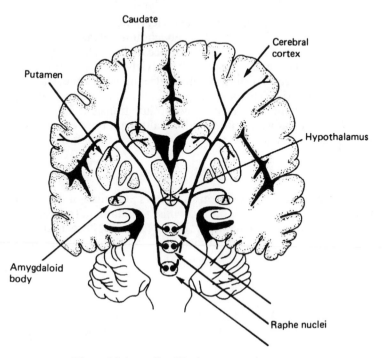

Figure 5.3 Ascending 5-hydroxytryptamine tracts

anxiety and disorders of appetite. The role of 5-hydroxytryptamine in such diverse and complex behaviours can be explained by it having multiple kinds of receptor in the CNS, which have been identified by pharmacological and molecular techniques.

5-Hydroxytryptamine nerve terminals in the CNS have an uptake transporter which removes the transmitter from the ECF. A new class of effective antidepressant drugs are the selective serotonin reuptake inhibitors (SSRIs) which include **fluoxetine**.

Adrenaline and histamine may have roles as neurotransmitters or neuromodulators in the CNS.

Acetylcholine

Neurones that release acetylcholine and that contain the synthesizing enzyme choline acetyltransferase are distributed widely in most areas of the CNS, together with the inactivating enzymes, cholinesterases. High densities of acetylcholine neurones occur in the thalamus, basal ganglia, brain stem and spinal cord. Nicotinic acetylcholine receptors occur in the CNS and molecular techniques have identified a family of muscarinic receptor subtypes, designated M_1, M_2, etc.

Acetylcholine usually functions as an excitatory neurotransmitter. Acetylcholine-releasing interneurones in the caudate nucleus/putamen of the basal ganglia have excitatory functions in movement control and antagonists at muscarinic acetylcholine receptors are useful in the management of Parkinson's disease. There is a clear involvement of acetylcholine in pain perception.

Experimental studies implicate acetylcholine in cognitive processes. Many kinds of neurones, including acetylcholine-releasing cells, disappear with the severe neurodegeneration that occurs in Alzheimer's disease, but there is some sparing of muscarinic acetylcholine receptors. The long-acting inhibitor of cholinesterase, tetrahydroaminoacridine, was developed to activate muscarinic acetylcholine receptors indirectly. Some patients with Alzheimer's disease have shown mild, transient improvements in cognition with tetrahydroaminoacridine, although they experience acetylcholinergic side-effects.

Amino acid neurotransmitters

Several amino acids are neurotransmitters. Gamma-aminobutyric acid (GABA) and glycine are inhibitory, whilst L-glutamate (glutamate) and L-aspartate (aspartate) are excitatory. Between them, these amino acids, and perhaps others, are the neurotransmitters produced by the majority of CNS neurones.

GABA

Concentrations of GABA in the brain are relatively high because it is both an abundant inhibitory neurotransmitter and a metabolite linked with the Krebs cycle (Figure 5.4). Very few GABA neurones are found in the periphery.

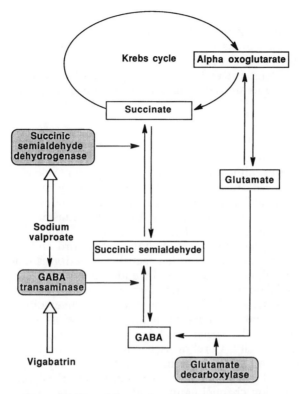

Figure 5.4 Sites of drug action on GABA metabolism

GABA is synthesized from glutamic acid (glutamate) by a decarboxy-lase. There is a CNS uptake system (transporter) into both nerve termi-nals and glia as well as the metabolizing enzyme, GABA transaminase, producing succinic semialdehyde. GABA receptors are of the GABA$_A$ and GABA$_B$ kinds.

GABA is invariably inhibitory on neuronal activity.

GABA neurones are involved in the control of movement by virtue of the presence of GABA neurone tracts within the basal ganglia and cerebellum, where Purkinje cells are GABAergic. Mimics of GABA, both directly and indirectly acting, are effective in the treatment of epilepsy. **Phenytoin** and *phenobarbitone* enhance GABA transmission by a mecha-nism that is unclear. *Vigabatrin* is an irreversible inhibitor of GABA transaminase and whilst **sodium valproate** also inhibits this enzyme, it inhibits succinic semialdehyde dehydrogenase more effectively (Figure 5.4). Whenever GABA breakdown is inhibited, the amino acid accumu-lates in the brain. This ability to increase GABA concentrations by enzyme inhibition is used to treat epilepsy by depressing cortical motor functions and reducing seizure spread.

In contrast, the benzodiazepines have a specific benzodiazepine recep-tor, which is coupled to a GABA$_A$ receptor and which, when activated, enhances GABA transmission by increasing chloride ion flux through

STAFFS UNIVERSITY LIBRARY

neurone membranes (see Figure 5.14). This indirect mechanism via a GABA receptor is probably how benzodiazepines exert their anticonvulsant actions. Antagonists at $GABA_A$ receptors (bicuculline, picrotoxin) are powerful convulsant poisons.

Baclofen, an agonist at $GABA_B$ receptors, which occur in the spinal cord, is effective in alleviating muscle spasm, but may cause sedation and hypotonia.

Excitatory amino acids

Many CNS neurones release glutamate, an excitatory amino acid (EAA) neurotransmitter, although there are also aspartate-releasing brain cells. Glutamate and aspartate occur in high concentrations in the CNS but their close similarity and involvement in neuronal metabolism complicate the identification of cells utilizing EAA neurotransmitters. Glutamate neurones are highly abundant in neocortex (including pyramidal neurones), in hippocampus, cerebellum, spinal cord and elsewhere. The importance of glutamate lies in the fact that it performs much of the fast cell-to-cell signalling in the CNS. In addition, the role of glutamate in ischaemic (stroke-induced) brain damage and its putative role as an excitotoxic substance in some neurodegenerative diseases, such as Huntington's disease and motor neurone disease, is of great interest. Overactivation of the specific EAA receptors causes neurone damage through excitotoxicity. Cerebral ischaemia causes local release of glutamate in the brain and the resulting excitotoxicity may cause some of the brain damage. The CNS contains several classes of EAA receptor, including ionotropic (ion channel gating) and metabotropic (second messenger producing) kinds. Antagonists at ionotropic EAA receptors would have therapeutic potential in treating the consequences of stroke but, despite much research, clinically acceptable compounds have yet to be found.

Glycine

Glycine is an inhibitory amino acid neurotransmitter primarily in the spinal cord.

A collateral of the α-motor neurone synapses with the Renshaw cell within the ventral horn of the spinal cord as shown in Figure 5.5.

This collateral releases acetylcholine, which depolarizes the Renshaw cell (via nicotinic acetylcholine receptors). The induced Renshaw cell activity liberates glycine, which causes hyperpolarization of the α-motor neurone. This forms a negative feedback loop, which limits activity in the α-motor neurone. Tetanus toxin prevents the release of glycine from the Renshaw cell, causing the uncontrolled spasm of skeletal muscle seen after tetanus infection. Strychnine is an antagonist of glycine at its receptors on the α-motor neurone, which explains why spasm of skeletal muscle is the main feature of strychnine poisoning.

Peptides

Dozens of peptides have been implied to have neurotransmitter function. Peptide transmission seems to differ from that of other neurotransmitters,

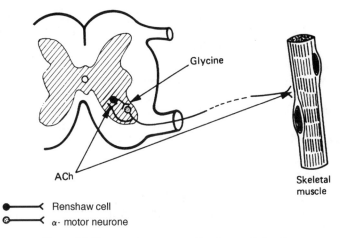

Figure 5.5 The α-motor neurone–Renshaw cell circuit

in that peptides are released from precursors at the nerve ending (cf. axonal transport of other neurotransmitters to the nerve ending). Many coexist with other neurotransmitters and may participate in co-transmission. Their action is terminated by metabolism. Many of them also exist in the periphery in neurones, especially in the enteric system. Some related peptides have hormonal in addition to neurotransmitter function.

The opioid peptides

There are three families of opioid peptides – the enkephalins, endorphins and dynorphins.

The enkephalins are derived from a single precursor. They have the amino acid sequences of:

Tyr.Gly.Gly.Phe.Met – met-enkephalin
Tyr.Gly.Gly.Phe.Leu – leu-enkephalin

They are widely distributed throughout the CNS, including those regions involved in pain perception – the substantia gelatinosa of the spinal cord, peri-aqueductal grey matter of the mid brain and the limbic system. They are also found in the periphery, in sympathetic ganglia, and enkephalin neurones are found in the intestinal tract.

There are also several endorphins, though it is not clear which are neurotransmitters or hormones and which are metabolites. The most widely studied is β-endorphin, a peptide (31 amino acids) fragment of the anterior pituitary hormone, β-lipotrophin. The N-terminal five amino acids of β-endorphin are the same as those of met-enkephalin.

β-Endorphin is essentially a pituitary hormone and is released along with ACTH in stress (they share a common precursor). It is also present in a very limited number of CNS nuclei (hypothalamic and solitary tract).

The dynorphins are of intermediate size – typical is dynorphin-A, which has 17 amino acid residues. The N-terminal five amino acids are the same

as the sequence of leu-enkephalin. The dynorphins are as widely distributed as the enkephalins, but their concentrations are lower. However, they
are more potent than the enkephalins.

Structural correlations

Figure 5.6 compares the structures of **morphine** and the enkephalins. The
terminal tyrosine of enkephalin corresponds to the phenol group of
morphine and the amino groups are held in the same spatial plane. The
NH_2-terminal end of all endogenous opioid peptides commence:
Tyr.Gly.Gly.Phe.

Opioid receptors

It is clear that there are multiple kinds of opioid receptor; the situation
becomes progressively more complicated with over 10 receptor kinds
currently mooted.

The enkephalins are thought to interact preferentially with δ-opioid
receptors, the dynorphins with κ-opioid receptors. The receptors for the
endorphins may differ.

There is considerable overlap between these receptors, and every opioid
peptide or drug has at least some affinity for each kind of receptor.
Similarly **naloxone** is active at each, though it is more effective at the μ-
opioid receptor. More selective antagonists are available.

Physiological role of opioid peptides

Instrumental in the discovery of these peptide neurotransmitters and
the research into their physiological role has been the existence of at
least two peripheral neuroeffector junctions at which opioids and endor-

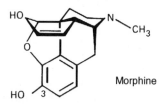

Morphine

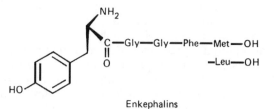

Enkephalins

Figure 5.6 Structural analogy between **morphine** and the enkephalins

phins inhibit neurotransmitter release. These are the guinea-pig ileum and mouse vas deferens (neurotransmitters being acetylcholine and noradrenaline respectively). These two sites have been extensively used as peripheral models of the central mechanism of action of opioids since:

(1) Potency ratios between agonists are the same as those for analgesic activity in people.
(2) Antagonist as well as agonist activity can be demonstrated for some compounds at both peripheral sites, as in the CNS.

It is known that in the CNS the opioid peptide neurotransmitters can act presynaptically to inhibit neurotransmitter release (though not necessarily of acetylcholine or noradrenaline).

Evidence for the physiological role of these peptides comes from our knowledge of the pharmacology of **morphine** and, more importantly, **naloxone**, the distribution of the peptides in the brain and the consequences of their local application.

In addition to pain perception, the peptides apparently have a role in modulation of hormone release, mood, consciousness and brain stem function – respiration, cough and vomiting. Coexistence with several other neurotransmitters has been reported in various brain regions. In the future, opioid derivatives with actions not obviously related to those of **morphine** may have clinical use in the control of appetite, hypertension and psychotic disease.

Other peptides

Substance P is quite widely distributed, with high concentrations in the dorsal horn where it has been suggested to be involved in sensory perception. It coexists with 5-hydroxytryptamine in the medullary raphe and with acetylcholine in the pontine neurones.

A number of other peptides, many of which are well known for their hormonal activity, have been localized in CNS neurones. Neurotensin and neuropeptide Y commonly coexist with monoamines and thus their pharmacology may be associated with overall control of central monoamine transmission. Similar neuromodulator roles have been suggested for cholecystokinin, somatostatin, vasoactive intestinal peptide (VIP) and thyroid releasing hormone (TRH).

Bradykinin and angiotensin may have neurotransmitter function but they remain a more important target for drug action outside the CNS.

Summary

(1) Classical neurotransmitters in the CNS (amino acids, monoamines, acetylcholine) occur in specific neurones, and they interact with each other.
(2) There is some understanding of their normal functions and the consequences of disturbed function.
(3) Peptide-releasing neurones have modulatory roles on CNS activity.

(4) Individual targets (e.g. receptors, enzymes, uptake carriers) afford opportunities for drugs selectively to modify the functions of neurotransmitters.

Extrapyramidal disorders of movement

There are two important neuronal pathways involved in motor coordination that originate in the cerebral cortex. One, including the corticospinal system, descends to the brain stem passing through a region of the medulla oblongata called the pyramids. The other makes multiple synaptic contacts within the basal ganglia before descending to the brain stem, bypassing the pyramids laterally – hence the terms extrapyramidal tracts and extrapyramidal disorders.

The bilaterally represented basal ganglia are considered to comprise the caudate nucleus, the lentiform nucleus (putamen and globus pallidus), the subthalamic nucleus and the substantia nigra. The caudate and the putamen together are known as the striatum.

Major neurotransmitters in the basal ganglia are dopamine and GABA (which are inhibitory) and glutamate and acetylcholine (which are excitatory).

Because of clearly defined motor disorders that have been shown to be related to changes in specific neurotransmitter functions, and an understanding of the drugs effective in the treatment of such disorders, more is known about this aspect of brain function than any other.

Parkinson's disease

This disease provides a good example of a neurological disorder that can be attributed to a defect in a central neurotransmitter system. It is also of interest because it demonstrates how investigations of chemical transmission processes in the CNS ultimately led to the development of a rational therapy for the disease.

Parkinson's disease is characterized by tremor and rigidity in skeletal muscle, akinesia (lit. lack of movement – hypokinesia would be a more accurate description) and bradykinesia (slowness of movement). There is a characteristic posture and gait, and absence of facial expressions. Severe depression commonly accompanies these motor changes. When the disease is first recognized the signs and symptoms may be mild, but the disease progresses and may ultimately lead to total incapacitation.

Treatment

Originally empirical medical treatment involved the use of antagonists at muscarinic acetylcholine receptors. These drugs were more effective against tremor than against rigidity and a high proportion of cases showed little or no improvement. Synthetic atropine derivatives (*orphenadrine, benzhexol*) are used to supplement **levodopa** (see below).

Levodopa

In 1960 therapy was introduced based on the dopaminergic nature of the nigrostriatal tracts in animals and the loss of dopamine in the striatum of brains taken from parkinsonian patients post-mortem. It was postulated that in Parkinson's disease there was a functional deficiency of dopamine in the basal ganglia and that correction of that deficiency should lead to an improvement in the condition. Dopamine administration could not achieve this because it does not pass the blood brain–barrier and has a very short $t_{1/2}$. Therefore the precursor amino acid **levodopa** (L-DOPA) was used. This crosses the blood–brain barrier and can be converted to dopamine within the brain by the enzyme aromatic L-amino acid decarboxylase. **Levodopa** is the drug of choice in the medical treatment of Parkinson's disease.

This has led to the postulate that in the striatum there is a functional balance between acetylcholine and dopamine and that any change causing a decrease in the activity of dopamine relative to acetylcholine (Figure 5.7) will produce the parkinsonian condition. The balance may be restored either by reducing the influence of acetylcholine (by antagonists at muscarinic acetylcholine receptors) or by increasing that of dopamine (**levodopa**).

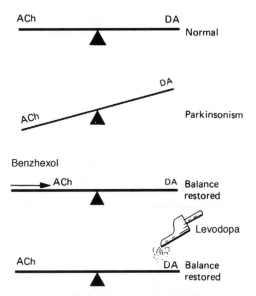

Figure 5.7 The functional balance between acetylcholine (ACh) and dopamine (DA) in the striatum, the imbalance in parkinsonism and its restoration by either antagonists at acetylcholine receptors or agonists at dopamine receptors

Four of the undesirable actions of **levodopa** may also be explained in terms of overactivity in dopaminergic systems:

(1) Vomiting – the chemosensitive trigger zone (CTZ) of the medullary vomiting centre (situated in the area postrema on the floor of the fourth cerebral ventricle close to the CO_2 sensing elements).
(2) Involuntary movements (dyskinesias).
(3) Psychosis.
(4) Some of the gastrointestinal and cardiovascular (hypotension, tachy-dysrhythmias) disturbances that occur during **levodopa** therapy may be peripheral in origin and related to the high doses required.

Since **levodopa** has a low therapeutic index, partly because relatively little dopamine is rendered available to the striatum, two drug combinations are currently used to enhance drug availability where it is needed.

In combination with an inhibitor of decarboxylase
Significant reduction in dosage is obtained by combining **levodopa** with an inhibitor of aromatic L-amino acid decarboxylase that does not pass the blood–brain barrier (*carbidopa, benserazide*). In this case little of the **levodopa** is metabolized in the periphery so that more is available for conversion to dopamine after penetrating the brain. Consequently, lower oral doses are required.

In combination with an inhibitor of MAO-B
MAOs are divided into two groups dependent on specificities of substrates and inhibitors; that which exists in the striatum and oxidizes dopamine is termed MAO-B.

Selegiline is a selective inhibitor of MAO-B and enhances striatal dopamine availability when used in combination with **levodopa**. It does not share with inhibitors of MAO-A the adverse interactions with drugs or tyramine-containing foodstuffs that elicit dangerous hypertensive crises (see p. 87).

Other agonists at dopamine receptors

Amantadine and *bromocriptine* are agonists at dopamine receptors. Neither appears to be as effective as **levodopa**. In most cases of Parkinson's disease selected for medical treatment, **levodopa** and an antimuscarinic agent used together produce better results than either alone.

Parkinson's disease, along with the other extrapyramidal disorders, is an unpleasant, debilitating and progressive disease. The patient benefits from only a small improvement in condition but drug treatment does not slow the disease progression.

Huntington's chorea

In this hereditary disease there is a progressive impairment of motor coordination with grimacing, distorted speech and bizarre movements of the limbs conveying a dance-like gait (hence chorea). Dementia may follow the motor symptoms.

On examination post-mortem, there is atrophy of components of the basal ganglia, especially the caudate nucleus, and a deficiency in GABA and the enzyme responsible for its synthesis, glutamic acid decarboxylase. There is also a deficiency of choline acetyltransferase and a functional excess of dopamine.

Treatment

Whilst the symptoms can be treated with antipsychotic drugs (*haloperidol*), the drug of choice is *tetrabenazine*.

Tetrabenazine causes a reserpine-like depletion of dopamine. Reserpine itself depletes catecholamines in the central and peripheral nervous systems and also drastically depletes brain 5-hydroxytryptamine, and because of this non-electivity it is a toxic drug that has no clinical use. In contrast, *tetrabenazine* causes more selective depletion of dopamine in the CNS without interfering with peripheral catecholamines or central 5-hydroxytryptamine. It does not cause the hypotension, and suicidal depression characteristic of reserpine, but its use may be limited by the development of depression.

Drug-induced extrapyramidal disorders

Iatrogenic motor disorders are common.

Drug-induced parkinsonism

From consideration of Figure 5.7, it is clear that drugs that either enhance central acetylcholinergic activity or reduce dopamine activity will cause a parkinsonian state.

No centrally acting mimic of acetylcholine has had any long-term clinical use, which may cause drug-induced parkinsonism as a side-effect. However, physostigmine is known to cause tremor.

In contrast, there is widespread use of antagonists at dopamine receptors, mainly in psychiatry.

The antipsychotic drugs are all capable of inducing such extrapyramidal disorders, though the incidence and severity differs within the group. The incidence is greatest with *fluphenazine* and *haloperidol*, moderate with **chlorpromazine** and least with *thioridazine*.

Treatment of extrapyramidal effects is by reduction of dose and addition of antimuscarinic drugs.

Drug-induced tardive dyskinesia

This is another characteristic adverse effect of the antipsychotic drugs. The characteristics of tardive dyskinesia are a delayed impairment of motor coordination with typical abnormal involuntary movements, notably of the face, tongue and neck. Paradoxically this is due to excess dopaminergic activity. During prolonged antagonism at dopamine receptors, there is compensatory supersensitivity to dopamine, perhaps mediated by proliferation of dopamine receptors (cf. denervation supersensitivity).

STAFFS UNIVERSITY LIBRARY

Whilst it is clear that this extrapyramidal disorder could theoretically be treated by increasing the dose of the antipsychotic drug, in the long term this only aggravates the problem since it precipitates further supersensitivity.

Extrapyramidal disorders caused by drugs other than the antipsychotic agents

Antagonism at dopamine receptors is also the mechanism of action of many antiemetic drugs and these are also capable of causing extrapyramidal disorders. Some of these are prescribed either as antiemetic or antipsychotic agents (*perphenazine*), others are used solely as antiemetic agents (*metoclopramide*).

Summary

(1) There is some understanding of how specific neurotransmitters are abnormal in diseases of the basal ganglia. For example, dopamine deficiency seems to be the underlying defect in Parkinson's disease.
(2) This knowledge underlies some rational drug treatments of the movement disorders. For example, the precursor of dopamine, **levodopa**, and agonists at dopamine receptors are useful in treating the symptoms of Parkinson's disease.

Antidepressant drugs

Depressive illness falls broadly into two categories:

(1) Neurotic (reactive) depression: depression as a response to stress or problems particularly those involving loss of an emotional attachment (e.g. bereavement).
(2) Psychotic (endogenous) depression: manic-depressive psychosis is characterized by sustained phases of either excitement (hypomania, mania) or, more commonly, severe depression.

In contrast with psychotic depression, neurotic depression rarely requires drug therapy, but between these extremes there may be a continuous spectrum of depressive illness. The use of drugs alone to treat depression is rarely sufficient; counselling, psychotherapy and electroconvulsive therapy may be required.

There is strong evidence to suggest that depressive illnesses arise from a functional lack of noradrenaline and/or 5-hydroxytryptamine within the limbic system.

The aim of chemotherapy in depressive illness is restoration of normal function by facilitating or stimulating transmission at central monoaminergic synapses.

Drugs that prevent enzymatic destruction of neurotransmitters

MAO exists as two distinct isoenzymes – MAO-A and MAO-B. Noradrenaline and 5-hydroxytryptamine are preferential substrates for MAO-A, dopamine for MAO-B.

The older non-selective inhibitors of MAO are structurally related to amphetamine and may be slowly reversible (*tranylcypromine*) or irreversible (**phenelzine**); both inhibit MAO-A and MAO-B. These drugs affect both noradrenaline and 5-hydroxytryptamine. *Selegiline* selectively inhibits MAO-B but is ineffective in depression.

The ability of inhibitors of MAO to attenuate the sedation and hypothermia induced in animals by reserpine can be used as an indication of the therapeutic potential of antidepressant drugs.

Inhibitors of MAO elevate the mood of depressed patients and this forms their primary use, but there is a 7–10 days delay before their clinical effect is seen, although inhibition of the enzyme is apparent within a few hours of administration. These drugs suppress paradoxical sleep (see p. 256) but alleviate the sleep problems associated with depression.

It is still not certain that the antidepressant actions of these compounds rely solely on their ability to inhibit MAO.

Adverse effects

Acute overdosage may cause excitement, insomnia, pyrexia and convulsions. Chronic toxicity includes hepatotoxicity, orthostatic hypotension and excessive CNS stimulation that manifests itself as hypomania, tremor, insomnia and, in some instances, convulsions.

An important problem is the change produced in the response to exogenous substances present in food or administered as drugs (see pp. 86, 444). The potentiation of tyramine in foodstuffs is the best publicized effect where, because of the inhibition of gut and liver MAO, dietary tyramine is not inactivated and achieves a high concentration in plasma. Tyramine is an indirectly acting sympathomimetic agent. **Phentolamine** is an effective antidote but patients receiving inhibitors of MAO must be told which foodstuffs and drugs to avoid to obviate such a crisis. It is largely this problem that has led to the virtual disuse of these drugs in depressive illness. However, the recent development of reversible and selective inhibitors of MAO-A (*moclobemide*) that do not appear to exhibit such a marked toxic interaction with tyramine has reawakened interest in inhibitors of MAO.

Drugs that prevent monoamine re-uptake into the nerve terminal

Antidepressant drugs such as **imipramine** and **amitriptyline** are effective inhibitors of neuronal re-uptake of both noradrenaline and 5-hydroxytryptamine. These drugs, which are often referred to as tricyclic antidepressant drugs, are structurally derived from the phenothiazine antipsychotic drugs

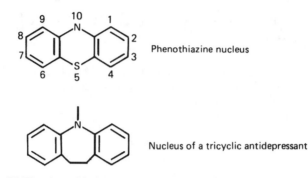

Figure 5.8 The phenothiazine antipsychotic and tricyclic antidepressant drug nuclei

(Figure 5.8). All compounds in this category prevent the re-uptake of noradrenaline and 5-hydroxytryptamine by inhibition of the active uptake process that is in part responsible for the inactivation of these neuronally released monoamines.

Tricyclic compounds are broken down quickly in the body by demethyl-ation. Their metabolites (desmethylimipramine, nortriptyline) also have antidepressant properties and have approximately twice the potency of the parent compounds. Although the action of these drugs within the synapse may be observed within 30 min of administration, the clinical effects, as with the inhibitors of MAO, develop only slowly over 2–3 weeks. The explanation for this is not known but may involve autoregulatory feedback mechanisms acting via presynaptic receptors.

Imipramine and **amitriptyline** also produce a competitive antagonism at central muscarinic acetylcholine receptors. Such antagonism may contribute to the elevation of mood and awareness. Other effects due to this property (dry mouth, urinary retention, blurred vision) are troublesome but may be minimized by giving a large single daily dose of the drug at night without loss of antidepressant effect. The antimuscarinic effect of **amitriptyline** in particular has been exploited to treat nocturnal enuresis in children.

Imipramine and **amitriptyline** frequently give rise to serious cardiovas-cular problems. These arise from the inhibition of uptake of noradrena-line and adrenaline (potentiating these agents), the antimuscarinic effect, an antagonism at α-adrenoceptors and a direct quinidine-like effect on cardiac cell membranes.

Amitriptyline and *nortriptyline* are sedative and are used in psychotic depression accompanied by severe anxiety and agitation. **Imipramine** and compounds related to it are less sedative. Protriptyline, on the contrary, has stimulant properties and is used to treat 'somnolent' psychotic depres-sion where motor retardation and inertia form part of the illness.

Drugs that preferentially prevent the uptake of noradrenaline or 5-hydroxytryptamine

Drugs that preferentially inhibit the re-uptake of noradrenaline or 5-hydroxytryptamine offer the possibility of selective action in the treatment of depressive illness, although there is little clinical evidence to support this notion. Selective inhibitors of noradrenaline re-uptake include mapro-tiline and *lofepramine*. SSRIs include **fluoxetine**. SSRIs lack antimus-carinic unwanted effects and have little effect on noradrenaline re-uptake and may be more safely prescribed in patients taking antihypertensive agents and in those with cardiac disease.

Central agonists and antagonists at 5-hydroxytryptamine receptors

Iprindole has a chemical structure bearing slight similarities to 5-hydroxy-tryptamine and it may act in part as an antidepressant by an agonist action at central 5-hydroxytryptamine receptors. Its efficacy in both mild neurotic depression and less severe psychotic depression suggests that it may also have an action at central adrenoceptors. It is less sedative than the tricyclic antidepressant drugs and has weak antimuscarinic activity but it is hepato-toxic and is contraindicated in liver disease.

Buspirone is an agonist at 5-HT_{1A} receptors with antidepressant and anxiolytic activity.

Mianserin and *trazodone* are antidepressant drugs whose mechanism of action is obscure. They have little effect on the re-uptake of noradrena-line or 5-hydroxytryptamine, but they may enhance noradrenaline release by blocking pre-synaptic α-adrenoceptors.

Drugs acting on electrolytes

Many patients suffering from affective illness show a grossly elevated concentration of neuronal intracellular Na^+. In depression this is typically doubled; in mania neuronal Na^+ retention is even higher. A **lithium** salt, given as a slow-release preparation, displaces the Na^+ and the intracellu-lar concentration of Na^+ returns towards normal. This is an effective way of treating mania, but in depression, the illness must first be eliminated using a tricyclic or other compound, following which a **lithium** salt may be given prophylactically. By this means, recurring bouts of depressive illness, which often become part of the lifestyle of a patient, can be entirely elimi-nated. The use of this compound is limited by its acute nephrotoxicity; dosage must be determined for each patient and regular checks on Li^+ clearance should be maintained.

Future developments

It has been suggested that the failure of noradrenergic transmission that is believed to underlie psychotic depression may be due to overactivity or oversensitivity of presynaptic α-adrenoceptors. Similar mechanisms may operate to cause reduced 5-hydroxytryptamine transmission. Presynaptic receptors may offer novel targets for drug treatment (antagonists).

Summary

(1) Most effective antidepressant drugs enhance monoaminergic transmission in the brain by preventing re-uptake or preventing breakdown of the monoamines.
(2) Enhancement of both noradrenaline and 5-hydroxytryptamine transmission are important, with some drugs showing selectivity for one or the other.
(3) Therapeutic responses are slow to develop, indicating that the acute biochemical changes are not the whole story.
(4) Bipolar (manic) depression may be treated additionally with lithium, which normalizes intracellular Na^+ concentrations.

Antipsychotic drugs

Psychosis

Psychosis is a major mental disorder characterized by derangement, loss of contact with reality and often delusions, illusions and hallucinations.

In organic psychosis (e.g. alcoholism, senility) damage is evident macroscopically in the brain post-mortem. In contrast, in functional psychosis the brain appears macroscopically normal at examination post-mortem.

Schizophrenia embodies a group of functional psychotic disorders characterized by retreat from reality, bizarre or regressive behaviour, auditory hallucinations and commonly delusions of grandeur or persecution (paranoia).

Antipsychotic drugs are useful in the treatment of psychoses and in pre-anaesthetic medication. In the past they have misleadingly been termed neuroleptic agents (mood regulating) or major tranquillizers.

Antipsychotic drugs

Current antipsychotic drugs originate from different chemical classes.

Phenothiazines

Phenothiazine has a tricyclic structure (Figure 5.8) and is the nucleus of numerous derivatives with antipsychotic activity (**chlorpromazine**).

Thioxanthenes

Substitution of the N in position 10 of phenothiazine (Figure 5.8) by C produces thioxanthene. Some derivatives of thioxanthene have antipsychotic activity similar to that of **chlorpromazine** – *flupenthixol*.

Butyrophenones

Butyrophenones are tricyclic compounds but are unrelated chemically to either the phenothiazines or thioxanthenes. Some butyrophenones have antipsychotic activity similar to that of **chlorpromazine** – *haloperidol*.

Diphenylbutylpiperidines

Pimozide causes less sedation than **chlorpromazine** and may be the antipsychotic of choice in schizophrenia in apathetic withdrawn patients.

Dibenzodiazepines

Clozapine has low propensity to produce extrapyramidal adverse effects and may be useful in treatment-resistant patients.

Antipsychotic drugs of different chemical classes produce qualitatively similar effects on mood and behaviour, differing only in potency. Butyrophenones are generally the most potent.

These drugs exert a relatively selective depressant effect on conditioned responses. In people, they reduce defensive hostility, attention and emotional responses. Intellectual activities are not altered appreciably. The most obvious effect of **chlorpromazine** is a dose-related depression of behaviour. In aggressive animals with low doses there is a taming effect. As the dose is increased there is reduced locomotor activity and at higher doses the animals become immobile and catatonic. In the catatonic state the animal has increased muscle tone and will for a time maintain an abnormal posture imposed on it. Induction of catatonia distinguishes **chlorpromazine** from the barbiturates (see p. 264) and the anxiolytic agents (see p. 260). It is also possible to demonstrate inhibition of conditioned behaviour (e.g. escape behaviour in response to a bell) with doses too low to modify an unconditioned response (e.g. escape behaviour in response to a mild noxious stimulus). This again is in contrast to the effects of non-specific depressant agents with which both conditioned and unconditioned responses are similarly affected.

These antipsychotic agents are the drugs of choice in the treatment of both functional psychoses (notably schizophrenia) and organic psychoses. Antipsychotic agents are also effective antagonists of the centrally acting sympathomimetic agents and hallucinogens and are the drugs of choice in poisoning from these drugs.

Mechanism of antipsychotic action

The similar effects of chemically different antipsychotic agents on behaviour and mood are ascribed to their common ability to block dopamine receptors in the mesolimbic system, a part of the brain controlling emotion, behaviour and mood. The antipsychotic action correlates significantly with antagonism at D_2 and not at D_1 dopamine receptors (see p. 221). This antipsychotic property suggests that psychoses are manifestations of excess dopaminergic activity in the mesolimbic system but such an abnormality has not been substantiated by non-pharmacological means.

Other effects due to dopamine antagonism

Blockade of D_1 and D_2 dopamine receptors in the brain by antipsychotic agents is not restricted to the mesolimbic system.

Antagonism of dopamine in the caudate and putamen causes rigidity and tremor of skeletal muscle (see p. 231, Figure 5.9). These extrapyramidal motor effects are most prominent with butyrophenones (*haloperidol*) and phenothiazines with a piperazine group at position 10 in the phenothiazine nucleus (Figure 5.8, *fluphenazine, prochlorperazine, trifluoperazine*).

Centrally acting antimuscarinic agents (benzhexol) that relieve Parkinson's disease (see p. 228) reduce antipsychotic drug-induced motor effects. Tranquillization with a piperidine-substituted phenothiazine (*thioridazine*) may be preferable therapy, because this kind has a lower incidence of extrapyramidal motor disturbances. This is attributable to the ratio of antimuscarinic : antidopaminergic activity being greater in piperidine phenothiazines than in other antipsychotic agents.

Since dopamine is an important neurotransmitter within the vomiting reflex, antagonists at dopamine receptors are important antiemetic drugs (see p. 241).

Antipsychotic agents antagonize dopamine-mediated inhibition of prolactin release from the anterior pituitary gland and may cause an excess flow of milk (galactorrhoea, see p. 157). Elevated dopamine content may cause increased libido in women and decreased libido and depression in men. Appetite can be stimulated with resultant obesity.

Effects not due to dopamine antagonism

Antipsychotic drugs can block central and peripheral receptors other than those for dopamine. Receptors that may be affected include muscarinic

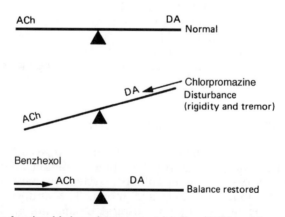

Figure 5.9 The functional balance between acetylcholine (ACh) and dopamine (DA) in the striatum, its disturbance by antipsychotic agents and its correction by antagonists at muscarinic acetylcholine receptors (Figure 5.7)

acetylcholine receptors, α-adrenoceptors and H_1 histamine receptors. Blockade of non-dopamine receptors is most marked with phenothiazines and least with butyrophenones.

Clinically useful effects

Numerous effects can result from blockade of non-dopamine receptors by phenothiazines, and some of these are clinically useful, including:

(1) Antagonism at muscarinic acetylcholine receptors – alleviating motion sickness (*promethazine*).
(2) Antagonism at H_1 histamine receptors – alleviating allergic reactions (*promethazine*).
(3) The sedative activity in suppressing restlessness caused by mental disturbances or alleviating itching (pruritus) associated with jaundice (*promethazine*).
(4) The potentiating effect on the action of other central depressant agents, particularly opioid analgesic agents (**chlorpromazine**).

Unwanted effects

Some effects resulting from blockade of non-dopamine receptors are unwanted – on the cardiovascular system (orthostatic hypotension), the gastrointestinal tract (constipation) and the eye (blurring of vision).

Sensitization reactions to phenothiazines occur as blood dyscrasias, cholestatic jaundice and skin rashes.

Choice of antipsychotic drug

There is no convincing evidence that combinations of antipsychotic drugs are more beneficial than one drug alone. The choice of drug depends on the acceptability of a particular unwanted effect in individual patients. The differing abilities of antipsychotic drugs to induce extrapyramidal motor effects (see p. 231) and autonomic disturbances (see above) have been noted. Outpatient treatment of psychotic or agitated patients who may not take their tablets regularly is facilitated by the use of long-acting preparations (*fluphenazine decanoate* injection deep i/m), despite the common occurrence of extrapyramidal motor effects with piperazine-substituted phenothiazines.

Summary

(1) Antagonists at D_2 dopamine receptors are the mainstay of treatment of psychosis.
(2) Parkinsonian adverse effects are common, and prolonged therapy may result in tardive dyskinesias.
(3) The phenothiazine group of antipsychotic drugs are antagonists at several other receptors – H_1 histamine and muscarinic acetylcholine receptors and α-adrenoceptors.

Vomiting, emetic and antiemetic agents

The output of the medullary vomiting centre, which lies laterally in the reticular formation, near the solitary tract, passes:

(1) To high centres to be perceived as the sensation of nausea.
(2) By parasympathetic outflows to the gut (relaxation of the cardiac or oesophagogastric sphincter) and the exocrine glands (sweating and salivation).
(3) By somatic efferent pathways to the expiratory (retching) and inspiratory (expulsion) muscles of respiration and postural muscles.

Linked with the vomiting centre is the CTZ. This area is sited on the floor of the fourth cerebral ventricle in the area postrema. It lies outside the blood–brain barrier and so can detect toxic substances in the blood.

Important neurotransmitters associated with the vomiting reflex are 5-hydroxytryptamine (particularly mediated by 5-HT$_3$ receptors), dopamine (agonists at dopamine receptors are emetic) and acetylcholine (note the increased parasympathetic activity that precedes and continues during vomiting).

Vomiting is usually preceded by parasympathetic activation and is effected by respiratory muscles.

There are parallel mechanisms for the initiation of the vomiting response to any stimulus. All therapeutically useful antiemetic drugs seem to act on the input circuitry of the emetic centre. The neural and humoral inputs are of four origins (at least) as follows:

(1) Psychic – bombardment from higher centres generated by, for example, the sight, sound and smell of someone else vomiting or conditioned anticipation of a noxious stimulus, for example, cancer chemotherapy.
(2) Gastrointestinal afferent nerves – excited by, for instance, pharyngeal mechanical stimulation, chemical damage, irritation or disease in the gut.
(3) Motion – which is only partly of vestibular (labyrinthine) origin, a significant part is visual and disagreement between the visual and proprioceptive versions of the position of the body in space is a particularly potent cause.
(4) Chemical – many drugs can directly (CTZ) or indirectly (from gut) cause nausea and vomiting as a part of their acute toxicity: agonists at dopamine receptors (**levodopa**), agonists at opioid receptors (which may be related to dopaminergic activity), oestrogens, **digoxin**, *cisplatin* and the other alkylating agents used in cancer chemotherapy.

Antiemetic agents

Antiemetic agents are generally antagonists of 5-hydroxytryptamine, dopamine, acetylcholine, or all of these.

As with coughing, clinical situations in which vomiting serves a protective function should not be suppressed by drugs. In most clinical situations, however, emesis serves no useful purpose and may exacerbate the condition of the patient – early pregnancy, travel sickness, postoperative period, migraine, radiotherapy, cancer chemotherapy and drug therapy (e.g. **morphine**).

Motion sickness

Hyoscine (see p. 69) is most effective, though sedative and producing all the expected antimuscarinic peripheral side-effects. Better tolerated (though still sedative) but less effective are some antagonists at H_1 histamine receptors (*cyclizine, promethazine*). The neural pathway carrying vestibular impulses to the emetic centre actually passes through the CTZ, though its neurones are not those excited by apomorphine and other chemical triggers. These two pathways converge on the emetic centre later. Not surprisingly, drugs effective in motion sickness are effective in middle ear disease and, to a lesser extent, in Menière's disease. These drugs also have some effect in postoperative (or postanaesthetic) vomiting and in the vomiting of early pregnancy. The opioids are much more emetic in ambulant than bedridden patients and this (vestibular) component is countered by the drugs for motion sickness.

Other conditions

In most other situations the phenothiazines (**chlorpromazine**, *trifluoperazine*) are effective, notably postoperatively, in radiotherapy, uraemia, carcinomatosis and pregnancy. In pregnancy drugs should be avoided if at all possible (see p. 412). They are also very effective against vomiting induced by ergot alkaloids, sympathomimetic agents and **levodopa** and at high doses against **digoxin** and opioid analgesic agents.

Metoclopramide, an antagonist at dopamine D_2 receptors and a weak antagonist at 5-HT_3 receptors, is an antiemetic relative of *procainamide* with both peripheral and central mechanisms of antiemetic action. The peripheral actions include increased gastric emptying and reduced reflux that probably arise from action at prejunctional receptors that promote acetylcholine release. It has been found effective in the vomiting associated with migraine, pregnancy, Menière's disease, motion sickness, opioid analgesic agents, radiotherapy and postoperatively, but it is not potent against cytotoxic chemotherapy. *Metoclopramide* also shows extrapyramidal adverse effects, worse in children, that summate with those of phenothiazines. It causes prolactin release (galactorrhoea).

Anticipatory nausea and vomiting, for instance before cancer chemotherapy, may be alleviated by the benzodiazepines. Nausea and vomiting during chemotherapy may be partially relieved by high-dose *metoclopramide* in combination with *dexamethasone*. The recently discovered selective antagonists at 5-HT_3 receptors (**ondansetron**) show great promise in this area, and in postoperative vomiting.

Summary

(1) Vomiting may be induced directly, by stimulation of the vomiting centre, or indirectly, by stimulation of the CTZ by endogenous or exogenous chemicals.
(2) Dopamine-, acetylcholine- and 5-hydroxytryptamine-containing pathways are involved in vomiting and antagonists at their receptors are useful antiemetic agents.
(3) Antagonists at muscarinic acetylcholine receptors, acting on the vomiting centre, are particularly useful for motion sickness.
(4) Antagonists of dopamine, acting on the CTZ, are particularly useful for chemically induced vomiting.
(5) Antagonists at 5-HT$_3$ receptors are useful for postoperative vomiting and that induced by cancer chemotherapy.

Opioid analgesic agents and their antagonists

All are structurally related to **morphine**, the most important of the alkaloids extracted from the latex of the opium poppy (*Papaver somniferum*). The term opioid means acting like opium but they are also called opiates (derived from opium) or narcotic analgesic agents, because high doses can cause narcosis – a state of stupor and insensibility. They produce their effects by interacting with the G-protein-linked receptors for the peptide neurotransmitters, enkephalins, endorphins and dynorphins (see p. 225).

Opioid analgesic agents

Derivatives of **morphine** possess two kinds of activity:

(1) They can act as agonists causing the well-known effects of analgesia, respiratory depression, cough suppression, vomiting and constipation.
(2) They can act as antagonists of these agonists.

Some derivatives (**morphine**) are termed pure or full agonists, whilst others are pure antagonists (**naloxone**). Yet further derivatives have both agonistic and antagonistic actions. The spectrum of agonist/antagonist activity at three of the kinds of opioid receptor is summarized in Table 5.1.

Opioid actions are both central and peripheral.

Central opioid agonist actions

The narcotic analgesic agents have very selective actions upon centres throughout the CNS. The receptors responsible for these different actions

Table 5.1 Three kinds of opioid receptor

	mu (μ)	kappa (κ)	delta (δ)
Agonist	**Morphine**	**Pentazocine** (ketocyclazocine) dynorphin	Leucine enkephalin
Antagonist	**Pentazocine** **Naloxone**	Norbinaltorphimine **Naloxone**	Naltrindole **Naloxone**

Note: **pentazocine** possesses both agonist and antagonist activities, but at different receptors.

are currently being elucidated. Actions include analgesia, sedation, anaesthesia, respiratory depression and cough suppression, hallucinations, convulsions, miosis and vomiting. The opioid analgesic agents also cause euphoria. Which of these factors predominates depends on the drug and the animal species. *Pethidine* is more likely to cause convulsions than is **morphine** whilst *methadone* causes less sedation than **morphine** in people. **Morphine** is sedative in people but convulsant in cats.

Analgesia

Analgesia is produced both by an effect on the pain pathways, at the spinal level (pain threshold), and on the reaction to the stimulus within the limbic system (pain tolerance). The latter is associated with the euphoriant action of the drug. Patients state that pain is still perceived but that it does not matter so much. Opioid drugs may also exert a local analgesic action if inflammation is present. Activation of μ-opioid receptors can explain the analgesic action of most therapeutically useful opioid analgesic agents.

Opioid analgesic agents are more effective against dull constant pain, although sharp stinging pain can be reduced. Their analgesic action is enhanced by salicylates (summation) and antipsychotic drugs (unknown mechanism) but reduced by barbiturates, which lower pain threshold when given alone.

The individual drugs differ in the ways detailed below.

Maximum analgesic efficacy

Diamorphine (heroin), **morphine** (and *methadone* and *dextromoramide*) have the greatest analgesic efficacy, then, in descending order, *pethidine*, *dihydrocodeine*, **codeine** and *dextropropoxyphene*.

Systemic bioavailability after oral administration

This is a function of lipid solubility. Note that **morphine** (Figure 5.6) has two hydroxyl groups and is relatively insoluble in lipid and therefore shows moderate oral efficacy, whilst *pethidine* is less polar and is more effective orally.

STAFFS UNIVERSITY LIBRARY

Duration of action

Diamorphine and *fentanyl* are short acting, most others act for longer.

Incidence of undesirable side-effects at satisfactory analgesic doses

Sedation may or may not be clinically desirable. Vomiting is always undesirable in an analgesic. **Codeine** is capable of causing the same degree of analgesia as 10 mg **morphine** (i/m), but this would be accompanied by excessive vomiting.

Respiratory depression

Analgesia caused by any opioid is accompanied by depression of respiratory rate (changes in tidal volume may be variable). There is an elevation in the threshold of the medullary centres to the excitatory effects of CO_2, consequently $Paco_2$ increases. The resultant periodic breathing (Figure 5.10) is characteristic of narcotic poisoning.

  Although respiratory depression is the cause of death in **morphine** poisoning, people can tolerate the consequences of severe respiratory depression caused by an opioid because it can occur without significant cardiovascular depression. This contrasts with that caused by most general anaesthetic agents when vasomotor depression and hypotension accompany hypoventilation.

Cough suppression

The derivatives of **morphine** are the only clinically useful drugs that depress the cough centre (situated in the medulla near the respiratory centres). Some derivatives of **morphine** possess similar antitussive activity relative to analgesic activity. Quantitative separation is seen in derivatives with bulky substituents at position 3 (Figure 5.6), hence **codeine** and pholcodine, which are effective antitussive agents at subanalgesic doses.

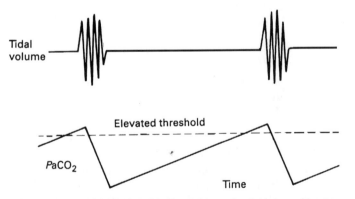

Figure 5.10 Periodic breathing induced by large doses of opioid drugs (due to an elevated threshold for the respiratory stimulant action of CO_2)

Qualitative separation has also been achieved. Only those stereoisomers equivalent to (–)-**morphine** possess opioid-like activity (generally these are also (–)-rotatory but there are some exceptions). **Dextromethorphan** possesses no analgesic or respiratory depressant activity yet retains antitussive activity, being equipotent with **codeine**.

Emetic action

All the derivatives of **morphine** can cause vomiting. The mechanism is by stimulation of the CTZ. Vomiting can be especially troublesome if the patient is ambulatory. Subsequently, opioids can depress the vomiting centre. Thus if vomiting is going to occur it will happen soon after injection. Vomiting can be controlled by antagonists at dopamine receptors (phenothiazines, *metoclopramide*).

Selectivity of emetic action is seen with **apomorphine**, which has few other **morphine**-like actions. **Apomorphine** is known to be a mimic of the neurotransmitter dopamine (see p. 240).

Miotic action

Most opioids stimulate the oculomotor centre and cause pupillary constriction (parasympathetic innervation). This may complicate the use of pupil size as an index of depth of anaesthesia (see p. 257), though it is a useful symptom of opioid poisoning. Tolerance to this excitatory action occurs slowly, thus miosis is still present in addicts.

Peripheral agonist actions

Morphine causes an increase in tone of the stomach, duodenum, small intestine and colon, leading to decreased intestinal propulsion. Sphincters throughout the tract are particularly sensitive. Opioids also have a direct effect on mucosal ion transport, reducing fluid accumulation in intestinal contents. Both these mechanisms contribute to the constipative action of opioids. Hence the use of kaolin and **morphine** for diarrhoea of assorted causes. A selective opioid constipative agent is **loperamide**. This drug is poorly absorbed and acts locally in the intestine, so it lacks analgesic and respiratory depressant actions at constipative doses. It is available as an over-the-counter preparation.

Histamine release

Morphine, in common with other basic drugs (**tubocurarine, atropine**), can displace endogenous histamine from its binding site. This is of clinical importance if the patient has a history of allergic conditions. The consequences are irritation at the site of injection, bronchospasm (which may be fatal in an asthmatic patient) and peripheral vasodilatation leading to postural hypotension.

Tolerance

Tolerance is a decreased response to continued drug use, which is generally surmountable by increasing the dose of the drug. Tolerance develops to some actions of **morphine** with remarkable speed and to a considerable extent. An addict may tolerate 500 times the clinical dose of **morphine**. Generally, tolerance develops quickest to the depressant actions, there being little tolerance to the miotic, emetic and convulsant actions. Whilst tolerance may be apparent after single injections of opioids in a person and certainly after approximately six consecutive injections (as in postoperative pain), this may be of little clinical significance (see below). The mechanism of tolerance is unknown but is not due to increased biotransformation.

Physical dependence

Physical dependence is defined on page 446. It cannot occur unless the subject has developed tolerance. The withdrawal symptoms are generally opposite to the original effects of agonists (diarrhoea, hyperventilation, mydriasis), though vomiting occurs.

The symptoms develop at the time the next regular dose is due, reach peak severity in 36–72 h and last for approximately a week.

If opioids are used to relieve acute pain (e.g. six injections), withdrawal symptoms, though detectable, may pass unnoticed if the patient is not anticipating any reaction.

The treatment of dependence is theoretically simple and effective. Hospitalization is essential. The injected addictive drug (commonly *diamorphine*) is withdrawn and a derivative that has a longer duration of action, that causes less euphoria and has adequate oral bioavailability is substituted (commonly *methadone*). The dose given is just sufficient to prevent withdrawal symptoms. Over a period of weeks (governed by the severity) the dose of the substitute is reduced gradually, during which time whatever biochemical imbalance was responsible for the syndrome returns to normal (see p. 447). Intense psychiatric supervision is necessary. Following this the patient is clinically cured. The difficult part is the rehabilitation that must follow.

It should be stressed that the risk of inducing severe dependence in a patient during treatment for acute pain (the therapeutic addict) is remote. Treatment of dependence is more relevant to illicitly obtained drugs and in these instances there are complicating factors – pathological, psychological and sociological.

Antagonists at opioid receptors

The antagonists of opioids should be considered from two viewpoints:
(1) Their use in the treatment of agonist overdose.
(2) The use of mixed agonist–antagonist drugs as analgesic agents in their own right.

Use as antagonists

Naloxone is a more potent antagonist at μ-opioid receptors than at κ- or δ-opioid receptors. Thus ten times less **naloxone** is needed to inhibit μ-opioid-receptor-mediated effects than to inhibit κ-opioid-receptor-mediated effects. The characteristics of the antagonism in all cases are competitive. The major use of **naloxone** is in reversal of postoperative respiratory depression, notably in the neonate. **Naloxone** has a short duration of action (30 min).

All derivatives possessing antagonist activity will precipitate the withdrawal syndrome in opioid addicts. The symptoms thus precipitated will appear within seconds and last for 24 h (cf. the withdrawal syndrome precipitated by abstinence).

Use of mixed agonist–antagonist drugs as analgesic agents

The antagonist analgesic agents (**pentazocine**) share with the pure agonists analgesic, respiratory depressant, cough suppressant, constipative and emetic activities. They differ in that they normally cause dysphoria, they can cause hallucinations (which are normally of a persecutory nature) and they do not cause dependence of the pure μ-opioid receptor agonist type.

Several derivatives are currently available. The two most commonly used are **pentazocine** and *buprenorphine*.

Pentazocine

Pentazocine, reputedly an agonist at κ-opioid receptors and an antagonist at μ-opioid receptors, has analgesic efficacy similar to *pethidine* and causes dysphoria though hallucinations are uncommon. These effects are mediated via a σ-receptor that is not **naloxone** sensitive and hence is not classified as an opioid receptor. A very rare form of dependence has been described – it is different from that to pure agonists at μ-opioid receptors (even weak agonists like **codeine**). Withdrawal symptoms are abdominal pain, sweating, lacrimation and rhinorrhoea, and can be tolerated without medication.

Buprenorphine

Buprenorphine differs from **pentazocine** in that it has a greater efficacy and a much longer duration of action. In addition, both the agonist and antagonist actions of *buprenorphine* appear to be mediated at a single kind of opioid receptor, the μ-opioid receptor. It is therefore a partial agonist. It is strongly sedative and causes neither euphoria nor dysphoria. Psychotic effects have not been reported. Vomiting (especially in the ambulatory patient) may be more frequent than that characteristic of the group. The drug may be administered parenterally, sublingually and orally. **Naloxone** is not an effective antagonist when injected after *buprenorphine*, though it can prevent its action when given before. *Doxapram* (see p. 249) is an effective antidote to *buprenorphine* overdosage.

Summary

(1) Opioid analgesic agents mimic the endogenous opioid peptides, enkephalins, endorphins and dynorphins.
(2) Although several kinds of opioid receptor exist (μ, κ, δ), most clinically useful effects occur through activation of μ-opioid receptors.
(3) The most serious adverse effects are respiratory depression and vomiting.
(4) Some opioids have selectivity for a particular opioid effect, e.g. **dextromethorphan** as a cough suppressant and **loperamide** for the treatment of diarrhoea.

Stimulant and hallucinogenic agents

Although a particular neurotransmitter may be excitatory at one site and inhibitory at another, it is possible to generalize that some neurotransmitters are more likely to be excitatory and others inhibitory – glycine and GABA generally inhibit, while glutamate and aspartate increase neuronal activity in the CNS.

Stimulant agents either enhance excitation or antagonize inhibition. Following drug-induced excitation there is commonly a phase of depression.

Stimulant agents

Centrally acting sympathomimetic agents

Amphetamine causes stimulation throughout the CNS, particularly of the reticular formation. This, in combination with other actions (see below), results in prolonged alertness, postponement of fatigue, motor stimulation, suppression of appetite (anorexia), confusion and anxiety. Hallucinations are rare. It is a potent peripheral sympathomimetic amine (see p. 82).

Its central mechanisms of action include release of noradrenaline and dopamine (it causes a behaviour pattern characteristic of other agonists at dopamine receptors), release of 5-hydroxytryptamine, inhibition of monoamine uptake and inhibition of MAO.

Whilst the (+)- and (–)-isomers have equal potency in the periphery, dexamphetamine [dextroamphetamine] is twice as potent as a central stimulant.

Acute poisoning is characterized by delirium and autonomic symptoms. Treatment involves acidification of urine to promote excretion (see p. 401) and **chlorpromazine** (its antipsychotic and α-adrenoceptor blocking actions are of benefit). Death is due to cardiovascular collapse.

Chronic toxicity poses problems of tolerance, severe psychic dependence and a psychosis almost identical to paranoid schizophrenia.

Current clinical use is restricted to the rare condition of narcolepsy.

Structural manipulation of the amphetamine molecule affords more selective derivatives. *Tranylcypromine* is an inhibitor of MAO but causes less stimulation of the autonomic and central nervous systems than amphetamine.

Convulsant agents

Drugs can cause convulsions by many different mechanisms at sites between the spinal cord and cerebral cortex.

Strychnine

Strychnine poisoning is treated with short-acting neuromuscular blocking agents and sedative agents (the mechanism of action of strychnine is described on p. 224).

Bicuculline and picrotoxin

Bicuculline is a competitive antagonist of the inhibitory neurotransmitter GABA at $GABA_A$ receptors (see Figure 5.14), while picrotoxin causes functional opposition.

Nikethamide

The mechanism of action of nikethamide is not known. Since the respiratory stimulant dose is lower than the convulsant dose in conscious subjects, it was once used in the treatment of barbiturate poisoning. However the dose necessary to stimulate respiration in a comatose subject is a convulsant dose and this has led to the abandonment of such drugs. Since then the prognosis for barbiturate poisoning has significantly improved.

Doxapram

Unlike nikethamide, the ratio between respiratory stimulant and convulsant doses is acceptable and *doxapram* is used as a respiratory stimulant when no more specific method is available. Its relative selectivity of action may be related to peripheral stimulation of chemoceptors.

Whilst some of the above drugs have negligible clinical use, several are valuable in neurophysiological and pharmacological research.

Methylxanthines

The related alkaloids *caffeine* and *theophylline* have useful central and peripheral actions. They stimulate the CNS, skeletal and cardiac muscle, relax smooth muscle and cause diuresis.

For central stimulation *caffeine* is much more potent than *theophylline*. At oral doses of 200 mg, *caffeine* postpones fatigue, with no adverse effects. A cup of strong tea or coffee contains approximately 150 mg *caffeine*. The lethal dose in people is so high as to be unknown but physical and psychic dependence can occur.

For cardiac stimulation, smooth muscle relaxation and diuresis, *theophylline* is more potent than *caffeine*. See p. 130 for a further description of the peripheral actions and mechanisms of action of methylxanthines.

Appetite and centrally acting anorectic drugs

The complex control of appetite involves many regions of the brain but is integrated from the hypothalamus. Of the neurotransmitters that have direct or indirect involvement in feeding behaviour, the most studied are the catecholamines and 5-hydroxytryptamine, but more recently attention has been focused on some peptides, notably the opioid peptides.

In the past amphetamine was widely used to suppress appetite. It is a potent and effective drug. Now its use is not recommended because it causes pronounced peripheral noradrenergic stimulation, often unsurmountable difficulties in sleep and chronic CNS toxicity, notably dependence and psychosis. A few derivatives of amphetamine are available that are less effective though are proportionately safer. Their mechanism of anorectic action is mediated by catecholamines.

The anorectic action of **fenfluramine**, though it is chemically related to amphetamine, is mediated by the release of 5-hydroxytryptamine. **Fenfluramine** is almost as effective as amphetamine but causes negligible noradrenergic change (acute poisoning is unaccompanied by significant cardiovascular change) and the drug has a generally sedative profile.

If a drug is deemed necessary to assist a patient to follow a reducing diet, **fenfluramine** remains the only recommended drug.

Appetite stimulation is produced as an adverse effect by the antipsychotic drugs (antagonism of catecholamines and 5-hydroxytryptamine) and by the anxiolytic agents (which may imply a role for GABA in the feeding centres).

Hallucinogens

A hallucination is a sense perception not based on objective reality. Though normally thought of as visual, drugs can also alter all other sensory perceptions (tactile, auditory, taste, pain).

Many drugs cause hallucinations by affecting various neurotransmitters. In few cases is the mechanism of action fully understood. In effect, however, hallucinogens cause a failure of sensory input control resulting in a flooding of the perception and stimulation, via collateral branches, of the reticular formation but note that not all hallucinogens in the following list can be classified as stimulant agents. Hallucinogens also enhance attentional processes (Figure 5.11).

Centrally acting sympathomimetic agents

Whilst amphetamine (see p. 248) can occasionally cause hallucinations following parenteral administration, its methoxylated derivatives (mescaline,

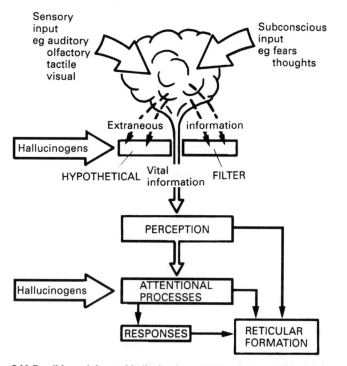

Figure 5.11 Possible aetiology of hallucinations: in this model for the processing of information in the brain, hallucinogens cause both a breakdown of the input filter and heightened attentional process

dimethoxymethylamphetamine) are potent hallucinogens. They cause vivid visual hallucinations, though the mechanism is unknown.

Lysergic acid diethylamide

LSD causes vivid visual hallucinations. The mechanism is presumed to stem from its ability to interact with central neurotransmitter 5-hydroxytryptamine.

Cocaine

Cocaine causes euphoria, indifference to pain and tactile hallucinations. The mechanism is presumed to be related to inhibition of central monoamine uptake (see p. 88).

Narcotic antagonist analgesic agents

Pentazocine causes dysphoria and visual hallucinations that are commonly persecutory.

Nitrous oxide

Nitrous oxide lowers the sensory threshold causing notably auditory distortion. The mechanism may involve interaction with endorphins and enkephalins.

Cannabis

The main active constituent of cannabis is Δ^9-tetrahydrocannabinol. It lowers the sensory threshold and causes euphoria and time distortion.

Hallucinogens have no therapeutic use as such.

Acute toxicity

Bizarre behaviour occurs; further toxicity is specific for drug group.

Chronic toxicity

Psychoses may occur at any time after drug taking.

Summary

(1) Stimulant and hallucinogenic agents have little valid clinical use but are frequently abused.
(2) Exceptions are **fenfluramine** as an anorectic agent and methylxanthines for their cardiovascular and bronchodilator effects.
(3) Caffeine is a widely used and socially accepted stimulant to postpone fatigue.

Antipyretic analgesic agents

Drugs of this group usually combine antipyretic, analgesic and anti-inflammatory actions. Their anti-inflammatory properties and peripheral adverse effects are presented on page 213. In this section the antipyretic and analgesic properties of **aspirin** and **paracetamol** will be covered.

Thermoregulation and fever

Body temperature is controlled primarily by the hypothalamus, which acts like a thermostat and also as an integration centre for sensory information from deep body (core) and environmental (cutaneous) thermoceptors. Hypothalamic outflow to peripheral effector systems controls body temperature. Thermoregulation is initially by changes in vasomotor tone – either cutaneous vasoconstriction to conserve heat or vasodilatation for heat loss.

If further adjustment is necessary to maintain body temperature, increased thermogenesis (voluntary exercise, shivering) and piloerection in animals, or active heat loss (sweating, and panting in animals) is initiated. Autonomic effectors may be supplemented by behavioural changes to gain or lose heat.

In fever (e.g. as a result of infection or after injection of pyrogenic substances) the hypothalamic thermostat behaves as if it had been reset at a higher temperature. Thus effectors increase the core temperature so that it is higher than normal (febrile state). Peptides (e.g. interleukin-1, interleukin-6 and tumour necrosis factor), released from macrophages involved in the immune response to infection, mediate fever. These endogenous pyrogens increase synthesis of PGs of the E series, which appear to be the final chemical mediators of fever. PGs have been detected in the cerebrospinal fluid (CSF) of febrile animals and hypothalamic injection of PGEs causes fever.

Pain

The role of the various central neurotransmitters in the response to pain is as yet poorly understood. Enkephalins (see p. 225) may be involved but other substances, including substance P and the PGs, particularly when the pain involves a peripheral inflammatory response, have been implicated.

Aspirin

Antipyretic action

Aspirin acts as though to reset the central thermostat to its prefebrile level so that the abnormally high core temperature is now detected and heat loss mechanisms (e.g. sweating) are activated. **Aspirin** does not reduce core temperature when the thermostat is operating normally or when the body temperature is elevated for reasons other than disturbed hypothalamic function (e.g. during excessive physical exercise).

Aspirin inhibits a febrile response and at the same time prevents the appearance of PGs in the CSF. Thus it is thought that by inhibiting cyclooxygenase, **aspirin** prevents the production of the PG mediators of fever.

Analgesic action

Aspirin analgesia has an important peripheral component, particularly when inflammation is the cause of the pain, but a central component also seems likely (see **paracetamol**). **Aspirin** is useful for the relief of many kinds of mild pain.

Other CNS actions

In high doses **aspirin** first causes stimulation and then depression of the CNS. Stimulation of respiration leads to a decrease in Pa_{CO_2} (respiratory alkalosis). Compensation occurs by bicarbonate loss in the urine so that

STAFFS UNIVERSITY LIBRARY

the plasma bicarbonate concentration is reduced. Later in more severe poisoning lactic and ketoacids accumulate in the blood due to interference with normal carbohydrate and fat metabolism (metabolic acidosis). Confusion, dizziness, tinnitus (ringing in the ears) and high-tone deafness can occur, and as the dose is increased delirium, psychosis, stupor and coma may ensue. Nausea and vomiting may occur, and though there is a peripheral component (gastric irritation), a central effect is also involved since i/v **aspirin** can cause vomiting that is abolished by ablation of the medullary CTZ. Salt and water depletion from vomiting, sweating and over-breathing is severe.

Aspirin is thought to cause a rare, but often fatal, syndrome (Reye's) of liver and brain damage in children with chicken pox or influenza. Consequently **paracetamol**, not **aspirin**, is the antipyretic analgesic drug of choice in children aged under 12 years, and **aspirin** is used only when the anti-inflammatory action is specifically indicated (e.g. juvenile rheumatoid arthritis).

Paracetamol

Antipyretic and analgesic actions

Paracetamol is approximately equipotent with **aspirin** as an antipyretic and analgesic agent but differs from **aspirin** in that it lacks anti-inflammatory action. This is because **paracetamol** inhibits peripheral cyclo-oxygenase less than it does the central enzyme. This indicates that **paracetamol** has a central component to its analgesic action. The mechanism of the central action is not known but differs from that of opioid analgesic agents.

Other CNS actions

In some individuals relaxation, drowsiness and euphoria have been reported following ingestion of **paracetamol** but this may be related to relief from pain rather than a direct action on the CNS. After very high doses CNS stimulation, excitement and delirium may occur, followed by sedation and stupor.

Other toxic effects are mainly peripheral in origin with delayed liver damage being the most serious consequence of acute overdosage and renal damage being possible after chronic abuse. Liver damage may be less with concurrent administration of *acetylcysteine* (alternative source of –SH groups for toxic metabolite of **paracetamol**, see p. 355).

Many proprietary mixtures that include **aspirin** or **paracetamol** are available, as are preparations in which **aspirin** is presented in a soluble form. The application of such preparations is discussed on pages 499 and 536.

Summary

Antipyretic analgesic agents:

(1) Combine antipyretic, analgesic and anti-inflammatory actions.

(2) Inhibit cyclo-oxygenase and decrease PG production.
(3) Are commonly used to reduce fever but have no effect on hyper-
    thermia.
(4) Are commonly used to reduce pain, particularly that associated with
    peripheral inflammation.

The state of consciousness and the general anaesthetic agents

When given in large enough doses the structurally non-specific drugs are
capable of depressing the activity of all excitable cells. Some general observations concerning the activity of structurally non-specific drugs are
outlined elsewhere (see p. 4). The state of general anaesthesia, which
occurs with lower doses of these agents, involves a loss of consciousness
with minimal depression of other brain functions. A simplistic approach is
to say that anaesthesia is a depression of neuronal functions, those responsible for consciousness being the most vulnerable. However, there is a lack
of understanding of the basic mechanisms of consciousness and thus of its
modification by drugs. It may be that recent developments identifying
enhanced neurotransmission by the inhibitory neurotransmitter GABA, or
antagonism of excitatory transmission as selective actions of some agents
in this group, are relevant to the mechanism of anaesthetic action.

The physiological basis of sleep and consciousness

The reticular formation contains areas responsible for the sleep/wake
cycle (reticular activating system). The sleep and wake centres have inherent rhythmicity and are mutually inhibitory. The wake centre is dominant.
Their regular control of the cycle is influenced by many factors, which can:

(1) Maintain wakefulness – unusual sensory stimuli (noise, light, pain),
    excessive limbic activity (anxiousness), mental disorders (anxiety,
    depression), a will to stay awake and various unsatisfied urges.
(2) Encourage sleep – absence of the above.

Consciousness, on the other hand, is believed to be the responsibility of the
cortex. Sleep/wake cycles are still observed in animals or children in which
the cortex is absent or virtually destroyed. Automatic responses occur but
no signs are shown of awareness of self and environment. It is likely, but
impossible to prove, that such animals or people lack consciousness.

Sleep and insomnia

The depth of sleep can be measured by electroencephalogram recordings
(Figure 5.12 illustrates typical records), although behavioural changes do

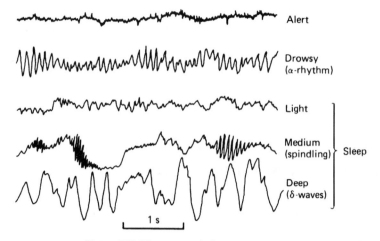

Figure 5.12 Electroencephalogram patterns

not always correlate with the EEG record. Note the fast electrical activity typical of alertness, the α-rhythm (approximately 10/s, typical of drowsiness, eyes closed), the bursts of activity (spindling) during sleep and the δ-waves (high voltage, low frequency) of deep sleep.

There is an additional stage of sleep called paradoxical sleep. This is characterized by rapid eye movements (REM sleep), an increase in electrical activity, difficulty in arousing the subject and dreaming.

The course of a night's sleep is usually constant with deep sleep occurring early and the incidence and duration of paradoxical sleep increasing as the course of sleep progresses. Paradoxical sleep is thought to be a psychological necessity and its reduction (by drugs) undesirable.

Anxiety is the most common cause of insomnia characterized by difficulty in getting to sleep, followed by ingestion of caffeine-containing drinks and then pain. The pattern of insomnia in patients suffering from depression is, instead, early awakening.

There is no drug that causes natural sleep. The drugs usually used to treat insomnia are the relatively selective anxiolytic agents (**temazepam**), which reduce the cause of insomnia and encourage more natural sleep. Insomnia due to pain can rationally be treated with analgesic agents and that due to depression responds to antidepressant drugs.

Anaesthesia

Anaesthesia refers to a reversible drug-induced absence of all awareness and sensation.

General anaesthetic agents reduce the overall activity of all parts of the brain in a predictable order. A progressive depression descends through the CNS, the cortex (loss of inhibition leading to excitation), the mid brain (sedation leading to anaesthesia), the spinal cord (loss of reflexes) and finally the medulla (respiratory and vasomotor depression leading to death).

Stages and planes of anaesthesia

These were defined many years ago for diethyl ether without premedication and were based on observations of peripheral manifestations of the progressive depression of the CNS, notably change in pupil size, skeletal muscle tone, respiratory pattern, eye movements and the presence or absence of various reflexes (corneal, laryngeal, pharyngeal). With the replacement of diethyl ether by other anaesthetic agents and the use of pre-anaesthetic medication, the historic stages and planes are less relevant to modern anaesthesia.

The most useful index of the stage of surgical anaesthesia is the absence (or near absence) of autonomic responses to pain (increased BP, heart rate, pupil size). Pupil size (constricted) and respiratory pattern (diaphragmatic assuming the patient is breathing spontaneously) are also confirmatory indices.

Each anaesthetic agent produces a different pattern of EEG changes. However, in general there is an increase in electrical activity equivalent to the stage of excitation, a distortion of rhythm equivalent to surgical anaesthesia and electrical silence indicating brain death. The distortion of rhythm during anaesthesia may range from cortical depression to something resembling seizure activity. It has been suggested that there may be a number of different non-conscious CNS states.

General anaesthetic agents

Since the site of action of these agents is within a lipid phase in the brain, a most important consideration is their ability to reach that phase. This governs the speed of induction of, and the recovery from, anaesthesia (see p. 390). Since most lipid-soluble compounds (organic solvents) are potentially anaesthetic agents, the only difference between clinically useful and useless agents is whether anaesthesia is or is not accompanied by undesirable effects – petrol is a general anaesthetic agent but causes bronchial irritation, liver and kidney damage.

Inhalational anaesthetic agents

The most commonly used inhalational anaesthesia employs a mixture of **nitrous oxide** (50–70%) and **halothane** (1%), although the use of alternatives to **halothane** (*enflurane, isoflurane*) is increasing.

Though a homogeneous group, the clinically useful anaesthetic agents differ in the properties described below.

Physical properties

Nitrous oxide is a gas at normal temperature and pressure. Some agents are highly inflammable (diethyl ether). **Halothane**, *enflurane* and *isoflurane* are non-inflammable volatile liquids that are chemically inert (Figures 1.3 and 5.13).

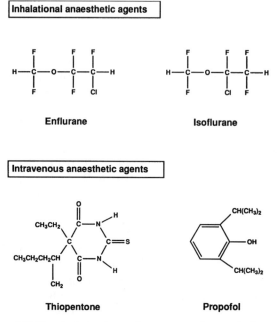

Figure 5.13 Chemical structures of some general anaesthetic agents

Speed of induction

Nitrous oxide is the fastest (the least soluble in blood, see p. 391), diethyl ether the slowest, and **halothane**, *enflurane* and *isoflurane* are intermediate.

Potency

This is expressed as the minimal alveolar concentration for anaesthesia (see p. 393). The volatile anaesthetic agents are more potent than the gases.

Analgesic activity

It is not an inevitable property of an anaesthetic agent that it is also an analgesic at subanaesthetic concentrations. **Nitrous oxide** is a potent analgesic, while **halothane**, *enflurane* and *isoflurane* have no selective analgesic properties. Alone among anaesthetic agents, **nitrous oxide** is used as an analgesic (e.g. in labour and in emergency pain relief before hospital admission) at concentrations of approximately 50%. The mechanism of its analgesic action is release of endogenous opioid peptides.

Muscle relaxation

While deep anaesthesia produces muscle relaxation, it also depresses many of the reflexes that protect the patient from the shock of surgery.

For this reason a relatively light level of anaesthesia is usually employed and neuromuscular blocking agents (see Table 2.3) are used as adjuncts in order to achieve the required degree of muscle relaxation.

Production of cardiac dysrhythmias

Most anaesthetic agents containing a halogen can sensitize the myocardium to the actions of catecholamines and thus cause dysrhythmias. However, *enflurane* and *isoflurane* are less likely to cause dysrhythmias than **halothane.**

Hypotension and respiratory depression

Medullary depression occurs with high doses of all anaesthetic agents, though if respiration is maintained artificially, medullary depression is usually unimportant.

Liver damage

Liver damage is a common toxic action of organic solvents. Modern anaesthetic agents are relatively free from this toxicity but those that are extensively metabolized (**halothane** – 15%) may be hepatotoxic, particularly following repeated administrations. *Isoflurane* is not extensively biotransformed (>1%) and is often used as a substitute for **halothane** when there is a requirement for repeated administration of a general anaesthetic agent.

Intravenous anaesthetic agents

The advantages of i/v anaesthesia are: rapid (a few seconds) and pleasant induction, simple equipment, little postoperative vomiting, short duration, no respiratory irritation.

The disadvantages are: inability to control depth of anaesthesia easily, severe respiratory and vasomotor depression (especially in the shocked patient) and local irritation at the injection site.

Note that the anaesthetic agents must be both lipid in nature (to act) and be miscible with blood. Some unusual formulations are necessary to effect blood miscibility and these may contribute to local inflammation or more general toxicity (anaphylaxis).

Thiopentone sodium and *methohexitone sodium* are barbiturate derivatives (Figure 5.13) that are water soluble at alkaline pH but become lipid soluble at physiological pH. *Propofol* is a hindered phenol (Figure 5.13) that is incorporated into a lipid emulsion for injection. They are widely used. Specific disadvantages of barbiturates are necrosis on extravascular injection and possibly fatal exacerbation of acute intermittent porphyria (see p. 430). This disease is an absolute contraindication to administration of any barbiturate. *Propofol* may cause pain on injection. Recovery from the i/v anaesthetic agents currently available is due to drug redistribution (see p. 386). The speed of subsequent metabolism is *propofol > methohexitone sodium* > **thiopentone sodium.**

Diazepam (see below) and *midazolam* are not really classified as anaesthetic agents but are used extensively by the i/v route to cause deep sedation. *Midazolam*, unlike **diazepam**, is water soluble at acidic pH and causes less irritation at the injection site.

Pre-anaesthetic and postanaesthetic medication

Drugs commonly used before, during and after anaesthesia include: antagonists at muscarinic acetylcholine receptors (**atropine**) to reduce secretions and to prevent excess bradycardia; anxiolytic agents (**temazepam**) to allay anxiety and cause amnesia; antipsychotic drugs (droperidol) to sedate and minimize the risk of vomiting; neuromuscular blocking agents (**suxamethonium**, *vecuronium*) to cause skeletal muscle relaxation; opioid analgesic agents (**morphine**, **pentazocine**) and, upon completion of surgical procedures, antagonists of some of the above (**neostigmine**, **naloxone**).

Neuroleptanalgesia

This is a technique of preparing a patient for major surgery using a combination of a potent short-acting opioid analgesic (*fentanyl*) with an antipsychotic (neuroleptic) agent (droperidol). Whilst the patient remains conscious and can (up to a point) follow instructions, the level of indifference to circumstances is such that surgery can be performed.

Anxiolytic, sedative and hypnotic agents

Derivatives of the benzodiazepines constitute the vast majority of anxiolytic agents that are, in increasing dose, clinically useful as sedative and hypnotic agents.

Benzodiazepines

These drugs enhance the activity of the inhibitory neurotransmitter GABA at the GABA$_A$ receptor, which is situated on a chloride channel. The benzodiazepines act on another receptor on the chloride channel which is distinct from the GABA$_A$ receptor site (see p. 223 and Figure 5.14). Several endogenous ligands for this receptor have been proposed. Endogenous benzodiazepines have been detected in several animal species and it is clear that plants, if not animals, can synthesize these structures. Some proposed ligands (those related to β-carboline and a large protein known as diazepam binding inhibitor) bind to benzodiazepine receptors but exert pharmacological actions generally opposite to those of the benzodiazepines (inverse agonists).

Diazepam has a relatively selective action on components of the limbic system (septum, amygdala and hippocampus), thereby reducing anxiety at

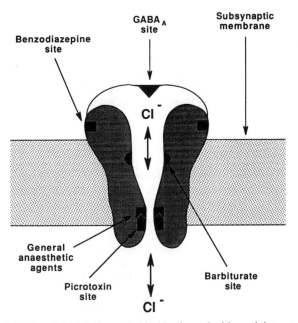

Figure 5.14 Ligand (GABA) gated chloride channel with modulatory sites for
benzodiazepines, barbiturates, general anaesthetic agents and picrotoxin

doses that have little effect on the reticular activating system (that is, little
sedative effect). It also has a relaxant effect on skeletal muscle (mediated
centrally) of value in the treatment of anxiety in which skeletal muscle
tone is increased.

Diazepam causes amnesia and whilst this is undesirable in patients
taking the drug long term, it can be valuable in pre-anaesthetic medication (e.g. in dentistry).

Diazepam possesses anticonvulsant activity (see p. 519). It has a long
$t_{1/2}$ and the drug can accumulate.

As is characteristic of the drug group, **diazepam** has neither antidepressant nor antipsychotic properties.

Unwanted effects are common to similar drugs: lapses in attention,
drowsiness and sedation (caution – performance in use of machinery or
driving may be adversely affected). Its actions summate with similar drugs.
Psychic and physical dependence can develop (see p. 446).

More than a dozen benzodiazepine depressant agents are currently
available. The pharmacodynamic differences between these are negligible. The custom of using some (chlordiazepoxide) for day-time alleviation of anxiety and others (*nitrazepam*) for night-time sedation probably
reflects either marketing policy or the relative doses in available preparations (see p. 504).

Actual differences are as follows.

Duration of action

For anxiolytic use long durations of action are generally preferred (**diazepam**, chlordiazepoxide). For insomnia drugs with shorter durations are generally preferred, causing less hangover effect and less motor impairment the following morning (**temazepam**). This distinction is important in the elderly with impaired liver function.

Cost

The longer established derivatives (**diazepam**) are approximately ten times less expensive than the newer drugs. This difference is important in view of the twenty million or so prescriptions for the drugs dispensed each year.

Antagonists at benzodiazepine receptors

Antagonists at the benzodiazepine receptor antagonize both the benzo-diazepine agonists and the inverse agonists. The most widely studied is **flumazenil**. It antagonizes **diazepam** in volunteers and has been used clinically in the management of benzodiazepine poisoning, although caution should be used as convulsions with a fatal outcome have been reported. It also finds a use in reversing the deep sedation of i/v benzodiazepines used in anaesthesia. **Flumazenil** virtually lacks pharmacological activity when given alone, although a minority of patients may experience weak partial agonist or even partial inverse agonist activity.

The alcohols

The alcohols are general anaesthetic agents, ethanol being the derivative with fewest adverse effects. It is widely used in self-medication, for social purposes and as an anxiolytic. In addition, it has vasodilator effects which may be beneficial in patients with peripheral vascular disease when taken in moderation.

Ethanol has a dose-dependent effect on performance and behaviour which has led many countries to place legal restrictions on its use when driving vehicles. Although there is considerable between-subject variation, the sequence of events relative to blood concentrations is shown in Table 5.2. This sequence of events applies to all CNS-depressant drugs (anxiolytic, sedative, hypnotic and general anaesthetic agents). The only differences are speed of induction and margin of safety. The terms anxiolytic, sedative, hypnotic and anaesthetic have been used as adjectives describing drugs, but it is more accurate to think in terms of anxiolytic, sedative, hypnotic or anaesthetic doses of drugs.

Excessive consumption of ethanol leads to dependence (see p. 446), psychosis and liver damage.

Table 5.2 Correlation between plasma concentration of ethanol and clinical state

Plasma ethanol concentration (mg/dL)	Effect
0–50	Reduced inhibitions
50–100	Slowed reaction time; unstable emotions
100–150	Slurred speech; behavioural changes
150–300	Ataxia; visual disturbances
300–400	Memory loss; hypothermia; stupor
400–700	Medullary depression (respiratory and vasomotor centres); death

*In some countries the legal limit is 50 mg/dL, and in a few countries it is zero. In the UK, the legal limit is defined as 35 mg/100 mL of expired (alveolar) air. This is equivalent to 80 mg/dL of blood.

Dose of ethanol in available beverages

Approximately the same amount of ethanol (7 g or 1 unit) is contained in a half pint of bitter beer, a single measure of spirits, a glass of sherry or of wine. Five units of ethanol on an empty stomach would produce a blood concentration peak of over 50 mg/dL in most individuals. V is approximately 0.7 L/kg, being greater in males than in females. Elimination is normally by zero-order kinetics at a rate of 15 (mg/dL)/h (approximately 1 unit/h).

The drug is oxidized in the liver by the route shown in Figure 7.11. Note the toxic acetaldehyde in the pathway, but as the aldehyde dehydrogenase step is normally rapid it does not accumulate.

Some drugs (**metronidazole**, p. 313, and *chlorpropamide*, p. 190) are inhibitors of aldehyde dehydrogenase and ethanol consumption is contraindicated during therapy with them. Disulfiram is an inhibitor of aldehyde dehydrogenase and is useful in the aversion treatment of ethanol addiction. During disulfiram treatment, if the patient takes ethanol, acetaldehyde accumulates and causes unpleasant effects including nausea and vomiting.

The central pharmacodynamics of methanol is identical to that of ethanol. It is also metabolized via the same pathway (see Figure 7.11) but the enzymes are less capable of handling formaldehyde and formic acid. These accumulate and cause blindness (chronic toxicity) or severe acidosis (acute toxicity).

Poisoning by a third commercially available alcohol, ethylene glycol (antifreeze), is characterized by CNS depression (coma, respiratory depression) and severe nephrotoxicity.

Chloral and its derivatives

The pharmacological properties of chloral and its derivatives are due to their biotransformation to trichloroethanol. They are used at sedative and hypnotic doses, are relatively safe and are useful as sedative agents in children.

Chloral hydrate is potentially an anaesthetic agent but its safety margin is too low for this usage. Gastric irritation often occurs and the drug should always be taken in dilute form and never on an empty stomach. Allergic reactions (urticaria, erythema) sometimes occur.

Triclofos sodium is a more palatable complex of *chloral hydrate* and gastric irritation rarely occurs.

Patterns of dependence on chloral derivatives are similar to ethanol dependence. Poisoning is treated in the same way as barbiturate poisoning.

Barbiturates

Structural modification of barbituric acid (itself without CNS activity) leads to hypnotic, sedative and anaesthetic agents that differ only in their time to onset and duration of activity.

The only justifiable clinical uses of barbiturates are:

(1) The specific use of *phenobarbitone* as an anti-epileptic drug (see p. 516).
(2) The use of **thiopentone sodium** and *methohexitone sodium* as i/v anaesthetic agents (see p. 259).

Although many barbiturate derivatives of intermediate duration of action have been used as sedative and hypnotic agents in the past and are still commercially available (amylobarbitone, butobarbitone), they are no longer recommended. Since 1985 these barbiturates have been included in the Misuse of Drugs Act.

Barbiturate poisoning and its treatment

The characteristics of barbiturate poisoning are: coma; hypothermia; shallow, regular and infrequent breathing; hypotension, imperceptible pulse. Death is usually due to inhalation of vomit.

The treatment of poisoning is artificial ventilation, forced diuresis and intensive care. The practice of using non-specific CNS stimulant agents (*nikethamide*, amphetamine) has virtually been abandoned.

Antagonists at β-adrenoceptors

In patients in whom acute anxiety might impair performance drastically and crucially, the reduction in noradrenergic symptoms can cause welcome relief. This particularly applies to intermittent occasions (e.g. interviews, examinations, auditions). In these instances antagonists at β-adrenoceptors are preferable to benzodiazepines if medication is deemed necessary.

Buspirone

Buspirone, an agonist at 5-HT$_{1A}$ receptors, has been marketed as an anxiolytic agent. It takes some weeks to exert its effects but causes little sedation.

Antagonists at H_1 histamine receptors

Phenothiazine antagonists at H_1 histamine receptors with sedative action are used as sedative agents. *Promethazine* is available without prescription. Antimuscarinic side-effects, such as dry mouth, are common.

Tolerance and dependence

The definitions of tolerance and dependence are given elsewhere (see pp. 246 and 446).

Tolerance is due to two components:

(1) Induction of liver MFO enzymes that accelerate drug biotransformation – most of the depressant agents are biotransformed to an appreciable extent, even if this is not the mechanism of recovery (**thiopentone sodium, halothane**).
(2) An unknown mechanism other than the above, which is presumably at the level of the biophase in the CNS. Alteration in the number of receptors, dissociation of signal transduction mechanisms from receptors, and activation of negative feedback mechanisms have all been suggested for various drugs. Note that tolerance may be apparent during the time-course of action of a single dose. For instance, the blood ethanol concentration at recovery of normal gait is significantly higher than that at the onset of observable intoxication (e.g. ataxia). On full recovery from massive **diazepam** overdose, very high plasma concentrations of drug may persist.

Cross-tolerance exists between all members of the group, though it is most marked between members of the same chemical group (e.g. barbiturates).

All of the members of the anxiolytic, sedative, hypnotic group are drugs of psychic and physical dependence and are the most common cause of addiction in the UK (there are approximately 500 000 ethanol addicts). The severity of dependence is a function of the potency of the drugs (barbiturates the greatest, benzodiazepines the least); the incidence is a function of availability (ethanol the greatest). Over a million people in the UK have been taking benzodiazepines for over a year.

Symptoms of dependence are tolerance, adjustment of lifestyle around periods of drug taking, anxiety, amnesia, sluggishness, nutritional deficiencies and ataxia.

Symptoms of withdrawal are craving, tremor, anxiety, hallucinations and, if severe, grand mal convulsions. Deaths have occurred during withdrawal.

Assuming regular drug taking, the time for development of dependence is a function of potency (barbiturates a few months, ethanol and benzodiazepines longer).

Treatment involves hospitalization, gradual reduction in drug intake (and where applicable switching to a less potent drug) and intensive psychiatric supervision.

Anticonvulsant drugs

Epileptic seizures are due to the presence in a part of the brain of unstable neuronal membranes (an ectopic focus) that can fire off spontaneously at high frequency (100 Hz). The attack is self-potentiating by positive feedback (post-tetanic potentiation). The result depends on the location of the lesion – momentary loss of consciousness, restricted movement of a limb, pain (trigeminal neuralgia) or generalized motor and autonomic changes.

The electrical activity of the brain is a balance between excitation and inhibition. Thus convulsant activity can be the result of too little inhibition or too much excitation. Many drugs with anticonvulsant activity either enhance inhibition or reduce excitation within the CNS. Some (**carbamazepine**, **phenytoin**, *lamotrigine*) block the reactivation of sodium channels and so discourage depolarization and the release of the excitatory neurotransmitter glutamate. Others (**sodium valproate**, *ethosuximide*) block T-type calcium channels, which are believed to have a pacemaker role in neuronal activity. Others favour hyperpolarization by enhancing the inhibitory neurotransmitter GABA action in opening chloride channels (**sodium valproate**, *vigabatrin*, benzodiazepines). Benzodiazepines act by a receptor-mediated action (see p. 260), while **sodium valproate** is an inhibitor of GABA metabolism.

The kinds of epilepsy and methods of treatment are described in detail on page 513.

Summary

(1) The biochemical basis of consciousness is poorly understood.
(2) The enhancement of inhibitory neurotransmission via the $GABA_A$ receptor is a mechanism common to many anaesthetic, anxiolytic and anticonvulsant agents.
(3) Drugs in this group have a potential for abuse.

6

Antiparasitic chemotherapy

Aims

After studying this section you should be able to:

- Name each of the principal current agents useful in antiparasitic chemotherapy and chemoprophylaxis.
- Describe the mechanism of its cytotoxic action.
- Describe the basis of its selectivity (a) towards parasite rather than host cells and (b) towards some parasites rather than others.
- Indicate something of its useful place in therapeutics.
- Indicate something of its adverse effects and disadvantages.

Introduction

The first part of this section deals with how the selectivity of action of agents useful in antiparasitic chemotherapy has been achieved. On pages 269–281 those antiparasitic chemotherapeutic agents showing biochemically based selectivity are classified according to their mechanisms of primary cytotoxic action, with cross-reference to their therapeutic use. On pages 281–285 those antiparasitic chemotherapeutic agents showing selectivity based on drug distribution are classified according to their mechanisms of differential disposition, with cross-reference both to their mechanism of primary cytotoxic action and to their therapeutic use. The remainder of the section places these same drugs (and others found empirically to be selective, but by as yet unknown mechanisms) in a therapeutic context. This has been done by classifying the parasitisms with back reference to the mechanisms of bacterial toxicity and selectivity of the useful antiparasitic drugs.

Definitions

Antiparasitic chemotherapy is the treatment of symptomatic parasitism with chemicals of known constitution. Human parasitisms fall into three groups:

STAFFS UNIVERSITY LIBRARY

(1) Infestation of organs with metazoa (insects, arachnids, worms).
(2) Infection of tissues or cells with unicellular organisms (protozoa, fungi, bacteria, Rickettsiae, Chlamydiae, viruses).
(3) Invasion of organs or tissues by aberrant human cells (malignant neoplasms).

Cytotoxicity means direct injury to, or disturbance of function of cells. The injury may be reversible or irreversible, structural or functional. The cytotoxic action may result in the death of cells (cytocidal effect) or prevention of their multiplication (cytostatic effect) without cell death. In the latter case the chemical (antibody) and cellular (phagocytic) defence mechanisms of the body can usually clear the residual static infecting population. Most antiparasitic drugs can be cytocidal in high concentration and cytostatic in lower concentration. Which is seen in practice depends on the body concentration attained with normal therapeutic doses.

The scale of measurement of cytotoxic action is really a continuous quantitative one (median cytotoxic concentration) but is often expressed less numerically as sensitivity or resistance of a parasite to clinically attainable concentrations of a chemotherapeutic agent. Resistance to a drug can be inherent (the drug is initially without effect) or acquired (resistance develops after initial susceptibility to the drug). If a parasite population acquires increased resistance (reduced sensitivity) to a chemotherapeutic agent it also shows cross-resistance to other agents sharing the same mechanism of cytotoxic action.

When we say that the cytotoxic action of a drug shows selectivity we mean that the drug affects one kind of cell more than another. The cytotoxic action of a drug is said to be qualitatively selective when that drug affects one kind of cell but does not affect a second kind of cell. This often occurs when the cellular target of the drug is present in the parasite but absent from the host cells. The cytotoxic action of a drug is said to be quantitatively selective when the drug at a given dose injures one kind of cell more than a second kind of cell or the drug injures one kind of cell at a dose lower than that required to injure a second kind of cell. Here both parasite and host cells possess the cellular target of the drug, but the amount of the drug target, the affinity of the drug for its target, or the access of the drug to its target may be greater in the parasite cell.

The scale of measurement of selective toxicity is the chemotherapeutic index, which, in animal models of parasitism, is equal to

$$\frac{\text{the median toxic dose to the host}}{\text{the median curative dose}}$$

More conservatively expressed in patient terms, the chemotherapeutic index =

$$\frac{\text{the threshold dose toxic to some patients}}{\text{the minimum dose curative for most patients}}$$

The basic assumption of human antiparasitic chemotherapy is that parasite cells differ from human cells. By chemical exploitation of these differences, toxicity to the parasite can be achieved without harm to the host. There are many ways of classifying these differences (and hence the origin of selectivity). Here, a two-way classification into biochemical and distributional bases of selectivity will be adopted.

Biochemical selectivity

The action of a chemotherapeutic agent shows biochemical selectivity when that agent is more toxic to parasite than to host cells, even when the sites of toxic action in both are exposed to the same drug concentration. This may be a qualitative difference (inhibition of cell wall synthesis, see below; dihydropteroate synthetase, see p. 272; anaerobic energy metabolism, see p. 280) or only a quantitative one (e.g. inhibition of dihydrofolate reductase, see p. 273; thymidine kinase, see p. 274; DNA-polymerase, see p. 276; RNA-polymerase, see p. 277; damage to cytoplasmic membrane, see p. 279).

Mechanism of toxic action

This may be one that makes the chemotherapeutic agent cytotoxic to all phases of the life cycle of the parasite, including the adult resting phase (damage to cytoplasmic membrane, see p. 279; inhibition of energy-yielding metabolism, see p. 280; inhibition of muscle function, see p. 280).Alternatively, it may be one that makes the chemotherapeutic agent cytotoxic only to parasites in the rapid growth and multiplication phase of their lifecycle (e.g. inhibition of cell wall synthesis, see below; nucleic acid synthesis, see p. 273; protein synthesis, see p. 277).

Mechanisms of cytotoxicity in cells undergoing rapid growth and multiplication

Inhibition of cell wall synthesis

Bacterial and fungal, unlike mammalian, cells provide themselves with an exoskeletal cell wall. The cell wall confers the characteristic shape on a cell and performs the important function of protecting the cell from osmotic damage. When cell wall synthesis is prevented, dividing bacterial cells swell and lyse if growing in a hypotonic medium. Drugs that interfere with the synthesis of cell wall material therefore show a qualitative, biochemically selective antibacterial action.

The β-lactam antibacterial agents (penicillins and cephalosporins) and **vancomycin** inhibit the formation of the insoluble peptidoglycan, which is a major constituent of the cell wall of all Gram-positive bacteria. In many Gram-negative bacteria a thinner peptidoglycan layer is present, surrounded by a lipophilic capsule.

Synthesis of the soluble precursors of peptidoglycan (two aminosugars and three small peptides, including D-alanyl-D-alanine = D-Ala-D-Ala) occurs in the cytoplasm, and they are then delivered to the inner face of the cytoplasmic membrane (Figure 6.1a). There assembly into the repeating unit of the linear peptidoglycan strand occurs, linked to a phospholipid membrane carrier. The carrier transports the unit to the outer face of the cytoplasmic membrane where it is cleaved (Figure 6.1b). Enzymes located on the outer face cross-link the strands to create a three-dimensional lattice (Figure 6.1c) of insoluble polymer. This is achieved by peptide bond formation (transpeptidation), using the D-Ala-D-Ala terminal as one-half of the substrate and cleaving it in the process. Other similar enzymes are present that remodel the lattice.

Penicillins (**benzylpenicillin** [penicillin G], see p. 307) and the closely related cephalosporins (**cephradine**, see p. 307) are structural analogues of D-Ala-D-Ala. They act exterior to the cell membrane, inhibiting the processes of transpeptidation and remodelling by combining covalently with the active centres of the enzymes (transpeptidases and other penicillin binding proteins). During the process the β-lactam bond is cleaved and the enzyme acylated. The penicillins are the most biochemically selective antimicrobial agents available. **Benzylpenicillin** has a narrow spectrum of bactericidal activity. All Gram-positive bacteria and gram-negative cocci are sensitive. Resistant bacteria usually secrete a β-lactamase enzyme (penicillinase or cephalosporinase) that hydrolyses and inactivates the drug. Some resistant bacteria show reduced affinity for the drug of the transpeptidase and other cell wall remodelling enzymes. Individual members of this group of antibiotic agents exhibit significant differences in properties and use, based on differences in structure and hence absorption (route of administration), distribution (penetration of the capsule of Gram-negative bacteria), affinity for the individual penicillin binding enzymes and affinity for β-lactamases.

Clavulanic acid is a potent inhibitor of β-lactamases that itself is without antibacterial activity. It is given in combination with penicillins to treat infection with bacteria that are resistant to penicillins due to production of β-lactamase.

Vancomycin is a water-soluble glycopeptide antibiotic that binds to the D-Ala-D-Ala terminal of the emerging peptidoglycan strand extracellularly (Figure 6.1b) and prevents its enzymatic modification by transpeptidase. **Vancomycin** is bactericidal to Gram-positive organisms.

Interference with the supply of precursors of nucleic acids

Pteridine co-enzymes are essential for the one-carbon transfer reactions during synthesis of purine and pyrimidine bases. Because cells have stores of preformed intermediates, there is a long lag time between an attack upon an early stage of this replicative metabolic pathway and the resulting inhibition of growth and multiplication.

Many bacteria, unlike mammalian cells, cannot absorb folate and instead utilize aminobenzoate to synthesize dihydrofolate (DHF) (Figure 6.2).

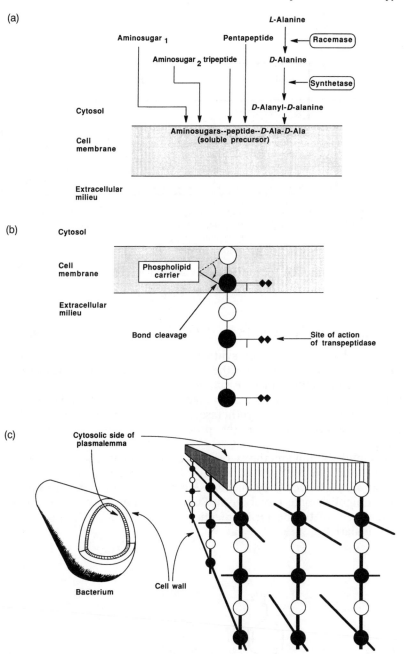

Figure 6.1 The stages of peptidoglycan synthesis in the formation of the bacterial cell wall: (a) intracellular stages; (b) intramembranous stages; the filled and open circles represent the two different aminosugars that alternate in a single strand of peptidoglycan; the T-shaped projections from alternate (filled circles) aminosugars represent a peptide of that shape and the filled diamonds represent the D-Ala-D-Ala terminal residue of that peptide; (c) extracellular stages – polymerization; the thicker vertical lines represent the strands of alternating aminosugars, the thinner lines represent the peptide cross links

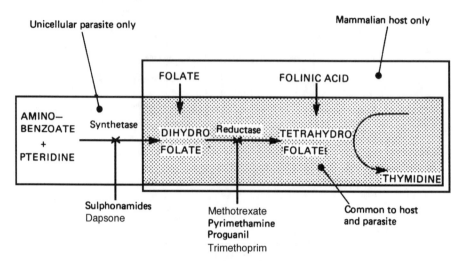

Figure 6.2 The folate pathway and its inhibitors

Interference with the synthesis of DHF from aminobenzoate

Since mammalian cells do not synthesize DHF from aminobenzoate, inhibitors of dihydropteroate synthetase necessarily show biochemical selectivity. Such inhibitors include sulphonamides and sulphones.

All are structural analogues of aminobenzoate (Figure 6.3) and compete with it for dihydropteroate synthetase. Using a sulphonamide as the substrate, the enzyme catalyses the production of a functionless DHF analogue.

Sulphonamides (sulphamethoxazole) have an extensive patchy spectrum of bacteriostatic and antimalarial activity that has been narrowed by the acquisition of resistance. They may cause renal toxicity unrelated to their effect on aminobenzoate metabolism. Sulphones (*dapsone*) are exploited in the treatment of the bacterial infection, leprosy, and of the protozoal infection, malaria.

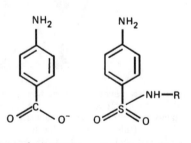

Para-aminobenzoate   A sulphonamide

Figure 6.3 Structural analogy of sulphonamides to para-aminobenzoate

Interference with the synthesis of tetrahydrofolate from DHF

Trimethoprim, *proguanil* [chloroguanide], *pyrimethamine* and **methotrexate** can only show a quantitative biochemical selectivity. They are all structural analogues of DHF that inhibit DHF reductase (Figure 6.2).

Trimethoprim is a small diaminopyrimidine analogue of DHF that is able passively to diffuse into parasite cells. It inhibits the bacterial form of DHF reductase (and that in malaria parasites) very much more potently than it inhibits the mammalian form of DHF reductase (it shows large quantitative biochemical selectivity). It has a spectrum of bacteriostatic activity similar to the sulphonamides. Adverse effects are rare but, used alone, resistance develops readily. It can also be combined with a sulphonamide (sulphamethoxazole) as *co-trimoxazole* to achieve efficient synergism by sequential blockade of the tetrahydrofolate (THF) synthetic pathway (Figure 6.2).

Pyrimethamine is another diaminopyrimidine analogue that passively diffuses into parasite cells. It inhibits the DHF reductase isoenzyme from malaria parasites much more than the homologous enzymes from mammalian or bacterial sources. The ready development of resistance of malarial parasites, when it is used alone, and its slowness of onset of action limit its usefulness. Like **trimethoprim**, it synergizes with a sulphonamide or sulphone. Folate deficiency anaemia (see p. 534) is a predictable adverse effect of high doses.

Proguanil is a prodrug. The active principle formed from *proguanil* in the body has properties very like those of *pyrimethamine*. Its slowness of onset of action make it useless in the treatment of clinical malaria but it is a valuable prophylactic agent for non-immune persons in an area where malaria is endemic (see p. 296).

Substituting –OH and –H in folic acid with $-NH_2$ and $-CH_3$ respectively yields **methotrexate**. This large analogue of DHF cannot penetrate into bacteria and protozoa. However, it enters mammalian cells by the active uptake mechanism for folate, and is poly-glutamated (thus increasing its cellular half-life). It only shows quantitative selectivity for cells with the highest THF turnover (most rapid cell division). It has a 100 000 times higher affinity for DHF reductase than does the natural substrate DHF, so it is virtually an irreversible inhibitor. Folic acid cannot compete successfully and thereby surmount its effects but folinic acid, by supplying THF directly, can (Figure 6.2). The host toxicity of **methotrexate** is typical of drugs acting on cell populations with rapid multiplication (see p. 321). When used alone resistance of neoplastic cells develops readily. Multiple mechanisms are involved in such resistance; decreased drug uptake, decreased intracellular half-life, alteration of DHF reductase resulting in decreased drug affinity, increased production of DHF reductase via gene amplification (see p. 287).

Interference with the supply of nucleoside and nucleotide precursors

Some structural analogues of purines (adenine, guanine) and pyrimidines (cytosine, thymine) are incorporated into the metabolic pathways of the cell to cause the synthesis of functionless intermediates that suppress nucleic acid synthesis.

Purine analogues

Acyclovir is a guanine analogue (acycloguanosine). It is a prodrug that is activated by phosphorylation by the form of thymidine kinase that is encoded by herpes virus. The reaction between **acyclovir** and the mammalian form of thymidine kinase is minimal, hence a selective toxicity to the herpes virus is shown. Thymidine kinase is the enzyme that catalyses the first step in the phosphorylation of deoxyguanosine to dGTP. Thus acycloGTP (derived from **acyclovir**) accumulates within the virus-infected cells and inhibits viral DNA-polymerase (in preference to mammalian DNA-polymerase, thus adding to the selectivity of action) and becomes incorporated into functionless DNA precursors. **Acyclovir** is the most selective antiviral agent available but its spectrum of activity is narrow, and it is only really useful to treat herpes virus.

Mercaptopurine inhibits many steps in the synthesis and interconversion of purines. Like **methotrexate**, its cytotoxic effects are greater in more rapidly dividing cells. *Azathioprine* is a prodrug from which mercaptopurine is released in the body.

Pyrimidine analogues

Zidovudine (AZT) is a thymidine analogue. It is a prodrug that is activated by host cell kinases to generate a triphosphate active species. Its mechanism of action is the inhibition of reverse transcriptase, the retrovirus enzyme that catalyses the conversion of viral RNA to DNA. *Zidovudine* is used in the treatment of patients infected with human immunodeficiency virus (HIV), the cause of AIDS. This antiviral agent has the adverse effect of severe bone marrow toxicity, which is thought to stem from its action on mammalian DNA-polymerase β (the form of this enzyme found in mitochondria). Mammalian DNA-polymerase α (the nuclear form) is resistant to *zidovudine*, allowing the relatively selective action against HIV.

Cytarabine is a prodrug that generates derivatives that compete with cytidine derivatives and cause profound inhibition of DNA synthesis. Its cytotoxic effects are greater in more rapidly dividing cells.

Fluorouracil is incorporated into a false nucleotide that blocks deoxyribonucleotide (especially thymidylate) synthesis. Its cytotoxic effects are greater in more rapidly dividing cells.

Flucytosine is a prodrug deaminated intracellularly to fluorouracil. It shows distributional selectivity (see p. 282) for fungi.

Interference directly with nucleic acid synthesis

Alkylation

All effective antineoplastic drugs in the class of drugs known as nitrogen mustards (e.g. **cyclophosphamide**) possess two alkylating groups (cf.

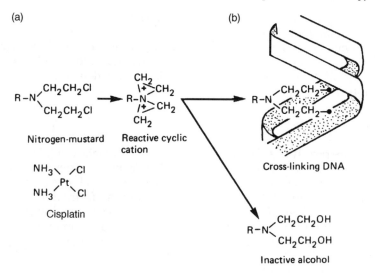

Figure 6.4 (a) The chemical changes in a nitrogen mustard which lead to alkylation and cross-linking of DNA; (b) *cisplatin* also can cross-link adjacent DNA strands

phenoxybenzamine, see p. 98). Highly reactive cyclic cations are formed spontaneously in aqueous solution (Figure 6.4a) and then bind covalently to side-chains of large molecules, especially the guanine base of DNA. This causes functional damage to the DNA, by cross-linking it to itself, another nucleic acid chain or other macromolecule. Any unbound cyclic cation is spontaneously hydrolysed to an inactive alcohol. The members of this group differ in their rate of production and inactivation of the cyclic cation. They are toxic to rapidly dividing cells, are widely useful in cancer chemotherapy, but produce the expected problems for the host (see p. 321). **Cyclophosphamide** is a prodrug that is activated by enzymatic ring cleavage in the liver. Further non-enzymatic reactions (see above) then occur to generate the active species, phosphoramide mustard.

The metal complex *cisplatin* diffuses into cells. The molecule dissociates, yielding Cl⁻ ions and revealing two reactive sites (Figure 6.4b) that bind particularly to the guanine base of DNA, cross-linking both within, and between, strands.

Intercalation

Doxorubicin is a basic antibiotic. Its structure comprises a flat, four-membered aglycone ring linked by a glycosidic bond to an aminosugar (daunosamine). The aglycone ring intercalates into the minor groove of DNA between layers of base pairs of the double helix. This disturbs the structure and function of the starter DNA employed by DNA-polymerase. It inhibits DNA and RNA synthesis at the same high concentration in isolated systems from all cells. However, the mechanism of cytotoxicity is more likely to result from the generation of protein-associated DNA

double-strand breaks. The molecular mechanism involved in the generation of these DNA strand breaks is incompletely understood but involves
the enzyme topoisomerase II (see below). Intercalating drugs such as
doxorubicin interfere with the DNA breakage and DNA rejoining
reactions of topoisomerase II. **Doxorubicin** is widely useful in cancer
chemotherapy.

Inhibition of DNA topoisomerase II

Topoisomerase II is an enzyme that covalently attaches to DNA. It catalyses strand breakage and rejoining of DNA during strand passage and
replication. *Etoposide* is a semisynthetic chemical analogue of podophyl-
lotoxin that inhibits topoisomerase II, causing the formation of double-
stranded DNA breaks. This confers useful anticancer activity. Resistance
to *etoposide* results from tumour cells with decreased amounts of topoisomerase II or tumour cells with an altered topoisomerase II (see p.
287).

Inhibition of DNA-gyrase

The quinolone *nalidixic acid* and the fluoroquinolone **ciprofloxacin**
inhibit DNA-gyrase. This bacterial enzyme cuts (and reseals) each strand
of bacterial DNA to remove the excess supercoiling that develops when
the strands separate to allow replication or transcription. In eukaryotic
nuclei a different enzyme, DNA topoisomerase II, performs the homologous function (see above). Quinolones show some, and fluoro-
quinolones substantial, quantitative selectivity. **Ciprofloxacin** is
bactericidal to a broad spectrum of aerobic bacteria, including intracellular pathogens.

Inhibition of DNA-polymerase

Acyclovir can be regarded as a prodrug from which is generated the active
principle acycloGTP. This selectively inhibits the viral form of DNA-
polymerase.

Inhibition of mitosis

The vinca alkaloids (**vincristine**, *vinblastine*) bring about an arrest of
mitosis in metaphase. In each case this is due to specific and reversible
combination with the globular protein tubulin, though the binding sites
differ. This prevents polymerization of tubulin into (and promotes depolymerization of) microtubules and hence prevents formation of a mitotic
spindle. Abnormal nuclear structures result and cell function is so
disturbed that cell death often ensues. Cells with the highest replication
rate are the most and earliest affected. These drugs are widely useful in
cancer chemotherapy and produce peripheral somatic and autonomic
neuropathy.

Interference directly with RNA synthesis

Inhibition of RNA-polymerase

Rifampicin combines with and inhibits the DNA-dependent RNA-polymerase isoenzyme in bacteria but not the homologous enzyme in mammalian cell nuclei. It is bactericidal to many bacteria, including *M. tuberculosis* and *M. leprae*, and has low host toxicity. One-step resistance develops readily. It is largely reserved for use in tuberculosis (see p. 313) and leprosy (with other drugs).

Inhibition of protein synthesis

To help in the understanding of this section you should revise the stages of protein synthesis on ribosomes. Most mammalian protein turnover is slow (fibrinogen apart) compared with that associated with cellular multi-plication. Quantitative biochemical selectivity, for bacterial rather than mammalian protein synthesis, is possible because bacteria contain only 70S (the S unit is a measure of density) ribosomes whereas most mammalian ribosomes are 80S. Mammalian mitochondria, however, do contain 70S ribosomes.

Inhibition of initiation of protein synthesis

Aminoglycoside antibiotic agents (**gentamicin**, *amikacin*) bind irreversibly to the acceptor part of the 30S subunit (Figure 6.5a) and distort it so that the initiation of protein synthesis is disrupted and accurate reading of codons is prevented. Aminoglycoside antibiotic agents are highly polar water-soluble bases. They diffuse through the water-filled pores in the outer capsule of Gram-negative bacteria and are then actively transported across the cytoplasmic membrane, linked to the electrical charge transport that establishes the membrane potential. Progressive disruption of the bacterial cell membrane develops. Aminoglycosides also damage cell membranes in the patient that are exposed to high concentrations, causing ototoxicity (damage to the hair cells of the inner ear) resulting in impaired balance and hearing and nephrotoxicity (damage to the tubular cells of the kidney). They have a fairly broad spectrum of bactericidal activity that includes many Gram-negative (including *Pseudomonas*) and some Gram-positive bacteria. Resistance develops readily.

Gentamicin is most useful in treating life-threatening infections by aerobic Gram-negative bacilli.

Amikacin is less susceptible than **gentamicin** to the bacterial enzymes that inactivate aminoglycosides.

Inhibition of peptide bond formation

Chloramphenicol is a relatively simple dipeptide. One molecule binds reversibly to each 50S subunit (Figure 6.5b) to block peptidyl transferase activity (and also to interfere with the binding of *clindamycin* and

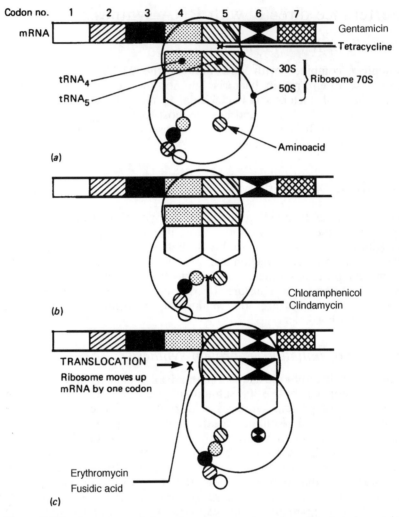

Figure 6.5 The three stages of elongation of the growing polypeptide chain in protein synthesis on the ribosome

erythromycin). It has a broad spectrum of bacteriostatic activity but, used by the systemic route, is reserved for life-threatening *H. influenzae* meningitis and typhoid fever. A dose-related reversible anaemia is a common toxic effect due to inhibition of protein synthesis on mitochondrial ribosomes. However, one patient in 40 000 is hypersensitive and suffers total, irreversible bone marrow depression (see p. 432).

Clindamycin is also a dipeptide that binds reversibly to the 50S subunit to block peptidyl transferase (and also to interfere with the binding of *chloramphenicol* and **erythromycin**). It is active on all isolated bacterial ribosomes, but in vivo is mainly bacteriostatic to Gram-positive bacteria and anaerobes (including *Bacteroides*).

Inhibition of translocation

Macrolide antibiotic agents (**erythromycin**): one molecule binds reversibly to the donor site of each 50S subunit (Figure 6.5c) to block translocation (and also to interfere with the binding of *chloramphenicol*). It is bacteriostatic to a narrow spectrum of microbes that includes many Gram-positive bacteria, Gram-negative cocci and anaerobes. The clearest indication for its use (see p. 310) occurs in a patient who requires **benzylpenicillin** but is allergic to it.

Sodium fusidate also blocks the ribosomal translocation step in bacterial protein synthesis. It is a narrow-spectrum antibiotic. It is useful systemically in infection by penicillin-resistant staphylococci, especially of bone. Resistance develops readily.

Mechanisms of cytotoxicity effective in all phases of the cellular growth cycle

The foregoing mechanisms operate on actively growing and multiplying parasites only, while the following mechanisms also operate on non-multiplying parasites.

Increased permeability of the cytoplasmic membrane

Damage to the cell membrane allows leakage of vital intracellular solutes. This mechanism makes a wide spectrum of parasites susceptible, exerts a cytocidal effect on non-growing cells, but limits selectivity.

Polyene antibiotic agents

Amphotericin binds to sterols in the cell membrane. These are abundant in fungal membranes where they largely comprise ergosterol. Intermediate amounts of sterols are found in mammalian membranes and mainly comprise cholesterol. Sterols are absent from bacterial membranes. The drug molecules enter the membrane to form an artificial pore or ionophore, increasing the outward permeability of the membrane to low MW intracellular solutes, especially ions. The drugs show useful selectivity for certain fungi (not those of ringworm) but also substantial host toxicity (see p. 301).

Inhibition of ergosterol synthesis

The azole compounds, imidazoles (**miconazole**) and triazoles (*fluconazole*) impair the synthesis of fungal membrane ergosterol (by inhibition of one of the cytochrome P_{450}-dependent demethylase enzymes) more than of mammalian membrane cholesterol. Under the influence of an azole derivative, not only does the fungal cell membrane become deficient in sterols but also abnormal methylated precursors accumulate. The affected fungal cell membranes become disorganized and show secondary impairment of the uptake of nutrients.

Azoles show a broad spectrum of antifungal activity and are fungicidal at high concentrations.

The allylamine *terbinafine* inhibits squalene epoxidase, another enzyme that is important in ergosterol synthesis. It is fungicidal to dermatophytes.

Miscellaneous

Aminoglycosides, as well as inhibiting protein synthesis, also damage cell membranes. This aspect of their action not only contributes to the bactericidal effect but also to the host toxicity.

Energy-yielding metabolism

Most aerobic organisms derive their energy by similar mechanisms, so that interference with this process has not been a fruitful source of selectively toxic drugs. Anaerobes differ significantly from the human host so selective interference with their anaerobic pathways is possible.

Nitroimidazoles (**metronidazole**) interfere with the function of ferredoxin (a Fe–S-protein acting as an electron transfer agent in plants, anaerobic bacteria and protozoa) by acting as an electron acceptor. **Metronidazole** is thus a prodrug activated by reduction to combine with ferredoxins. It is lethal to obligate anaerobic protozoa and facultatively anaerobic protozoa growing under anaerobic conditions (trichomonas, see p. 298; giardia; entamoeba, see p. 296) and also to obligate anaerobic bacteria (some streptococci, *Bacteroides*, *Cl. difficile* and *Borrelia vincenti*, see p. 313). Under the influence of nitroimidazole derivatives the cell is also deprived of reducing power by the diversion of electrons from their normal recipient. **Metronidazole** shows little host toxicity.

Muscle

Roundworms (*Ascaris*) and threadworms (*Enterobius*) need their motility to maintain their position in the lumen of the intestine of the host; paralysis therefore leads to worm expulsion (see p. 291). **Piperazine** causes relaxation of worm muscle and functional opposition to acetylcholine at worm neuromuscular junctions with little effect at those of mammals. It is well absorbed from the gut and host toxicity is negligible.

Summary

(1) Curative treatment of parasitic infestations or infections depends upon the selection of chemotherapeutic agents possessing the property of selective toxicity.
(2) The basis of the mechanism by which selective toxicity is achieved is either biochemical or distributional.

(3) Biochemical selectivity of toxicity can occur because a drug acts on a biochemical pathway that is specific to the parasite, or that is, though common to parasite and host, more susceptible to interference in the parasite. Isoforms of drug targets often underlie such differences in susceptibility.

(4) The biochemical sites of toxic action include inference with cell wall metabolism, replicative metabolism (nucleic acid synthesis, mitosis, protein synthesis), cell membrane metabolism, energy-yielding metabolism or the functioning of muscle.

Distributional selectivity

Even a drug that is equally toxic at its biochemical sites of action in host and parasite cells may nevertheless be useful as a chemotherapeutic agent if the sites of action in the parasitizing cells can be exposed to a higher concentration than those in the host cells. There are four ways in which this can be achieved.

Selective accumulation by the parasite

Tetracyclines

Tetracyclines (**tetracycline**) are cytotoxic to a wide range of parasites. Those affected include many bacteria (but not *Pseudomonas* or *Proteus*), Rickettsiae and Chlamydiae. These organisms accumulate tetracyclines to a high intracellular concentration by an active transport process. One way in which microbes acquire resistance to tetracyclines is by losing the net accumulation of the drugs, by developing an extrusion process that counters the accumulation.

After selective intracellular accumulation, tetracyclines bind reversibly to the acceptor part of the smaller subunit of the ribosome and inhibit the binding of aminoacyl-tRNA and therefore protein synthesis (Figure 6.5a). Unlike aminoglycoside antibiotic agents, tetracyclines do this in both 70S and 80S isolated ribosomes.

Tetracyclines are broad-spectrum, bacteriostatic, antibiotic agents with low host toxicity (see p. 311). However, this host toxicity does include increased blood concentration of nitrogenous waste compounds in patients with renal failure by inhibition of protein synthesis, shifting the balance towards catabolism.

4-Aminoquinolines

Chloroquine (and other 4-aminoquinolines and 4-quinolinemethanol derivatives) are selectively accumulated by malaria parasites infecting red blood cells. **Chloroquine** resistance in malaria is associated with a loss of this active uptake mechanism.

These are the drugs of choice for patients clinically ill with malaria. They clear the blood though they do not clear the liver of malaria parasites (see p. 293). **Chloroquine** shows little toxicity in antiparasitic doses; large doses have an anti-inflammatory action utilized in rheumatoid arthritis (see p. 215).

Selective activation of a prodrug

Acyclovir is a prodrug selectively activated in cells infected with herpes virus. It is in this sense that the drug formed from it, acycloGTP, accumulates in the viral parasite and also within infected host cells – that is, the environment of the parasite.

Flucytosine is a pyrimidine analogue prodrug that permeates certain fungi. Once within the fungal cell it is selectively activated by deaminating enzymes present in susceptible fungi (but not mammalian cells) to yield the pyrimidine analogue, fluorouracil (see p. 274). The active principle, fluorouracil, is thus selectively accumulated. It has a narrow spectrum of antifungal activity and resistance develops readily.

Malathion is a prodrug activated to the organophosphorus anticholinesterase compound malaoxon selectively by insects. Parasitic insects also inactivate malaoxon more slowly than mammals. Thus it is the malaoxon rather than the prodrug that is selectively accumulated by the parasite. **Malathion** is useful in treating louse infestations (see p. 288).

Selective distribution into a limited compartment that forms the parasites' environment

Skin

Griseofulvin is very poorly absorbed from the gut. However, that small proportion of the dose that is absorbed is selectively taken up by the skin cells synthesizing the precursors of keratin. As these differentiate, their **griseofulvin** content is strongly bound to keratin. Ringworm fungi growing among the keratin plates (of skin, nails, hair) concentrate the drug by absorption of **griseofulvin**-containing keratin. The **griseofulvin** then binds to tubulin, preventing polymerization and promoting depolymerization. The drug thus damages microtubule structure and function, and so interferes with the fungal cytoskeleton, cytoplasmic streaming and mitosis. It is thus fungistatic. It is only used for treatment of fungal infections of hair and nail (see p. 300).

Urinary tract

Most antibacterial drugs employed systemically for the treatment of urinary tract infection are concentrated in the urine by the processes of salt and water reabsorption. Penicillins and cephalosporins achieve particularly high urine concentrations because they are actively secreted by the renal tubules.

Urinary antiseptic agents

Nalidixic acid is rapidly and completely absorbed from the gut. Healthy kidneys clear the drug quickly by glomerular filtration. Normal therapeutic doses do not produce accumulation to an antibacterial blood concentration but renal tubular abstraction of water from the nascent urine results in concentration in the urine, to reach a bactericidal concentration.

Nalidixic acid shows minor biochemical selectivity for Gram-negative bacilli, which is reinforced in use by distributional selectivity based on the concentrating activity of the kidney. Bacterial resistance develops readily.

Selective administration to a limited compartment that forms the parasites' environment

Lumen of gut

Drugs that, when swallowed, are poorly absorbed from the gut (either because they are water but not lipid-soluble, or because they are water insoluble) contact lumen-dwelling parasites at high concentration.

The aminoglycoside antibiotic agent *neomycin* is toxic to bacteria but when given systemically is toxic to the host too. Gut absorption is negligible because it is highly polar (see p. 330). It is used in bowel preparation for intestinal surgery to reduce the bacterial content of any spills and of wall seams with the intention of reducing postoperative infective complications. Along with dietary protein restriction, it reduces the bacterial ammonia and amine production that is responsible for the encephalopathy (disturbance of consciousness, coma) of liver failure (Figure 6.6).

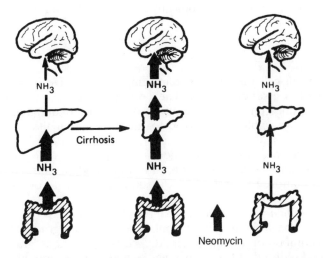

Figure 6.6 The liver normally clears the portal blood burden of ammonia-compounds arising from gut commensal bacteria. In liver failure the brain is reached and affected; neomycin restricts the gastrointestinal production of ammonia-compounds

STAFFS UNIVERSITY LIBRARY

Nystatin is a polyene antibiotic that is too toxic for systemic use. It is not absorbed because it is only slightly soluble in water. It is useful orally for candidiasis (see p. 301) of the gut.

Mebendazole is a water-insoluble drug that kills intestinal metazoa, probably by interference with glucose uptake. It is useful for threadworm infestations (see p. 291).

Pyrantel is a water-insoluble agonist at nicotinic receptors of skeletal muscle, causing depolarizing neuromuscular blockade (like **suxamethonium**, see p. 55) and spastic paralysis of worms (see p. 291), whose skeletal muscle resembles the multiply innervated kind found in vertebrates (see p. 58).

Skin

Many drugs showing good biochemical selectivity of action based on the foregoing principles are useful by topical routes of administration and thus have their selectivity reinforced by this distributional mechanism.

Antibacterial antibiotic agents

So little of a drug applied to the unbroken skin is absorbed into the systemic circulation that the more systemically toxic antibiotic agents can safely be used on the skin (e.g. *framycetin, neomycin, chlortetracycline*). The advantages of such a reliance on distributional selectivity are that pathogens are less likely to develop resistance to systemically valuable antibiotic agents, and it avoids the need for penicillins, sulphonamides, *streptomycin* or *chloramphenicol* to be applied to the skin (all have a strong tendency to induce skin allergy, see p. 426).

Mupirocin inhibits the formation of just one of the aminoacyl-tRNAs, thus depriving protein and other macromolecule synthesis of that amino acid (isoleucine). It is effective topically against most Gram-positive bacteria.

Antiseptic agents

Most act on all cell membranes, damaging the selective impermeability property that is essential to life. They rely for any selectivity they may have for microbes on poor penetration of the unbroken skin. On open wounds they are liable to be toxic to the granulation tissue and delay healing.

Chlorhexidine is a cationic detergent.

Povidone-iodine is an iodophore, in which iodine is solubilized by complex formation. It is less irritant to skin than tincture of iodine.

Cetrimide is a quaternary ammonium compound.

Hexachlorophane is a chlorinated bis-phenol that is bactericidal to Gram-positive bacteria. Regularly applied to the skin it gradually accumulates; the number of organisms in the surface layers is gradually but substantially reduced. Misuse, by whole body immersion of babies in strong solutions, has allowed sufficient to be absorbed through the skin to lead to CNS toxicity, even death.

Antifungal drugs

The polyene antibiotic *nystatin* is useful for mucocutaneous candidiasis (see p. 301).

Imidazoles (**miconazole**) and allylamines (*terbinafine*) can be applied locally in fungicidal doses. The morpholino derivative, *amorolfine*, also inhibits ergosterol synthesis in dermatophyte fungi, but by inhibiting a different enzyme in the synthetic pathway to the two foregoing drugs. It is applied locally to nails and is fungicidal.

Antiviral drugs

Idoxuridine is a pyrimidine analogue that shows slight biochemical selectivity based on metabolic acceptance as a pyrimidine and incorporation into a functionless DNA. Its main selectivity is based on this distributional mechanism (site of administration). It inhibits the replication of certain DNA viruses (see p. 316).

Arachnicides and insecticides

These include *carbaryl* (see p. 000), *lindane* and pyrethroids (*permethrin*). Selectivity is great and, while some show a biochemical component, the dominant basis is distributional. Spread on the skin as powder or emulsion, the dose per unit of body mass received by the ectoparasite is much greater than that received by the host. This is due both to the differing body mass : surface area ratios of the host and parasite, and also to the more ready penetration of the chitinous exoskeleton of the ectoparasite than of the intact human skin. In addition, the parasite ingests some of the drug.

Pyrethroids (see p. 288) cause a depolarization and hyperexcitability of nerve membranes. They are rapidly inactivated in mammals (but not fish).

Eye

The choice of antibiotic agents for use in the conjunctival sac is governed by considerations similar to those governing use on the skin. *Framycetin, neomycin* and *chlortetracycline* are examples.

Idoxuridine is also of some value in treating herpes virus infections involving the conjunctiva.

Summary

Distributional selectivity of toxicity can occur because a drug is selectively accumulated by the parasites (including selective activation of a prodrug by the parasites), distributed into a limited compartment containing the parasites, or administered to such a compartment.

Acquired drug resistance in parasites

Drug resistance in microbes

Origin

The development of drug resistance in microbial parasites usually has its origins in random spontaneous mutation. This occurs at a frequency of one per 10^6–10^7 cell divisions.

Selection

Mutants have no advantage, and may be at a disadvantage compared with the wild type, in a drug-free environment. However, they are better able to survive and multiply in a drug-containing environment, having been naturally selected by the administration of a drug to which the wild type is sensitive but the mutant strain is resistant. A single mutation may confer a high degree of resistance (one step) or just a small increment of resistance to which others can be added (multi-step) with selection to a high degree of resistance by prolonged or repeated inadequate drug dosage.

Spread

Spread of drug resistance between microbes is by transfer of genetic material (usually extrachromosomal DNA in the form of plasmids) by:

(1) Transduction, by a bacteriophage (e.g. *Staph. aureus*): plasmids are carried from one (resistant) bacterium to another (that was sensitive but becomes resistant on receipt and expression of the plasmid).
(2) Conjugation (e.g. Shigellae and *E. coli*): plasmids are conveyed between bacteria along with the donated chromosomal DNA during sexual reproduction. Transfer of resistance by conjugation does occur between bacteria of different species.

Mechanisms

(1) Enzymatic inactivation of the drug:
   (a) β-lactamase inactivation of penicillins and cephalosporins; *Staph. aureus* is most often discussed but β-lactamase production occurs in other species too, including Gram-negative bacteria, but not in streptococci (Strep.) or gonococci. The gene confers the ability to synthesize the β-lactamase enzyme; production of the enzyme is induced by contact with the antibiotic;
   (b) acetylation of *chloramphenicol*;
   (c) acylation of aminoglycoside antibiotic agents underlies acquisition of resistance by some bacteria.
(2) Loss of permeability to, or net accumulation of, the drug:
   (a) bacterial resistance to tetracyclines (see p. 281);
   (b) plasmodial resistance to **chloroquine** (see p. 281)

(3) Increased production of a metabolite that competes with the drug: aminobenzoate production is increased in some sulphonamide-resistant cells; DHF production is increased in Plasmodia resistant to pyrimethamine (see p. 296).

(4) Reduced affinity of the drug-sensitive site:
   (a) penicillin binding enzymes have decreased affinity in *Strep. pneumoniae* and *N. gonorrhoeae*;
   (b) dihydropteroate synthetase affinity for sulphonamides is reduced in some sulphonamide resistant cells;
   (c) DHF reductase affinity for **trimethoprim** is reduced;
   (d) DNA-dependent RNA-polymerase ability to bind **rifampicin** is reduced;
   (e) ribosome binding site for **gentamicin** or **erythromycin** is lost in some resistant bacteria.

Resistance in neoplastic cells to cancer chemotherapeutic agents

Mechanisms

(1) Reduced intracellular drug concentration:
   (a) by increased drug efflux (the multi-drug resistance phenotype); **doxorubicin**, *actinomycin D*, vinca alkaloids, *etoposide*;
   (b) by decreased inward transport; **methotrexate**.
(2) Decreased conversion to active form of drug; antimetabolites.
(3) Increased amount of target enzyme; **methotrexate**.
(4) Decreased affinity of drug for target enzyme; **methotrexate**, hydroxyurea, *etoposide*.
(5) Increased repair of drug-induced DNA damage; alkylating agents.
(6) Increased detoxification of drug; alkylating agents.
(7) Decreased activity of enzyme required for drug-induced cell death; **doxorubicin**, *etoposide*.
(8) Suppression of drug-induced cell death by apoptosis; most anticancer drugs.

Chemotherapy of metazoal infestations

Ectoparasites

Scabies

Scabies is a highly contagious infestation by the skin-dwelling mite (an acarid arachnid) *Sarcoptes scabiei* (Figure 6.7). The fertilized females burrow into the horny layer of the skin. This is symptomless at first but

STAFFS UNIVERSITY LIBRARY

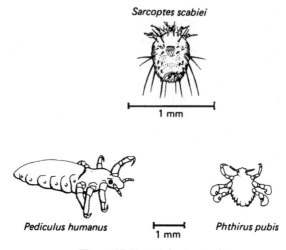

Figure 6.7 Metazoal ectoparasites

an allergic, itching rash develops later. Fortunately scabies infestation rarely involves the head.

Treatment involves completely covering the body surface (except the head) with a preparation containing *lindane, malathion* or *permethrin*. The treatment should be repeated on several days and should be extended to all members of the patient's household. The mites are killed by this process but the rash takes several weeks to clear. Renewal of symptoms is due to reinfestation.

Permethrin is an insecticide/acaricide developed from compounds (pyrethroids) that occur naturally in the pyrethrum flower. By prolonging the opening of Na^+ channels in neuronal cell membranes, *permethrin* induces repetitive action-potential discharge and hence the convulsive death of the scabies mite. The selectivity of this action has a strong distributional basis.

Lindane similarly damages neuronal cell membranes.

Louse infestation

Pediculosis is infestation with the head or body louse (*Pediculus humanus*, races *capitis* and *humanus*; Figure 6.7) whilst phthiriasis is infestation with the crab louse (*Phthirus pubis*; Figure 6.7). Pediculosis is transmitted by bodily contact or by the sharing of combs, hair-brushes or clothing. The lice infest head or body hair in circumstances of poor personal hygiene and are the vector of typhus. Phthiriasis is transmitted during sexual intercourse and the lice generally infest the pubic hair.

Head and body louse infestation can be eradicated using a lotion containing *carbaryl, malathion* or *permethrin*. Ideally the treatment should be extended to all members of the patient's household. During treatment the infested hair should be assiduously combed to remove the dying lice and their eggs (nits).

In view of the ability of head and body lice to develop resistance rapidly to insecticidal drugs, most health districts in the UK operate a policy of rotating the chemotherapy of such infestations.

Lotions containing *carbaryl, lindane* or *malathion* are effective against infestations with crab lice.

Carbaryl and the prodrug *malathion* (see p. 282) act to inhibit cholinesterase enzymes. When used topically to eradicate lice, both drugs show a high degree of distributional selectivity.

Endoparasites – worms

Classification of parasitic worms:

(1) Flatworms:
   (a) tapeworms;
   (b) flukes (includes schistosomes).
(2) Roundworms:
   (a) Ascaris (often called roundworm);
   (b) threadworms;
   (c) hookworms;
   (d) filariae.

Infestation with adult worms can occur in two basic sites:

(1) The worms live in the tissues of the host:
   (a) lymphatic vessels, skin, connective tissue – filariae;
   (b) liver, bile ducts, lungs – flukes and some schistosomes;
   (c) blood vessels – schistosomes.
(2) The worms live in the lumen of the alimentary canal (which has a low Po_2) and are therefore anaerobes:
   (a) tapeworms;
   (b) all roundworms except filariae.

Infestations with tissue-dwelling worms (Table 6.1) are not endemic in the UK and present great problems in the design of efficacious drugs or vaccines, the creation of a laboratory model of the infestation and field trials (including worm counts). Some effective, if rather toxic, drugs have been developed empirically but their mechanisms of vermicidal activity have been little studied.

Anaerobic worms inhabiting the gut lumen are more readily controlled by chemotherapy. Most worms in the infesting population are

Table 6.1 Metazoal infestations not endemic in the UK

Worm	Vector	Drug
Tissue infestation		
Schistosoma (bilharzia)	Fresh-water snail	*Praziquantel*
Filariae	Biting flies	*Diethylcarbamazine*
Filariae causing onchocerciasis	Biting flies	*Ivermectin*
Intestinal infestation		
Ancylostoma (hookworm)		*Pyrantel*
Strongyloides		*Thiabendazole*

adult, so interference with nucleic acid or protein synthesis, which so successfully achieves selective toxicity in bacteria (because they are rapidly growing and multiplying), is an inappropriate mechanism of vermicidal action. Since intestinal worms depend on muscular activity to maintain their position in the gut, biochemically selective interference with the function of worm musculature (**piperazine**) is valuable. However, distributional selectivity underlies the action of most useful vermifugal drugs because:

(1) The worms are located in a limited compartment (the gut lumen).
(2) The factors limiting absorption of chemicals from this compartment into the systemic circulation are known.
(3) Unlike the intestinal mucosa, the pellicle of the worm is highly permeable.

Infestation with beef tapeworm

In the UK beef tapeworm (*Taenia saginata*; Figure 6.8) infestation is of low incidence and in most cases is asymptomatic. The adult tapeworm clings to the intestinal mucosa (upper jejunum) by means of suckers found on its scolex (head). Successful treatment depends on the scolex being made to relinquish its hold on the mucosa.

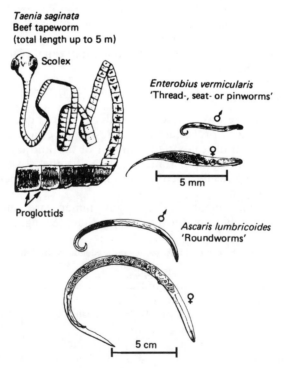

Figure 6.8 Metazoal endoparasites

Niclosamide kills the tapeworm, possibly by interfering with its anaerobic production of ATP. Since *niclosamide* is not absorbed from the gut, this biochemical selectivity receives great distributional reinforcement. Since the killed worm is not passed whole but partially digested, the scolex may be unrecognizable. The criterion of cure is 12 weeks without recurrence of segments in the stool.

Praziquantel is a taenicide of similar efficacy to *niclosamide*.

Roundworm infestation

Threadworms (*Enterobius vermicularis*; Figure 6.8) inhabit the colon and rectum. Threadworm infestation is very common in the UK (particularly in children), causing perianal irritation and sleeplessness when the female worms emerge from the anus at night to lay eggs. Reinfestation is common, so good hygiene practice (to break the ano-oral transmission process) and chemotherapy should be adopted by all members of the patient's household.

Roundworm (*Ascaris lumbricoides*; Figure 6.8) infestation is less common in the UK. Ingestion of contaminated food or water leads to egg hatching in the intestinal lumen. Microscopic larval worms burrow through the intestinal wall and are carried in the blood stream to the lungs. Worm larvae enter the alveoli, ascend to the glottis, are swallowed and develop as adults in the small intestine. The pathological consequences of Ascaris infestation are variable (very mild to fatal), may depend on the number of infesting worms and can include tissue damage caused by larval invasion.

Enterobius and Ascaris both hold their position in the intestinal lumen by swimming against intestinal peristalsis. Enterobius may also anchor to the intestinal mucosa using the fluke-like appendages located near its mouth.

Mebendazole is effective against both Enterobius and Ascaris. It kills the worms by interfering with their uptake or utilization of glucose. Interference with blood glucose concentration is not seen in the human host, so *mebendazole* may show some biochemical selectivity. However, *mebendazole* is poorly absorbed from the gut so that its selectivity as a vermifuge undoubtedly has a large distributional component.

Piperazine is effective against both Enterobius and Ascaris. It acts as an inhibitory agonist on the musculature of the worms, directly evoking relaxation. The living, flaccidly paralysed worms are then expelled from the intestine of the host by peristaltic activity. **Piperazine** is well absorbed from the gut. However, it has little or no relaxant activity in human muscle (see p. 280) and is relatively free from unwanted effects. **Piperazine** is thus biochemically selective as a vermifuge.

Pyrantel is effective against both Ascaris and Enterobius. *Pyrantel* acts as an excitatory agonist at the nicotinic acetylcholine receptors of the muscle of Ascaris and Enterobius causing spastic paralysis of the worms. Tested on isolated mammalian muscle, *pyrantel* has significant **suxamethonium**-like activity. *Pyrantel* is water insoluble, so little is absorbed by the host. Hence its vermifugal action shows distributional selectivity.

Summary

(1) Scabies or louse infestations can be eradicated by topical administration of drugs that cause the repetitive discharge of nerve action potentials (e.g. *lindane, permethrin*) or that inhibit cholinesterases (e.g. *carbaryl, malathion*).
(2) Beef tapeworm infestation can be eradicated by *niclosamide* or by *praziquantel*. The taenicidal action of *niclosamide* exhibits selectivity with both biochemical and distributional bases.
(3) Threadworm and roundworm (*Ascaris lumbricoides*) infestations can be eradicated by attention to hygiene and the oral administration of a vermifugal drug (e.g. *mebendazole*, **piperazine**, *pyrantel*).
(4) The vermicidal action of *mebendazole* involves inhibition of glucose uptake or utilization and exhibits selectivity with both biochemical and distributional bases.
(5) The vermifugal action of **piperazine** involves relaxation of worm musculature and exhibits selectivity with a biochemical basis.
(6) The vermifugal action of *pyrantel* involves spastic paralysis of worm musculature and exhibits selectivity with a distributional basis.

Chemotherapy of protozoal infections

Malaria

Tens of millions of people world wide are infected by the malarial parasite. Approximately 2250 cases of malaria are reported annually in the UK, with an increasing proportion being due to infection with *Plasmodium falciparum* (see below). Several of these patients die because of delayed or incorrect diagnosis or treatment.

Human malaria is caused by four species of the protozoon Plasmodium (Table 6.2) transmitted by the female anopheline mosquito. Approximately 50% of cases are due to *P. falciparum* and 40–45% to *P. vivax*.

The main clinical features of malaria are fever, anaemia, enlarged spleen and jaundice. In *P. falciparum* malaria the sequestration of parasitized red blood cells in the cerebral capillaries leads to cerebral malaria, which has a high mortality rate. The fever is due to the periodic rupture of red cells containing parasites. The older names for the various forms of malaria are derived in part from the periodicity of this rupture and fever, namely tertian malaria, as for *P. vivax* and *P. ovale* when the fever occurs on every third day (counting the onset of fever as day 1) and quartan as for *P. malariae* where the fever occurs on every fourth day. In *P. falciparum* infections the fever may be tertian but it is often continuous or irregular.

Table 6.2 The characteristics of human malaria infections

Infecting species	P. falciparum	P. vivax	P. ovale	P. malariae
Time to onset of symptoms	6 days	8 days	9 days	14 days
Fever cycle	2 days or	2 days irregular	2 days	3 days
Severity of attack	Severe	Mild/severe	Mild	Mild
Relapse (due to hypnozoites)	No	Yes	Yes	No
Recrudescence (due to persistent blood forms)	Yes	Yes	Yes	Yes
Older name	Malignant malaria	Benign tertian	Benign tertian	Benign quartan

The lifecycle is depicted in Figure 6.9. When an infected female mosquito takes a blood meal, sporozoites are inoculated from the saliva. These are rapidly transferred from the blood to the liver parenchymal cells (hepatocytes) where they divide (tissue schizogony) to form multinucleated tissue schizonts. On completion of this pre- or exo-erythrocytic cycle, several thousand merozoites are released into hepatic capillaries by rupture of the hepatocytes. Some of these enter red blood cells and undergo a series of divisions and periods of growth to form trophozoites and subsequently schizonts (erythrocytic schizogony). It is the rupture of the red cells containing these schizonts and the release of merozoites,

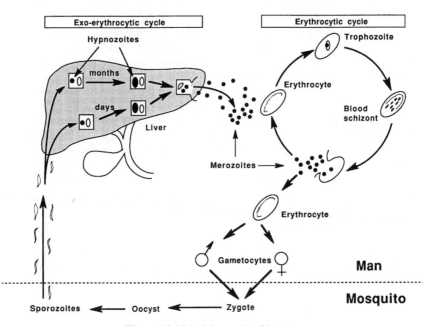

Figure 6.9 Malarial parasite: life cycle

malaria pigment (haemozoin, a haem polymer) and other cellular contents that induces the fever (see above). Each released merozoite is capable of infecting another erythrocyte to repeat the process of schizogony. Some of the trophozoites develop into male and female gametocytes. These are transferred to the mosquito (primary host) during a blood meal and undergo a sexual phase of division (sporogony) yielding sporozoites.

In *P. vivax* and *P. ovale*, but not *P. falciparum* and *P. malariae* malaria, some parasites (hypnozoites) remain dormant in the liver cells (exo-erythrocytic). Reactivation of these over varying periods is responsible for clinical relapses. In falciparum and malariae malaria the development of immunity or treatment with a drug that clears the blood (**chloroquine**) can genuinely rid the body of the parasites (radical cure). In vivax and ovale malaria, however, the symptoms are temporarily suppressed (clinical cure) but parasites can subsequently emerge from the liver causing relapse. Recrudescence, reappearance of the clinical disease due to the persistence of erythrocytic forms, can occur in all four forms of malaria.

Drugs providing clinical cure of malaria

Clinical cure implies clearing the blood of parasites and thus suppressing symptoms. Since *P. falciparum* and *P. malariae* display no exo-erythrocytic hypnozoites, clinical cure provides radical cure. For other Plasmodia it does not and relapse can occur.

Rapidly acting blood schizonticides

These include **chloroquine** (a 4-aminoquinoline), *quinine* and *mefloquine* (4-quinolinemethanols) and *halofantrine* (a 9-phenanthrenemethanol), which can clear the blood of parasites within 24 h. The members of this group are generally thought to act by the same mechanism, although the details of this action are not clearly understood. A number of mechanisms have been suggested, particularly for **chloroquine**, including intercalation into DNA, suppression of DNA replication, inhibition of polyamine synthesis and formation of haemolytic complexes with ferriprotoporphyrin derived from host cell haemoglobin. More recent work suggests that **chloroquine** inhibits the enzyme haem polymerase, which catalyses the conversion of haem to haemozoin. The resultant accumulation of haem within the red blood cell is toxic to the malarial parasite. For **chloroquine** and *quinine* the mechanism of selectivity is distributional. These drugs are selectively concentrated by the erythrocytic parasites, therefore only in these is a concentration adequate to produce the toxic effect achieved.

Resistance to **chloroquine**, particularly in *P. falciparum*, due to failure of the parasite to concentrate the drug is now widespread, probably as a consequence of its prophylactic use. Resistance to *quinine* and *mefloquine* does occur but these drugs are still effective in many **chloroquine**-resistant strains and provide alternative (albeit more toxic in the case of *quinine*) treatments.

Antiparasitic doses of **chloroquine** do not usually produce serious unwanted effects (but see pp. 215 and 537). *Quinine* exhibits unwanted effects collectively known as cinchonism. These include depression of muscular force (unwanted hypotension but relief of nocturnal leg cramps), tinnitus, visual disturbances, rashes, abdominal pain and nausea. *Mefloquine* causes a number of unwanted effects, including dizziness, loss of balance and, more rarely, neuropsychiatric disturbances. On prolonged treatment or frequent use there may be accumulation because of the long $t_{1/2}$. The major hazard with *halofantrin* is its potential to induce cardiac dysrhythmias in susceptible patients.

Drug combinations providing sequential inhibition of DHF synthetase and DHF reductase

Combinations of pyrimethamine with either sulfadoxine or dapsone are slow acting schizonticides. This action is too slow to be used alone in clinical cure (see Prophylaxis below) but may be used as an adjunct to *quinine* in the treatment of malaria caused by *P. falciparum* that is resistant to **chloroquine**. The antimalarial action represents sequential inhibition of nucleic acid synthesis with biochemical selectivity (see p. 272).

Resistance to pyrimethamine (see p. 296) is widespread, and is observed in many **chloroquine**-resistant strains of *P. falciparum*. High doses or long-term use of pyrimethamine may cause bone marrow depression.

Drugs providing radical cure of malaria: tissue schizonticides

Radical cure of malaria implies clearing the liver of exo-erythrocytic parasites (hypnozoites) in infections caused by *P. vivax* and *P. ovale*. Since the only drug available (**primaquine**) is potentially toxic (see below), radical cure should not be attempted until a clinical cure has been achieved (using a blood schizonticide) and the patient is fit enough to withstand the treatment.

Primaquine, an 8-aminoquinoline, is rapidly absorbed from the gut but neither the antimalarial activity nor the host toxicity is directly related to the blood concentration of **primaquine**. It is a prodrug that is transformed in the liver to oxidizing agents (quinoline-quinone derivatives). These oxidizing agents are cytotoxic and may be responsible for both the antimalarial effect and host toxicity. The malarial parasite and human erythrocytes depend on the activity of the pentose-phosphate biochemical pathway for the production of reduced glutathione, which protects cellular proteins from oxidation. If this pathway is compromised the cells become very vulnerable to oxidative damage. Gametocytes and the liver-dwelling (but not blood-dwelling) forms of the malarial parasites have a deficiency of an enzyme or co-factor in the pentose-phosphate pathway and are thus killed by the oxidizing action of **primaquine** metabolites. It has also been suggested that the metabolites may interfere with the functioning of the co-factor, ubiquinone, in mitochondrial respiration. Selectivity for the parasite depends on differences between the parasite and host co-factor.

In most patients the antimalarial action of **primaquine** shows moderate biochemical selectivity. However, in patients with a genetically determined deficiency of glucose-6-phosphate dehydrogenase (see p. 431), the pentose-phosphate pathway of erythrocytes is compromised and the cells become very susceptible to oxidative damage. **Primaquine** thus evokes intravascular haemolysis. Glucose-6-phosphate dehydrogenase deficiency has a high incidence in areas where malaria is endemic. This abnormality may have been naturally selected there because it is speculated to confer some natural immunity to malaria. The labile erythrocytes of persons with glucose-6-phosphate dehydrogenase deficiency are severely damaged by parasite entry and are destroyed by the reticuloendothelial system before the parasite can grow to maturity.

In all patients, **primaquine** can cause methaemoglobinaemia. Patients deficient in methaemoglobin reductase (see p. 429) are especially prone to this problem, as they cannot rapidly reduce methaemoglobin.

Prophylaxis of malaria

No drugs or vaccines provide true causal prophylaxis (prevention of pre-erythrocytic liver infection), against all four species of infecting sporo-zoites. **Primaquine** is too toxic for routine prophylactic use.

Drugs currently available provide imperfect suppressive treatment. They do not stop the contraction of malaria, or its establishment in the liver, but act to prevent the establishment of the erythrocytic cycle. Signs and symptoms of malaria may break through during the treatment course or may appear after termination of therapy.

Drugs for prophylaxis include **chloroquine**, *mefloquine*, pyrimethamine combined with dapsone, and proguanil (which has the same mechanism of action as pyrimethamine, see p. 273). Resistance to proguanil develops readily and there is cross-resistance to pyrimethamine. The mechanism of this resistance involves increased synthesis of DHF, so resistant parasites are more dependent on DHF synthetase and hence more susceptible to sulphones. In this situation the pyrimethamine and dapsone combination is valuable. The pyrimethamine and sulphonamide combination is no longer recommended for prophylaxis because of bone marrow depression.

Prophylaxis should be commenced before visiting a malaria-endemic area and should be continued for at least 1 month after returning from it. Increasing emphasis is placed on *mefloquine* in areas of **chloroquine**-resistant *P. falciparum* but it should be limited to 3 months use. The choice of an appropriate agent should take into account a number of factors, including the risk of exposure to malaria, the extent of drug resistance, the efficacy and unwanted effects of the drug and patient-related-criteria such as age, pregnancy, hepatic and renal function. Specialist centres listed in the BNF can provide up to date advice.

Entamoeba histolytica amoebiasis

Entamoeba histolytica (Figures 6.10b, 6.11) is one of several species of anaerobic amoebae that can colonize the lumen of the human intestine. Distribution of the infection is world-wide and approximately 10% of the world population harbour Entamoebae as harmless commensal organisms. Symptoms of the infection are infrequent in the UK but occur when, for

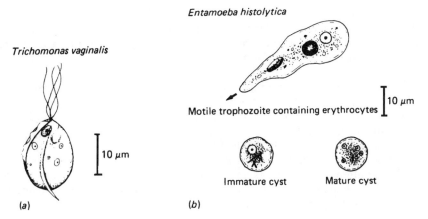

Figure 6.10 Protozoal parasites: (a) *Trichomonas vaginalis*; (b) *Entamoeba histolytica*

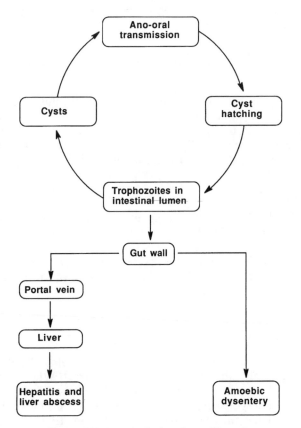

Figure 6.11 *Entamoeba histolytica*: life cycle

STAFFS UNIVERSITY LIBRARY

an unknown reason, the entamoebae invade the wall of the large intestine, causing ulcers and phagocytosing red blood cells (amoebic dysentery). Amoebae may also be carried via the portal vein to the liver. Here they cause tissue necrosis (bacteriologically 'sterile' abscesses) and hepatitis.

When conditions in the intestine are unfavourable, the amoebae form cysts, which are excreted in the faeces. Ingestion of food or water contaminated with cysts completes the ano-oral transmission process and cysts hatch in the small intestine.

Good sanitation and hygienic food preparation successfully prevents transmission of Entamoebae. Amoebicidal drugs can eradicate infection, both in patients exhibiting symptoms and in asymptomatic cyst-passers. Amoebicidal agents may be classified according to the body compartments from which the parasite is removed.

Drugs active against amoebae invading the gut wall and liver

Oral **metronidazole** is the agent of choice for acute amoebic dysentery, hepatitis or liver abscess. It is poorly effective against amoebae dwelling in the intestinal lumen of asymptomatic patients, probably because it is present in insufficient local concentration following its rapid and almost complete absorption higher up the gut.

Drugs active only against amoebae dwelling in the intestinal lumen

Diloxanide furoate is used after all signs and symptoms of infection have subsided to prevent or terminate the carrier state. It is directly amoebicidal to the luminal trophozoites but the mechanism is unknown; it is presumed to be biochemically selective since most of the oral dose is absorbed and excreted in the urine but causes little host toxicity.

Antibiotic use

Incompletely absorbed antibiotic agents (tetracyclines) may be used as an adjunct to **metronidazole** in the treatment of intestinal amoebiasis. The antibacterial action leads to less favourable conditions for development of the amoebae and reduces secondary bacterial infections of lesions. Additionally, tetracycline has some minor direct amoebicidal activity.

Trichomoniasis

Trichomonas vaginalis (Figure 6.10a) is an anaerobic flagellated protozoon that commonly inhabits the genitourinary tract. When conditions are favourable (e.g. suppressed vaginal flora, more alkaline vaginal mucus), Trichomonas undergoes opportunist overgrowth causing vaginal inflammation. In men the infection is usually symptom free though urethritis may occur. Transmission of infection results from sexual intercourse.

Nitroimidazole derivatives (**metronidazole**) orally are safe and effective trichomonacides. They are prodrugs selectively activated to short-lived cytotoxic intermediates (which possibly release superoxide anions) in anaerobic cells (see p. 280).

Recurrence of trichomonal vaginitis is usually the result of reinfection, so that it is wise to treat the sexual partner even if he/she is symptom free. **Metronidazole** shows an interaction, like *disulfiram*, with ethanol (see p. 263). Metabolites of **metronidazole** may cause dark coloration of the urine.

Summary

(1) Drugs are used in malaria to effect a clinical cure (removal of parasite from the blood), radical cure (removal of parasite from the liver) or for prophylaxis.
(2) Drugs used in clinical cure. **Chloroquine** (and other rapidly acting blood schizonticides) are selectively accumulated by the parasites and clear sensitive parasites from the blood in 24 h. Sequential inhibitors of the folic acid pathway (pyrimethamine plus sulfadoxine or dapsone) are slowly acting schizonticides used in combination with *quinine* in **chloroquine**-resistant *P. falciparum* malaria.
(3) The drug used in radical cure (**primaquine**): is a prodrug metabolized to cytotoxic oxidizing agents in the liver; shows moderate biochemical selectivity; causes methaemoglobinaemia in patients deficient in methaemoglobin reductase; causes haemolysis in patients deficient in glucose-6-phosphate dehydrogenase.
(4) Drugs used in prophylaxis: include **chloroquine**, *mefloquine*, proguanil and pyrimethamine with dapsone; only prevent the establishment of the erythrocytic cycle; are chosen after consideration of the risk of infection, extent of drug resistance, efficacy and toxicity of drug- and patient-related factors.
(5) Drugs used in amoebiasis: oral **metronidazole** is the drug of choice in acute amoebic dysentery, hepatitis or liver abscess; *diloxanide furoate* clears parasites from the intestinal lumen and terminates the carrier state.
(6) Drugs used in trichomoniasis: nitroimidazole derivatives (**metronidazole**) are selectively activated to cytotoxic intermediates; **metronidazole** interacts, like *disulfiram*, with alcohol.

Chemotherapy of fungal infections

Compared with the development of antibacterial chemotherapy, the development of antifungal chemotherapy has been slow. There are two main reasons for this:

(1) Unlike bacteria, fungal cells are eukaryotic – biologically much more akin to mammalian cells. This similarity militates against selective toxicity, and the currently available antifungal drugs are, in general, more toxic than antibacterial agents.
(2) The stimulus for antifungal drug research has only become powerful within the last few decades, since radiotherapy and the use of immunosuppressant drugs has created an immunocompromised population of patients whose lives are threatened by systemic fungal infections.

Infections of keratin (dermatophytoses)

Various microscopic fungi (dermatophytes) utilize keratinized tissue (skin, hair, nail) as a medium for growth. The initial skin infection may result from contact with infected domestic or farm animals or from contact with surfaces (e.g. bathroom and changing room floors) contaminated with fungi. The initial infection tends to spread outwards as a disc. The centre of the disc may heal so that the lesion takes on the appearance of a ring – hence the name ringworm. Ringworm is often named according to the locus of the infection, for example, tinea pedis (athlete's foot).

Localized ringworm infection of skin

Superficial infection is controlled by removal of any animal source of the infection and by attention to personal hygiene reinforced by topical administration of antifungal agents.

Imidazole derivatives (**miconazole**) have a broad spectrum of fungicidal activity, being effective against both dermatophytes and yeast-like fungi. For mechanisms of toxicity and selectivity see pages 279 and 285.

Terbinafine (see p. 280) is an effective treatment for fungal skin infections.

Amorolfine (see p. 285), applied as a lacquer, is useful in the treatment of dermatophyte infection of the fingernails or toenails.

Compound benzoic acid ointment (Whitfield's Ointment) contains benzoic acid and salicylic acid. Salicylic acid is keratolytic and assists both the shedding of fungus-laden tissue from the horny (keratin) layer of the epidermis and the penetration of the fungistatic agent benzoic acid to deeper-lying tissues. In topical treatment of ringworm, *compound benzoic acid ointment* has efficacy comparable to that of the preparations containing imidazoles but is cosmetically less acceptable.

Undecanoates; this fungistatic acid, and its esters (methyl) or salts (zinc), can be used in the topical treatment of ringworm but is less effective than the imidazoles.

Widespread or intractable ringworm

Widespread ringworm infection of the skin or infection of hair or nails are best treated systemically.

Griseofulvin is the agent of choice when hair or nails are involved. It has a narrow spectrum (dermatophytes only) of fungistatic activity. For mechanisms of toxicity and selectivity, see page 282. The keratin formed during treatment resists invasion by fungal hyphae. Since treatment must be continued until all infected keratin has been shed (can be more than 1 year in the case of toe nails), unwanted effects (headache, skin rashes, nausea, impairment of memory, increased porphyrin excretion), although uncommon, assume greater significance.

Intravenous **miconazole** and oral *ketoconazole* are effective in widespread ringworm infection. However, the injection vehicle for **miconazole** (polyethoxylated castor oil) may give rise to hypersensitivity reactions. Furthermore, *ketoconazole* has been associated with fatal hepatotoxicity and the potential benefits of oral *ketoconazole* should be carefully weighed against this risk.

Mucocutaneous infections by yeasts

The yeast *Candida albicans* is a normal inhabitant of the skin and mucous membranes of the gut and genitourinary tract. Opportunist overgrowth (candidiasis) occurs when competitive flora are suppressed (broad-spectrum antibiotic agents), when normal defences are suppressed (gluco-corticosteroids, cytotoxic drugs) or when biochemical changes occur in the fungal habitat (pregnancy, diabetes, debilitation). Candidiasis most frequently occurs in the mouth and throat (thrush) and in the vagina.

The polyene antibiotic *nystatin* is fungicidal to many species of fungus. For mechanisms of toxicity and selectivity, see pages 279 and 284. It is too toxic for systemic use but it is useful against mucocutaneous candidiasis. It is not absorbed from the gut so the oral route is useful for alimentary tract infection (enteritis due to Candida) and local application for oral thrush (pastilles, suspensions) or for vaginitis (pessaries).

Imidazole or triazole derivatives may be administered topically (**miconazole**) or orally (**miconazole**, *fluconazole*) in the treatment of superficial candidiasis.

Fungal infection of deep tissues

This tends to occur only in patients whose defences have been seriously impaired by glucocorticosteroids or cytotoxic drugs. The pathogens are a wide variety of fungi of low pathogenicity in immunocompetent patients.

The polyene antibiotic **amphotericin** is a close chemical relative of *nystatin* but sufficiently less toxic to allow its slow i/v infusion. Unwanted effects are common and include irritation at the injection site (pain and thrombophlebitis), nausea, vomiting, tinnitus and blurred vision. Renal toxicity is dose related, reversible at lower doses and seen in 80% of patients. The toxicity of **amphotericin** can be significantly reduced by the use of formulations in which the drug is encapsulated in liposomes.

Flucytosine is a prodrug with a narrow spectrum (yeasts) of antifungal activity. For mechanisms of toxicity and selectivity, see pages 274 and 282. Following oral administration it is well absorbed from the gut. Blood counts are necessary during prolonged administration.

Simultaneous administration of **amphotericin** and *flucytosine* can widen the antifungal spectrum of the chemotherapy and reduce the likelihood of fungal resistance.

Imidazole or triazole derivatives, too, are useful in the therapy of systemic fungal infections; *ketoconazole* can be given orally and **miconazole** by i/v infusion.

Summary

(1) Localized ringworm infection may be controlled by the topical administration of imidazoles (e.g. **miconazole**), *terbinafine* or *amorolfine*, which interfere with ergosterol synthesis.

(2) Widespread ringworm infection may be controlled by oral **griseofulvin** or azole derivatives. **Griseofulvin** is fungistatic and exhibits selectivity with a strong distributional basis.

(3) Candidiasis may be controlled by the topical administration of **nystatin** or by the use of azole derivatives.

(4) Fungal infections of deep tissues may be controlled by systemic administration of **amphotericin**, *flucytosine* or azole derivatives. **Amphotericin** has an antifungal action similar to that of **nystatin**, but is sufficiently less toxic to permit its systemic administration.

Chemotherapy of bacterial infections

Principles of treatment

Before committing a patient to a course of antibiotic therapy ask, is it necessary?

The basis of rational treatment is the bacteriological diagnosis. The clinical diagnosis from the patient's history and physical signs often points towards a particular bacterial pathogen (lobar pneumonia – *Strep. pneumoniae* (pneumococcus); urinary tract infection – *E. coli*; wound infection – *Staph. aureus*), and on this basis an antibacterial drug is chosen. A definitive bacteriological diagnosis requires isolation of the organism responsible. An initial Gram stain takes less than 1 h, culture and provisional identification 24 h, and sensitivity testing with confirmed identification 24–48 h. The patient's chemotherapy can be reviewed in the light of the bacteriological results and may be altered if clinically (inadequate resolution of temperature, pulse rate and other signs of inflammation) and bacteriologically indicated. Table 6.3 lists some important bacterial pathogens and appropriate antibacterial agents.

The object of chemotherapy is to produce a sufficient concentration of antibacterial drug at the site of an infection to kill (bactericidal action) or

Table 6.3 Important pathogenic bacteria, infections and drugs of choice

Genus/species	Infection	Antibacterial agents 1st choice	2nd choice
Gram-positive cocci			
Staph. aureus	Wound	**Flucloxacillin**	**Erythromycin**
	Osteomyelitis	**Vancomycin**	
Strep. pyogenes	Throat	Phenoxymethyl	**Erythromycin**
	Skin	penicillin	
Strep. pneumoniae	Pneumonia	**Benzylpenicillin**	**Erythromycin**
	Meningitis	**Benzylpenicillin**	**Cefotaxime**
Gram-positive bacilli			
Corynebacterium	Diphtheria	Antitoxin	**Erythromycin**
diphtheriae		**Benzylpenicillin**	
Listeria monocytogenes	Septicaemia	**Ampicillin**	Co-trimoxazole
	Meningitis	**Amoxycillin +**	
		gentamicin	
Gram-negative cocci			
N. meningitidis	Meningitis	**Benzylpenicillin**	**Cefotaxime**
N. gonorrhoeae	Gonorrhoea	**Amoxycillin**	Ciprofloxacin
Gram-negative bacilli			
E. coli	Urinary tract	**Trimethoprim**	**Cephradine**
Klebsiella	Urinary tract	**Cephradine**	**Gentamicin**
	Pneumonia	**Cefuroxime**	
Proteus	Urinary tract	**Ampi-/amoxycillin**	**Cephradine**
Pseudomonas aeruginosa	Urinary tract	**Gentamicin**	**Ciprofloxacin**
	Septicaemia	**Gentamicin +**	
		ceftazidime	
Salmonella typhi	Typhoid	**Ciprofloxacin**	Chloramphenicol
H. influenzae	Respiratory tract	**Amoxycillin**	**Trimethoprim**
	Meningitis	**Cefotaxime**	Chloramphenicol
Legionella pneumophila	Pneumonia	**Erythromycin**	**Rifampicin**
Anaerobes			
Bacteroides	Abscesses	**Metronidazole**	Clindamycin
Cl. perfringens	Gas gangrene	**Benzylpenicillin**	**Metronidazole**
Cl. difficile	Pseudomembranous colitis	**Vancomycin**	**Metronidazole**
Others			
Treponema pallidum	Syphilis	**Benzylpenicillin**	**Erythromycin**
M. tuberculosis	Tuberculosis	**Rifampicin**	Ethambutol
		Isoniazid	Streptomycin
		Pyrazinamide	
Mycoplasma pneumoniae	Pneumonia	**Erythromycin**	**Tetracycline**
Chlamydia	Genital tract	**Tetracycline**	**Erythromycin**
Pneumocystis	Pneumonia	Co-trimoxazole	

effectively to inhibit the multiplication (bacteriostatic action) of the responsible bacterium without damaging the tissues of the host. In general, the serum concentration should exceed by a factor of four the minimum inhibitory concentration (MIC) determined in the laboratory. Table 6.4 summarizes prescribing information on some commonly used antibiotic agents.

Table 6.4 Prescribing of some commonly used antibiotic agents

Drug	*Serum $t_{1/2}$ (h)	Elimination	Route of administration	Dosage interval (h)
Benzylpenicillin	0.5	ts	i/m i/v	6
Phenoxymethyl-penicillin	0.5	ts	oral	6
Flucloxacillin	0.5	ts	oral i/m i/v	6
Ampicillin	0.5	ts	oral i/m i/v	6
Amoxycillin	2	ts	oral i/m i/v	8
Cephradine	1	ts	oral i/m i/v	8
Cefuroxime	1	ts	oral i/m i/v	8
Cefotaxime	1	ts	i/m i/v	8
Gentamicin	2.5	gf	i/m i/v	8
Erythromycin	3	m	oral i/v	8
Vancomycin	6	gf	i/v	6
Tetracycline	8.5	gf m	oral	8
Ciprofloxacin	4	gf ts	oral i/v	12
Trimethoprim	8	gf	oral	12
Metronidazole	8	m gf	oral i/v rectal	12

gf = glomerular filtration; m = metabolism; ts = tubular secretion. *Mean values for normal individuals.

Routes of administration

Antibacterial drugs are administered by mouth in mild infections that do not require hospital treatment. In severe infections they are given parenterally (i/v or i/m) at a dose rate that rapidly achieves subtoxic peak and antibacterial trough serum concentrations. Intravenous administration ensures that the necessary dose is received with less discomfort for the patient. Intravenous antibacterial drugs can be given by bolus injection or continuous infusion; to avoid chemical neutralization take care in mixing one antibiotic solution with another or with i/v infusion fluid (see BNF Appendix 6).

Inadequate doses and infrequent administration encourage the emergence of resistant organisms.

Duration of therapy

This depends on a number of factors including the infecting organism, the site of infection, the host response and the kind of drug. Some severe infections (infective endocarditis, tuberculosis) always require prolonged antibacterial drug therapy.

Concurrent therapy

Additional measures may be at least as important in the treatment of infections, even when the antibacterial drug used is appropriate and at a sufficient dose. Abscesses must be drained, devitalized tissue and foreign bodies removed and obstruction to drainage (e.g. of the urinary tract) overcome. Resolution of chest infections is assisted by physiotherapy.

Prophylactic use

This is permissible only in a restricted range of clearly defined circumstances. There must be a specific target infection to be prevented, due to a specific organism that is reliably sensitive to the proposed prophylactic antibacterial drug. Objective methods should have demonstrated effectiveness of the prophylaxis in reducing the incidence of the target infection. See pages 307–308, 310 and 313 for examples. The risks of prophylaxis include the selection of resistant bacteria, superinfection with more resistant organisms and adverse drug reactions.

Failure to respond

If the patient does not improve, consider the following factors.

Pharmacokinetic factors

(1) Inadequate dosage.
(2) Wrong antibacterial drug – if there is a mixed infection.
(3) Incorrect route – oral antibacterial drugs may be ineffective in a patient who has vomiting or malabsorption or a severe infection.
(4) Inadequate duration of therapy may lead to early relapse.
(5) Use of inappropriate antibacterial drug combinations – a combination of two β-lactam antibiotic agents may result in antagonism, as one drug may induce enzymes that inactivate the other.
(6) Inadequate penetration into site of infection – aminoglycosides penetrate poorly into the CSF and would not be appropriate sole agents for the treatment of meningitis.

Pharmacodynamic factors

(1) Failure of the patient to take the drug (poor compliance) commonly occurs in patients on long-term therapy (tuberculosis).
(2) Additional measures required – drainage of pus.
(3) Poor host immune response due to coexisting disease (diabetes, anaemia, immune deficiency) or drug therapy (glucocorticosteroids, cytotoxic drugs).
(4) Development of antibacterial drug resistance (see p. 286) or superinfection by an organism that is resistant to the antibacterial drug.
(5) Fever due to a cause other than bacterial infection (malignancy) or to an organism that does not respond to conventional antibacterial drugs (viruses, protozoa).

Laboratory factors

(1) Inadequate, inappropriate (taken after antibacterial drug therapy has been commenced) or delayed specimens may not allow the laboratory to identify the pathogen.
(2) Insufficient clinical details on the requesting form may result in appropriate techniques (extra culture media) being omitted.
(3) Laboratory error.

Factors modifying the response

(1) Age: newborn infants, especially those delivered preterm, have immature livers and cannot detoxify certain drugs (*chloramphenicol*). Adverse reactions to antibacterial drugs are more common in the elderly (**isoniazid** and liver damage).
(2) Pregnancy: the fetus is at risk (deposition of tetracyclines in developing bones and teeth).
(3) Renal and hepatic function: poor renal excretion may result in accumulation of drugs (**gentamicin**). Renal function declines in old age and dose adjustment may be necessary. Drugs that are excreted or detoxified by the liver (**erythromycin**, *chloramphenicol*, **isoniazid**) should be used with caution in patients with poor liver function.

Antibacterial drug combinations

There are certain rules governing use of antibacterial drug combinations. Three are possible:

(1) A bacteriostatic with a bactericidal drug – this combination should be avoided. Bactericidal drugs act best against growing bacteria. If growth is prevented by a bacteriostatic drug, antagonism of the bactericidal drug may be important, for example there is a higher mortality in pneumococcal meningitis when **benzylpenicillin** (bactericidal) and **tetracycline** (bacteriostatic) are used in combination.
(2) A bacteriostatic with another bacteriostatic drug – these are simply additive, with the exception of **trimethoprim** and sulphamethoxazole (*co-trimoxazole*) in which the combination of two bacteriostatic agents produces a synergistic drug.
(3) A bactericidal with another bactericidal drug – can be synergistic, for example **benzylpenicillin** plus **gentamicin** in the treatment of infective endocarditis. Synergistic combinations are useful in the management of neutropenic (low blood neutrophil concentration) fevers, seen in patients after treatment with anticancer chemotherapy.

The advantages of combination therapy include:

(1) Reduction in the emergence of resistant strains during long-term therapy (tuberculosis).
(2) Improvement of the antibacterial spectrum (severely ill patients, patients with impaired host defences, multiple infecting organisms).
(3) Production of synergism (**ampicillin** plus **gentamicin** in *Enterococcus faecalis* endocarditis or neutropenic fevers).

Penicillins

All penicillins are made up of a fused β-lactam and thiazolidine ring and a side-chain (Figure 6.12). An intact β-lactam ring is essential for antibacterial activity. The side-chain is important in determining the pharmacodynamic (antibacterial spectrum) and dispositional properties of the penicillin drug. It has been altered so that it:

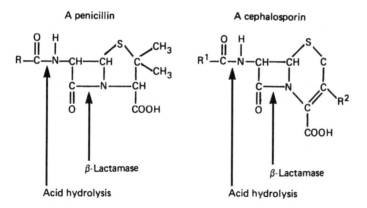

Figure 6.12 The penicillin and cephalosporin nuclei: the bonds susceptible to acid hydrolysis and β-lactamases

(1) Becomes resistant to hydrolysis by gastric acid, although absorption from the gut remains incomplete although adequate for most clinical purposes.
(2) Is made resistant to β-lactamase.
(3) Has a broader spectrum of antibacterial activity.

For mechanisms of bacterial toxicity and selectivity, see page 269.

Parent penicillins

Benzylpenicillin (penicillin G) is very potent and remains the drug of choice in some infections. It is hydrolysed by gastric acid and so inactivated and is therefore given parenterally. After i/m or i/v injection absorption is rapid and the drug is widely distributed in body tissues and fluids. Penetration into the CSF is minimal unless the meninges are inflamed, as in meningitis. There is very little metabolism. Elimination is by renal tubular secretion, and 60–90% of the administered dose is eliminated in 1 h. *Probenecid* can block this excretion and thus increase serum and CSF concentrations.

Benzylpenicillin shows bactericidal activity against a spectrum of pathogens, including Gram-positive cocci, Gram-negative cocci and Gram-positive bacilli (Table 6.3). The drug is inactivated by hydrolysis of the β-lactam ring by bacterial β-lactamase enzymes.

Procaine penicillin (combines equimolar amounts of benzylpenicillin and procaine) is an i/m depot preparation that provides adequate tissue concentrations of **benzylpenicillin** for up to 24 h. It is useful in the treatment of syphilis.

Phenoxymethylpenicillin (penicillin V) is acid stable. It is indicated for streptococcal tonsillitis and is useful for prophylaxis against streptococcal infections that would cause recurrence, in patients who have suffered rheumatic fever and against pneumococcal disease in patients who have had a splenectomy or have sickle cell disease.

STAFFS UNIVERSITY LIBRARY

Penicillinase-resistant penicillins

Flucloxacillin is resistant to the action of staphylococcal β-lactamase and gastric acid. Food interferes with its absorption, but even in the fasting state this is incomplete. In serious staphylococcal infections **flucloxacillin** should be given i/v. It should be reserved for infections caused by staphylococci that produce β-lactamase and should not be used to treat infections due to organisms that are sensitive to the more potent **benzylpenicillin**.

Broad-spectrum penicillins

Ampicillin has more activity against selected Gram-negative bacilli than **benzylpenicillin**. It is acid stable and adequate serum concentrations are obtained after oral administration (though absorption is incomplete). It is, however, susceptible to β-lactamase and, like **benzylpenicillin**, is rapidly eliminated by renal tubular secretion. It may be given parenterally if required. **Amoxycillin** is better absorbed and achieves a peak blood concentration approximately twice that of **ampicillin**. Its antibacterial activity is virtually identical to **ampicillin**. Food does not interfere with the absorption of **amoxycillin** and the incidence of diarrhoea is less than with **ampicillin**. High-dose **amoxycillin** is useful for short course therapy of urinary tract infections, otitis media and gonorrhoea. **Amoxycillin** is also useful for prophylaxis in patients with heart valve disease undergoing dental treatment. This produces a transient bacteraemia, which leads to infection of, and further damage to, congenitally or rheumatically damaged endocardium.

Extended-spectrum penicillins

Piperacillin is susceptible to β-lactamase, acid labile and given i/v. It is useful to treat serious infections due to *Pseudomonas aeruginosa*, usually in combination with an aminoglycoside.

Imipenem is a member of the β-lactam family of antibiotic agents but it is distinguished by a unique structure that gives it a very broad spectrum of activity. It has activity against Gram-negative and Gram-positive aerobic and anaerobic bacteria. It is best given i/v and its use is therefore restricted to the treatment of serious infections. Adverse effects resemble those of other β-lactams – hypersensitivity and CNS toxicity including seizures, particularly in the elderly.

Host toxicity of penicillins

Penicillins are less toxic than any other group of antibiotic agents. Their major unwanted effect is the production of hypersensitivity reactions (see p. 424). Reactions are either:

(1) Immediate (within 30 min) or accelerated (within 72 h) – erythema, angio-oedema, wheezing, shock, hypotension, death.
(2) Late (more than 72 h) – urticaria, rash, serum sickness syndrome (rash + fever + joint pain).

Maculopapular rashes occur commonly with **ampicillin** or **amoxycillin**, usually in patients with infectious mononucleosis. Therefore *phenoxymethylpenicillin* is preferred for the management of a suspected streptococcal sore throat. These **ampicillin** rashes do not usually signify true penicillin allergy.

The severity of allergic symptoms increases on re-exposure to penicillin. All patients should be asked if they are allergic to penicillin before any of the above drugs is prescribed. Treatment consists of *adrenaline* i/m, **chlorpheniramine** slowly i/v and *hydrocortisone sodium succinate* i/v (see p. 425).

Less common adverse effects of penicillin are neurotoxicity (which usually occurs when very high doses are used, especially in patients with renal failure), interstitial nephritis, hypokalaemia and diarrhoea.

Cephalosporins

The cephalosporins resemble the penicillins as they have a β-lactam structure but the five-membered thiazolidine ring of the penicillins is replaced by a six-membered dihydrothiazine ring (Figure 6.12). They thus have the same mode of action. Addition of different side-chains has modified the activity of the original drug and there are now numerous members of the cephalosporin family. The cephalosporins are classified into first, second and third generation groups according to their spectrum of antibacterial activity. First generation cephalosporins (**cephradine**) are the most active cephalosporins against Gram-positive cocci, but are less active against Gram-negative bacilli. Second generation cephalosporins (**cefuroxime**) have a broader spectrum of activity, especially against some species of Gram-negative bacilli. Third generation cephalosporins (**cefotaxime**, **ceftazidime**) have, broadly speaking, sacrificed their Gram-positive activity for increased Gram-negative activity. **Ceftazidime** is active against *Pseudomonas aeruginosa*.

As with the penicillins, hypersensitivity is the commonest adverse effect of the cephalosporins. Approximately 10% of patients allergic to penicillins are also allergic to cephalosporins. They also cause diarrhoea.

The most important mechanism of resistance to cephalosporins is the production of various β-lactamases by bacteria.

Cephradine and **cefuroxime** can be given orally; the other members must be given parenterally. Most cephalosporins are excreted by active secretion by the kidney tubules. *Ceftriaxone* is a third generation cephalosporin that is eliminated by the liver. Its dose does not need to be reduced in renal failure.

Cephalosporins are expensive and some members of the group are very valuable in treating hospital-acquired infections due to more resistant Gram-negative bacilli. It is preferable to use agents with a narrower spectrum where they would suffice.

Macrolides

For mechanisms of bacterial toxicity and selectivity, see page 279. The major member of this group is **erythromycin**. It is available in a variety of topical, oral and parenteral forms. Although inactivated by gastric acid, it is normally adequately absorbed, but food delays the absorption of **erythromycin** base. The drug is widely distributed throughout the body with the exception of the brain and CSF. It is metabolized by the liver and is mainly excreted in bile. It is a bacteriostatic agent, except when used in high doses or against low numbers of bacteria when it can be bactericidal. The spectrum of activity is similar, but not identical, to that of **benzylpenicillin** and it is often used in treatment of patients allergic to penicillin. In addition, it has activity against β-lactamase-producing *Staph. aureus* and is useful in the management of atypical pneumonias because of its activity against Legionella, Mycoplasma and Chlamydia. Host toxicity is minimal; unwanted effects include mild gastrointestinal upset, thrombophlebitis at the site of i/v injection and allergy. If it is used for more than 2 weeks it may produce a cholestatic jaundice.

Azithromycin produces higher tissue concentrations than **erythromycin**; it can be given once daily, as opposed to the four times daily dosing of **erythromycin**.

Aminoglycosides

For mechanisms of bacterial toxicity and selectivity, see page 277. This group has several members with similar pharmacological characteristics, leading to characteristic dispositional features (see p. 377). Absorption of hydrophilic aminoglycosides from the gut is negligible. Distribution is predominantly extracellular – there is poor penetration into the CSF, prostate, biliary tract and pulmonary secretions. There is no significant metabolism and elimination is by glomerular filtration. Aminoglycosides accumulate in patients with renal failure. Persistent high serum concentrations produce deafness (high tone) by damaging the outer hair cells of the organ of Corti, as well as producing vestibular damage; in addition renal tubular damage can occur. These adverse events can be avoided by monitoring of serum concentrations of aminoglycosides in order to maintain therapeutic concentrations without producing toxicity (see p. 380).

Gentamicin is the most generally useful aminoglycoside. It has a wide spectrum of activity particularly against Gram-negative bacilli (including *Pseudomonas*). It is useful in the management of serious infections including endocarditis when it is combined with **benzylpenicillin**.

Amikacin is active against some Gram-negative bacilli that are resistant to **gentamicin** because it is susceptible to fewer aminoglycoside inactivating enzymes (see p. 286). It is usually held in reserve for infections due to these organisms.

Streptomycin is the oldest aminoglycoside and is now mainly useful as a second line agent in the management of tuberculosis.

Neomycin is too toxic to be given systemically. It is used topically or is given orally to reduce bowel flora before surgery or in the management of liver failure. Some systemic absorption can occur with toxicity as a result.

Vancomycin

For mechanisms of bacterial toxicity and selectivity, see page 269. **Vancomycin** is ototoxic and nephrotoxic and therefore requires serum concentration monitoring. It is useful in the treatment of pseudomembranous colitis (given orally). **Vancomycin** is also indicated in the management of serious Gram-positive infections (mainly staphylococcal). It is useful in patients who are allergic to penicillin, and against staphylococci (both *Staph. aureus* and coagulase-negative staphylococci) that are resistant to **flucloxacillin**. **Vancomycin** is given intraperitoneally to treat Gram-positive peritonitis in patients on continuous ambulatory peritoneal dialysis (CAPD).

Tetracyclines

For mechanisms of bacterial toxicity and selectivity, see page 281. Tetracyclines (**tetracycline**) are bacteriostatic agents. They have a broad spectrum of antibacterial activity, although their usefulness is limited by acquired bacterial resistance. They remain important in the management of infections due to Mycoplasma and Chlamydia. Absorption from the gut is incomplete but adequate. Two factors account for variability in absorption:

(1) The hydrochloride derivatives are soluble in water, giving an acid solution; in a neutral or alkaline medium (the intestine) they tend to precipitate out or do not dissolve.
(2) They are chelating agents and complex with the divalent ions Ca^{2+}, Al^{2+}, Mg^{2+} (milk, antacid mixtures) and *ferrous sulphate* significantly reducing bioavailability.

Tetracyclines are both metabolized in the liver and excreted in the urine. They are widely distributed in tissues but achieve only 10% of the serum concentration in the CSF. They complex with calcium in growing long bones and in the enamel of developing teeth (impairing their development) and should never be prescribed in pregnancy or in children aged under 12 years.

Doxycycline is well absorbed and can be administered once daily. It is excreted mainly in bile and is therefore the tetracycline of choice in renal failure.

Unwanted effects of tetracyclines include rashes and allergic reactions, gastrointestinal upset (most severely pseudomembranous colitis), hepatic toxicity, aggravation of renal failure and benign intracranial hypertension.

Clindamycin

For mechanisms of bacterial toxicity and selectivity, see page 278. *Clindamycin* is a member of the lincosamide group of antibiotic agents. It can be bacteriostatic or bactericidal. It is adequately absorbed by mouth and is well distributed in tissues but does not penetrate into the

CSF. It is metabolized in the liver and excreted in the urine. It is used mainly in staphylococcal bone and joint infections and as an alternative to **metronidazole** in the treatment of infections due to anaerobic bacteria. Its major unwanted effect is diarrhoea, including pseudomembranous colitis, and therefore it should be stopped immediately if diarrhoea occurs.

Fusidic acid and its salts

For mechanisms of bacterial toxicity and selectivity, see page 279. *Sodium fusidate* is only recommended for use in staphylococcal infections, particularly osteomyelitis as it penetrates well into bone. It must always be used in combination with another anti-staphylococcal agent as resistance develops rapidly if it is used alone. Its oral absorption is variable, it is highly protein bound and it is inactivated in body tissues. Unwanted effects include gastrointestinal upset and rashes and it can cause jaundice, so regular monitoring of liver function tests is recommended.

Chloramphenicol

For mechanisms of bacterial toxicity and selectivity, see page 277. *Chloramphenicol* is bacteriostatic and well absorbed when administered by mouth. Its wide distribution includes the CSF. It is metabolized in the liver and a small proportion of the active drug along with its inactive metabolites is eliminated in the urine. Its conjugation mechanism in the liver is immature in the newborn and therefore it easily accumulates to toxic concentrations. Its inhibition of protein synthesis is responsible for its major adverse effect – depression of the bone marrow. As a result, the full blood count (including platelets) of patients receiving the drug should be performed every 48 h. Rarely *chloramphenicol* administration results in idiosyncratic aplastic anaemia – a complication that was fatal before the advent of bone marrow transplantation. Due to this significant toxicity, *chloramphenicol* is now only used in life-threatening infections (meningitis, typhoid fever) where use of an alternative agent is not possible.

4-Quinolones

For mechanisms of bacterial toxicity and selectivity, see page 276. **Ciprofloxacin** is derived from the urinary antiseptic *nalidixic acid*. **Ciprofloxacin** has a wide spectrum of activity, particularly against Gram-negative bacteria. It is a valuable drug for the management of severe hospital acquired infections, including those due to *Pseudomonas aeruginosa*, and is also indicated in serious salmonella infections (typhoid fever) and as single-dose therapy for gonorrhoea. Unwanted effects include gastrointestinal upset, allergic reactions and CNS disturbance. The 4-quinolones have been associated with joint damage in animals and therefore are avoided in childhood and pregnancy.

Metronidazole

For mechanisms of bacterial toxicity and selectivity, see page 280. **Metronidazole** is well absorbed after oral or rectal administration. It is active against anaerobic bacteria and some protozoa. It is widely distributed throughout the body, including into the CSF and abscesses. It is useful in surgical prophylaxis and is an alternative to **vancomycin** in the treatment of pseudomembranous colitis.

Sulphonamides and trimethoprim

For mechanisms of bacterial toxicity and selectivity, see page 272. Sulphonamides have been largely superseded due to increased acquired bacterial resistance and toxicity.

Co-trimoxazole is a synergistic combination of sulphamethoxazole and **trimethoprim**. Toxicity of *co-trimoxazole* is mainly attributable to the sulphamethoxazole component. *Co-trimoxazole* is definitely indicated for *Pneumocystis carinii* pneumonia, seen most usually in patients infected with the HIV virus.

Trimethoprim alone is suitable therapy for simple urinary tract infection and acute or exacerbation of chronic bronchitis. **Trimethoprim** can cause haematological unwanted effects particularly in patients who are folate deficient, e.g. the elderly or debilitated.

Superinfection

Any antibacterial drug with a wide bacterial spectrum and either incomplete absorption or partial gut elimination may reduce commensal organisms in the bowel, allowing the overgrowth of, or colonization with organisms naturally resistant to them (*Cl. difficile*, *Candida albicans*, resistant staphylococci, *Pseudomonas*). Overgrowth of *Cl. difficile* can in its most severe form result in pseudomembranous colitis. This is treated with oral **vancomycin** or **metronidazole**.

Tuberculosis

Most patients infected with *M. tuberculosis* can be effectively treated by prolonged administration of combination antibacterial drug therapy. Current antituberculosis chemotherapy involves administration of **isoniazid**, **rifampicin** and **pyrazinamide** for 2 months, followed by **isoniazid** and **rifampicin** for a further 4 months. This regimen is modified in the light of susceptibility data, and if drug resistance is thought to be likely *ethambutol* is included in the initial 2 months.

Isoniazid is bacteriostatic against *M. tuberculosis* in its resting phase but bactericidal against dividing bacilli. It penetrates cells to reach intracellular organisms. It inhibits a bacterial enzyme essential for the manufacture of a component of the organism's cell wall. The drug is well absorbed and crosses the blood–brain barrier. It is acetylated in the liver at a rate that is genetically determined (see p. 428). Hence some unwanted effects are more likely in slow acetylators. Adverse effects include peripheral neuropathy, which can be prevented by pyridoxine replacement, and hepatitis, which can be fatal.

Rifampicin has a wider spectrum of antibacterial activity (see p. 277), but is a crucial part of any tuberculosis treatment regimen. It cannot be used alone due to the rapid development of resistance. It can cause gastrointestinal unwanted effects. Liver function tests should be checked before therapy and monitored during therapy in alcoholics and those with pre-existing liver disease. Abnormal liver function tests are common but usually transient. Hepatic microsomal enzyme induction results in reduction of the efficacy of oestrogen oral contraceptives, corticosteroids, sulphonylureas, **warfarin** and *phenytoin*. Secretions including urine and tears are coloured orange-red.

Pyrazinamide is bactericidal and is maximally active under acid conditions. It may cause hepatic dysfunction, arthralgia and hyperuricaemia.

Ethambutol is a bacteriostatic agent. It is prescribed on a weight basis as high doses may cause visual toxicity. Patients should be warned to report any change in vision early as initial changes are reversible on withdrawal of the drug. Approximately 80% of *ethambutol* is excreted unchanged in the urine and therefore it should be avoided in renal failure or the dose should be reduced.

Chlamydia

Chlamydiae are bacteria that can only reproduce inside other cells. They possess both DNA and RNA. Chlamydiae are susceptible to **tetracycline** and **erythromycin**. They cause eye infection, including trachoma, psittacosis, pneumonia and non-specific genital tract infection.

Summary

(1) Rational selection of an antibacterial drug for systemic chemotherapy depends upon an explicit or provisional bacteriological diagnosis, including the sensitivities of the pathogen to the drugs.

(2) Dose, route, frequency and duration of administration are chosen to attain and maintain antibacterial concentrations in the infected tissues, to assist host defences in eradicating infection.

(3) Prophylactic use or combination of antibacterial drugs should not be undertaken outside of clearly defined criteria.

(4) The inhibitors of the synthesis and remodelling of cell walls (penicillins, cephalosporins, *vancomycin*) form an invaluable range of bactericidal drugs, providing narrow-spectrum members with very specific indications, and members resistant to enzymic inactivation, through broader- to extended-spectrum members.

(5) The aminoglycoside family are bactericidal to Gram-negative pathogens. Though useful, they have a small therapeutic index,

producing inner ear and renal toxicity that may necessitate therapeutic drug monitoring.
(6) Other families of antibacterial drugs are bacteriostatic but still useful – macrolides, tetracyclines, 4-quinolones, **metronidazole** and **trimethoprim**.
(7) *Clindamycin*, *fusidic acid* and *chloramphenicol* are of more restricted usefulness, in specialized circumstances.
(8) Tuberculosis requires prolonged administration of a combination of drugs – **isoniazid**, **rifampicin** and **pyrazinamide** are the commonest initial therapy.

Chemotherapy of viral infections

Viruses are obligate intracellular parasites having the genetic information for reproduction but no mechanism for carrying it out. They comprise a core of nucleic acid surrounded by a protein coat. The protein coat protects the virus when it is outside cells and it confers host cell affinity and antigenicity.

Viruses contain only one kind of nucleic acid and hence are classified into:

(1) DNA viruses – herpes simplex (cold sores), varicella-zoster (chicken pox, shingles), adenovirus (conjunctivitis, respiratory tract infections).
(2) (a) RNA viruses – enteroviruses (including poliovirus), influenza, rabies;
(b) RNA retroviruses – human immunodeficiency virus (HIV).

The viral replication process

(1) Virus particles exist free in the environment or host ECF.
(2) Adsorption onto specific cell surfaces.
(3) Penetration into cell.
(4) Lysosomal digestion of the protein coat.
(5) Transcription of the DNA of the viral genome by host or viral enzymes (preceded by reverse transcription of the RNA of RNA retroviruses).
(6) Synthesis of:
(a) early proteins (mainly enzymes for replication);
(b) viral nucleic acids;
(c) late proteins (mainly coat proteins).
(7) Assembly of virus particles.
(8) Release from the host cell with cell damage or death, induction of release of interferon, inflammation (gives localizing symptoms) and repair.

STAFFS UNIVERSITY LIBRARY

Development of effective antiviral chemotherapy is rendered difficult because the virus becomes integrated into the biochemical mechanisms of the host cell. Antiviral drugs are therefore often toxic to the host. In addition, viral replication is completed before symptoms appear. In general, viral diseases are best controlled by immunization.

Immunization

Antiviral antibodies are directed against the protein coat of the virion. Vaccination produces active immunity. Viral vaccines may contain live attenuated virus (e.g. the Sabin poliovirus vaccine, the combined measles + mumps + rubella (MMR) vaccine), killed virus (e.g. the Salk poliovirus vaccine, rabies vaccine) or subunits of virus (e.g. hepatitis B vaccine, influenza vaccine).

Immunoglobulins provide passive immunity. *Normal immunoglobulin* is prepared from the pooled plasma of blood donors. It is useful to protect patients at risk from measles and hepatitis A. Specific immunoglobulins are prepared from the blood of convalescent or recently immunized donors. They are useful to protect patients against hepatitis B, varicella-zoster and rabies.

Antiviral drugs

Antiviral drugs may be classified according to their mechanism of action.

Inhibition of viral nucleic acid synthesis

This group mainly includes nucleoside analogues that interfere with the synthesis of viral DNA.

Idoxuridine is an analogue of thymidine. It is incorporated into the growing DNA chain and acts as a chain terminator. It also inhibits the formation of host cell DNA (see p. 285) and is therefore too toxic for systemic use. It is used topically to treat herpes simplex and varicella-zoster infections but has been largely replaced by **acyclovir**.

Acyclovir is both a guanosine analogue and a prodrug. Because **acyclovir** is so selective (see pp. 274 and 282) it is a very valuable antiviral agent. It is useful systemically to treat varicella-zoster infections, systemically and topically for herpes simplex infections including herpes simplex encephalitis and dendritic ulcer (branching, thread-like ulcer of the epithelial layer of the cornea). It has also been used as prophylaxis against herpes virus infections in immunocompromised patients. **Acyclovir** does not eliminate the virus.

Ganciclovir is related to **acyclovir** but is more active against cytomegalovirus. This virion may be transmitted by respiratory secretions, sexual intercourse, blood transfusion or organ transplantation. Like other herpes viruses, cytomegalovirus remains latent in the body after primary infection. It may reactivate if the host becomes immunocompromised. This may cause serious illness, such as pneumonia, sight-threatening retinitis, gastroenteritis, CNS disorders and blood dyscrasias. In the treatment of infection by cytomegalovirus, *ganciclovir* is phosphorylated by host cell thymidine kinase but has some selectivity for viral DNA-polymerase. It is very toxic and is therefore reserved for life- or sight-threatening cytomegalovirus infections in immunocompromised patients.

Zidovudine (AZT) is a nucleoside analogue that is phosphorylated by host cell thymidine kinase (see p. 274). It is used in treatment directed against HIV. It inhibits viral reverse transcriptase more effectively than it inhibits host cell DNA-polymerase. In patients with AIDS, treatment with *zidovudine* partially improves immune function and reduces the incidence of opportunistic infections, such as with *Pneumocystis carinii*, and increases survival. Treatment of individuals, who test positive for HIV but as yet do not show signs of AIDS, with *zidovudine* may prolong survival. Its most significant adverse effect is bone marrow depression.

Inhibition of synthesis of late proteins and assembly

Amantadine is used occasionally as prophylaxis in outbreaks of influenza A. It has a beneficial effect in Parkinson's disease (see p. 230) due to its dopamine-like effects. Unwanted effects include gastrointestinal disturbances, insomnia and nervousness.

Summary

(1) Viruses, being obligate intracellular parasites, produce disease that is easier to prevent with vaccines (where available) than it is to treat with chemotherapeutic agents.
(2) **Acyclovir** is the most selectively toxic and valuable antiviral drug, which can be useful against herpes simplex and varicella/zoster infections.
(3) *Ganciclovir* and *zidovudine* are more toxic but useful for cytomegalovirus and HIV infections respectively.

Chemotherapy of malignant neoplasms

Next to heart disease, cancer (malignant neoplastic disease) is the major cause of death. Cancer can arise in all tissues. Although new tissue growth can be regarded as a common factor, each kind of tumour must be considered as a separate disease. The biology of the tumour, the clinical symptoms and treatment are diverse. Some tumours may be cured (many cancers of the blood, leukaemias, are particularly sensitive to chemotherapy) but treatment of others (the common carcinomas such as those of colon and lung) hardly affects tumour growth and dissemination. Colonic and lung cancers grow slowly and are only terminally associated with gross bodily changes. In contrast, pancreatic tumours grow quickly and secrete hormones that produce early and dramatic secondary changes. The incidence of the different cancers also varies and may have a biological basis (sex organ and breast cancers) or may be related to social and industrial conditions (cigarette smoking and lung cancer, aniline dyes and bladder cancer). In general, the age-corrected incidence of cancer is decreasing; however the incidence of malignant melanoma, breast and cervical cancers is increasing.

In the past, due to poor therapeutic responses and a high incidence of adverse effects, chemotherapy was considered only as a last resort, after the apparently more successful treatments, surgery and radiotherapy, had failed. Recent progress (particularly with intermittent combination chemotherapeutic schedules) holds considerable promise and chemotherapy is now the preferred form of treatment of the leukaemias, lymphomas, choriocarcinomas and certain other tumours.

Some tumours are more resistant to chemotherapy (e.g. those of the lung and colon) but progress is being made, particularly with the introduction of adjuvant therapy. This is the administration of anticancer drugs immediately after surgery, when the metastatic tumour burden is small (that is, less than 10^6 cells). This approach has resulted in increased survival in node-positive breast cancer and Duke's C colon/rectal cancer.

Metastasis of the tumour via the blood and lymph gives rise to secondary tumours throughout the body. When this has occurred radiation and surgery are impractical and chemotherapy must be used.

The main problem in cancer chemotherapy is the lack of highly selectively toxic agents. Cancer cells arise from normal cells and, unlike the situations described for viral, bacterial and fungal infections, there is a paucity of obvious selective drug targets. With currently used antiproliferative anticancer drugs, many rapidly dividing normal cells (bone marrow, gut epithelium, spermatogenic cells, lymphoid tissue, hair follicles, fetus) are also killed. In addition, delivery of drugs into solid tumours is particularly problematical. Cancers are also characterized by intrinsic or acquired drug resistance profiles (see p. 287).

As the therapeutic index of these drugs is low, doses should be optimized for each patient. Drugs are prescribed per square metre of body surface area, the latter being computed from the height and weight of the patient. The therapeutic index can be increased by using high doses, followed by bone marrow rescue using peripheral blood progenitor cells harvested from the patient before treatment. This has improved the proportion of patients cured with leukaemia, Hodgkin's disease and non-Hodgkin's lymphoma.

Chemotherapy can cure a minority of cancers (e.g. Hodgkin's disease, testicular cancer). Anticancer drugs either inhibit cell proliferation or kill sensitive tumour cells by a mechanism called apoptosis (programmed cell death). One form of drug resistance is the suppression of this cell suicide mechanism, and genes such as bcl-2 prevent drug-induced apoptosis (see p. 287). Another is the induction of the multiple drug resistance gene.

For the majority of patients, palliation of the symptoms or modest prolongation of survival is all that is usually achieved. The limited success (enhanced tumour regression, longer remission periods, decreased adverse effects) of intermittent combination therapy has been obtained by rather empirical clinical methods. Developments in knowledge of cell-cycle kinetics (and pharmacokinetics) provide some understanding of the mechanisms involved.

Transformation of a normal cell to a neoplastic cell that produces a tumour is associated with changes in the expression of oncogenes (e.g. the myc and ras genes). Oncogenes promote uncontrolled cell division and de-differentiation to a more primitive cell type. Cellular transformation is also frequently associated with the mutation or loss of tumour suppressor genes (anti-oncogenes, e.g. the p53 gene). The p53 protein allows the cell to detect DNA damage from natural, chemotherapeutic or radiation sources. The cell repairs the damage or, if it is too great, initiates apoptosis. Understanding the functions of oncogenes and tumour suppressor genes will help the design of future, and hopefully more selective, anticancer drugs.

Cell kinetics and dose strategy

Cellular replication involves passage through a cell cycle (Figure 6.13). In general, anticancer drugs may be described as being either cell-cycle phase dependent or phase independent.

Cell-cycle phase-dependent drugs

Cell-cycle phase-dependent drugs act chiefly on cells in certain phases of the cell cycle (but not G_0). When a cell culture is treated with drugs in this group the percentage of surviving colony-forming cells declines steeply at first with increasing dose but reaches a plateau where further

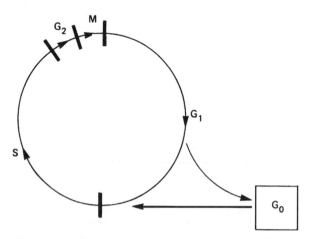

Figure 6.13 G_0 = non-proliferating cells which can re-enter the cell cycle; G_1 = variable (usually long) interphase period prior to DNA synthesis (cells grow in size); S = period (6–8 h) of DNA synthesis; G_2 = period (approximately 2 h) prior to mitosis (tetraploid); M = mitosis

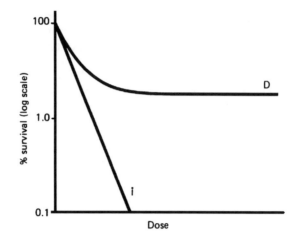

Figure 6.14 Tumour colony-forming cells in culture: D = cell-cycle phase-dependent drug; I = cell-cycle phase-independent drug

increase in dose produces no further increase in cell death (Figure 6.14, curve D). **Methotrexate**, *mercaptopurine*, *fluorouracil* (S) and vinca alkaloids (M) are phase-dependent drugs.

The cell kill is greater if the drug is given in repeated fractions rather than as the summated single dose. Most are antimetabolites, each producing a particular biochemical blockade. They are most effective in those tumours with a large proportion of the cells that are actively dividing.

Cell-cycle phase-independent drugs

Cell-cycle phase-independent drugs act on cells in any phase of the cycle, including a slight effect on the G_0 phase. Survival of cells in culture declines progressively with increasing dose (Figure 6.14, curve I). **Cyclophosphamide, doxorubicin** and *cisplatin* are phase-independent drugs.

They are equally effective in tumours where the growth fraction and mitotic index are low. Their effects are also dose dependent – the degree of cell kill is proportionate to the dose given and a bolus dose is as effective as a fractionated dose of the same amount.

Large solid tumours are less responsive to drugs because they are not well vascularized. Also many cells are in G_0. However, some cancers respond to the use of cell-cycle phase-independent drugs first, both to reduce cell numbers and promote recruitment of cells into the growth phase of the cell cycle, thus rendering them susceptible to cell-cycle phase-dependent drugs. If exposure to cell-cycle phase-independent drugs is prolonged (say more than two cell cycles, approximately 48 h in man), many normal cells would also be drawn out of G_0 and killed.

Cell kinetic studies have provided a logical basis for the fact that high dosage intermittent combination therapy is the most effective treatment mode. Drugs and timings are selected that allow maximal tumour cell killing, recovery of normal tissue during the drug-free interval and minimal emergence of drug resistance.

Cell-cycle nomenclature

Cell-cycle time: the time for a proliferating cell to pass through the cell cycle to produce a daughter cell. It is very variable between kinds of tumour but fairly constant for a single kind of tumour.
Doubling time: the time required for the cell population to double (typically acute leukaemia – 2 days; breast cancer – 200 days).
Growth fraction: the overall proportion of proliferating tumour cells.
Mitotic index: the fraction of cells in mitosis in a steady-state situation.

Principal adverse effects of cancer chemotherapy

When compared to other drug therapy, adverse effects are severe and may necessitate supportive drug therapy and intensive nursing care. Their appearance may be life threatening and may limit the further use of the drugs.

Immediate

(1) Nausea and vomiting, such as that induced by *cisplatin*, are relieved by *metoclopramide* and other antiemetic agents, especially **ondansetron**, a highly selective antagonist at $5-HT_3$ receptors, acting on the area postrema and possibly on vagal efferent fibres in the gastrointestinal tract. It is usually delayed after bolus injection: the maximum effect occurs 8–10 h after treatment. It is a central action exerted on the CTZ.
(2) Irritancy. Extravasation at the injection site, such as that provoked by **doxorubicin**, leads to pain and inflammation.

Delayed

(1) Bone marrow depression occurs 7–14 days after a single dose of many anticancer drugs. Neutrophils are the most susceptible. Myelosuppression is indicated by decrease in platelet and leucocyte counts and may be used as an indicator of the efficacy of treatment (may lead to bleeding disorders, increased susceptibility to infection and even marrow aplasia). Severe myelosuppression and septicaemia can be reduced by the concurrent administration of granulocyte colony stimulating factor (G-CSF).
(2) Immune suppression is related to marrow depression and to a direct effect on lymphocytes and other 'immunocytes'. There is a low resistance to infection and there may be a reduced immunological response against the neoplasia itself.
(3) Gastrointestinal tract disturbances (e.g. induced by **methotrexate**) are mucosal ulceration (easiest to see in the mouth), bleeding and diarrhoea.

(4)   Alopecia or epilation (hair loss) (commonly seen with **doxorubicin**) is often complete but reversible.
(5)   Neurotoxicity (commonly with vinca alkaloids) is seen as peripheral neuropathy that leads to constipation and ileus, and loss of sensation in the fingers and toes.
(6)   Hepatic damage may be due to toxic metabolites.
(7)   During pregnancy, cancer chemotherapeutic drugs must be avoided as animal studies have shown them to be teratogenic.
(8)   Impaired growth in children.
(9)   Infertility (often irreversible) occurs, associated with premature menopause in women and azoospermia in men. Banking of sperm is wise in male patients prior to receipt of chemotherapy.
(10) Mutagenesis – alkylating agents are associated with an increased incidence of secondary malignancies, for example, acute myeloid leukaemia after combination therapy and bladder cancer after treatment with **cyclophosphamide**.

Many of the anticancer drugs (*azathioprine*, **cyclophosphamide**) are also immunosuppressive agents, useful alone and in relatively low doses for longer periods after organ transplantation and for the treatment of certain autoimmune diseases (e.g. systemic lupus erythematosus).

Antimetabolites

Drugs in this category interfere either with the supply of purines and pyrimidines or, by competitive inhibition or substrate competition, with their utilization in the synthetic metabolism of nucleic acids.

Methotrexate inhibits DHF reductase (see p. 273). It can cure choriocarcinoma. It is effective against a wide variety of solid and blood tumours but is particularly prone to produce gastrointestinal lesions. Excessive toxicity to normal cells can be overcome by the concurrent administration of folinic acid.

Fluorouracil (see p. 274) is useful in the palliative treatment of malignant neoplasms. It is one of a very few drugs that provides benefit in the treatment of colon cancer. *Cytarabine* (see p. 274) is useful in inducing remission in acute leukaemia.

Mercaptopurine (see p. 274) is metabolized in the liver by xanthine oxidase; this can be prevented by **allopurinol**, which is occasionally used to increase the cytotoxic action. It is useful (with other agents) in the maintenance treatment of acute leukaemias.

Drugs directly or indirectly affecting DNA

Hydroxyurea is a specific inhibitor of ribonucleotide reductase, which results in inhibition of DNA synthesis and blocks the cell cycle at G_1. It is well absorbed. Clinical usefulness is restricted to the treatment of the chronic leukaemias (particularly chronic myeloid leukaemia) which are generally resistant to alkylating agents.

Doxorubicin produces double-stranded DNA breaks (see p. 275). It has potent effects on bone marrow and is effective in acute myeloid leukaemia, and in a variety of solid tumours, particularly as a single agent in the treatment of breast cancer. It is highly toxic to normal tissue and is administered i/v in a fast-running infusion. Cardiac muscle is particularly susceptible and latent cardiomyopathy may be produced. Related drugs are *mitozantrone* and *epirubicin*, both with a similar spectrum of activity but less cardiotoxic.

Etoposide acts by inhibiting topoisomerase II to generate DNA double-strand breaks (see p. 276). It has a wide spectrum of activity, particularly in lung, testes, lymphoreticular disorders and Hodgkin's disease. It may be given both by mouth or by injection but the oral route produces erratic absorption and the i/v route is to be preferred. After repeated treatments peripheral neuropathy may develop.

Actinomycin D [dactinomycin] is the most potent cytotoxic drug on a molar basis. It inhibits DNA-dependent RNA-polymerase, thus preventing transcription. It is reserved for certain paediatric tumours, such as Wilm's tumour and Ewing's sarcoma.

Bleomycin is a generic name for a group of anticancer antibiotic agents. It inhibits cell proliferation and prevents DNA replication by selective DNA inhibition, so that progression of cells through the S-phase of the cycle is inhibited. It is active against squamous cell carcinoma, particularly of head and neck, cervix and lung. It is also used in the lymphomas and testicular cancer. Its main advantage is that it does not produce myelo-suppression and therefore can be given in patients whose bone marrow function is compromised. However it has a propensity to cause pulmonary fibrosis and therefore the total dose must be restricted.

Nitrogen mustard alkylating agents

Nitrogen mustards are all derivatives (different R-groups) of the basic structure given in Figure 6.4. They form etheyleniminium ions (see p. 274) and replace hydrogen in the DNA molecule by an alkyl group. Cross-linking of DNA chains disrupts cell replication.

Cyclophosphamide is a wide spectrum antitumour drug given either by mouth or injection. It is a prodrug that requires activation by liver (MFO, see p. 353) enzymes. A metabolite (acrolein) is irritant to the bladder, causing haemorrhagic cystitis that is avoided by hydration and simultaneous administration of the neutralizing antagonist *mesna*. One of its active metabolites may denature cytochrome P_{450}, thus impairing the biotransformation of various drugs including **cyclophosphamide** itself.

Ifosfamide is structurally similar but has different pharmacological and toxicological properties. The dose-limiting toxicity is damage to the bladder and therefore the uroprotector *mesna* must be given concurrently.

Lomustine is a lipid-soluble nitrosourea, which is useful in the treatment of brain tumours.

Chlorambucil is the slowest-acting nitrogen mustard and the treatment of choice in chronic lymphatic leukaemia. Orally active, it is considered by many to be a 'mild' agent, but in the correct dosage is as toxic as

STAFFS UNIVERSITY LIBRARY

cyclophosphamide – particularly prone to produce thrombocytopenia when given continuously.

Melphalan (R = L-phenylalanine) is usually reserved for myeloma and occasionally breast and ovarian carcinoma.

Other alkylating agents

The alkane sulphonate *busulphan* has two reactive sulphonic acid groups separated by a methylene bridge of the same length as in nitrogen mustards. It is the least toxic of the alkylating agents. Platelet depression is unusual but it may produce marrow aplasia, so frequent monitoring of the blood count is necessary. It has been useful, given orally, for chronic myeloid leukaemia. Fibrosing alveolitis is an adverse effect (<u>busulphan lung</u>) peculiar to this agent.

Cisplatin is an organometal compound (see p. 275) that causes intra- and inter-strand DNA cross-links. It has a wide spectrum of clinical activity, including ovarian and testicular cancer, head and neck cancer, lung cancer. The main problem is nephrotoxicity, and therefore it must be given with hydration. It causes considerable emesis, which can be controlled with **ondansetron**. Should sepsis result from therapy, aminoglycosides must not be given as their adverse interaction with *cisplatin* may precipitate acute renal failure.

Carboplatin is an expensive organic analogue of *cisplatin* that is less emetic, not nephrotoxic and has the same spectrum of activity. Dose is directly related to renal clearance.

The methylating agent *procarbazine* is a hydrazine prodrug whose derivative binds covalently to DNA and promotes single-strand breaks. It is used in the combination chemotherapy for the treatment of Hodgkin's lymphoma. A *disulfiram*-like effect is produced if ethanol is ingested.

Tumour cells may become resistant to alkylating agents with time, perhaps as a result of enhanced DNA repair mechanisms (animal studies indicate that agents that inhibit DNA repair processes, *caffeine* and **chloroquine**, tend to lessen this resistance when given concurrently).

Vinca alkaloids

These consist of two plant alkaloids with only a small difference in structure but rather different biological and physical properties. Administration is by i/v injection only.

Vinblastine is effective against Hodgkin's disease, sarcomas, testicular cancer and non-Hodgkin's lymphoma.

Vincristine is effective against acute lymphatic leukaemia, Hodgkin's disease and non-Hodgkin's lymphoma.

Cells accumulate the vinca alkaloids, probably due to their capacity to bind tubulin and interfere with microtubule assembly within the cell. Microtubules are associated with spindle formation before mitosis and axoplasmic flow, the latter may account for the neurotoxic adverse effects.

The taxane *paclitaxel* shows promise in the treatment of ovarian and breast cancers. Like the vinca alkaloids it binds to microtubules and induces a cell-cycle arrest in phase G_2/M. Its mechanism of action is distinct from that of the vinca alkaloids in so much as it stabilizes microtubules.

Hormones

Prednisolone is widely used in combination chemotherapy. The lymphosuppressive action of glucocorticosteroids is exploited in the treatment of leukaemias and lymphomas; there is also antitumour activity against some solid tumours. They promote a sense of well-being. Immunosuppression does not appear to compromise treatment.

Specific hormonal therapy started in 1939 with the treatment of prostate cancer with oestrogens. The tumours that respond are generally less anaplastic (more highly differentiated) than those that do not. Hormones are often used in preference to other drugs because of the undesirable effects of the latter on the immune response.

Androgen-dependent prostate cancer regresses in response to pharmacological manipulation of androgenic activity (oestrogens, antagonists at androgen receptors, *goserelin*).

Advanced breast cancers are routinely screened for oestrogen receptors. Tumours lacking these receptors are only treated by chemotherapy. Twothirds of tumours possess receptors and half of these respond to hormonal manipulation – removal of ovaries, **tamoxifen** (see p. 166), *goserelin*, *aminoglutethimide*, removal of adrenal glands or, paradoxically, large doses of oestrogens or androgens.

With the antagonist at oestrogen receptors **tamoxifen**, it is not clear whether its partial agonist property at oestrogen receptors contributes to its cytostatic effects on breast tumour cells. It is relatively free of adverse effects. It has become the hormonal agent of first choice in postmenopausal women with metastatic breast cancer and is often chosen as the initial treatment in premenopausal women. **Tamoxifen** is also being evaluated as prophylaxis for women at high risk of developing inherited breast cancer.

Progestogens are used for endometrial and renal tumours.

Radiotherapy

Radiotherapy (X-rays, neutrons) is an extremely effective way of treating localized tumours by the generation of highly reactive free radicals that react with DNA: a second course of radical treatment cannot be given, as this would damage normal tissues. It is often used in combination with cytotoxic drugs.

^{32}P is as effective as *busulphan* in chronic myeloid leukaemia. ^{131}I is the treatment of choice for elderly patients with thyrotoxicosis. It is selectively concentrated in the thyroid tissue (see p. 178) and therefore useful in the treatment of differentiated tumours of the thyroid gland.

Manipulation of immunity

The interleukins (including interferons; see p. 209), act as immunomodulators and may also have therapeutic potential as anticancer agents.

Summary

(1) Cancer is the general name given to a variety of diseases that result from the uncontrolled growth of cells in a primary tumour, which can arise in most tissues. Consequently both symptoms and treatments differ.

(2) Malignant neoplasms present a difficult target for selective toxicity because the 'parasites' are the patient's own cells. The therapeutic index of anticancer drugs is often low and, except for certain tumours, the cure rate is disappointing.

(3) Most effective drugs are cytocidal to rapidly replicating cells. Hence selectivity is only achieved against rapidly multiplying neoplastic cells and cells of some normal tissues are also damaged (e.g. mucosae, gonads).

(4) Cell-cycle phase-dependent drugs are most effective when a large proportion of cells is dividing, and include the antimetabolites, which inhibit the synthesis of DNA, as well as the vinca alkaloids, which prevent the separation of the mitotic chromosomes.

(5) The action of some drugs is not dependent upon the phase of the cell cycle and these are effective when the mitotic index is low. This group includes those drugs that directly interact with DNA (e.g. **doxorubicin**, *cisplatin*).

(6) Antimetabolites (e.g. **methotrexate**, *fluorouracil*) interfere with the supply of purines or pyrimidines, or with their utilization in the synthesis of DNA.

(7) DNA is also targeted by other drugs, *hydroxyurea* inhibits ribonucleotide reductase and prevents synthesis, **doxorubicin** and *etoposide* produce double-strand breaks (but by different mechanisms) and *actinomycin D* prevents DNA-dependent transcription.

(8) Alkylating agents are a diverse group of reactive chemicals that donate alkyl groups to DNA, disrupting its replication. **Cyclophosphamide** requires activation by hepatic MFOs. *Cisplatin* is an organometal compound. *Procarbazine* is a particularly useful component of many intermittent combination chemotherapies. Tumour response is often very similar to that to radiotherapy.

(9) The plant derivatives, vinca alkaloids and *paclitaxel*, interfere with the role of microtubules during mitosis.

(10) Lymphomas, leukaemias and some solid tumours are sensitive to the cytotoxic affects of high doses of glucocorticosteroids.

(11) Breast cancers that contain oestrogen receptors are often sensitive to hormone manipulation. The mixed antagonist and agonist, **tamoxifen**, is the treatment of choice as it is relatively free of adverse effects.

(12) Adverse effects related to cytotoxicity are common. Nausea and vomiting may be controlled by antiemetic agents. Delayed toxicity includes bone marrow depression, immunosuppression and gastrointestinal disturbances, all of which may be life threatening. The drugs are mutagenic, which can be expressed as new primary cancers or fetal damage in the pregnant woman.

7

Drug disposition and metabolism

Aims

- To explain the entry of drug molecules into body tissues and their subsequent removal in terms of familiar physical, chemical and biological processes.
- To introduce the concepts underlying the quantitative description of drug handling.
- To focus attention on the entry and removal of particular drugs, which serve as type substances for broad groups with similar physicochemical properties.
- To provide the scientific basis underlying the therapeutic choices of routes of administration and dosage regimens of drugs.

Introduction

The relationship between drug concentration and tissue response and the nature of that response are studied in the science of pharmacodynamics. Several processes collectively determine the concentration of drug at its site of action and how the concentration alters with time (Figure 7.1). These dispositional processes are studied quantitatively in the science of pharmacokinetics.

Disposition is a comprehensive term that includes the processes of absorption, distribution and elimination.

Absorption is the term used to describe the entry of drug molecules into the systemic blood via the mucous membranes (of, for example, the alimentary or respiratory tracts), via the skin or from the site of an injection.

Distribution is the term used to describe the movement of drug molecules between the water, lipid and protein constituents of the body.

Elimination is the term used to describe the removal of the original drug molecule from the body by excretion or by metabolism (alteration of the structure of the molecule).

Designing dosage regimens to optimize therapy and to minimize toxicity is greatly assisted by an understanding of the pharmacokinetic properties of drugs. Also, variability in responses to drugs and selectivity of drug

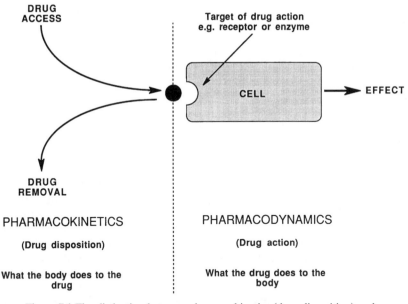

Figure 7.1 The distinction between pharmacokinetics (drug disposition) and pharmacodynamics (drug action)

actions between tissues can have dispositional as well as pharmacody-namic causes. Many unwanted effects of single drugs (see p. 416) or inter-actions between drugs (see p. 438), have a dispositional basis.

Drug movement through membranes

Plasma membranes consist of a bimolecular lipid sheet (10 nm thick) with polar (hydrophilic) groups outside and non-polar (hydrophobic) groups inside. Most membranes behave as if they have very small water-filled pores (1 nm diameter). Drugs pass through membranes either by diffusion (passive) or occasionally by specific carrier systems.

Therefore, the major determinants of the disposition of drugs are the physical properties of membranes and the physicochemical properties of drugs.

Lipid diffusion

Most drugs move through the lipid part of the membrane by passive diffu-sion. The rate can be expressed by Fick's law:

$$\frac{dQ}{dt} = P_k \frac{A}{w} (C_1 - C_2)$$

where: dQ = amount of drug diffusing within the time interval dt; P_k = permeability constant; A = membrane area; C_1 and C_2 are the drug concentrations on either side of the membrane; w = thickness of membrane. The driving force is the concentration gradient $(C_1 - C_2)$. The permeability constant is closely related to the lipid/water partition coefficient of a drug.

The lipid/water partition coefficient is a physicochemical property that expresses the relative solubility of the drug in lipid compared with water. To measure the lipid/water partition coefficient, a small amount of drug is added to a mixture of an oily solvent (usually *n*-octanol, the physico-chemical properties of which mimic those of cell membranes) and water. The mixture is shaken until equilibrium is reached and the two layers are allowed to separate. The lipid/water partition coefficient is the concentration of the drug in the oily phase divided by its concentration in the aqueous phase. Drugs with high lipid/water partition coefficients are often described in pharmacokinetic short-hand as being lipid soluble. Drugs with lipid/water partition coefficients markedly less than 1.0 are described as water soluble. This jargon can easily confuse unless it is realized that it is quite common for lipid-soluble drugs (that is those with high lipid/water partition coefficients) to dissolve readily in water. Lipid-soluble drug molecules or species penetrate membranes rapidly, whereas water-soluble drugs or species (that is those with small lipid/water partition coefficients) do not.

An increase in molecular weight, with constant lipid-solubility, results in a decrease in membrane permeability.

Many drugs can be ionized in aqueous solution. However, only the non-ionized species of such drugs is lipid soluble. The proportions of ionized and non-ionized species are determined by the pH of the medium (Figure 7.2) and the ionization constant of the drug (the pK_a = acid dissociation constant = the pH at which one-half of the drug molecules are ionized). This relationship is expressed in the Henderson–Hasselbach equation:
Acid form:

$$HA = A^- + H^+$$
$$pH = pK_a + \log ([A^-]/[HA]) \tag{7.1}$$

Basic form:

$$BH^+ = B + H^+$$
$$pH = pK_a + \log ([B]/[BH^+]) \tag{7.2}$$

In most circumstances, where permeability is the rate-limiting factor, the rate of drug movement is thus proportional to both the concentration gradient and lipid solubility of the non-ionized, readily diffusible species. Consequently the rate of drug movement depends on the pH of the media on each side of the membrane.

Table 7.1 summarizes the important physicochemical properties of drugs considered so far.

Aqueous diffusion

Drugs can also pass through water-filled pores in the membrane if their molecules are small enough (MW less than 100 Da). This is the mechanism by which some highly water-soluble molecules pass rapidly through membranes (e.g. ethanol, MW = 46 Da; urea, MW = 60 Da). In general,

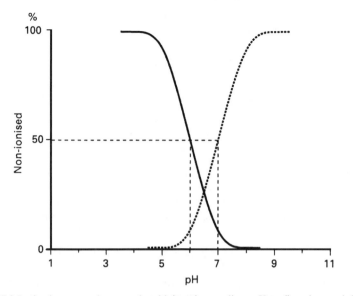

%

Figure 7.2 Ionization curve for a weak acid (continuous line, $pK_a = 6$) and a weak base (dashed line, $pK_a = 7$)

Table 7.1 Important physicochemical properties of drugs

Solubility in water
Lipid/water partition coefficient
pK_a

drugs are too large to pass through these water-filled pores as most drugs have molecular masses in excess of 100 Da, typically 100–400 Da.

Specific carrier systems

Some membranes possess active transport or facilitated diffusion systems, which exhibit substrate specificity, stereospecificity, saturability and competition between analogues; for example, natural amino acids and their analogues (e.g. **levodopa** and *methyldopa*), *thyroxine sodium*, antimetabolites (e.g. purines and pyrimidine analogues). Few drugs meet the structural requirements for carrier transport.

Diffusion across a membrane is rarely rate limiting for highly lipid-soluble drugs and those moving by aqueous diffusion. For these compounds, the rate of blood flow is usually the limiting factor – their movement across membranes is described as <u>perfusion rate limited</u>. The rate of absorption of ethanol from the stomach, for example, is limited by gastric mucosal blood flow.

The cells of some membranes (e.g. endothelia of capillaries, glomeruli) adjoin one another loosely, with gaps between cells of approximately

STAFFS UNIVERSITY LIBRARY

10 nm. These gaps effectively offer no barrier to most drugs, unless the drug is bound to plasma protein (see p. 340).

Absorption

Formulations and routes of administration

Most drugs are administered as a medicine, formulated along with other materials known as excipients, which are pharmacologically inactive. The formulation serves some or all of the following purposes:

(1) To enable the administration of an accurately measured dose.
(2) To improve drug stability.
(3) To present the drug in a convenient form for administration.
(4) To regulate the rate of disintegration and/or solution of the medicine.

Oral formulations

Disintegration and dissolution

These two processes must precede absorption for most oral formulations. Tablets often contain excipients that cause them to swell on contact with water and to disintegrate into fine particles. The active drug then dissolves from the surface of the particles. The rate of dissolution is generally faster the smaller the particles, because the surface area/mass ratio increases as the size of the particles decreases.

Many drugs are weak acids or bases and so exhibit pH-dependent dissolution. Such drugs can be formulated with a buffering agent (e.g. **aspirin** with sodium bicarbonate) to help the acid to dissolve. When exposed to the environment in the gastrointestinal lumen, the drug reprecipitates but as very small (micronized) particles that dissolve very readily.

Rate of absorption

The rate of absorption from the gut can be influenced by many factors.

Drug absorption can occur from the stomach but the small intestine is quantitatively much more important because of its vastly greater surface area and blood flow. If gastric emptying is delayed (e.g. by taking a drug with food), then the rate of absorption of the drug is usually decreased.

If the drug dissolves out of the formulation at a slower rate than the rate of drug absorption, then absorption is described as dissolution rate limited. However, if dissolution is relatively rapid, it is the permeability characteristics of the drug that determine the rate of absorption.

Sustained and delayed release oral formulations

Rapid dissolution of drug may produce very large local concentrations of the drug which may cause damage to the gut mucosa (**aspirin**, potassium chloride, iron salts). Rapid dissolution can also lead to systemic adverse effects due to a brief, large peak of concentration in the blood (*aminophylline* producing CNS stimulation). Alternatively, the duration of response to the drug may be too short for practical day to day treatment (*quinidine*). These problems are sometimes solved by producing pharmaceutical formulations that release the drug slowly or after a delay. Not all these formulations are justified but all are more expensive than the standard formulation of the drug. A variety of techniques is employed as described below.

Enteric-coated tablets

The coating does not dissolve until the tablet reaches a non-acid medium. Enteric coatings are used to protect the drug from acid (e.g. **erythromycin**) or to protect the stomach from the drug (e.g. **aspirin**, **prednisolone**). The thicker the coating, the slower it dissolves.

Modified-release capsules

Smoothly sustained release may be obtained by filling capsules with a mixture of granules that dissolve at different rates (e.g. *aminophylline*). A thin or readily soluble coating to the granules gives immediate release of the active drug. A thick or relatively insoluble coating delays release.

Mucous membranes other than stomach and small intestine

These membranes can be used as routes of administration for drugs that are required to provide a local effect or to provide systemic absorption for drugs that are susceptible to intestinal or liver metabolism. Since the venous drainage of these membranes occurs into the systemic circulation rather than the hepatic portal system, gut and liver enzymes are bypassed. The rate of systemic absorption is determined by the area of the surface to which the drug is applied and/or blood flow to the area.

Buccal mucosa

The buccal mucosa provides a convenient site for highly lipid-soluble compounds (**glyceryl trinitrate** in the prophylaxis of effort angina and the treatment of heart failure – there are short-acting sublingual and sustained-release buccal tablets available).

Respiratory mucosa

Bronchial mucosa and alveoli provide the largest surface area of any mucous membrane and are accessible to gases, vapours and aerosols (liquid or solid particles). Particle size is of critical importance as only small particles reach the smallest airways.

Examples:	Uses:
Halothane, nitrous oxide	Anaesthesia
Salbutamol	Relief of bronchial asthma (local effect)

Nasal mucosa

The nasal mucosa provides an inefficient (because a large proportion of the dose is wasted) but convenient route of entry for some small peptides which can be administered as a nasal spray.

Examples:	Uses:
Desmopressin	Diabetes insipidus
Sodium cromoglycate	Allergic rhinitis (local effect)

Rectal mucosa

The rectal mucosa provides a useful absorptive surface when the patient is unconscious, asleep, vomiting or suffering local gastric adverse effects. The absorption of lipid-soluble drugs can be delayed if the drug is given in a fatty suppository, as the drug partitions preferentially into the fatty medium of the suppository.

Examples:	Uses:
Rectal **diazepam** solution	Serial seizures
Sulphasalazine suppositories	Ulcerative colitis (local effect)
Prednisolone foam	Ulcerative colitis (local effect)
Metronidazole suppository	Prophylaxis of surgical wound infection

Skin

Healthy skin

Healthy skin is a highly specialized protective envelope that prevents uncontrolled water loss. Skin is several millimetres thick and normally has a small blood flow. Thus, the entry of water-soluble compounds is limited. However, many lipid-soluble drugs can enter the body via the skin and produce therapeutic or unwanted effects.

Examples:	Effects:
Glyceryl trinitrate skin patch	Prophylaxis of effort angina
Nicotine skin patch	Treatment of dependence
Glucocorticosteroid esters	ACTH suppression

Infants and toddlers are specially vulnerable to the undesired effects of substances absorbed through the skin because of their large surface area/mass ratio (Table 7.2).

Table 7.2 Changing average surface/mass ratio with age

	Child (1 month)	Child (5 years)	Adult
Height (m)	0.50	0.90	1.8
Surface area (m²)	0.25	0.67	1.9
Weight (kg)	5.00	20.00	70.0
m²/kg × 100	5.00	3.40	2.7

Diseased skin

In diseased skin, for example due to extensive burns, wounds or dermatitis, the waterproof barrier is lost; even water-soluble drugs can enter and fatal accidents have resulted. Occlusive dressings, by increasing the hydration of the skin, augment transdermal absorption.

Examples:
Sulphonamides
Neomycin

Unwanted effects:
Crystalluria
Deafness

Parenteral routes

Parenteral (injection) routes are necessary when the proportion of the orally administered drug that is absorbed is small or if effective blood concentrations of the drug need to be achieved rapidly. The absorption rate is determined by the blood flow at the site of injection unless sustained release (e.g. depot) formulations are used.

Intravenous

Absorption is complete when injection is complete unless part of the dose is injected accidentally outside the blood vessel. The intravenous (i/v) route is used if a rapid effect is required, if the drug is too irritant by other routes or if the use of the oral route is prevented (e.g. by disease or abdominal surgery).

Intramuscular

Skeletal muscle has a rich capillary plexus. The capillary endothelium has large water-filled pores that are freely permeable even to water-soluble drugs with large molecular weights. The intramuscular (i/m) route is the standard one for injections by nurses. Many emergency drugs (analgesic, antiemetic or oxytocic agents) are given by this route (deltoid, gluteal and quadriceps muscles). The rate of absorption is proportional to the dose, the extent of dispersion through the muscle and the rate of tissue blood flow – exercise promotes absorption.

Subcutaneous

Subcutaneous tissues are poorly perfused, especially when the cardiac output is small (e.g. haemorrhagic shock, acute diabetic ketoacidosis). The subcutaneous (s/c) route is the standard route for self-injection (e.g. in diabetes). Convenient sites are the upper arm, thigh and abdomen. Absorption is relatively slow, even in healthy subjects, and may be deliberately delayed by administration of sustained-release formulations (depot insulins) or by co-administration of a vasoconstrictor agent (*adrenaline* with **lignocaine**).

Sustained- and delayed-release parenteral formulations

Solution in oil

Esters of drug (drug combined with a long-chain fatty acid, e.g. *fluphenazine decanoate*) can be injected dissolved in a non-toxic oil. The drug diffuses out from an injection site very slowly over a period of weeks. The rate-limiting step is hydrolysis of the ester to release the active drug, e.g. fluphenazine at the interface between the oil and the aqueous phase of body tissue. This formulation is used for maintenance dosage in psychotic patients who would otherwise fail to take prescribed treatment regularly.

Soluble colloid complex in water

The drug is held in a micelle by weak, hydrogen bonds. Release from the complex occurs slowly in the circulation after absorption (e.g. *iron sorbitol* given i/m).

Suspension of insoluble complex

A complex between soluble drug and a relatively inert molecule is almost insoluble. Soluble drug is slowly released from such suspensions at the site of i/m or s/c injection. This extends the duration of action of the drug, e.g. *procaine penicillin* compared to **benzylpenicillin** or *isophane insulin* compared to *soluble insulin*.

Suspension of crystals

Notably *insulin zinc suspension* – the smallest particles (*insulin zinc suspension amorphous*) give most rapid absorption. The largest crystals (*insulin zinc suspension crystalline*) give the slowest absorption and longest duration of action. A mixture of amorphous : crystalline *insulin zinc suspension* in the ratio of 3 : 7 has a duration of action of 4–24 h.

Systemic bioavailability

Systemic bioavailability can be defined as the fraction (F) of the dose of drug administered that reaches the systemic circulation. For i/v injection

Table 7.3 Reasons for small systemic bioavailability of drugs after oral administration

Mechanism	Examples
Incomplete solution	**Aspirin** in enteric-coated tablets
Breakdown in gut lumen	**Benzylpenicillin**
Binding in gut lumen	Tetracyclines with divalent cations
Negligible absorption	**Gentamicin**
Metabolism by gut wall	*Isoprenaline*, **levodopa**
Metabolism by liver	**Glyceryl trinitrate, morphine**

F equals 1.0, but by other routes, particularly after oral administration, F may be less than 1.0 (Table 7.3). After oral administration, some drugs may be extensively metabolized on their <u>first pass</u> through the liver. All of the drug absorbed form the gastrointestinal tract is carried in the hepatic portal vein to the liver. After a drug has entered the general circulation, only a proportion of the drug passes through the liver on second and subsequent circulations.

Where systemic bioavailability after oral administration is small, drugs may need to be given via other mucous membranes or parenterally. The oral route may still be suitable, despite extensive metabolism, if the metabolites are pharmacologically active (e.g. **aspirin** is converted to salicylic acid).

Summary

(1) The processes of absorption, distribution and elimination together determine the amount of a drug in the body.
(2) Most drugs pass through membranes by passive diffusion.
(3) Absorption is the entry of drugs into the systemic blood.
(4) Absorption from the gut commonly occurs in the small intestine.
(5) Absorption is influenced by the area of the absorbing surface and/or blood flow to the area.
(6) Formulations can be used to delay and sustain absorption from the gut and injection sites.
(7) Systemic bioavailability is the fraction of the dose of drug administered that reaches the systemic circulation.

Distribution

Distribution involves the movement of drug molecules from the circulating blood to other areas of the body, including the sites of action, of binding and of elimination. Drug action at one site and not another may be due to selective access of drug (pharmacokinetic selectivity) rather than differences in the sites of action (pharmacodynamic selectivity). For drugs applied to the site of action (e.g. local anaesthetic agents injected for nerve block, bronchodilator agents inhaled as aerosols for local action in airways), absorption and distribution reduce drug effects.

Once a drug has entered the blood it mixes rapidly (circulation time = 20 s). The rate and extent of distribution depend upon the relative arterial blood perfusion rates of different organs and the permeability characteristics of cell membranes towards different drug molecules. The initial driving force is the concentration gradient between plasma and the site to which distribution is occurring.

Haemodynamic (perfusion) factors

The whole of the right heart output (and therefore of the absorbed dose) is passed through the lungs to the left heart. The bulk of the absorbed dose is then carried rapidly to the vessel-rich group of organs (brain, myocardium, liver, kidneys, adrenal glands and thyroid), which receive approximately 80% of the cardiac output at rest. During late pregnancy this includes the uterus and placenta.

A few minutes after a drug is injected as an i/v bolus it is relatively concentrated in these organs. Drug is more slowly distributed to skeletal muscle, which has a relatively small blood flow at rest. It reaches skin and adipose tissue more slowly still and it reaches avascular structures (tendon, cartilage) only very slowly indeed.

Permeability factors

Arterial blood flow determines the rate at which drug reaches the interstitial fluid of a given organ or tissue. The capillary endothelia of most tissues contain large pores (50–100 nm diameter) and therefore present no barrier to diffusion to even water-soluble drugs/ionized species (Figure 7.3). Non-protein-bound drugs diffuse readily into interstitial fluid. Therefore, virtually all drugs can gain access to the interstitial fluid/cell surface. This may be their site of action (e.g. penicillins). The fractional quantity of the drug that is bound to plasma proteins remains within the vascular system.

The rate of penetration into cells and across special tissue barriers is, however, dependent on the physicochemical properties of the drug molecule, as the barrier is composed of lipid membranes (Figure 7.3). Highly water-soluble drugs (e.g. **gentamicin**) behave like inulin; that is they penetrate into cells slowly or not at all. Conversely, highly lipid-soluble drugs (e.g. **thiopentone** and inhalational anaesthetic agents) penetrate very rapidly.

Rate and extent of distribution

For any one drug and one organ the rate of distribution can be perfusion limited or permeability rate limited.

Perfusion limits the rate of distribution for highly lipid-soluble drugs traversing most membranes and for most drugs crossing membranes with

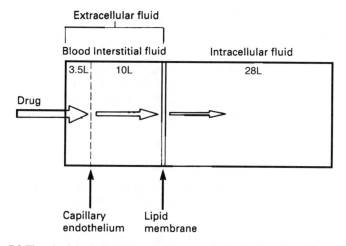

Figure 7.3 The physiological fluid spaces in man and the distribution of drug molecules across these membranes

large pores. For example, **thiopentone** is so lipid soluble that its rate of entry into the CNS is determined solely by cerebral blood flow (Table 7.4). If a drug has a large affinity for the tissue (high tissue/plasma partition coefficient), then much drug needs to be delivered before equilibrium is reached. Therefore, the time to equilibrium is long when tissue perfusion is small and the drug has a high tissue/blood partition coefficient.

Permeability limits the rate of distribution for water-soluble drugs crossing membranes with small pores. Here the time to equilibrium increases as the permeability of the drug decreases and as the proportion of drug present as the ionized, non-diffusible species increases. The factors dictating removal of drug from an organ are the same as those regulating its access.

The differences in times to onset of effect of drugs after i/v administration due to their different physicochemical properties are illustrated in Table 7.4.

Table 7.4 Effect of physicochemical property of a drug on the time to the onset of action

Drug	Physico-chemical property	Effect	Time to onset	Rate-limiting process
Thiopentone	Lipid soluble	Anaesthesia	15 s	Circulation time CNS perfusion
Morphine	Weak base	Analgesia	10 min	Diffusion into CNS
Digoxin	Intermediate solubility	Increased ventricular force	30 min	Diffusion into cardiac cell

STAFFS UNIVERSITY LIBRARY

Binding of drugs by proteins (and other macromolecules)

Virtually all drugs are adsorbed to macromolecules in tissues and in plasma in a readily reversible manner involving non-covalent bonds. These drug/macromolecule complexes associate and dissociate with a half-time ($t_{1/2}$) measured in milliseconds. Rarely, therefore, is the dissociation of the complex rate limiting.

Binding of drugs to plasma proteins

The total drug concentration in plasma at any time (C) is the sum of the free drug concentration ($C \times f_u$) and that bound ($C \times f_b$) to plasma proteins, where:

f_u = fraction unbound and $f_b = (1 - f_u)$ = fraction bound.

Few drugs exist in plasma solely in the free form. Drug adsorption to plasma proteins can be considered to be of two kinds:

Simple partitioning into a lipid phase

Many lipid-soluble drugs (e.g. **thiopentone**) partition preferentially into the non-aqueous phase of plasma. The unbound fraction, f_u, is constant over the therapeutic range of plasma concentrations (Figure 7.4).

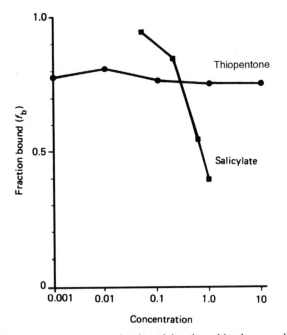

Figure 7.4 Relationship between fraction of drug bound in plasma and total plasma concentration of drug (on a log scale) for **thiopentone** (●, μg/mL) and salicylate (■, mg/mL)

Association with specific ionic binding sites

Many acidic drugs (e.g. salicylic acid, sulphonamides, **warfarin**) bind to one (the same) specific site on each albumin molecule and some basic drugs (e.g. **diazepam**, **propranolol**) bind to α_1-acid glycoprotein and lipoproteins. Usually the number of binding sites considerably exceeds the number of drug molecules, therefore, f_b is constant over a wide range of total drug concentrations.

A few drugs (e.g. salicylic acid, **sodium valproate**) have such large affinities for these specific binding sites that as the total drug concentration in plasma increases within the clinically encountered range, the binding sites become saturated. Above this saturating concentration, f_b declines (Figure 7.4) and the concentration of unbound drug increases much more steeply as the total concentration of drug in the plasma increases than at non-saturating concentrations.

Binding of drugs to tissue macromolecules

Most drugs equilibrate to a larger concentration in tissues than in plasma. Such drug adsorption is reversible. For **digoxin** (see p. 381), this binding dominates its pharmacokinetics. Non-reversible binding can also occur.

Examples:

Drug	Site	Mechanism
Tetracyclines	Bones, teeth	Binds when blood flow moderate associated with growth Later blood flow very small Also chelation to Ca^{2+}
Cyclophosphamide	Nuclei	Covalent bonding to purine and pyrimidine bases

Dispositional significance of protein binding

(1) The plasma protein/drug complex is a pharmacologically inactive mass transit system, carrying drugs to tissues. Protein binding often causes the total plasma concentration of a drug to exceed its aqueous solubility (e.g. **phenytoin**, **propranolol**, **benzylpenicillin**). As a result, distribution is more rapid.

(2) The drug/protein complex (plasma/tissue) acts as a reservoir, that both smooths fluctuations in the concentration of free drug in plasma water and at the site of action, and prolongs the action of the drug. If the plasma albumin concentration is small (as in nephrotic syndrome, liver failure, malabsorption, starvation), this effect is reduced.

(3) Two acidic drugs can compete for specific binding sites on plasma albumin. As a result, the free plasma concentration of one of these drugs may be much larger than when there is no competing drug present, so that the pharmacological effect is exaggerated (see p. 441).

(4) At large plasma concentrations a few drugs can saturate the binding sites.

Special compartments and special barriers

The rate and extent of distribution of a drug to and from these tissues can be limited either by perfusion or permeability factors. For tissues with a lipid membrane between plasma and the site of drug action and a large blood flow (e.g. brain, placenta), drug permeability across the membrane is usually the limiting factor. Only for the most lipid-soluble drugs (e.g. **thiopentone**) is blood flow the limiting factor. Distribution into tissues with a small blood flow is usually perfusion limited.

Brain

Unlike the peripheral capillary endothelium, capillary endothelia of blood vessels of the CNS have continuous tight junctions that provide a gap-free lipid membrane between blood and CSF.

Highly polar, water-soluble drugs (e.g. **gentamicin**) penetrate slowly, if at all. Non-polar, lipid-soluble drugs (e.g. **thiopentone** and inhalational anaesthetic agents) penetrate rapidly, and drugs with intermediate solubility (e.g. tetracyclines) penetrate at an intermediate rate.

The stronger an acidic drug (the smaller the pK_a) the smaller the concentration of unionized molecules at pH 7.4 and the slower the rate of penetration into brain – salicylic acid (pK_a 3) penetrates slowly. Similarly, the stronger a basic drug (the larger the pK_a) the smaller the concentration of unionized molecules and the slower the rate of penetration into brain – **morphine** (pK_a 8) penetrates slowly. The penetration of acidic and basic drugs depends also on the lipid solubility of the unionized molecules – *adrenaline* has few CNS effects but the less polar amphetamine (no –OH groups) has marked CNS effects.

Several drugs are transferred from the CSF to the plasma across the choroid plexus against a concentration gradient. This mechanism resembles the transport system in the renal tubule.

Examples:

Anions	*Cations*
Benzylpenicillin	**Tubocurarine**
Probenecid	

This process reduces the concentration of penicillins in the CSF and, therefore, impairs their effectiveness against bacterial infections within the CNS. As a consequence, very large doses of these antibiotic agents are required to treat infection of the CNS.

Essential nutrients (amino acids, glucose, purines, pyrimidines) are actively transported into the CSF and brain. **Levodopa** (which is a naturally occurring amino acid) and its analogue *methyldopa* also enter by this means.

Placenta

Lipid-soluble drugs cross the placenta readily. Hence general anaesthetic agents can interfere with respiration in the newborn child after administration to the mother during delivery. **Morphine** and related analgesic agents cause the same problem. All drugs penetrate into the fetal circulation at some rate. Even highly polar water-soluble drugs (e.g. **gentamicin**) penetrate to the fetus slowly. Slow penetration only protects the fetus if delivery is imminent.

Breast

The breast is an example of a pharmacokinetic <u>deep</u> compartment with a moderate blood supply. Most drugs enter breast milk by passive diffusion through lipid membranes. Compounds with a MW less than 100 Da (ethanol) enter by passive diffusion through water-filled pores in the membrane. Iodine is actively transported and, therefore, administration of radioactive iodide to the mother is an absolute contraindication to breast feeding. For most drugs concentrations in milk are similar to those in plasma at equilibrium. However, as the amount of drug in plasma is usually small in relation to the total amount in the body, so the total amount of drug delivered to the infant during breast feeding is small in relation to doses recommended for therapeutic purposes in infants. Hence breast feeding can be continued when the mother is taking **digoxin**, tricyclic antidepressant drugs, **paracetamol**, **phenytoin**, diuretic agents and even **warfarin**.

Breast feeding should be discouraged where the mother is taking drugs for prolonged periods and where the drugs could have serious adverse effects on the infant (radioactive iodide, cytotoxic drugs, **carbimazole**, *theophylline*, sulphonylurea oral hypoglycaemic drugs).

Eye

Anterior compartment

The conjunctiva, sclera, iris and ciliary muscle receive a moderate blood supply but the cornea and lens are avascular (see Figures 2.6 and 2.7). Drugs can penetrate to these structures and the aqueous humour from the conjunctival sac (e.g. *chloramphenicol*). As there is little perfusion of either side of the membranes, the rate of drug movement is mainly proportional to the lipid solubility of the drug and the proportion that is non-ionized. As the stroma of the cornea has a large water content, relatively water-soluble drugs (*pilocarpine*) can penetrate into aqueous humour.

Note: **benzylpenicillin** is extruded from the aqueous humour as it is from the CSF.

Posterior compartment

The sclera, choroid and retina are moderately vascular but the vitreous humour is avascular. Drugs cannot reach these structures by diffusion from the conjunctival sac as the diffusion distance is too great. Instead drugs reach these structures from the systemic circulation.

Serous cavities

In general, all drugs enter and leave serous cavities (pleural, pericardial, peritoneal sacs, joint spaces) slowly. Water-soluble drugs penetrate slowly and lipid-soluble drugs more rapidly. Acute inflammation facilitates the penetration of drugs, as the movement of water through the capillary epithelium increases during inflammation. Chronic inflammation, however, leads to fibrosis and this impedes penetration.

Bones and teeth

Drug access is proportional to the local blood flow. Infection produces oedema, ischaemia and avascular necrosis so that only prompt treatment is effective. The growth region of bone is moderately well perfused. Blood flow becomes very small when growth ceases. Certain drugs and ions form complexes with bone salt, especially in growing bone (e.g. lead, fluoride, tetracyclines).

Skin and nails

These are avascular and thus penetration of drugs from the systemic circulation is very slow. **Griseofulvin**, an antifungal agent, has a large affinity for keratin and so achieves selectively large concentrations in skin and nails.

Abscess cavities

Acute abscesses are thin walled and have an increased local blood flow. Consequently antibiotic agents penetrate readily. Chronic abscesses have thick avascular walls and drugs do not penetrate. Similarly penetration into sputum is slow. In acute (but not chronic) otitis media (infection of the middle ear) the organisms are accessible.

Extent of distribution – apparent volume of distribution

After a dose of drug is administered distribution equilibrium will eventually be reached. The extent of distribution can be defined as the apparent volume of distribution (V).

$$V = \frac{\text{Amount of drug in body at equilibrium}}{\text{Plasma drug concentration}}$$

The concept can be illustrated with a dye model (Figure 7.5). A known dose (D) of dye is injected into a beaker of water, stirred well and a sample taken. Measurement of dye concentration enables calculation of compartment volume (Figure 7.5a), which is the same as the actual volume. This is the situation for a few drugs, which are either restricted

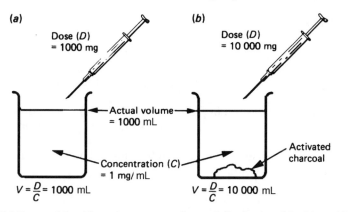

Figure 7.5 Dye model to illustrate apparent volume of distribution: (a) with no 'tissue binding' and homogeneous concentration; (b) with 'tissue binding' simulated by activated charcoal

Table 7.5 Examples of apparent volumes of distribution (V)

Substance	V (L)	Equivalent physiological space
Evans blue, **heparin**	3.5	Plasma water
Inulin, **gentamicin**	13.5	ECF
Tritiated water, ethanol	41.5	Total body water
Digoxin	350	None

to plasma (very large molecules or plasma protein bound), restricted to ECF (highly water-soluble) or distributed evenly throughout the body (Table 7.5). Most drugs, however, have a tissue/plasma partition coefficient much greater than one, that is, they exhibit some tissue binding. These drugs therefore 'appear' to have a V greater than total body volume (Figure 7.5b).

Problem:
Assuming the activated charcoal occupies 100 mL, calculate the partition coefficient between the charcoal and water.

Answer:

Volume of water	$= 1000 - 100 = 900$ mL
Amount of drug in water	$= 900$ mL $\times$ 1 mg/mL $= 900$ mg
Amount of drug bound to charcoal	$= 10\,000 - 900 = 9100$ mg
Concentration of drug in charcoal	$= 9100$ mg $\div$ 100 mL $= 9.1$ mg/mL
Concentration of drug in water	$= 1$ mg/mL
Partition coefficient	$= 9.1 : 1$. Hence the reason why, in Figure 7.5, the volume of distribution is apparently 10 000 mL.

Summary

(1) Distribution is the movement of drug from the blood to other areas of the body.
(2) The rate of distribution can be limited by the rate of perfusion or permeability.
(3) Many drugs are carried in plasma reversibly bound to plasma proteins.
(4) The rate of distribution of most drugs into the CNS is proportional to their lipid solubility.
(5) The extent of distribution at equilibrium is known as the apparent volume of distribution.

Elimination

Elimination is achieved by excretion of the unchanged drug or its metabolism (Figure 7.6). Excretion of drugs is mainly by the kidney but can also occur through other organs that communicate with the exterior. Excretion in the urine is important for water-soluble drugs and water-soluble metabolites of the more lipid-soluble drugs.

Clearance is used as a measure of elimination and applies to both excretion and metabolism. The concept of clearance can be illustrated

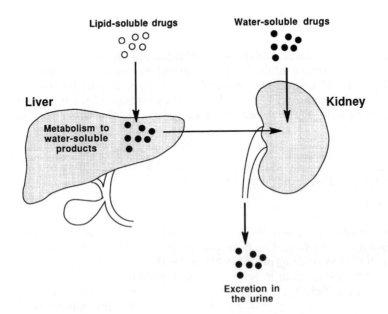

Figure 7.6 The two principal pathways of drug elimination

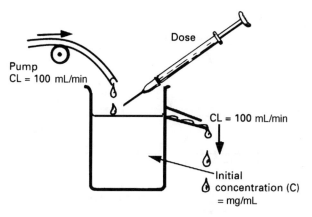

Figure 7.7 Dye model to illustrate clearance

with a dye model (Figure 7.7). Dye solution is pumped from a beaker and clean water is replaced at the same rate to keep the volume of distribution constant. As the concentration decreases, so the rate of elimination decreases in direct proportion. Clearance (CL) is the proportionality constant between the rate of elimination and concentration.

Rate of elimination of dye = CL × C mg/min

Hence:

$$CL = \frac{\text{Rate of elimination (mg/min)}}{C \text{ (mg/mL)}}$$

Consequently the units of clearance are mL/min. In the dye model (Figure 7.7), CL = 100 mL/min.

A convenient definition of clearance is the volume of blood effectively stripped of drug in unit time. Clearance can be expressed in terms of the effects of a particular organ. For example, renal plasma clearance is the volume of plasma effectively stripped of drug by the kidney per unit time. Total clearance is the sum of the renal plasma clearance and clearance by metabolism and by excretion through other organs, notably the liver.

Excretion by the kidney

The renal clearance of a drug is determined by the rate of filtration at the glomerulus and by the degree of tubular re-absorption (Figure 7.8).

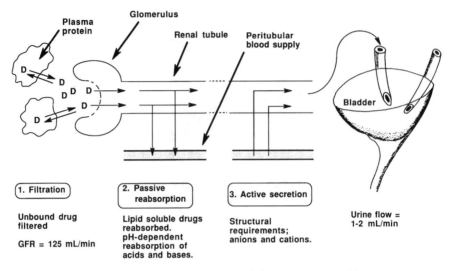

Figure 7.8 Processes influencing drug (D) excretion by the kidney

Rate of filtration at the glomerulus

Drug filtration is determined by the glomerular filtration rate (GFR, normally approximately 125 mL/min in man), the concentration of the drug in plasma water and the extent of protein binding of the drug. Drug bound to plasma does not enter the glomerular filtrate to any extent (e.g. **warfarin** $f_u = 0.03$). The drug concentration in the filtrate is equal to the unbound drug concentration in plasma, so there is no tendency for drug dissociation from adsorption sites on plasma proteins. The rate of filtration is independent of the lipid solubility or the degree of ionization of the drug.

Creatinine clearance

The clearance of creatinine is widely used to measure GFR when assessing renal impairment. Creatinine is a catabolic product of amino acid metabolism derived from muscle. Its rate of production is proportional to muscle mass and is fairly constant for an individual. Creatinine (MW 113 Da) is water soluble, distributes through ECF, exhibits limited binding to proteins and is eliminated by renal filtration with a clearance equal to GFR. There is some passive re-absorption of creatinine, which is matched by active secretion. Creatinine clearance can be determined in two ways:

(1) By collecting a 24 h urine sample, a blood sample at the midpoint of the 24 h period and assaying their creatinine contents.

$$\text{CL}_{cr} \text{ (mL/min)} = \frac{\text{Creatinine content of 24 h urine sample (mg/24 h)}}{\text{Serum creatinine content (mg/mL)} \times 60 \times 24}$$

(2) More commonly, by collecting and assaying a blood sample and by calculating creatinine production from an estimation of muscle mass using easily measured physical characteristics (height, weight, sex). At a <u>steady state</u>, the rate of elimination of creatinine equals its rate of production.

CL_{cr} in a young adult is approximately 125 mL/min. Serum creatinine concentration is relatively constant within an individual, as both creatinine production and CL_{cr} decrease with age. Renal clearance of a drug greater than 125 mL/min implies some active secretion, while renal clearance less than the CL_{cr} implies some re-absorption or plasma protein binding. Note that as urine flow is normally approximately 1 mL/min, whereas GFR is 125 mL/min, it can be deduced that more than 99% of water filtered at the glomerulus is re-absorbed. Consequently, less than 1% of a lipid-soluble drug filtered at the glomerulus finally appears in the urine.

Tubular re-absorption

Passive

As salt and water are removed (approximately 99% normally) from the filtrate in the renal tubules, there is a tendency for drug concentration in the tubules to raise and drug molecules diffuse back into the peritubular plasma down a concentration gradient. The rate of re-absorption depends on the same physicochemical properties of the drug that govern its absorption.

Highly polar water-soluble drugs (e.g. **gentamicin**, oxidized drug metabolites and conjugates) are too large to penetrate the water pores of cells and have negligible solubility in the membrane lipids. There is little re-absorption of such drugs and the renal clearance approaches the GFR. Their concentration in urine can approach 100 times that in plasma. Drugs with intermediate polarity (**digoxin**) resemble the water-soluble drugs. Non-polar, lipid-soluble drugs (**thiopentone**, **phenytoin**, inhalational anaesthetic agents) are re-absorbed from the tubular urine almost completely. Their renal clearance is negligible.

Acidic drugs (pK_a 2–7.4) (salicylic acid) show pH-dependent excretion. The lipid-soluble species (non-ionized form) is re-absorbed but the charged, polar species (anion) is not. The maximum renal clearance is obtained at the maximum attainable urine pH, usually 8 (Table 7.14). Basic drugs (pK_a 6–12) (**lignocaine**) also show pH-dependent excretion. The lipid-soluble species (non-ionized form) is re-absorbed but the charged, polar species (cation) is not. The maximum renal clearance is obtained at the minimum attainable urine pH, usually 5 (Table 7.17).

Active

This occurs for drugs that resemble essential metabolites (e.g. L-amino acids, *thyroxine*, *methyldopa*). The active re-absorption of uric acid is inhibited by another acid, *probenecid*.

Tubular secretion

Secretion implies active transport into the renal tubules against a concentration gradient. There are two distinct systems each with a small specificity. Each system shows competition and saturation kinetics. Compounds with small rates of transport can act as inhibitors. The transport is often bidirectional. Examples of actively secreted anions are penicillins, thiazides and loop diuretic agents, salicylates and drug conjugates. Actively secreted cations include **neostigmine** and **morphine**.

If there is active secretion, renal clearance usually exceeds GFR and renal clearance can equal the total renal plasma flow. Clearance can even exceed renal plasma flow if the drug is concentrated in red cells and if this store of drug is available for secretion (e.g. *prilocaine* in strongly acidic urine). Renal clearance of actively secreted drugs is not reduced by protein binding, as the drug/albumin complex dissociates very rapidly as free drug is secreted. Thus, although **benzylpenicillin** is approximately 50% bound, the renal clearance approximates to renal plasma flow.

Drug disposition in renal insufficiency

There is accumulation of unchanged water-soluble drug or metabolites in plasma until the concentration of the drug is so large that, despite the small volume of plasma cleared, the rate of elimination equals the rate of drug intake (or metabolite production). Non-renal elimination mechanisms may become more important.

Water-soluble and intermediate solubility drugs accumulate – **gentamicin** (toxic effects on inner ear and kidney) and **digoxin** (toxic effects on the heart).

Lipid-soluble drugs (**phenytoin**) do not accumulate but any water-soluble hydroxylated metabolites do, and their effects may be clinically detectable.

Actively transported drugs show intermediate accumulation. Large doses of the diuretic **frusemide**, which is actively secreted, can be given without evidence of systemic toxicity.

Where glomerular filtration is the predominant mechanism of drug elimination, there is a close correlation between drug clearance and CL_{cr}. In renal insufficiency, the loading dose required is similar to that of a healthy individual (V is unchanged) but the maintenance dose must be reduced. The maintenance dose rate can be calculated using nomograms (graphical representations between the variables, dose rate and CL_{cr}). Renal failure is important in deciding the dosage regimen when a large proportion of the drug is eliminated by the kidneys and the drug has a small therapeutic index.

Excretion – other routes

Liver

Bile flow is small, approximately 0.5 mL/min. Therefore, biliary clearance of unmetabolized drugs, which enter bile by simple diffusion, is negligible.

However, biliary excretion is significant for some drug metabolites. Active transport systems exist for polar compounds with a MW greater than 250 Da. These mechanisms are applicable for carbohydrates (e.g. dextran, inulin, sucrose, *mannitol*) and acidic compounds (e.g. bile acids, bilirubin, iodine contrast media, glucuronide, glycine and sulphate conjugates and penicillins).

Excreted compounds are often re-absorbed from the gut, usually after deconjugation brought about by the normal bacteria in the gut. The drug may be re-excreted by the liver to produce enterohepatic recycling (e.g. contraceptive steroids, phenothiazines, Figure 7.9). The re-absorbed drug, metabolite or conjugate is often finally excreted by the kidney.

Biliary obstruction and liver failure produce impairment of biliary excretion.

Lungs

Drug molecules may diffuse across alveolar membrane. The lungs are the major organ of elimination of volatile anaesthetic agents. Excretion in expired air may be obvious to smell but quantitatively insignificant (e.g. ethanol, *paraldehyde*, thiols).

Saliva, milk, sweat, sebum

The amounts of drug excreted are small but relevant to the breast-fed infant and to the treatment of acne with antibacterial drugs that partition into sebum (e.g. **tetracycline**).

Summary

(1) Elimination is the removal of the original drug molecule from the body by excretion or by metabolism.

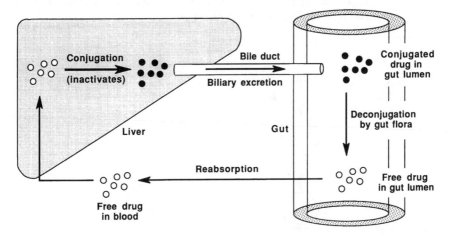

Figure 7.9 Enterohepatic circulation of steroids

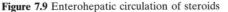
STAFFS UNIVERSITY LIBRARY

(2) Excretion in the urine is important for water-soluble drugs and metab-
     olism by the liver important for lipid-soluble drugs.
(3) Clearance is the volume of blood stripped of drug in unit time.
(4) Renal clearance of a drug is the sum of glomerular filtration plus
     active secretion minus re-absorption.
(5) Lipid-soluble drugs are passively reabsorbed from kidney tubules,
     while water-soluble drugs are not; acids and bases exhibit pH-depen-
     dent renal excretion.

Drug metabolism

Most lipid-soluble compounds are metabolized to more water-soluble
products. Drugs must possess some degree of lipid solubility to be able to
pass through liver cell membranes to gain access to enzymes. The metabolism (biotransformation) of foreign compounds (xenobiotics) occurs
mainly in liver, although kidney, adrenal cortex, lungs, placenta, skin and
even lymphocytes may be involved to a small extent.

Atracurium (see p. 56) is an unusual drug in that it breaks down in
peripheral blood to inactive products so that its neuromuscular blocking
action is terminated. *Atracurium* breaks down by spontaneous degradation (at pH 7.4, 37°C).

The metabolism of most drugs occurs in two phases (Figure 7.10):

Phase I – reactions that unmask or insert a hydrophilic functional group
            (e.g. –OH). Phase I reactions generally produce a more water-
            soluble and less active compound.
Phase II – conjugation reactions. The conjugation occurs at the site of a
            reactive group (often –OH, added perhaps by a phase I
            reaction). A phase II reaction renders a compound much more
            water soluble and totally inactive.

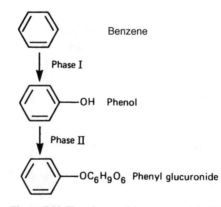

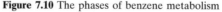

Figure 7.10 The phases of benzene metabolism

Metabolic pathways – phase I

Mixed function oxidase (MFO)

This enzyme system is the most important for Phase I reactions. It is located in the smooth endoplasmic reticulum (microsomal fraction), is relatively non-specific and is also known as mono-oxygenase (one atom of the O_2 molecule is incorporated into each molecule of product). A major component of the system is the haem protein cytochrome P_{450} (so called because in the reduced state it forms a complex with carbon monoxide that absorbs light at 450 nm). Cytochrome P_{450} comprises a superfamily of closely related isoenzymes. Some of the subfamilies of cytochrome P_{450} are involved in the metabolism of several endogenous substances (e.g. corticosteroids). Other subfamilies are involved in the metabolism of xenobiotics (foreign substances). The individual isoenzymes have evolved selectivity for particular substrates.

Examples:

Chemical reaction	*Example*
Hydroxylation of aromatic ring	of benzene to give phenol
Hydroxylation of alkyl chain	of toluene to give benzyl alcohol
Epoxidation	of benzopyrene to give benzo-pyrene epoxide
Oxidative deamination	of amphetamine to give phenyl-acetone

Other oxidations

Some are cytoplasmic (e.g. ethanol metabolism, Figure 7.11), others are mitochondrial, (e.g. MAO – substrates include noradrenaline, tyramine, see p. 85).

Reductions

Reductive metabolism of drugs (Figure 7.12) is less common than oxidation.

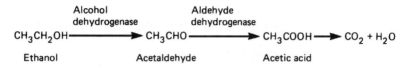

Figure 7.11 Oxidation of ethanol

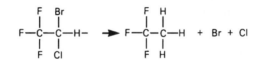

Figure 7.12 Reductive metabolism of **halothane**

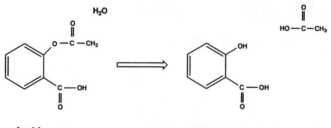

Figure 7.13 Hydrolysis of **aspirin** (acetylsalicylic acid)

Hydrolysis

Ester bonds (in **aspirin**, **atropine**, *pethidine*) and amide bonds (in **lignocaine**) can be hydrolysed (Figure 7.13). Esterases are present in gut, liver, plasma and other tissues.

Metabolic pathways – phase II

Glucuronide conjugates

Glucuronides are the most common conjugates. Glucose is oxidized to glucuronic acid. This in turn combines with alcoholic or phenolic hydroxy groups or amines groups on drug molecules to form glucuronide conjugates (Figure 7.10).

Other conjugates

Products from phase I metabolism or parent drugs can form addition compounds with sulphate (paracetamol sulphate), acetate (acetylisoniazid), glycine (salicyluric acid) or methyl groups (e.g. noradrenaline to adrenaline).

Pharmacological importance of drug metabolism

Usually liver metabolism involves the conversion of lipid-soluble to more water-soluble compounds, which diffuse into the blood and are excreted by the kidney. Some large MW conjugates are actively transported into the bile duct. The majority of metabolites are less pharmacologically active (potent) than the parent drugs.

Prodrugs

Some compounds (prodrugs) are themselves pharmacologically inactive but are converted by liver metabolism to products that are pharmacologically active. The term is also inaccurately used for pharmacologically active drugs that are metabolized to metabolites that are more potent than the parent drug. Metabolites of non-toxic drugs can be toxic, in which case the drug can be thought of as a protoxin.

Some prodrugs have different pharmacokinetic properties from their metabolites. *Pivampicillin* is an ester of **ampicillin**, and hence is more lipid soluble and with a larger oral bioavailability. *Pivampicillin* is de-esterified by the liver to ampicillin. **Diazepam** is metabolized to several other pharmacologically active benzodiazepines, including *N*-desmethyldiazepam, that have longer half-lives and contribute to the action of **diazepam**.

The therapeutic action of a drug may reside entirely in its metabolites (that is the drug is a true prodrug). **Cyclophosphamide** is converted by the liver to an alkylating derivative responsible for the cytotoxic effects. **Levodopa** is taken up by neurones in the CNS and metabolized to dopamine, resulting in improvement in Parkinson's disease. *Enalapril* is converted in the liver to the pharmacologically active enalaprilat, which is itself too water soluble to be absorbed after oral administration.

Conversion of a drug to active metabolites may be limited to one organ, so increasing selectivity of action. *Sulphasalazine* is metabolized by bacteria in the large intestine to 5-aminosalicylic acid, responsible for its anti-inflammatory action in ulcerative colitis. **Acyclovir** is selectively metabolized to the monophosphate by herpes viruses and then converted to the active triphosphate by the viral host cell.

Metabolites may be in whole or in part responsible for the toxic effects of the parent chemical. The blindness and peripheral neuropathy of methanol are a consequence of its conversion to formaldehyde. **Paracetamol** is mainly metabolized to inactive conjugates but a minor oxidized metabolite is a reactive quinone (Figure 7.14). Normally this derivative is conjugated with

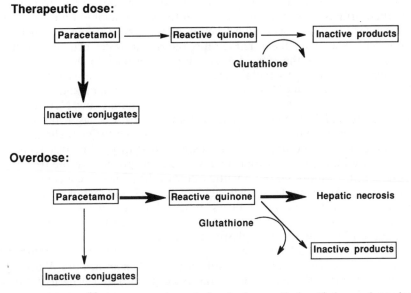

Figure 7.14 Pathways of paracetamol metabolism in therapeutic (small) dose and overdose

glutathione in the liver. However, glutathione stores are limited and in **paracetamol** overdosage the liver content of glutathione is soon consumed. The remaining reactive quinone covalently bonds to proteins, resulting in hepatic necrosis. Early treatment with *acetylcysteine*, which is converted to glutathione, can prevent liver failure in **paracetamol** overdose.

Metabolic rate

The concept of clearance can be equally applied to liver metabolism. An organ clearance can be defined in terms of an eliminating organ. Hepatic clearance equals liver blood flow (normally approximately 1500 mL/min) multiplied by the <u>extraction ratio</u> (= E = the fraction of the drug in the blood that is metabolized during a single passage through the liver). The extraction ratio can vary from 1 (virtually all drug presented is removed) to 0 (no drug metabolized).

> *Examples:*
> | *Small extraction ratio* | *Large extraction ratio* |
> |---|---|
> | **Phenytoin** | **Lignocaine** |
> | *Salicylic acid* | **Glyceryl trinitrate** |
> | **Warfarin** | **Morphine** |

For drugs with a large extraction ratio, the liver has such a large capacity for metabolism that clearance is unaffected by changes in enzyme activity or by the fraction of drug that is protein bound, but is proportional to blood flow (changes in amount delivered), that is metabolism is perfusion limited. Shock (with reduced hepatic blood flow) decreases metabolism. **Lignocaine** and **morphine** are unusually persistent in patients with cardiogenic shock. Drugs with large extraction ratios exhibit considerable first-pass metabolism. (After absorption from the gut all the drug is presented to the liver in the hepatic portal vein. Subsequently, only a fraction of the absorbed drug is presented to the liver in the systemic blood on each pass as the liver blood flow is only a fraction of the total cardiac output.)

For drugs with a small extraction ratio, the rate at which drug is delivered to the liver exceeds the rate of either drug diffusion into the liver or the capacity of the liver to metabolize. Therefore, clearance is sensitive to changes in the fraction of drug in the plasma that is unbound and to changes in enzyme activity, but is not sensitive to changes in blood flow. Nevertheless, the liver can still be the major route of elimination for drugs in this group.

The concept of extraction ratio can also be applied to renal elimination.

Most drug metabolizing systems exhibit <u>first-order</u> kinetics (rate of enzymatic elimination is proportional to the concentration of the free drug in the plasma) within the therapeutic range of drug plasma concentrations. A few drugs, for example, salicylic acid (see p. 397), **phenytoin** (see p. 388) and ethanol (see p. 390), exhibit saturation kinetics, which can approximate to <u>zero-order</u> kinetics (that is the rate of enzymatic elimination is constant and independent of plasma concentration).

There is a genetically determined variation in the rate of metabolism by some specific enzyme systems. The best studied examples are *N*-acetylation (see p. 428), plasma cholinesterase (see p. 430) and drug hydroxylation by MFO (see p. 429).

Metabolism and drug interactions

The activity of the MFO system can be increased by exposure to some drugs or foreign chemicals – the system is said to be inducible. As a result, there is an increased rate of elimination of the inducing drug itself and many other drug substrates (see p. 442). The therapeutic effect of drugs can therefore be reduced if their metabolism is induced.

Conversely, a number of the enzyme systems can be inhibited by drugs, leading to decreased elimination of other drugs or endogenous substrates. This can lead to excessive drug effects, although often the interaction is not of major clinical significance or can be taken into account by change in dosage (see p. 443).

When exposure to the inducing or inhibiting drug or chemical ceases, MFO activity returns to normal. This may mean that another dosage adjustment is needed to prevent overdosage (when an inducing influence is removed) or underdosage (when an inhibiting influence is removed).

Summary

(1) Metabolism of most drugs occurs in two phases, phase I unmasks or inserts a hydrophilic functional group while phase II involves conjugation.
(2) Many drugs are oxidized by the mixed function oxidase system. This system can be induced and inhibited by drugs.
(3) Prodrugs are pharmacologically inactive compounds metabolized to active products.

Pharmacokinetics

Pharmacokinetic knowledge contributes in many ways to the practice of therapeutics, which include:

(1) Distinguishing between pharmacokinetic and pharmacodynamic causes of variation in and unexpected responses to drugs.
(2) Evolving concepts that are common to all drugs; thus information gained about one drug helps in anticipating the pharmacokinetics of another drug.
(3) Often explaining the manner of use of a drug and 'occasionally suggesting a more convenient or effective dosage regimen.
(4) Often allowing anticipation of the likely outcome of a therapeutic manoeuvre.

A good strategy for understanding this topic is to read the following text and then to tackle the examples (see pp. 369–370).

One-compartment open model

The handling by the body of most drugs can be modelled by a stirred beaker of water that is continuously emptied and replenished by two identical pumps, which simulates the major processes of drug disposition. The rate and completeness of absorption are under the control of the operator when injecting a dose of a dye (representing drug) into the beaker. Immediate injection is equivalent to bolus i/v injection in a patient. This dose is then distributed throughout the volume of water in the beaker (or apparent volume of distribution, Figure 7.5) at a rate that is determined by the stirrer (equivalent to the heart). As the concentration is the same throughout the beaker it is called a <u>one-compartment model</u>. Most drugs, at distribution equilibrium, behave as if their concentration is homogeneous throughout the body. The compartments, and their volumes, for modelling drug handling rarely equate to physiological compartments (see p. 345). Elimination from the beaker (equivalent to the kidneys, liver, lungs, etc.) starts as soon as some dye has entered and is determined by the rate at which one pump removes coloured water and the other replaces it by clean water; that is the rate at which the pumps <u>clear</u> the water in the beaker.

It is characteristic of this model that the dye does not disappear at a steady rate. The dye disappears more rapidly when its concentration is large. In fact, the rate of elimination of dye (the slope in Figure 7.15a) is proportional to the concentration. Any process in which the rate of change of a variable is proportional to the magnitude of that variable is

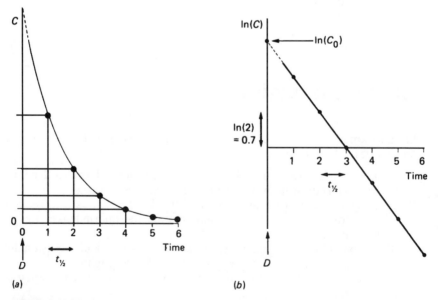

Figure 7.15 The exponential decay of concentration: (a) on an arithmetic scale; (b) on a logarithmic scale, with time after injection of a constant dose (D) into a one-compartment open model

said to be an <u>exponential</u> process. An important characteristic of an exponential process is that the variable changes by the same fraction (or multiple) in a given period of time, irrespective of the magnitude of the variable or the length of time for which the process has been running. This means that any exponential process can be described simply and conveniently by a single time value, expressing the time it takes for the variable to change by a particular fraction. For drug elimination, the value usually used is known as the elimination half-time, often shortened to half-life $(t_{1/2})$.

This simple model adequately describes the handling of most drugs used in patients, although it is sometimes necessary to postulate more than one distribution compartment (see p. 368) and an elimination process that can be saturated at large concentration (see p. 370). In what follows, this simple model is used to illustrate the principles of pharmacokinetics.

Intravenous bolus dose

If a dose (D) of drug is injected slowly i/v the average patient behaves towards the drug as though composed of a well-stirred single open compartment of volume (V) (see Figure 7.5a). There is a very short delay before the peak plasma concentration is reached. The peak concentration that would have been reached if the drug could have been distributed instantaneously after instantaneous injection, that is the concentration at zero time (C_0), can be deduced by assaying the plasma concentration (C) at various times (t) and extrapolating back to zero time (see Figure 7.15).

From this value and a knowledge of the amount of drug injected (D), the apparent volume of distribution of the drug (V) can be calculated from the relationship $C_0 = D \div V$.

The compartment, with apparent volume of distribution V, loses drug by a process of elimination to the outside world (hence <u>open</u>). This loss results in the decay of the drug concentration in the compartment in a time-dependent (kinetic) fashion. The rate of decay (dC/dt) is proportional only to the concentration (that is it is exponential), so the process is described as first order:

$$dC/dt = -k_{el}C \qquad \text{(differential form)}$$

$$C = C_0 \, e^{(-k_{el}t)} \qquad \text{(integral form)}$$

C is an exponential function of time and three interrelated parameters can be used alternatively to describe the rate of the decay of C with time:

(1) Half-life (or half-time) $t_{1/2}$.
(2) Elimination rate constant k_{el}.
(3) Elimination clearance CL.

The term first order is used to describe exponential elimination processes, because the rate of decay is proportional to the drug concentration raised to the power 1:

$$dC/dt = KC^1$$

where K is the proportionality constant.

STAFFS UNIVERSITY LIBRARY

For some processes the rate of elimination is constant. In these rare cases the rate equation is a special form of the equation above and can be written:

$$dC/dt = KC^0$$
$$= K$$

This is because any number raised to the power zero = 1. Hence such elimination processes are called zero-order processes.

The time taken for the concentration to halve ($t_{1/2}$ – dimensions = time) is constant, irrespective of the concentration or the elapsed time. Another characteristic of an exponential process is that re-plotting the same data on the same abscissa (time), but a logarithmic ordinate (concentration), produces a straight line (Figure 7.15b). (This is how the peak concentration, C_0, and hence V, could be deduced by back extrapolation to $t = 0$).

Using natural logarithms (ln; dictated by the 'e' in the integral form of the equation), the negative slope of this semi-logarithmic plot is the elimination rate constant, k_{el} (dimensions = /time). A k_{el} of 0.1/h implies that 10% of the drug is eliminated per hour. Because the elimination constant is the negative slope of the plot of ln C versus time, we can express k_{el} as:

$$-k_{el} = slope = \frac{\ln C_1 - \ln C_2}{t}$$

We can rewrite $\ln C_1 - \ln C_2$ as $\ln (C_1 \div C_2)$, and when the time interval is equal to the half-life ($t_{1/2}$), $C_1 \div C_2 = 2$ (that is the concentration is halved). As $\ln 2 \approx 0.7$, the relationship between k_{el} and $t_{1/2}$ is as follows:

$$k_{el} = 0.7 \div t_{1/2} \tag{7.3}$$

The third way of describing the elimination process is by the elimination clearance, CL (dimensions = volume/time). This is defined as the proportionality constant in the relationship between rate of drug elimination (dimensions = mass/time) and its driving force, the plasma concentration (dimensions = mass/volume). Clearance can also be understood as the volume of plasma that would contain the mass of drug eliminated in unit time.

$$Rate\ of\ elimination = \frac{mass\ of\ drug\ eliminated}{time}$$

Because concentration = mass/volume,

$$Rate\ of\ elimination = volume \times \frac{concentration}{time}$$

Hence the rate of elimination can be rewritten as:

$$Rate\ of\ elimination = V \times dC/dt \tag{7.4}$$

As the rate of elimination is proportional to concentration (for exponential processes),

$$Rate\ of\ elimination = Constant \times C \tag{7.5}$$

Hence:

$$V \times dC/dt = CL \times C \qquad (7.6)$$

where CL is the proportionality constant, the clearance. From this equation it can be seen that clearance has the dimensions of volume per unit time.

It can be shown that:

$$k_{el} = CL \div V \qquad (7.7)$$

Therefore, combining Equations 7.7 and 7.3:

$$t_{1/2} = 0.7V \div CL \qquad (7.8)$$

Drugs can have a $t_{1/2}$ varying from approximately 10 min (e.g. *soluble insulin*) to days (e.g. 36 h for **digoxin**). Note (Figure 7.16a, b) that an empirically observed long $t_{1/2}$ can have two independent causes – either a small CL or a large V.

Intravenous infusion

If a drug were infused into a closed compartment (that is absorption occurs, but no elimination), then the drug concentration would increase linearly with time. However, normally elimination occurs from the compartment. Hence, the i/v infusion of a drug at a constant rate (D/T,

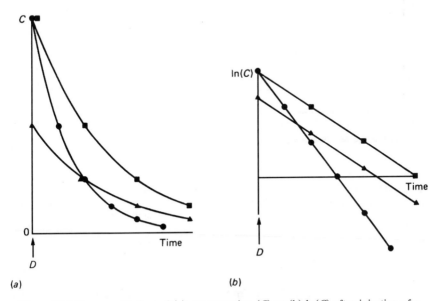

(a)   (b)

Figure 7.16 Change with time of (a) concentration (C) or (b) ln(C) after injection of a constant dose (D) into a one-compartment open model: the effect of altering volume of distribution (V) or elimination clearance (CL). ● = initial values of V and CL; ▲ = effect of doubling V and hence doubling $t_{1/2}$ or halving k_{el}; ■ = effect of halving CL and hence doubling $t_{1/2}$ or halving k_{el}

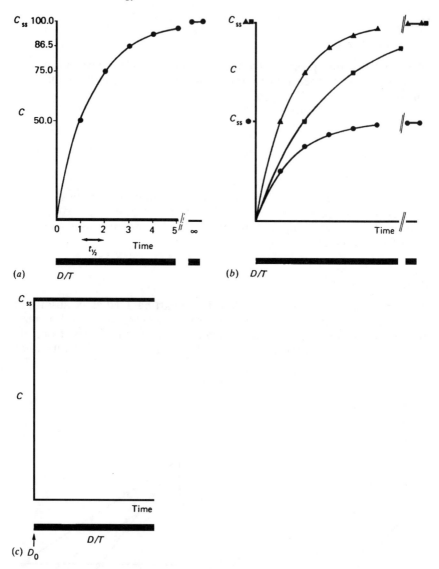

Figure 7.17 Change of concentration (C) with time after constant infusion (rate D/T) into a one-compartment open model: (a) accumulation asymptotic to C_{ss}; (b) the effect of altering infusion rate or elimination clearance (CL). ● = initial values of D/T and CL; ▲ = effect of doubling D/T; ■ = effect of halving CL and hence doubling $t_{1/2}$; (c) the effect of the loading dose D_0

where D is the dose given in time T) results in the accumulation of the drug in the compartment to a steady-state plateau concentration (C_{ss}) (Figure 7.17a). This is because the elimination process is exponential. Initially drug output is zero so that the rate at which the drug is infused exceeds the rate of elimination. As a result the concentration of the drug increases until the rate of output = the rate of input. This is described as the steady state.

The time-course of the growth of concentration is exponential and has a $t_{1/2}$ that is identical with the elimination $t_{1/2}$. The time to reach the plateau depends only on $t_{1/2}$. The shorter the $t_{1/2}$ the quicker the plateau is attained (Figure 7.17b). It is conventional and convenient to regard the steady state as effectively attained when more than 95% of the steady-state concentration (C_{ss}) is reached. It takes approximately five half-lives for the concentration to reach 95% of the eventual C_{ss} (Table 7.6).

The actual concentration at steady state (the plateau concentration) is determined by the rate of drug infusion and the clearance. Note that if the apparent volume of distribution for a drug (V) is large (and it therefore has a long $t_{1/2}$), the time it takes to reach steady state is longer, but the final C_{ss} is the same as for a drug with a small V, provided that both are infused at the same rate and that they have the same plasma clearance.

At a steady state the concentration of drug in the compartment does not change. The rate of drug input to the compartment is the infusion rate (D/T), the rate of output is the rate of elimination (CL $\times$ C_{ss}, from Equation 7.6). Hence

$$D/T = \text{CL} \times C_{ss} \tag{7.9}$$

Table 7.7 highlights the most important equation met so far.

Intravenous bolus dose and infusion

If it is important to achieve a steady-state concentration rapidly (e.g. when treating life-threatening conditions), a single large bolus dose (a <u>loading dose</u>) can be given and then the infusion is begun. Figure 7.17c shows the algebraic sum of Figures 7.17a and 7.15a.

Table 7.6 Time-course of approach to steady state

Time (in multiples of $t_{1/2}$)	Plateau concentration (% of C_{ss})
1	50
2	75
3	87.5
3.3	90
4	93.75
5	96.87
6.66	99
9.99	99.9

Table 7.7 Fundamental pharmacokinetic equations

$t_{1/2} = 0.7\ V \div \text{CL}$
$D/T = \text{CL} \times C_{ss}$

The loading dose (D_0) that is needed is that which produces a peak concentration (C_0) equal to the C_{ss} that would eventually be achieved by the infusion (maintenance dosing).

$$D_0 \div V = C_0 = C_{ss} = (D/T) \div CL$$

Hence from Equation 7.8

$$D_0 \div (D/T) = t_{1/2} \div 0.7 \tag{7.10}$$

That is, the greater the $t_{1/2}$ of a drug the larger the bolus dose that is needed in relation to the maintenance dose rate.

Regularly repeated intravenous bolus doses

If repeated bolus doses are given, the drug accumulates as it does during constant infusion, except that the concentration versus time curve is 'saw-toothed'. After each bolus dose the concentration increases rapidly before decreasing exponentially until the next bolus dose is given. The shape of the average compartmental concentration at steady state $(C_{ss,av})$ resulting from regular bolus dosing is no different from that resulting from infusion at the same drug input rate (D/T).

The rate of approach to steady state again depends only on the elimination $t_{1/2}$. The steady-state average concentration $(C_{ss,av})$ is determined by the dose rate and clearance (Figure 7.18). Large trough to peak fluctuations result from large infrequent dosing, and smaller fluctuations at the

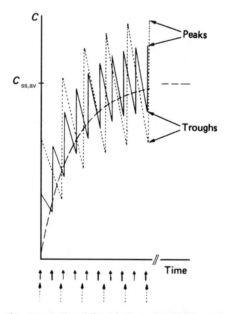

Figure 7.18 Change of concentration (C) with time after dosing a one-compartment open model with a constant dose rate (D/T) but varying interdose intervals (T). — — — — = smoothed average C with T near 0 as with i/v infusion: ⟶ = repeated bolus injections at significant dose intervals; - - - - ⟶ = repeated bolus injections at longer T

same dose rate can be achieved by giving smaller doses at more frequent intervals.

Intravenous bolus dose and repeated doses

As in the case of i/v bolus dose and infusion (see p. 363), the time it takes to reach steady-state can be reduced by starting the sequence with an appropriately sized loading dose (Equation 7.10 applies), followed by regular doses to maintain the steady-state concentration. When the dosing interval equals the $t_{1/2}$ the maintenance dose must be one-half of the loading dose to make good the loss (Figure 7.19). Note that this makes for simple relationships between doses, volume of distribution, peak and trough concentrations and dosing interval:

$$C_{ss,av} = C_0 \div (2 \times 0.7)$$

For other dosing intervals the general expression is:

$$C_{ss,av} \div (D/V) = t_{1/2} \div (0.7\ T) \tag{7.11}$$

or in mass terms

$$A_{ss,av} \div D = t_{1/2} \div (0.7\ T)$$

where $A_{ss,av}$ is the average amount of drug in the body at steady state.

Single oral dose

The oral route of administering drugs is much more convenient than i/v injection or indeed than any route requiring injection, and as in most

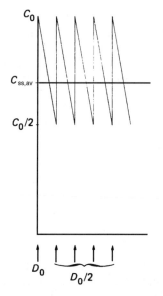

Figure 7.19 The early establishment of a steady state in discontinuous dosing by a loading dose

STAFFS UNIVERSITY LIBRARY
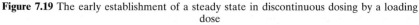

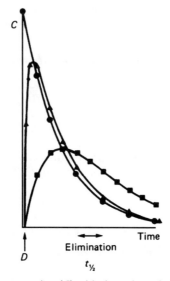

Figure 7.20 Change of concentration (C) with time after administration of a single dose (D) into a one-compartment open model: the effect of altering absorption $t_{1/2}$. ● = absorption $t_{1/2}$ near 0 as with i/v bolus; ▲ = absorption $t_{1/2}$ = elimination $t_{1/2}$; ■ = absorption $t_{1/2}$ = 10 × elimination $t_{1/2}$

circumstances it is equally effective, we must examine how these concepts and equations need to be modified to adapt them to this common form of clinical dosing.

Figure 7.20 shows the changes in the concentration/time curve that occur when a single dose reaches the compartment by first-order absorption occurring at different rates. These curves assume that absorption is complete (that is F, the fraction of the dose absorbed, = 1). You can describe the time for one-half of the drug to be absorbed as the absorption half-time.

Notice that as the absorption half-time increases (that is as absorption slows), the peak concentration declines, the peak concentration occurs later after dosing and that the compartment concentrations at each time after the peak time are larger.

Less obvious from the figure, but nevertheless true and useful, is the fact that the area under the concentration/time curve is unchanged. This is because the deficit early after the dose due to the delay in absorption is exactly matched by the later excess.

Repeated oral dosing

Repeated oral dosing leads to phasic accumulation of drug somewhere between the smooth ascent of Figure 7.17a and the extreme fluctuations of Figure 7.18. The average concentration increases asymptotically with a half-time that is usually dominated by the elimination $t_{1/2}$ but may be even longer if absorption is very slow. When absorption is very slow it may be incomplete, because defaecation occurs before all the drug has been absorbed.

The input dose rate is equivalent to that derived from i/v infusion (D/T) but needs to be multiplied by the bioavailability (F) which is often less than 1 when a drug is given orally. The $C_{ss,av}$ attained is determined by the input dose rate ($F \times D/T$) and clearance as in Equation 7.9.

The size of the fluctuations is determined by the dose interval and volume of distribution but the fluctuations are more damped as the absorption half-time increases.

Oral loading dose followed by regular maintenance dose

The therapeutically required $C_{ss,av}$ can be achieved quickly by giving a loading dose that is larger than the repeated maintenance dose (Figure 7.19). The size of the loading dose can be calculated by multiplying the maintenance dose by the factor established in Equation 7.11 that is $t_{1/2} \div (0.7\ T)$.

Summary of pharmacokinetic terms and symbols

Pharmacokineticists, who study the processes of drug handling in animals and man, have evolved a series of more or less standard terms and symbols (see Rowland and Tozer, 1995 in Suggested further reading, p. 548):

A (mg)	– the amount of drug in the body at a particular time.
$C_{ss,av}$ (mg/L)	– the mean plasma drug concentration when a steady state is attained.
C (mg/L)	– the concentration in the main/central/plasma compartment at a particular time after the previous dose.
C_0 (mg/L)	– the concentration at zero time, assuming complete absorption with no elimination; obtained by back extrapolation.
CL (L/h)	– drug clearance; the volume of fluid (blood, plasma or water) that contains the mass of drug eliminated in unit time.
CL_{cr} (L/h)	– clearance of endogenous creatinine; a useful measure of kidney function that approximates to GFR.
D (mg)	– dose of drug.
F	– fraction of dose absorbed from site of administration; the bioavailability.
k_a (/h)	– absorption rate constant; reciprocally related to the time for 50% absorption.
k_{el} (/h)	– elimination rate constant; reciprocally related to the time for 50% elimination.
$t_{1/2}$ (h)	– elimination half-time; the time for C to decrease by one-half or the time for 50% elimination.
T (h)	– interval between doses during a course of drug treatment.
V (L)	– apparent distribution volume; the size of the conceptual compartment in which the drug is distributed.

Two-compartment model

It is common for drugs with significant lipid solubility to show evidence of distribution into more than one compartment after i/v injection. The implication is that their concentration does not behave as though homogeneous in one compartment, but is better modelled by being considered homogeneous in each of two (<u>central</u> and <u>peripheral</u>) <u>compartments</u>. Intravenous injection into the two-compartment model of Figure 7.29 would produce a semi-logarithmic central compartment concentration/time curve (analogous to Figure 7.15b), like Figure 7.21.

Immediately after injection and mixing, the drug is restricted to the central compartment (volume V_1) so its peak concentration is large ($D \div V_1$). The concentration declines not only because elimination clearance is occurring from the central compartment, but also because distribution is occurring into the peripheral compartment. Immediately after injection the concentration in the peripheral compartment is zero but then increases to approach that in the central compartment. This redistribution can be described by a distribution clearance. Distributional steady state is attained when the concentrations in the two compartments are equal, and from now on the handling can be modelled by a single compartment. The time it takes for this to occur is determined by the ratio of the two clearances. Further decay of the central compartment concentration is controlled by elimination clearance and back extrapolation to time zero allows the total volume of distribution ($V_1 + V_2$) to be derived. It should be realized that elimination clearance from the cental compartment is occurring throughout.

If the same drug is administered orally the slowness of the absorptive processes masks the rapid simultaneous distribution processes and the system behaves for all practical purposes like a one-compartment model. Thus in therapeutics a firm grasp of the kinetics of the one compartment

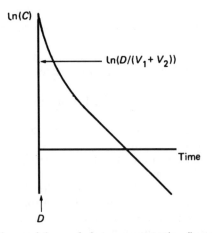

Figure 7.21 The two phases of decay of plasma concentration (logarithmic scale) with time revealing the need for a two-compartment model of drug disposition

open model allows rational manipulation of the doses and dose intervals of most drugs in most patients. Multicompartment models are needed with large rates of systemic delivery of lipid-soluble drugs – i/v **thiopentone** in the induction of general anaesthesia (see p. 386), inhalational anaesthetic agents (see p. 392).

Examples

In these examples the dye model has been scaled up to the dimensions that might apply to real drugs used in the treatment of an adult patient. Obtain a sheet of two or three cycle semilogarithmic graph paper and plot the concentration data of Table 7.8, example A, on the vertical (semilogarithmic) axis against time on the horizontal axis. Alternatively use normal graph paper and plot the $\log_{10}$ of the concentration against time.

The points lie on a straight line that, when back extrapolated to zero time, cuts the concentration axis (C_0) at 10.7 mg/L. From this it can be determined that the distribution volume (V) given by $D \div C_0$ is 160 ÷ 10.7 or 15 L.

The concentration decreases to one-half in 1.75 h $(t_{1/2})$. The clearance can be found by substituting into a rearranged form of equation 7.8, giving a CL of 0.7 × 15 ÷ 1.75 or 6 L/h.

If the dose were repeated every 12 h no accumulation would occur. Assuming complete absorption $(F = 1)$, the C_{ss} from Equation 7.9 would be 2.2 mg/L and the average amount of drug present during a dosage interval in the steady state is approximately one-fifth of a single dose from Equation 7.11.

Repeat this exercise for example data set B assuming partial absorption $(F = 0.6)$. If the dose were repeated every 24 h, what would be the value of the average steady-state concentration $(C_{ss,av})$ and the $A_{ss,av} \div (F\,D)$? (answers in Table 7.9).

Table 7.8 Three example sets of concentration/time data after the dose stated was given at zero time

	Concentration (mg/L) after dose given at time 0		
Time (h)	A 160 mg	B 500 µg	C 100 mg
0.5	8.74	–	0.74
1	7.14	–	0.55
2	4.80	–	0.30
4	2.14	–	0.09
6	0.96	0.77	0.03
8	0.45	–	0.01
10	0.19	–	–
12	0.10	0.70	–
24	–	0.56	–
36	–	0.46	–
48	–	0.38	–

Table 7.9 Answers to examples

	A	B	C
D (given)	160 mg	500 µg	100 mg
C_0	10.7 mg/L	0.84 µg/L	1 mg/L
V (L)	15	350	100
$t_{1/2}$ (h)	1.75	40.8	1.17
CL (L/h)	6	6	60
T (h) (given)	12	24	0.5
F (given)	1	0.6	1
$C_{ss,av}$	2.2 mg/L	2.1 µg/L	3.3 mg/L
$A_{ss,av} \div (F\,D)$	0.21	2.4	3.4

Repeat this exercise for example data set C assuming complete absorption $(F = 1)$. If the dose were repeated every half an hour, what would be the value of the average steady-state concentration $(C_{ss,av})$ and the $A_{ss,av} \div (F\,D)$? (answers in Table 7.9). Intravenous infusion would be a better way of achieving this.

These three examples represent different patterns of drug disposition observed with drugs that have different physicochemical properties (A, see p. 378, **gentamicin**; B, see p. 381, **digoxin**; C, see p. 399, **lignocaine**).

Kinetics of zero-order elimination

If the elimination of a drug is dominated by metabolism and if the enzymes responsible are saturated by the prevailing concentration, the concentration decays at a rate that is constant and independent of the concentration (a zero-order process). The time it takes for the concentration to decrease to one-half is not constant, but varies with the concentration of the drug in the blood. In other words, $t_{1/2}$ cannot be used as a statistic to describe a zero-order process. Similarly, other parameters that are constants for first-order processes depend on the blood concentration of the drug for zero-order processes.

A few drugs approach concentration that saturate their elimination processes in their therapeutic concentration ranges (**phenytoin**, see p. 388; ethanol, see p. 390; **aspirin**, see p. 397) and therefore have elimination kinetics that approximate to zero-order processes. Many more drugs exhibit these kinetics at toxic concentrations.

Near the foot of the plasma concentration decay curve, where the enzymes responsible for drug metabolism are unsaturated, the rate is dependent upon substrate concentration and the characteristic curvature of a first-order elimination process is revealed (Figure 7.22). The parameters describing the rate and point of inflection respectively are those of the Michaelis–Menten relationship commonly used in handling saturable phenomena.

$$dC/dt = \frac{-V_{max}\,C}{K_m + C}$$

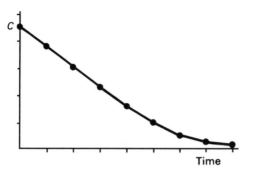

Figure 7.22 Decay of plasma concentration of a drug that displays zero-order kinetics at large concentrations and first-order kinetics at small concentrations

where dC/dt = rate of change of plasma concentration; V_{max} (mg/L)/h = maximal rate of decay of plasma concentration when elimination is saturated; K_m (mg/L) = plasma concentration at which elimination rate is 50% of the maximum. This can account for the apparent zero-order and first-order phases. At a small serum concentration, when C is very much smaller than K_m, the equation reduces to a form analogous to a first-order rate equation. Therefore, the rate of change of concentration is proportional to concentration:

$$dC/dt = -(V_{max} \div K_m) \times C = \text{constant} \times \text{concentration}$$

Conversely, at a large serum concentration, when C is very much larger than K_m, the equation reduces to a zero-order kind of relationship in which the rate of change of concentration is constant:

$$dC/dt = -V_{max} = \text{constant}$$

Drug dosage regimens

The objective of a dosage regimen in therapeutics is to prescribe doses, the size and timing of which will provide the maximum therapeutic benefit at the minimum cost in unwanted effects. Most drugs show orderly relationships between the dose rate and both the therapeutic and unwanted responses (except for allergic responses).

There are two significant boundaries:

(1) That between dose rates that are ineffective and those causing the desired response.
(2) That between dose rates causing the desired response and those causing toxic effects.

One way of defining the <u>therapeutic index</u>, which gives expression to the margin for error in dosing, is the ratio between these boundaries – the multiple by which the just toxic dose rate exceeds the just effective dose rate.

Attempts to determine optimal dose rates from observation, or even from measurement of therapeutic responses in patients, are complicated by the compounding of two sources of variability in the cause/effect chain.

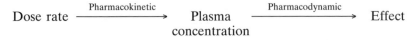

$$\text{Dose rate} \xrightarrow{\text{Pharmacokinetic}} \begin{array}{c}\text{Plasma}\\\text{concentration}\end{array} \xrightarrow{\text{Pharmacodynamic}} \text{Effect}$$

If an orderly relationship (in terms of both intensities of responses and times) holds between plasma concentration of drug and effects (both therapeutic and unwanted), optimal dose rates can be determined relatively easily using measurements of plasma drug concentration.

The maximal acceptable toxic and minimal useful effects (Figure 7.23) define a <u>therapeutic window</u> in the range of plasma concentrations. The therapeutic objective becomes the prescription of a dosage regimen that ensures the attainment and maintenance of plasma concentrations lying entirely within the therapeutic window.

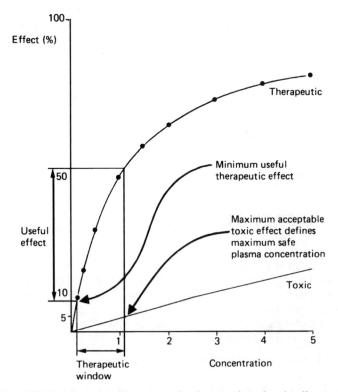

Figure 7.23 Concentration effect curves for therapeutic and toxic effects and the therapeutic window

To determine the dose rate (D/T) that will produce any target steady-state plasma concentration $(C_{ss,av})$ requires knowledge of the fraction absorbed (F) and elimination clearance (CL) (Equation 7.9). The clearance can be obtained from a knowledge of the volume of distribution (V) and either elimination half-life $(t_{1/2})$ or elimination rate constant (k_{el}).

To select a dosage regimen that achieves this dose rate requires three further considerations, providing that absorption and elimination are first-order exponential processes and that distribution is rapid.

Therapeutic index

If the therapeutic index is large (e.g. greater than 100, as with **benzylpenicillin**, see p. 308), wide fluctuations in concentration are tolerable. Consequently, relatively large doses can be given at long intervals (relative to the $t_{1/2}$). If the therapeutic index is small however (e.g. approximately 3, as with **gentamicin**, see p. 379; **digoxin**, see p. 383), the tolerable dosage regimen is narrow and fluctuations in the concentration must be minimized by giving relatively small doses at short intervals relative to the $t_{1/2}$.

Urgency of onset of effect

A second important consideration is the need for a loading dose. When clinical circumstances demand an immediate drug effect but the drug has a long $t_{1/2}$, it is necessary to give a larger first dose (loading dose; D_0) sufficient to produce a therapeutic concentration after distribution throughout the distribution volume (V). The effect of the drug is then sustained by giving a smaller maintenance dose (D_M) at intervals (T), sufficient to keep pace with clearance (CL).

Elimination half-life

A third consideration is the $t_{1/2}$, which may be short (less than 1 h), moderate (4–24 h) or long (more than 24 h).

Short $t_{1/2}$

If the $t_{1/2}$ is short and the therapeutic index is large (e.g. penicillins), a very large dose can be given at convenient intervals of 4, 6 or 8 h $(D_0 = D_M)$. The lack of toxicity allows us to compensate for the short $t_{1/2}$ by enlarging the dose – doubling the dose adds one $t_{1/2}$ to the time the plasma concentration spends in the therapeutic window. The effect persists long enough for a therapeutic response, although each dose is completely eliminated before the next is given.

When the therapeutic index is small, however, a sustained drug effect can only be attained by small, frequent doses (e.g. *soluble insulin*, $t_{1/2}$ less than 9 min, in diabetic ketoacidosis). An even better approach is continuous i/v infusion (e.g. *soluble insulin* as above; *oxytocin*, $t_{1/2}$ several minutes, for induction or augmentation of labour; **lignocaine** for suppression of ventricular ectopic foci after myocardial infarction).

Moderate $t_{1/2}$

If the $t_{1/2}$ is moderate it is convenient to give one half of the initial dose every $t_{1/2}$ ($D_0 = 2 \times D_M$). Then there is no accumulation (**trimethoprim** every 12 h or **tetracycline** every 8 or 12 h in infections, see Table 6.4, p. 000).

Long $t_{1/2}$

If the $t_{1/2}$ is longer than 24 h, a 24 h dosage interval (T) gives much the best patient compliance. The theoretical maintenance dose (D_M) corresponds with the proportion of the loading dose (D_0) that is eliminated during that time (from equation 7.10).

A patient receiving **digoxin**, for example, may show a $t_{1/2}$ of 2 days. 0.7 $T \div t_{1/2}$ = approximately one-third (from equation 7.11). Thus a daily dose of 250 µg would correspond with a loading dose of 750 µg. Even if no loading dose were given, the amount in the body would accumulate until the same steady-state concentration was attained.

Monitoring of plasma concentrations

Monitoring of plasma concentrations of a drug is of most value as an aid to therapy when the therapeutic effect itself is difficult to quantify over short time periods (**phenytoin** for epilepsy) or when the therapeutic window is narrow (**gentamicin** for serious infections with Gram-negative bacteria, **lithium carbonate** for prophylaxis of manic-depressive psychosis, **lignocaine** for cardiac dysrhythmias). It must be recognized that the therapeutic window is a guide to those plasma concentrations at which benefit generally outweighs hazard. The plasma concentration boundaries vary between individuals.

Concentration/effect and time/effect relationships

The magnitude of response of an isolated organ to a drug usually exhibits a sigmoidal relationship with the log of the drug concentration (see p. 2). The size of response to the drug in man often shows a similar relationship to log unbound plasma concentration (Figure 7.24a). For many drugs the position of the concentration/effect curve during both an increase and decrease in concentration is superimposable (e.g. during and subsequent to drug infusion). This is seen with neuromuscular blockade produced by **suxamethonium**. After i/v administration the drug rapidly gains access to the neuromuscular junction and the onset and offset of effect here is rapid.

Some drugs exhibit anticlockwise hysteresis. This means that the magnitude of effect for a given plasma concentration is greater during offset than during onset of the effect (Figure 7.24b). Reasons include:

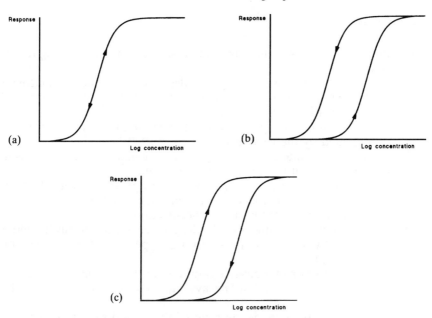

Figure 7.24 Plasma concentration–response relationships: (a) no hysteresis; (b) anticlockwise hysteresis; (c) clockwise hysteresis

(1) Delay in distribution – the site of action is in a deep tissue compartment (e.g. peak **digoxin** effect is approximately 6 h after peak plasma concentration).
(2) Delay in pharmacological response – there is an interval between drug reaching its site of action and its measured effect (e.g. peak **warfarin** concentrations are followed by rapid inhibition of prothrombin formation but there is a delay of approximately 1 day before there is a reduction in blood coagulation).
(3) Formation of active metabolites (e.g. **diazepam** metabolism to several pharmacologically active benzodiazepines).

The opposite phenomenon of clockwise hysteresis can also be seen. In this case the magnitude of effect for a given plasma concentration is greater during onset than offset of the effect (Figure 7.24c). Reasons include:

(1) Physiological homeostatic mechanisms – these return the perturbed system to normal but there is a delay in their onset (e.g. decrease in BP with a vasodilator drug countered by reflex tachycardia).
(2) Tolerance – the drug effect declines with time. This may occur over minutes, days or even weeks. Tolerance may have a pharmacokinetic basis (e.g. increased clearance with *phenobarbitone*) or a pharmacodynamic basis (e.g. change in sensitivity of neurones in the CNS to **morphine**).

STAFFS UNIVERSITY LIBRARY

Summary

(1) Pharmacokinetics is the quantitative science underlying drug disposition.
(2) The handling of most drugs can be described by a one-compartment model, with parameters of volume and elimination rate proportional to concentration (first-order process).
(3) The half-life of a drug = 0.7 times the apparent volume of distribution divided by the clearance.
(4) Continuous or intermittently repeated drug administration results in accumulation until a steady state is reached.
(5) At steady state, rate of drug input = rate of drug output. Rate of drug input is bioavailable dose per unit time and rate of drug output is clearance times steady-state concentration.
(6) The handling of a lipid-soluble drug given intravenously is better described by a model incorporating a peripheral and a central compartment.
(7) For some drugs metabolism is saturated at the prevailing concentration so the concentration decays at a constant rate (zero-order process).
(8) The therapeutic index is the ratio of the drug dose rate that is just toxic to the drug dose rate that just produces the desired response.
(9) The therapeutic window is bounded by the plasma concentrations that define the maximal acceptable toxic and minimal useful effects.
(10) A dosage regimen of a drug is dictated by its therapeutic index, desired urgency of onset of effect and elimination half-life.

Physicochemical groupings of drugs

It is the physicochemical properties, rather than the pharmacological actions of drugs, that determine how they are handled in the body. Five characteristic patterns of drug disposition are described, corresponding with five physicochemical groups (Table 7.10 and Figure 7.25).

There are two major properties of a drug that determine how it is handled by the body.

The degree of ionization of the drug molecules in solution

This is dependent on the pK_a of the drug and the pH of the fluid in which the drug is dissolved (see p. 330).

The lipid solubility of the unionized drug molecules

This is often measured as the lipid/water partition coefficient (see p. 330).

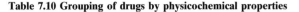

Table 7.10 Grouping of drugs by physicochemical properties

Groups	Examples
(1) Water-soluble drugs	**Gentamicin**
(2) Intermediate drugs	**Digoxin**
(3) Lipid-soluble drugs	**Thiopentone, phenytoin,** inhalational anaesthetic agents
(4) Acidic drugs (pK_a 2–7.4)	Salicylic acid
(5) Basic drugs (pK_a 6–12)	**Lignocaine**

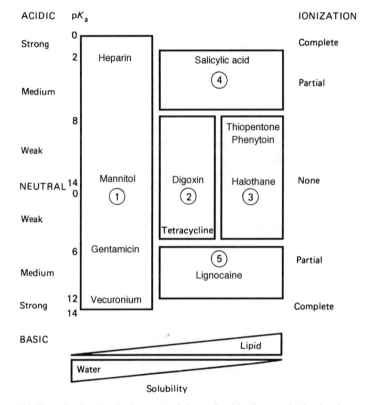

Figure 7.25 Five physicochemical groups of drugs. In this diagram ionization increases when moving up (acidic) or down (basic) from the middle. The lipid solubility of the unionized molecule increases when moving from left to right

Water-soluble drugs

Examples

(1) Highly ionized (strong) acids (pK_a less than 2) that are almost 100% ionized in all biological fluids. Drug conjugates – sulphates, glucuronides, glycine conjugates; *sodium cromoglycate.*

(2) Drugs with multiple polar groups. Polyhydric alcohols – *mannitol*, sorbitol; mucopolysaccharides – **heparin**; aminoglycoside antibiotic agents – **gentamicin**, *neomycin*; glycopeptide antibiotics – **vancomycin**.
(3) Highly ionized (strong) bases (pK_a more than 12) that are almost 100% ionized in all biological fluids. Quaternary amines ($R_4N^+OH^-$) – **tubocurarine, neostigmine, suxamethonium**.

Characteristic features

All water-soluble drugs are handled by the body in a similar way, that is:

(1) Absorption from the gastrointestinal tract is negligible and injection is usually necessary for systemic effects.
(2) Distribution is restricted to the ECF.
(3) The drugs poorly penetrate the CSF or brain.
(4) Binding to plasma proteins is not important, except for some strong acids.
(5) Elimination is mainly by excretion of the unchanged drug in the urine. The drug usually enters the urine by ultrafiltration but many anions and cations are also actively secreted into the urine and the bile. Non-renal excretion is relatively unimportant for these drugs unless they have a large MW (greater than 400 Da), when hepatic excretion becomes important.

The disposition of the aminoglycoside antibiotic **gentamicin** is representative of the group.

Gentamicin

This is a widely used antibiotic agent that is effective against Gram-negative bacteria, including *E. coli* and *Klebsiella pneumoniae*. It is important to understand how it is handled in the body because it has toxic effects on the inner ear (vestibular and auditory function) and on the kidney. The amount of drug required to produce damage is only a little greater than the amount required to treat infection (that is the drug has a small therapeutic index).

Chemistry

Gentamicin is a variable mixture of three very similar components giving an average MW of approximately 480 Da (Figure 7.26). Each component consists of two substituted aminosugar molecules linked through an aminocyclitol. There are several polar groups on the molecules (chiefly –OH), which make them much more soluble in water than in lipid or organic solvents.

Absorption

The drug is not absorbed from the gut and must be given by injection if a systemic effect is required. As with other drugs, the rate of absorption from the site of injection is proportional to the local blood flow.

Gentamicin

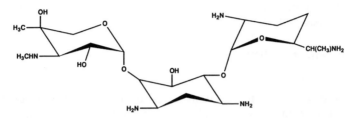

Figure 7.26 Structure of one of the aminoglycoside components of **gentamicin** to illustrate the numbers of ionizable groups

Distribution

The water-soluble antibiotic molecules cannot generally penetrate into mammalian cells. Therefore, like inulin, they are restricted to the ECF. The distribution volume (V) is approximately 15 L in an adult (Figure 7.3). Penetration across lipid membranes into brain, CSF, inner ear fluid, fetal circulation and sputum is slow.

Elimination

Excretion by the kidney is the major route and the clearance (CL) closely approximates to the GFR or creatinine clearance (CL_{cr}). Since gentamicin does not generally penetrate cells, there is little opportunity for contact with intracellular enzymes and consequent metabolism. Again the resemblance to inulin is strong. An exception to this generalization occurs in the renal tubular cells, some of which take up aminoglycoside antibiotic agents. This contributes to the nephrotoxicity of these drugs.

Persistence and accumulation

When kidney function is normal the handling resembles Figure 7.15a and the average $t_{1/2}$ is approximately 2 h. Thus 8 h after a dose more than 90% (50 + 25 + 12.5 + 6.25) of that dose has been eliminated; the dose can therefore be repeated without accumulation.

Renal impairment produces a very different state however. A reduction in CL causes a proportionate prolongation of $t_{1/2}$. It is then essential to scale down dosage in order to avoid accumulation and toxicity.

Plasma concentration and patient response

Concentration (C) of **gentamicin** 1 h after dosage usually needs to exceed 5 mg/L for a therapeutic effect in septicaemia, but can be as large as 12 mg/L without causing toxicity.

Trough concentrations (just before the next dosage) are more relevant to toxicity. With less than 2 mg/L there is little risk, but with more than 4 mg/L the risk is large. If the trough concentration is large the tiny but slowly penetrated compartment of the inner ear fluid gradually fills up with the drug.

A mean concentration ($C_{ss,av}$) of 3–4 mg/L represents a compromise avoiding inadequate peaks and excessive troughs.

Dosage requirements

In renal disease

The daily dosage rate to maintain a desired $C_{ss,av}$ is a linear function of CL_{cr}. It varies from approximately 20 mg/day (40 mg every 48 h) in anuric patients (which allows estimation of non-renal clearance) to 480 mg/day (160 mg every 8 h) in patients with normal kidney function. Thus the daily dosage rate required to produce a given $C_{ss,av}$ varies over a 24-fold range.

In children

CL_{cr} and **gentamicin** dosage requirements both regress with weight (or surface area) largely irrespective of age. The newborn is a special case, however, having immature kidneys and a CL_{cr} approximately one-third of the value appropriate to its size. Since ECF volume is relatively large in the newborn, the combined effect is a longer $t_{1/2}$ (Equation 7.8, p. 361). The principle that daily dosage rate for a given $C_{ss,av}$ parallels CL_{cr} is generally valid for drugs that are not lipid soluble (rearrangement of Equation 7.9, p. 363, demonstrates that dose rate per unit concentration has the same dimensions as clearance).

Individualization of the dosage regimen

(1) Estimate the parameters of the pharmacokinetic model (Figure 7.27, V and CL) from patient features (body mass, CL_{cr}) and known relationships between these variables for the population.
(2) Determine the dose that should produce a peak concentration in the range 5–12 mg/L and the dosage interval that should produce a trough concentration not greater than 2 mg/L.

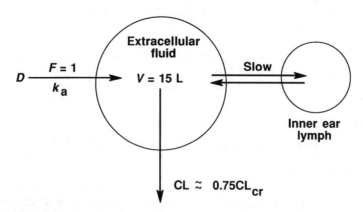

Figure 7.27 One-compartment open dispositional model for **gentamicin** in a 70-kg man

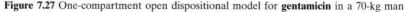

(3) Start treatment, sample plasma 1 h after a dose and assay for gentamicin concentration.
(4) Deviation from target peak (1 h) concentration represents deviation of the V of this individual from the population mean assumed. Adjust dose.
(5) Sample plasma immediately before a dose and assay for gentamicin concentration.
(6) Deviation from target trough concentration represents deviation of the CL of this individual from the population mean assumed. Adjust interval.

Aids to this process include calculation, tables, nomograms and computer programs.

Summary

(1) Water-soluble drugs either possess multiple polar groups or are strong acids or bases.
(2) The disposition of **gentamicin** is typical of the group. It is not absorbed orally and must be given by injection. Its distribution is restricted to the ECF. It is eliminated by renal excretion.
(3) Dosage of **gentamicin** must be reduced in renal failure and in children.

Drugs with intermediate solubility

Not all drugs have extreme physical properties. Many are intermediate between the highly water-soluble aminoglycoside antibiotic agents and the highly lipid-soluble i/v anaesthetic agents. **Tetracycline** is included but **digoxin** has been selected as an important example.

Characteristic features

(1) Absorption from the gut is adequate for clinical use but is often not complete.
(2) Distribution is not restricted to the ECF; the drug penetrates through cell membranes and into the intracellular water.
(3) Protein binding has an influence on the distribution and elimination of the drug.
(4) Elimination is predominantly by excretion of the unchanged drug in the urine; however, a proportion of the drug undergoes metabolism.

Digoxin

This drug has the useful effect of slowing ventricular rate in patients with atrial fibrillation and increasing the force of contraction in heart failure

STAFFS UNIVERSITY LIBRARY

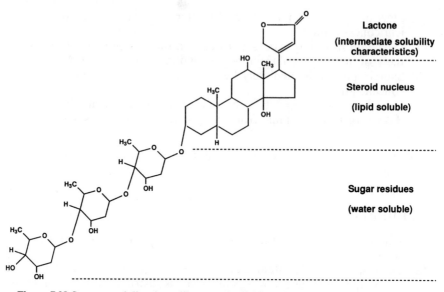

Lactone
(intermediate solubility
characteristics)

Steroid nucleus

(lipid soluble)

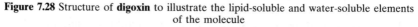

Sugar residues

(water soluble)

Figure 7.28 Structure of **digoxin** to illustrate the lipid-soluble and water-soluble elements of the molecule

(see p. 122). However, the toxic dose (heart block, ectopic ventricular activity) is very close to the therapeutic dose, so there is little safety margin.

Chemistry

The relatively lipid-soluble steroid nucleus carrying two OH groups is linked to a highly water-soluble trisaccharide (three digitoxose units) by a glycosidic bond (Figure 7.28). This structure probably favours accumulation at cell surfaces where the drug inhibits the Na^+/K^+-ATPase pump. The glycoside (MW 781 Da) dissolves more readily in ethanol than in water or other organic solvents.

Absorption

Digoxin is administered by mouth in tablet form. The dissolution standard that tablets are expected to meet is 75% in solution within 1 h. It is absorbed quickly but not completely. The fraction (F) absorbed or bioavailability is approximately 0.6 (mean) and rather variable (0.4–1.0). Reduction of particle size in the formulation increases the rate of dissolution and improves bioavailability. A solution for i/m or i/v injection is available for a more rapid response but at the cost of increased liability of acute toxicity.

Distribution

Digoxin is distributed throughout body water. It is bound to protein in plasma (f_b = approximately 0.3) and in tissues. When distribution is

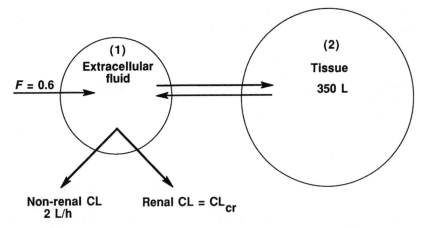

Figure 7.29 Two-compartment dispositional model for **digoxin** in a 70-kg man

complete most of the dose is located in skeletal muscle. **Digoxin** does not enter fat. V is much greater than body weight (approximately 5 L/kg) because of the large binding capacity of skeletal muscle. The distribution is best described by a two-compartment model (Figure 7.29, and example B, p. 369). The decay of plasma concentration with time is biphasic. The first phase is mainly associated with distribution to tissues and the second phase is a result of elimination.

Elimination

The total CL is greater than for the aminoglycosides but the $t_{1/2}$ is much longer (1–2 days) because of the large V.

Excretion

The renal CL is approximately equal to CL_{cr}: both glomerular filtration and tubular secretion contribute. Seventy per cent of the drug is excreted unchanged in the urine.

Metabolism

The non-renal CL is approximately one-half of the renal CL in normal subjects. Sugar molecules are split off and the steroid nucleus is further hydroxylated in the liver.

Persistence and accumulation

Approximately one-third of the dose is excreted per day. **Digoxin** therefore accumulates until the total amount of drug in the body is approximately three times the single daily dose. This process is 90% complete in approximately 1 week ($3-4 \times t_{1/2}$). Once the steady state has been attained the total amount of **digoxin** in the body fluctuates relatively little during the dosage interval (contrast **gentamicin**).

Plasma concentration and patient response

Absorption is more rapid than distribution so the magnitude of the peak plasma concentration and the time to peak is largely influenced by the rate of absorption. The brief large peak may be associated with nausea via an action on the CTZ but not with cardiac toxicity. The cardiac response parallels the hypothetical concentration in a deeper tissue compartment. $C_{ss,av}$ is probably the most relevant concentration, which is approximated by C at 6 h.

A concentration of 1–2 µg/L is usually adequate to control the ventricular rate in atrial fibrillation. However a concentration of more than 2 µg/L is associated with an increased frequency of ventricular ectopic beats. The therapeutic index approaches unity.

Dosage requirements in disease

The rapid attainment of a large therapeutic concentration (2 µg/L) would require i/v injection of $2 \times V$ µg or 10 µg/kg. V is approximately halved however in the elderly and in those with severe renal impairment. Both these states are associated with a relatively small skeletal muscle mass. Gradual accumulation is usually preferred.

Daily dosage requirement for a $C_{ss,av}$ of 1–2 µg/L in the adult varies from 62.5 µg (one paediatric/geriatric tablet) in the anuric to 500 µg in the patient with normal kidney function. Dosage requirement approximately parallels CL_{cr}.

Individualization of the dosage regimen

Assay of the plasma concentration of **digoxin** is less useful in dosage individualization (Figure 7.29 summarizes the pharmacokinetic model) than that of **gentamicin** (see p. 380).

When **digoxin** is compared with **gentamicin**, dosage individualization is:

(1) More necessary because of the long $t_{1/2}$ and the large incidence of potentially lethal cardiac toxicity.
(2) More difficult because there are more sources of variance – bioavailability, V, compliance, non-renal CL and serum albumin binding.

Dosing summary

Decide whether a loading dose is required. Its size is determined from the lean body weight of the patient. Administer it orally or slowly i/v.

Determine what maintenance dose is required, from the estimated GFR of the patient. Administer it once, or in two divided doses, daily.

Observe the patient for the slowly developing therapeutic and adverse effects and use these to guide adjustment of the maintenance dose. This is relatively easy in atrial fibrillation, because it is easy to determine whether an appropriate effect (reduction of ventricular rate, loss of pulse deficit) is being produced. It is much harder in congestive heart failure.

Assay of the plasma concentration of **digoxin** is most useful in distinguishing between cardiac disease and **digoxin** toxicity as the source of a patient's cardiac signs and symptoms.

Summary

(1) **Digoxin** is typical of a drug with intermediate solubility. It is partially absorbed from the gut. Its distribution volume is large. Its elimination is by renal and hepatic mechanisms.
(2) **Digoxin** has a long half-life due to a very large distribution volume, consequent on extensive binding in skeletal muscle.

Lipid-soluble drugs

Examples

This group of drugs is large and includes many drugs that act on the CNS. They have in common a high lipid (or organic solvent)/water partition coefficient. The group includes:

(1) Weakly acidic drugs (pK_a greater than 8) – **phenytoin** and other anticonvulsant agents.
(2) Virtually neutral drugs – **thiopentone** and other i/v anaesthetic agents, many sedative and inhalational anaesthetic agents, **glyceryl trinitrate**, steroids (**ethinyloestradiol**, **norethisterone**, *dexamethasone*).

Characteristic features

(1) Absorption from the gut is usually rapid and complete unless chemical inactivation occurs.
(2) Initial distribution of the drug is very rapid. Characteristically the drugs enter tissues, including brain, at a rate that is limited by the flow of blood, not by the rate of diffusion through the cell membranes.
(3) A large proportion of the drug is bound to plasma proteins and to intracellular proteins and lipids. The concentration of drug molecules free in the body water may be very small indeed.
(4) The concentration of drug in the glomerular filtrate is also very small and the drug molecules are so lipid soluble that they are re-absorbed from the renal tubule as quickly as the filtered water. Thus the unchanged drug is not effectively excreted in the urine.
(5) Some of the drugs in this group, that have a high vapour pressure, are excreted unchanged in the expired air

STAFFS UNIVERSITY LIBRARY

(6) Drugs of this group are oxidized in the liver, and to a lesser extent in other tissues, to more polar metabolites, which may be alcohols or phenols (phase I, see p. 353).
(7) Water-soluble metabolites resemble **gentamicin** in their elimination. Many are conjugated with sulphate, glycine or glucuronic acid prior to excretion (phase II, see p. 354).

Thiopentone

This very short acting barbiturate is administered i/v for the production of complete general anaesthesia of short duration or for the induction of sustained anaesthesia.

Chemistry

Thiopentone (MW 242 Da) is a highly lipid-soluble compound due to the presence of barbituric acid and an alkyl chain (see Figure 5.13). Although it has a pK_a of 7.6 and is therefore a very weak acid (it is used as the sodium salt), its predominant physicochemical property is its lipid solubility.

Distribution

Thiopentone is approximately 70% bound to serum albumin by 'hydrophobic bonds'. The binding of barbiturates increases with lipid solubility (Table 7.11).

A single i/v dose of **thiopentone** can produce almost instantaneous anaesthesia that only lasts for approximately 5 min. Large doses cause respiratory arrest.

An intermediate-acting barbiturate has a similar potency to **thiopentone** (approximately the same concentration in the brain is needed to produce anaesthesia). However, no dose of it can mimic the very short duration of action seen with **thiopentone**. This short duration of action is not due to rapid metabolism but to rapid distribution into skeletal muscle. Only after several hours is a substantial fraction of a single dose located in fatty tissue. Consciousness returns whilst a large proportion of the original dose is still in the body. Repeated doses are cumulative.

Two-compartment dispositional model

The bi-exponential decay in plasma **thiopentone** suggests that its pharmacokinetic properties should be considered in terms of a two-

Table 7.11 Protein binding of barbiturates to serum albumin is related to lipid solubility

	CH_2Cl_2/water partition coefficient	Proportion bound
Thiopentone	580	0.75
An intermediate-acting barbiturate	39	0.35
Phenobarbitone	3	0.20

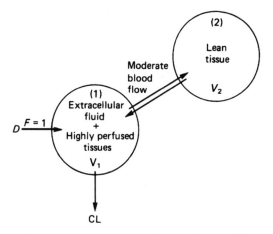

Figure 7.30 Two-compartment dispositional model for **thiopentone**

compartment (or more complex) model (Figure 7.30). Entry into various tissues (brain and liver) is so rapid that it appears to be limited solely by the rate of blood flow. Multicompartment 'physiological models' have been devised for **thiopentone**, which employ known blood flow rates to principal anatomical regions. One relatively simple model of this kind comprises:

(1) A highly perfused central compartment or vessel-rich group of organs including brain, liver, myocardium, adrenal glands, kidneys and receiving approximately 4 L/min.
(2) A lean tissue compartment (mainly skeletal muscle) and receiving approximately 1 L/min at rest. Adipose tissue is quantitatively less important, receiving approximately 0.3 L/min.

Metabolism

Thiopentone is cleared exclusively by metabolism from the central vessel-rich compartment; here the clearance concept is applicable in the same way as it is to the renal excretion of **gentamicin** or **digoxin**. Less than 1% is excreted unchanged in the urine over 48 h.

Some short-acting **thiopentone** is metabolized to the intermediate-acting pentobarbitone (that is the S is replaced by O). Both **thiopentone** and its pentobarbitone product are further metabolized by the addition of an OH group to the longer hydrocarbon side-chain. The MFO system is responsible for this metabolism (see p. 353).

Phenytoin

This anticonvulsant is widely used in epilepsy at a daily dose of 200–500 mg. It lacks the pronounced hypnotic action seen with barbiturates.

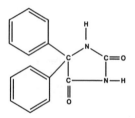

Phenytoin

Figure 7.31 Structure of **phenytoin** to illustrate features of the molecule responsible for its lipid solubility (benzene rings, lack of polar groups)

Chemistry

Phenytoin is mainly used as the sodium salt – MW (acid) = 252 Da; pK_a = 8.3. It is poorly soluble in aqueous solutions (14 mg/L) at pH less than 7 (Figure 7.31).

Distribution

The larger solubility in serum (75 mg/L) is due mainly to extensive protein binding, approximately 90% being bound to serum proteins *in vivo*. Concentrations in saliva and CSF are approximately 10% of the serum concentration.

Metabolism

Phenytoin is extensively metabolized by the MFO in the liver, less than 5% appearing in the urine as unchanged drug. The glucuronide conjugate of the para-hydroxylated product is the main metabolite in urine – **phenytoin** exhibits both phase I and phase II metabolism.

Non-linear kinetics

Generally, a **phenytoin** serum $C_{ss,av}$ less than 10 mg/L is only partially effective, whereas a $C_{ss,av}$ more than 30 mg/L is associated with toxic symptoms (ataxia, dysarthria, nystagmus). Monitoring of $C_{ss,av}$ is desirable, since the relationship between $C_{ss,av}$ and daily dose is non-linear. There is a disproportionate increase in $C_{ss,av}$ with increase in dose rate as a consequence of the distinctive dose-dependent pharmacokinetics of this drug. There is an apparent increase in $t_{1/2}$ with dose or C because the pharmacokinetics are not first order. The elimination of **phenytoin** from the body is best described in terms of Michaelis–Menten/enzyme/non-linear kinetics (see p. 370) – ethanol and salicylic acid are eliminated similarly.

The C/t curve (Figure 7.22) appears to be biphasic, approximating to zero order at large C (more than 30 mg/L of **phenytoin**), and becoming first order (exponential) at small C (less than 10 mg/L).

Table 7.12 Increments in dose rate producing equal increments in $C_{ss,av}$ vary inversely with $C_{ss,av}$

$C_{ss,av}$ (mg/L)	Increment in dose rate (mg/day)
<5	100
5–10	50
>10	25

Clinical applications

A progressive but slow (increment every 2–4 weeks) increase in dose rate is appropriate until control of seizures is obtained or further increase is prevented by toxicity. Non-linear kinetics demands diminishing increments (Table 7.12). Reductions in dosage necessitated by mild intoxication require similar adjustments.

Individual differences in D_M/T for any desired $C_{ss,av}$ are not accurately predictable. Surface area is the best guide but this only accounts for a part of the variation. Daily dose/surface area (mg/day per m^2) is greater in children than adults.

Renal functional impairment reduces the clearance of metabolites of **phenytoin** but does not reduce the rate of metabolism of unchanged drug. Protein binding is reduced in severe kidney disease and as a result the drug is metabolized more rapidly.

Ethanol

Chemistry

In a dispositional sense ethanol (ethyl alcohol, CH_3CH_2OH) belongs to group 3 (Table 7.10) but it is not a highly lipid-soluble drug. Ethanol is highly water soluble, but its small MW (46 Da) enables it to pass readily through the water-filled pores of cell membranes and behave as if it were a lipid-soluble drug.

Absorption

Ethanol is rapidly and completely absorbed through the mucosae of stomach and jejunum.

Distribution

Distribution is rapid throughout all aqueous regions of the body. The distribution volume is the total body water. Ethanol equilibrates rapidly across the blood/brain barrier.

Plasma concentration and effect

Progressive increments of plasma concentration (C) produce progressive general CNS depression varying from mild sedation to general anaesthesia and fatal respiratory depression. The effect of ethanol on the brain depends not only on C (Table 5.2) but also on the direction in which C is changing. The effect of a given C is greater when C is increasing and less when it is steady or decreasing. The same is true for other CNS-depressant drugs. This form of clockwise hysteresis (see p. 375) is due to acute tolerance.

Elimination

Metabolism

Hepatic parenchymal cells oxidize ethanol to acetaldehyde and then to acetate (by aldehyde dehydrogenase). The main enzyme responsible for the first stage is the cytoplasmic alcohol dehydrogenase, although a microsomal ethanol-oxidizing system is a minor contributor. Above a certain plasma concentration ($K_m \approx 100 \ \mu g/mL$), elimination of ethanol approximates to zero order, that is, is independent of C (see p. 370). In most people, this saturating concentration is reached after drinking a single unit of alcohol. The average maximum rate (V_{max}) equals 8 g/h or 10 mL/h, that is, 200 mL beer or 20 mL whisky/h. As elimination is constant irrespective of concentration, the time it takes for the concentration to decrease to one-half is not constant, so a meaningful $t_{1/2}$ cannot be calculated.

Excretion

Ethanol is re-absorbed from the renal tubule so that the urine concentration is only slightly greater than the concentration in the blood. Thus renal plasma clearance approximately equals the rate of urine flow (1–2 mL/min). After small or moderate doses, less than 10% of the dose is eliminated in the urine. Excretion in expired air occurs but represents less than 1% of the dose.

Inhalational anaesthetic agents

Inhalational anaesthetic agents are gases or volatile liquids that have a large solubility in lipid at normal atmospheric pressure (see p. 4). The differences in physicochemical properties between individual anaesthetic agents influence the rate of onset of and recovery from anaesthesia and the partial pressures necessary to induce anaesthesia.

Partial pressure

In general the response to a drug is a function of the concentration in the biophase (fluid in intimate contact with receptors). In the case of inhalational anaesthetic agents, it is more convenient to express concentration in terms of partial pressure than mass of gas per unit volume of liquid. This is because diffusion of a gas between phases occurs down a gradient of partial pressure, at a speed proportional to the gradient, until differences in partial pressure are eliminated.

Partial pressure is defined as the individual pressure exerted by a gas in a mixture of gases. In the gas phase the partial pressure of the anaesthetic agent can also be expressed as a proportion of the total pressure (normally 1 atmosphere).

Solubility in blood and tissues

Some anaesthetic agents have a greater affinity for blood than for the gas phase. This affinity is expressed as their solubility in blood.

Henry's law states that:

Mass of gas dissolved by unit volume of liquid =
solubility × partial pressure of the gas at constant temperature

Consequently the amount of anaesthetic agent that must be dissolved (and therefore the time it takes) to achieve a particular partial pressure in the blood is proportional to solubility, for example, a large mass for diethyl ether (and therefore slow induction and recovery), a small mass for **nitrous oxide** (and therefore rapid induction and recovery) (Figure 7.32). Contrast the soluble diethyl ether (solubility = 12) with the insoluble **nitrous oxide** (solubility = 0.5) (Table 7.13).

The partition coefficient (ratio of solubilities) for the inhalational anaesthetic agents between most tissues (including the brain) and blood is near unity. However, the partition coefficient between adipose tissue and blood may be much greater than unity (**halothane** = 60 : 1).

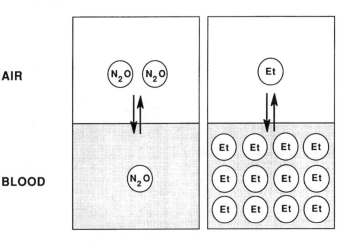

λ (Blood/gas)   0.5   12.0

Figure 7.32 The influence of blood/gas solubility on the partition of inhalational anaesthetic agent between air and blood at equilibrium (Et = diethyl ether; λ = partition coefficient)

STAFFS UNIVERSITY LIBRARY

Table 7.13 Blood solubilities and potencies of general anaesthetic agents

Anaesthetic agent	Solubility (blood/gas)	MAC (% v/v)
Diethyl ether	12	2
Halothane	2.3	0.8
Enflurane	1.9	1.7
Isoflurane	1.4	1.4
Nitrous oxide	0.5	>80

Kinetic models

Since these agents are highly lipid soluble, the pharmacokinetics must be modelled by several compartments (Figure 7.33) as described for **thiopentone**. As in that case, distribution is perfusion rather than diffusion limited:

(0) External air containing gas at a certain concentration.
(1) Central, rapidly equilibrating compartment consisting of functional residual lung capacity (less dead space) plus blood plus highly perfused tissues including the brain.
(2) Lean tissue compartment (mainly skeletal muscle).
(3) Adipose tissue compartment.

Transfer of anaesthetic agent into the lean tissue compartment is initially more significant than into the adipose tissue compartment because of the much greater blood flow in the former.

An anaesthetic agent can be considered to be distributed through an apparent volume of distribution (described for solid and liquid drugs with a low vapour pressure on p. 344) known as the <u>gas equivalent volume.</u>

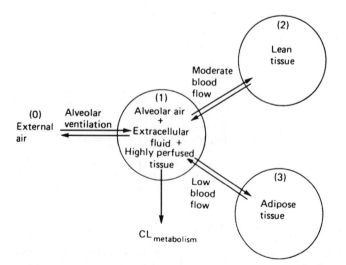

Figure 7.33 Three-compartment dispositional model for gaseous general anaesthetic agents

This volume is the sum of the compartment volumes multiplied by their respective partition coefficients.

Potency

An anaesthetic agent is potent if it produces a given depth of anaesthesia at a low partial pressure in the inspired air. This is expressed as minimal alveolar concentration (MAC) for anaesthesia, which is the proportion (percentage v/v) of anaesthetic agent in the inspired air that, at equilibrium, prevents the reflex response to skin incision in 50% of subjects. **Halothane** (MAC = 0.8) is potent, whilst **nitrous oxide** (MAC more than 80) is of small potency (Table 7.13). The potency of inhalational anaesthetic agents is positively correlated with lipid solubility (see p. 4).

Induction of anaesthesia

The time to induction of anaesthesia is dependent upon the rate of increase of partial pressure of the anaesthetic agent in the brain. This time is reduced when:

(1) Inspired partial pressure is high – consequently the concentration of anaesthetic agent should be larger than the MAC during induction of anaesthesia, with subsequent reduction once anaesthesia has been induced. This is equivalent to using a loading dose before a maintenance dose with solid or liquid drugs.
(2) Alveolar ventilation is large – this increases transfer of anaesthetic agent from external air to alveoli.
(3) Body weight is small – gas equivalent volume is reduced.
(4) Anaesthetic agent is of small solubility – time taken for equilibrium to be reached is directly proportional to solubility – diethyl ether has a large solubility and induction is slow while **nitrous oxide** has a small solubility and induction is fast (Figure 7.34).

Maintenance of anaesthesia

A near steady state may be reached in which the partial pressure in the brain approaches that in the blood and inspired air. However, there will still be a net transfer of anaesthetic agent to lean and adipose tissues, as it takes a considerable time to bring these tissues to distribution equilibrium due to their poor perfusion with blood. The mass of anaesthetic agent dissolved in these sites of loss is proportional to the duration of anaesthesia.

Recovery

The time from cessation of administration of a general anaesthetic agent to recovery is dependent on the rate of decrease of partial pressure in the central compartment. This time is short when the inspired partial pressure is zero and alveolar ventilation is large, body weight is small, the anaesthetic agent is poorly soluble and the duration of exposure was short. Unequilibrated muscles represent a sink unless blood flow is impaired by

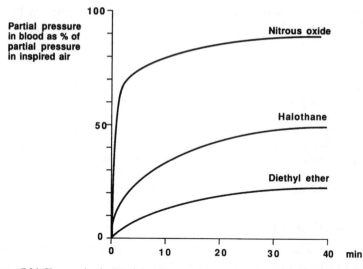

Figure 7.34 Changes in the partial pressures of three general anaesthetic agents in blood with time at a constant inspired partial pressure

shock. The converse applies – anaesthetic agent washing out of muscles (and adipose tissue) after long exposure delays recovery. There is some elimination of **halothane** by metabolism.

Summary

(1) Lipid-soluble drugs are well absorbed from the gut, distributed widely and eliminated by metabolism.
(2) The decay of plasma concentrations of **thiopentone**, after i/v injection, is due to distribution to a peripheral compartment, and this process terminates its effect.
(3) Ethanol has a small MW and behaves as if it was lipid soluble.
(4) **Phenytoin** and ethanol exhibit saturation kinetics.
(5) Inhalational anaesthetics are gases or volatile liquids and are lipid soluble.
(6) The time to induction of anaesthesia is reduced when inspired partial pressure is high, ventilation is large, body weight is small and blood/gas solubility is small.
(7) Potency is correlated with lipid solubility.

Acidic drugs

Acidic drugs (pK_a 2–7.4) with widely diverse pharmacological actions have similar modes of absorption, distribution and elimination.

Examples

(1) NSAIDs: **aspirin**, *naproxen*.
(2) Oral anticoagulant agents: **warfarin**.
(3) Penicillin antibiotic agents: **benzylpenicillin, ampicillin**.
(4) Sulphonamide antibacterial drugs: sulphamethoxazole.
(5) Oral hypoglycaemic drugs: **tolbutamide**.
(6) Diuretic agents: **bendrofluazide**.
(7) *Phenobarbitone* is the only common barbiturate with a pK_a significantly less than 8.
(8) Uricosuric agents: *probenecid, sulphinpyrazone*.

All these drugs are donors of H^+; they can be arranged in order, the strongest (low pK_a) at the top, the weakest (high pK_a) at the bottom (Table 7.14).

Characteristic features

(1) Many acidic drugs are present mainly as the uncharged acid (HA) at pH 3. The undissociated acid (HA) is more lipid soluble than the dissociated or ionized form (A^-, anion); thus, conditions in the stomach are favourable to absorption but surface area is small.
(2) In the plasma acidic drugs are present to a large extent as the charged anions (A^-). The anions of different acidic drugs compete for a common binding site on plasma albumin and for active secretion into bile and urine.
(3) The plasma clearance (CL) varies inversely with the extent of re-absorption from the renal tubule. If the urine pH is high, the drug in the urine is present mainly as the anion (A^-), re-absorption by non-ionic diffusion is discouraged and CL is large. Increase in CL causes a corresponding reduction in $t_{1/2}$.

Table 7.14 Ionization of acids

		Concentration ratio $[A^-]:[HA]$*			
Drug	pK_a	*Stomach* *pH 3.0*	*Urine* *(acid)* *pH 5.0*	*Plasma* *pH 7.4*	*Urine* *(alk)* *pH 8.0*
Benzylpenicillin	2.8				
Salicylic acid	3.0	$1:1$	$10^2:1$	$2.5\times10^4:1$	$10^5:1$
Aspirin	3.6				
	4.0	$0.1:1$	$10:1$	$2.5\times10^3:1$	$10^4:1$
Warfarin	5.0	$10^{-2}:1$	$1:1$	$2.5\times10^2:1$	$10^3:1$
Sulphamethoxazole	5.6				
	6.0	$10^{-3}:1$	$0.1:1$	$25:1$	$10^2:1$
	7.0	$10^{-4}:1$	$10^{-2}:1$	$2.5:1$	$10:1$
Phenobarbitone	7.4				

*Calculated from Equation 7.1 (see p. 330).

Note:
(1) Urine pH should be controlled when measuring excretion rates of acidic compounds.
(2) The usefulness of alkaline diuresis in acute poisoning by salicylates or phenobarbitone.

Salicylic acid

Aspirin is used for its analgesic, anti-inflammatory, anticoagulant and antipyretic properties (but see Reye's syndrome, p. 254). There are three main use situations: occasional, small dose utilizing the antipyretic and analgesic properties; chronic small dose utilizing the anticoagulant properties; chronic, large dose utilizing the analgesic and anti-inflammatory properties of **aspirin**. **Aspirin** (acetylsalicylic acid) is rapidly hydrolysed within the body ($t_{1/2}$ 15 min) to acetate and salicylic acid. Most of the pharmacological properties of **aspirin** are due to the metabolite, salicylic acid. **Aspirin** is, therefore, a prodrug although it may exert some therapeutic actions itself.

Chemistry

Aspirin is a weak acid (pK_a 3) and is soluble in water and organic solvents (see Figure 7.13).

Dosage form and absorption

Aspirin in solution is rapidly absorbed, mostly from the small intestine. Salicylates are poorly soluble at low pH. Dissolution of **aspirin** in intestinal fluids is the rate-limiting step in absorption. Simple **aspirin** tablets or dispersible formulations, with consequent rapid dissolution and absorption, are appropriate when rapid onset of effect is required (e.g. to treat a headache). For treatment of chronic diseases (e.g. joint inflammation), where rapid onset of effect is not required, enteric-coated or other slow-release preparations may be preferred as they minimize the local erosive action on gastric mucosa. Enteric-coated tablets can give erratic and incomplete absorption.

Distribution

Salicylic acid enters cells by diffusion through the lipid membranes. It is distributed throughout total body water and binds to sites on plasma albumin and tissue protein. At large salicylate doses its plasma concentration approaches that of albumin (0.6 mmole/L), and albumin binding sites become saturated with the drug. Consequently, there is a disproportionate increase in the fraction of free drug for any further increase in dose (Figure 7.4).

Plasma salicylate concentration and patient response

• Less than 100 mg/L: therapeutic – anticoagulant, analgesic and antipyretic effects. Unwanted effects include bleeding from gastric erosions (reduced platelet stickiness and hypoprothrombinaemia may contribute) and bronchospasm (an idiosyncrasy that is not due to allergy but to cyclo-oxygenase inhibition).

- 150–300 mg/L: therapeutic – anti-inflammatory effects. Adverse effects include tinnitus and deafness at maximum therapeutic concentrations.
- 300–750 mg/L: mild to moderate intoxication is manifest as hyperventilation, respiratory alkalosis, sweating, tachycardia, salt and water depletion. Toxicity increases with time. 500 mg/L at 48 h after overdose may represent severe intoxication. Treatment is by correction of salt and water depletion and by alkaline diuresis.
- More than 750 mg/L: severe intoxication is manifest as impaired utilization of pyruvate and lactate, metabolic acidosis, convulsions, circulatory arrest and renal failure. Haemodialysis may be required.

Metabolism and disposition kinetics

Hepatic metabolism is the major mechanism of elimination at small and moderate plasma concentrations (Table 7.15).

Salicylic acid displays the same non-linear elimination kinetics as **phenytoin** and ethanol. The process of conjugation to form salicyluric acid and phenolic glucuronide becomes saturated in the therapeutic dose range. The time it takes for plasma concentration to decrease to one-half therefore increases with the dose, that is $t_{1/2}$ cannot be used to describe the pharmacokinetics (Table 7.16).

Accumulation kinetics

Within the therapeutic range, increasing the dose produces a disproportionate increase in $C_{ss,av}$ and the time to reach steady state. For example, doubling the dose (1.5–3 g/day) in one experimental subject produced a four-fold increase in $C_{ss,av}$ (30–120 mg/L).

Table 7.15 Metabolic fate of aspirin

Fate	Metabolite	Urine (%)
Conjugated (Phase II) with		
Glycine	Salicyluric acid	45–55
Glucuronic acid	Phenolic glucuronide	15–25
Glucuronic acid	Acyl glucuronide	7–12
Hydroxylated (Phase I)		<3
Excreted unchanged (small dose)		5–25

Table 7.16 Saturation kinetics of salicylic acid, dependence of apparent $t_{1/2}$ on dose

Dose (g)	Apparent $t_{1/2}$ (h)
0.3	2.3
1	6
10	19
Overdose	>35 (untreated)

Renal clearance – increases with pH and urine flow

Renal excretion is a minor pathway at low concentrations but a major pathway at high concentrations (intoxication) due to saturation of metabolic elimination. CL increases approximately four-fold with each unit increase in urine pH. This explains the effective use of alkaline diuresis in salicylate intoxication.

Summary

(1) Acidic drugs can be absorbed from the stomach, mainly exist as the anion in bodily fluids, and their renal excretion is enhanced when tubular pH is high.

(2) **Aspirin** is rapidly metabolized to salicylic acid. Hepatic metabolism is the major route of elimination at low plasma concentrations but exhibits saturation. Renal excretion is important at high concentrations.

Basic drugs

Basic drugs (pK_a 6–12) with widely diverse pharmacological actions have similar modes of absorption, distribution and elimination.

Examples

(1) Opioid analgesic agents: **morphine**.
(2) Local anaesthetic agents: **lignocaine**.
(3) Antidysrhythmic drugs: **lignocaine**.
(4) Agonists at nicotinic acetylcholine receptors: nicotine.
(5) Antagonists at muscarinic acetylcholine receptors: **atropine**.
(6) Inhibitors of acetylcholinesterase: *physostigmine*.
(7) Sympathomimetic amines: **noradrenaline**.
(8) Antagonists at adrenoceptors: **phenoxybenzamine, propranolol**.
(9) Antipsychotic agents: **chlorpromazine**.
(10) Anxiolytic agents: **diazepam**.
(11) Tricyclic antidepressant drugs: **imipramine**.
(12) Antagonists at histamine receptors: **chlorpheniramine, cimetidine**.
(13) Antiparasitic drugs: **chloroquine**, *piperazine*.
(14) Smooth muscle relaxant agents: **theophylline**; blockers of L-type Ca^{2+} channels: **verapamil, nifedipine**.

All these drugs are acceptors of H^+; they can be arranged in order, the strongest (high pK_a) at the top and the weakest (low pK_a) at the bottom (Table 7.17).

Table 7.17 Ionization of bases

Drug	pK_a	Concentration ratio $[BH^+]:[B]$*			
		Stomach pH 3.0	Urine (acid) pH 5.0	Plasma pH 7.4	Urine (alk) pH 8.0
Guanethidine	11.4				
	11.0	$10^8:1$	$10^6:1$	$4\times10^3:1$	$10^3:1$
	10.0	$10^7:1$	$10^5:1$	$4\times10^2:1$	$10^2:1$
Amphetamine (amine group)	9.9				
Atropine, propranolol, imipramine	9.6				
Chlorpromazine, chlorpheniramine	9.3				
	9.0	$10^6:1$	$10^4:1$	$40:1$	$10:1$
Theophylline	8.6				
Morphine, lignocaine	8.0	$10^5:1$	$10^3:1$	$4:1$	$1:1$
Hydralazine	7.1				
	7.0	$10^4:1$	$10^2:1$	$0.4:1$	$0.1:1$
Cimetidine	6.8				

*Calculated from Equation 7.2 (see p. 330).

Characteristic features

(1) Basic drugs exist almost entirely as the non-lipid-soluble cation (BH^+) at pH 3; conditions do not favour absorption from stomach.
(2) Generally in plasma the fraction of bases bound (f_b) to protein is less than the f_b of acids; α_1-acid glycoprotein is involved rather than albumin.
(3) The concentration of total drug (cation plus base) in urine is greatly increased when the urine pH is reduced from 8 to 5 (Table 7.17).
(4) When excretion is a major factor in elimination (e.g. amphetamine), the plasma concentration $t_{1/2}$ is shortened if the urine is made acid.

Note:
(1) Urine pH should be controlled when measuring excretion rates of basic compounds.
(2) The usefulness of acid diuresis in poisoning by amphetamine.

Lignocaine

This is one of the most widely used antidysrhythmic agents in coronary care units. It has particular value in treatment of ventricular dysrhythmias after myocardial infarction (see p. 118).

Chemistry

Lignocaine is a weak base (pK_a 8) with limited solubility in water (7 mg/L) but very soluble in organic solvents (see Figure 3.1).

STAFFS UNIVERSITY LIBRARY

Absorption

Absorption is rapid ($t_{1/2}$ approximately 15 min) and complete from all sites except gut (discussed later). Absorption is more rapid from an alkaline environment and greatest from highly perfused tissues.

Distribution

Fifty per cent of **lignocaine** in the plasma is bound, not to albumin but to α_1-acid glycoprotein. Displacement is an unlikely phenomenon. The drug is so lipophilic that cell membranes are no barrier to its penetration. The rate of tissue uptake is a function of organ perfusion. This explains the rapid onset (approximately 1 min) and termination (approximately 20 min) of CNS and cardiac effects of **lignocaine** following a therapeutic bolus dose (1 mg/kg). Lipophilicity also explains the size of the 'reservoir' in muscle after prolonged administration. The volume of distribution in a 70 kg individual is approximately 120 L, as the drug lies mainly outside plasma in lung, kidney, brain, muscle and adipose tissue.

The arterial plasma decay curve of **lignocaine** after an i/v bolus dose is bi-exponential, as with **thiopentone**. The peak concentration in the rapidly equilibrating central compartment is established almost immediately. The initial exponential decay of plasma concentration with time occurs due to distribution into moderately perfused tissues (muscle). The second exponential decay phase is due to metabolism. Distribution is slow into fat (because it is so poorly perfused) and quantitatively less important.

Plasma concentration and effect

Lignocaine is generally ineffective at plasma concentrations less than 1.5 mg/L; the frequency and severity of adverse effects (convulsions) increase with plasma concentrations greater than 6 mg/L.

Metabolism and disposition kinetics

The hepatic MFO system removes one or both ethyl groups (*N*-dealkylation). Both products are biologically active. Aromatic C-hydroxylation and hydrolysis of the side-chain at the amide position also occur.

Clearance, bioavailability and $t_{1/2}$

Elimination of **lignocaine** is almost exclusively by hepatic metabolism and CL is very large (1 L/min in a 70 kg individual), approaching liver blood flow (1.5 L/min in a 70 kg individual). Large hepatic extraction (70%) explains the small bioavailability (30%) with oral dosage. Metabolites are active so the oral dose is more effective than the small bioavailability suggests. **Lignocaine** has a large hepatic extraction ratio so changes in liver perfusion affect CL. Consequently dosage requirements are diminished in diseases which depress circulatory function (cardiogenic shock, congestive heart failure) or hepatic metabolism (cirrhosis), where shunting of blood away from damaged areas can occur. **Propranolol** reduces cardiac output and hepatic blood flow and therefore reduces the CL of **lignocaine**.

Although CL is large, $t_{1/2}$ is not excessively short (1–2 h) because V is large (example C, see p. 369). There is a long delay (3–5 × $t_{1/2}$) between initiation of an infusion and attainment of the plateau concentration. Therefore, a bolus dose is given followed by an infusion to match metabolism.

Renal excretion is a minor pathway of elimination of **lignocaine** due to extensive re-absorption, so urine acidification has no significant influence on its elimination kinetics. This is in marked contrast with amphetamine, the $t_{1/2}$ of which is reduced from 16 h to 5 h by acidification of the urine from pH 7 to pH 5.

Summary

(1) Basic drugs are absorbed from the small intestine, exist at the cation in bodily fluids, and their renal excretion is enhanced when tubular pH is low.
(2) **Lignocaine** is a lipid-soluble base whose handling can be described by a two-compartment model when given by i/v injection.
(3) To attain and maintain therapeutic plasma concentrations it is given by a bolus dose followed by an infusion.

8

Clinical pharmacology

Aims

- To describe the principles in pharmacotherapeutics that are applicable to the treatment of many diseases or symptoms.
- To encourage a critical and informed approach to prescribing.
- To understand how extremes of age, or pregnancy or lactation, or kidney or liver disease in a patient should modify prescribing practice.
- To provide a framework for understanding adverse effects and interactions of drugs.
- To understand the use of the clinical trial in the process of new drug development.
- To emphasize that drug regimens employed in a treatment plan should have been validated by trial.

Introduction

Clinical pharmacology is the scientific study of the determinants of therapeutic drug efficacy. It draws together what is common to many therapeutic situations – both pharmacodynamics and pharmacokinetics.

(1) After rational drug selection (see Pharmacotherapeutics, p. 458), an effective concentration of drug must be achieved at the site of action, so the patient should take (ideas of principles of prescribing, consent, compliance) an appropriate dose, of a formulation, by a route, that leads to absorption and distribution to its site of action. Many diseases require a long continued exposure of the target of action to the effective concentration so repeated dosing is necessary – elimination determines the interdose interval.
(2) Doses of most medications are not included but you should recognize the situations in which dosage adjustment is necessary and those in which measurement of plasma concentration of drug is needed to guide dosage.
(3) If you remember the fundamental mechanism of action of a drug that underlies its therapeutic property, you may also be able to predict some of the unwanted effects.

(4) The principle tool for establishing the effectiveness of a medication is the controlled therapeutic trial. Scepticism is called for when confronted with pressure to prescribe any form of therapy that has not been validated by such means.

Principles of prescribing

(1) Drug therapy should be effective, safe and economical*.
(2) Prescribe a drug only when there is a clear indication.
(3) Exercise bias toward familiar, well-tried drugs.
(4) Prescribe dosage schedules that are clear and memorable.
(5) Define relevant measures of drug response.
(6) Adjust dose until the optimum is found, and only when this proves inadequate add a second drug.
(7) Review drug treatment regularly and withdraw what is no longer needed.
(8) Teach the patient about his/her drugs.

Prescribing in special groups – Elderly patients

Problems with drugs in the elderly

Elderly patients are more likely than younger adults to suffer from adverse drug reactions. Adverse drug effects are thought to be at least partly responsible for 5–10% of admissions to acute elderly care wards. Forty per cent of elderly patients in the community have experienced an adverse drug reaction.

Elderly patients are more likely than younger ones to suffer from multiple pathology because of the increased risk of many common diseases with advanced age (e.g. stroke, ischaemic heart disease, epilepsy, diabetes) and because chronic diseases accumulate with time. Increased occurrence of disease has two main consequences related to drug usage – more drugs are required for treatment and disease may affect the pharmacokinetic properties of or pharmacodynamic response to drugs. The polypharmacy that is common in elderly patients also occurs as a consequence of unchecked repeat prescriptions and widespread use of over-the-counter medication.

While some drugs are necessary, approximately one-half of all adverse drug effects responsible for hospital admission are due to inappropriate

---

*Expenditure on drugs in the UK was approximately £4.25 billion (1993) – 80% on NHS drugs (around 10% of the total NHS budget) and 20% on private prescriptions and over-the-counter drugs.

prescribing (drug treatment not indicated, wrong choice of drug for age group, wrong dose for age, predictable drug interactions). Many drug problems in older patients could be avoided, but this requires a knowledge of why elderly patients are different from younger adults, and good prescribing habits.

Why are the elderly different

Disease versus age

Altered response to a drug in an older patient could be due either to age itself or to one of the many diseases that occur in this age group. It can be difficult to distinguish the two effects. There is little difference between healthy elderly subjects and younger adults. The presence of disease such as renal impairment has more marked effects. Few studies have been performed in the very elderly (aged over 85 years). This age group is generally more frail, with higher disease frequency, than the 65–84 age group. Frail elderly patients seem to be particularly vulnerable to adverse drug effects, with more marked alterations in pharmacokinetics and pharmacodynamic response.

Pharmacokinetic changes with ageing

Absorption

Age has no effect on the extent of drug absorption by passive diffusion. The extent of drug absorption by active transport (e.g. *methyldopa*, **levodopa**) is reduced in older patients. The rate of gastric emptying declines with age. This results in a delay in reaching peak drug concentration but does not affect the extent of absorption for most drugs. The main clinical consequence is a slight delay in onset of effect for those drugs taken as a single dose for an acute symptom, such as an analgesic agent for headache. There is no problem with drugs taken on a regular basis once a steady state has been reached.

Pre-systemic metabolism

The general trend is for a reduction in presystemic metabolism with age with a corresponding increase in bioavailability. A 10% reduction in presystemic metabolism from 90% to 80% of a dose results in a doubling of bioavailability from 10% to 20% of the dose. For most drugs this takes place in the liver. For some (e.g. **levodopa**) it occurs in the bowel wall as well as the liver. The degree of reduction in presystemic metabolism of **levodopa** exceeds the reduction in active absorption, so that the net effect is an increase in bioavailability. The initial dose of all drugs that undergo extensive presystemic metabolism should be reduced in older patients, though because of wide interindividual variation, it is important to monitor the effect and adjust the dose to achieve the desired effect.

Distribution

Body composition changes with age, with a reduction in the proportions of body water and skeletal muscle but an increase in the proportion of fat. This affects the V of drugs, with a decrease in V for water-soluble and an increased V for lipid-soluble drugs. This is most important when a loading dose is being given (e.g. the loading dose of **digoxin** should be reduced in elderly patients).

The change in V also affects the $t_{1/2}$, with the increase in V for lipid-soluble drugs prolonging the $t_{1/2}$ (e.g. **diazepam**). The prolongation of $t_{1/2}$ may affect the dosing interval and duration of effect but does not alter the total maintenance dose.

Small changes in the concentrations of albumin (decreased; binding neutral and acidic drugs) and acute-phase reactant proteins (increased; binding basic drugs) may occur but are of little clinical significance.

Metabolism

There is a tendency for phase I drug metabolism to be reduced by approximately 20% in elderly patients, in line with the reduction in liver size. There seems to be no significant reduction in drug conjugation in most elderly patients.

For frail elderly patients and those with multiple pathology, the reduction in metabolism is greater and conjugation reactions are also affected. Drug dosage at onset of administration should be low in the dose range in most elderly patients, should be reduced further when treating frail individuals.

Renal excretion

Renal function shows a specific deterioration with age. This results in a reduction in CL of drugs excreted predominantly unchanged by the kidneys, proportional to the reduction in renal function. Relatively few drugs are affected (Table 8.1). The maintenance dose of renally excreted drugs should be reduced in proportion to the reduction in CL_{cr}. In addition, many drug metabolites are excreted in the urine. This may cause problems if the metabolites are active or if they accumulate and break down to regenerate the parent drug. Examples are: morphine-6-glucuronide, which is active and causes enhanced effects in patients with renal impairment; many of the NSAIDs are excreted as glucuronides, which accumulate in renal disease and result in increased concentrations of the parent drug.

Table 8.1 Examples of drugs mainly excreted unchanged by the kidney

atenolol, *sotalol*	**digoxin**
captopril	**gentamicin**
penicillins	**tetracycline**
acyclovir	**lithium**
vigabatrin	

Pharmacodynamic changes with ageing

The response to a given dose of drug in an elderly patient may be greater than in younger adults without a clear difference in plasma concentration. In addition, pharmacodynamic effects may occur that do not usually occur at a younger age. Suggested explanations are changes in receptor density, receptor sensitivity, transduction or effector mechanisms. Some examples of pharmacodynamic changes are considered below.

Selected examples of drugs showing changed pharmacokinetics or pharmacodynamics

From a clinical point of view it is important to realize how changes in pharmacokinetic and pharmacodynamic properties affect the response to a drug and to make compensatory changes in prescribing.

Diuretic agents

Loop diuretic agents (e.g. **frusemide**) are used mainly to treat cardiac failure. Elderly patients respond well to these if renal function is not significantly impaired. However, adverse effects such as hypokalaemia, hyponatraemia and postural hypotension are commoner than in younger patients. These changes appear to be due to pharmacodynamic mechanisms such as impaired cardiovascular homeostasis. Thiazide diuretic agents (e.g. **bendrofluazide**) in larger doses are also used to treat cardiac failure and cause similar difficulties to **frusemide**.

Smaller doses of thiazide are used to treat hypertension. The response to this is similar to that in younger adults and treatment has been shown clearly to reduce the risk of stroke and heart disease. Routine prescription of potassium supplements or potassium sparing diuretic agents is not necessary (the latter combination is more likely to cause hyponatraemia, which may be life threatening).

Antagonists at β-adrenoceptors

Because of the changed pharmacokinetic properties of these drugs, it is necessary to reduce the starting dose in elderly patients. To control hypertension or angina, antagonists at β-adrenoceptors seem to be as effective as in younger adults. A renally cleared drug selective for β_1-adrenoceptors (e.g. **atenolol**) is easier to use because unwanted effects are less and dosage requirements are easier to predict.

The disadvantage of antagonists at β-adrenoceptors is the frequent presence of contraindications to their use. Cardiac failure is much commoner in older patients. Many elderly patients have cardiomegaly without clinical evidence of cardiac failure before treatment, but prescription of an antagonist at β-adrenoceptors may precipitate cardiac failure. Other common contraindications are chronic obstructive pulmonary disease, asthma and peripheral vascular disease.

Digoxin

Problems in using **digoxin** arise partly from pharmacokinetic changes. The reduction in V means that a smaller loading dose is required than in younger adults. The maintenance dose needs to be reduced in line with any measured decline in renal function. All the typical **digoxin** adverse effects may occur as they do in younger adults. However, **digoxin** toxicity in elderly patients may present in even less specific ways, such as general deterioration in health, going 'off the legs' or confusion. **Digoxin** is a very useful drug for treating sustained atrial fibrillation and selected patients in cardiac failure with sinus rhythm. It is often misused and should particularly be avoided in the treatment of paroxysmal atrial fibrillation or slow atrial fibrillation.

Sedative agents

All sedative drugs cause problems in elderly patients that are mainly due to changed pharmacodynamic mechanisms. The most commonly used drugs are still the benzodiazepines. The biggest problem with these is their liability to lead to dependence in long-term use.

In addition, elderly patients show an increase in body sway due to impairment of neuromuscular reflexes that help keep the body upright. This leads to an increased risk of falling and of fractures (particularly neck of femur and wrist). Confusion is also a commoner problem than in younger adults. Great care is necessary when prescribing these drugs. There is now no excuse for starting long-term use of a benzodiazepine. A relatively short acting drug (e.g. **temazepam**) is usually best. Short courses should be used and compliance ensured by enlisting the help of a relative or friend where necessary.

Warfarin

The average dose of **warfarin** in elderly patients is 25% less than that in younger adults, though in both there is wide interindividual variation in dosage requirements. The increased sensitivity to **warfarin** with age is due to either an increased sensitivity of the drug target enzyme or a reduced capacity of the elderly liver to produce clotting factors.

This makes it easy to overdose, especially when starting treatment. The main adverse effect of **warfarin** is haemorrhage, which is dose related. Elderly patients have more potential bleeding sites, with increased risk of cerebral and gastrointestinal haemorrhage. There are also likely to be more contraindications to the use of **warfarin** in older patients, since conditions such as peptic ulcer, renal impairment, uncontrolled hypertension and haemorrhagic stroke are commoner in the over 65 age group. These factors are becoming increasingly important since it is now recommended that all patients over the age of 75 with atrial fibrillation should be anticoagulated as well as some aged 65–75, if they have other risk factors.

A nomogram is available that allows **warfarin** therapy to be started and adjusted to achieve over 90% of patients stabilized in 4–5 days and a small risk of overdosing. Prothrombin time (expressed as International Normalized Ratio – INR) must be measured before starting therapy and on a daily basis until stable. The dose of **warfarin** is adjusted each day according to the INR.

Antibacterial agents

Efficacy depends not only on the toxicity to microbes but also on the host's chemical and cellular responses and the immune response is impaired in elderly patients.

Care is necessary for those drugs that have a narrow therapeutic range with a risk of serious toxicity (e.g. **gentamicin**). Failure to adjust the dose in renal impairment (see p. 380) puts the patient at risk of further renal damage or deafness. This risk is critically dependent of the trough concentration so can be reduced if it is given as a single daily dose with adjustment made if the measured trough plasma concentration is too large.

Antihypertensive agents

Isolated systolic hypertension is predominantly a disease of those aged over 65, and in the more severe forms is often resistant to treatment.

Postural hypotension is more likely to occur than in younger patients, due to impaired cardiovascular reflexes. Headache and facial flushing with blockers of L-type Ca^{2+} channels seem to be less common in older patients, though leg oedema is more of a problem. Renal impairment with inhibitors of ACE is commoner in elderly patients since risk factors (peripheral vascular disease, cardiac failure) are more often present. Predictable pharmacokinetic changes with age occur with the inhibitors of ACE (mainly excreted by the kidneys) and the lipid-soluble antagonists at β-adrenoceptors and most blockers of L-type Ca^{2+} channels (extensive presystemic metabolism).

The evidence for benefit from treatment of hypertension is stronger in older patients. This arises because the elderly are more at risk of the complications of hypertension and thus smaller scale studies are able to establish benefit. Thiazide diuretic agents reduce the risk of stroke by approximately one-third and of cardiac events by approximately one-fifth. Antagonists at β-adrenoceptors are less effective for the same reduction in BP. There is no evidence yet whether new drugs (inhibitors of ACE, blockers of L-type Ca^{2+} channels) have any advantage. The treatment of choice in older patients should thus be a small dose of **bendrofluazide**, since it is effective, safe and economical.

Analgesic agents

Frail elderly patients metabolize **paracetamol** more slowly but there is a sufficiently wide safety margin to avoid difficulties.

The commonest difficulties are due to inappropriate prescribing – particularly of small dose opioid combinations and NSAIDs. Opioids (e.g. *codeine, dextropropoxyphene*) are often prescribed in combination with **paracetamol**. Most combinations do not contain an adequate analgesic dose of the opioid and are not better than **paracetamol** alone. Unfortunately, the dose that causes constipation and confusion is smaller than the analgesic dose and these unwanted effects are common in older patients. NSAIDs are frequently used when a simple analgesic would be better (most patients with osteoarthritis), thus putting patients at unnecessary risk of peptic ulceration, gastrointestinal haemorrhage and renal impairment. In addition, many NSAIDs are excreted as glucuronides (see p. 405).

Improving prescribing in the elderly

More effective treatment with reduced risk of adverse effects is an achievable goal. It requires some knowledge of pharmacokinetic and pharmacodynamic properties, evidence of potential benefit from treatment and a lot of common sense (sadly lacking in many cases when prescribing is audited).

Summary

Ten simple rules to improve prescribing in older patients are:

 (1) Know the drug – therefore become familiar with a small number of drugs you use on a regular basis.
 (2) Avoid reflex prescribing.
 (3) Check the correctness of the diagnosis.
 (4) Consider the risk/benefit ratio.
 (5) Use the smallest effective dose.
 (6) Keep the drug regimen simple.
 (7) Wonder whether any other drugs can be stopped.
 (8) Review all medication frequently.
 (9) Remember self-medication and drug hoarding.
 (10) Talk to the patients/carers about their drugs and involve the pharmacist in patient education.

Prescribing in other special groups

Renal disease

Pharmacokinetic problems

Some drugs excreted predominantly unchanged by the kidney are listed in Table 8.1. Whether or not the dose needs to be altered depends on the degree of renal impairment and the therapeutic index of the drug.

Benzylpenicillin has a wide margin of safety and doses only need to be reduced when using very large doses in patients with severe renal failure.

Atenolol is relatively safe but the dose should be reduced as renal function decreases – the dose should be halved when CL_{cr} declines below 40–50 mL/min or serum creatinine concentration is greater than 200–250 μmole/L.

Drugs with narrower therapeutic ranges must be used with great caution. The maintenance dose of **lithium** should be reduced and regular therapeutic drug monitoring used to keep the plasma concentration in the therapeutic range. Similarly with **gentamicin**, peak and trough concentrations should be measured to guide dose adjustment to keep the plasma concentrations at a safe level. **Digoxin** plasma concentrations also need to be monitored, but in the treatment of atrial fibrillation the pulse rate can be used as a dynamic end-point to guide dosage adjustment.

Impaired excretion of drug metabolites may assume importance. Firstly, if drug metabolites are active then the pharmacological effect is prolonged and the dose needs to be reduced (**diazepam**, which has several active metabolites; morphine-6-glucuronide, which is very unusual as virtually all other glucuronides are thought to be inactive). Secondly, if accumulated drug metabolite breaks down to release the active parent drug (NSAIDs), increased toxicity may ensue.

The other pharmacokinetic change that occurs in renal failure is reduced protein binding. This occurs because of a build up of endogenous substances that inhibit drug binding to albumin. It is not clear how many drugs are affected but increased toxicity with **warfarin** and **phenytoin** are thought to be at least partly due to this mechanism.

Pharmacodynamic problems

Diuretic and antihypertensive drugs may be less effective. **Warfarin** sensitivity is increased in addition to the reduced protein binding mentioned above. Drugs known to cause renal damage need to be used with great care in patients with existing renal insufficiency because of the risk of increasing the degree of renal impairment (e.g. inhibitors of ACE, NSAIDs, **gentamicin**, loop diuretic agents). Renal function must be monitored regularly so that the drug can be stopped if it causes deterioration.

Choice of drug in renal disease

Received wisdom is that drugs excreted unchanged by the kidney should be avoided in patients with renal impairment and that drugs metabolized by the liver should be prescribed instead. However, this is a simplistic view. The direct consequences of reduced excretion of metabolites have already been discussed. In addition, there is the possibility that accumulation of metabolites may result in a negative feedback, reducing the rate of metabolism by the liver. Drug metabolism has not been studied adequately in patients with renal disease. It is often easier to use a renally excreted drug in reduced dosage rather than deal with the uncertainties of a metabolized drug. Each case needs to be considered on an individual basis.

Liver disease

Pharmacokinetic problems

Unfortunately, there is no routine liver function test that allows us to predict the effect of liver disease on drug metabolism in a way that is clinically useful. Many liver diseases have minimal effects on drug metabolism in their mild or early stages. Clinically significant problems are more likely in severe disease and patients with liver failure.

First-pass metabolism tends to be reduced (e.g. in cirrhosis) with increased bioavailability. Dosages of the affected drugs (Table 8.2) should be reduced. CL from the systemic circulation is more variable but reduced for some drugs, particularly in end-stage liver failure. Conjugation tends to be less impaired than in phase I reactions. If in doubt, it is sensible to start with a small dose.

Albumin synthesis is reduced in liver disease. This leads to reduced protein binding for many drugs. The true clinical importance of this is difficult to establish, since metabolism may also be impaired. The V of affected drugs is increased and the $t_{1/2}$ prolonged even if CL is not affected.

Pharmacodynamic problems

The response to several drugs is increased in patients with liver disease even in the absence of significant pharmacokinetic changes. Patients tend to be more sensitive to all sedative drugs, including opioids, and these may precipitate hepatic coma. They are better avoided but if necessary, should be used in small doses initially. Sensitivity to **warfarin** is increased because of reduced synthesis of clotting factor precursors and alteration in vitamin K disposition.

Drugs with a risk of hepatotoxicity should be substituted with a risk-free alternative or used with caution if there is no alternative treatment. **Paracetamol** is safe in normal doses but the threshold for overdose hepatotoxicity is smaller. **Halothane** is best avoided. Drugs that cause obstructive jaundice (e.g. phenothiazines, oral contraceptive agents) need to be carefully assessed against the risks of not treating or alternative treatment.

Table 8.2 Examples of drugs subject to extensive pre-systemic metabolism

Liver	
Antagonists at β-adrenoceptors	**propranolol**, *oxprenolol, metoprolol, labetalol*
Antihypertensive agents	**nifedipine**, *hydralazine*
Antidysrhythmic agents	**verapamil**, **lignocaine**
Antidepressant agents	**imipramine**, **amitriptyline**, *nortriptyline*
Opioids	**morphine**, *pethidine, dextropropoxyphene*, **pentazocine**, **naloxone**
Others	*chlormethiazole, metoclopramide*, **levodopa**, **glyceryl trinitrate**, *isosorbide dinitrate*
Gut wall	oestrogens, **levodopa**, **chlorpromazine**

STAFFS UNIVERSITY LIBRARY

Choice of drug in liver disease

Received wisdom is that renally excreted drugs should be used where possible. However, liver disease may modify renal function and there are rather few drugs available that are excreted predominantly unchanged by the kidneys. Each drug needs to be considered individually depending on the kind and severity of the liver disease and other patient factors.

Pregnancy

The thalidomide disaster in the 1960s profoundly affected drug prescribing in pregnancy. It can be assumed that:

(1) The placenta is virtually no barrier to drug passage.
(2) The experience of many drugs during pregnancy is so limited that all drugs should be used with extreme caution.
(3) Fetal damage can occur at any stage of pregnancy, although the first trimester is the time of greatest risk.
(4) Safe drugs are very limited in number and they are likely to have been available for many years (e.g. penicillins, **paracetamol**).
(5) Only if the risk to the mother of not treating exceeds any risk to the baby, should drugs be prescribed (e.g. uncontrolled epilepsy is far more dangerous to both mother and child than the risk of fetal abnormalities).
(6) Before any agent is used, the *BNF* (Appendix 4) or some similar resource should be consulted.

See also Developmental toxicity, page 433.

Newborn children and infants

Neonates (first 30 days of life) differ from larger children not just in size, but also in having immature hepatic and renal function.

Older children are not just small adults; they proportionately have a much larger surface area, and a greater metabolic rate. Thus drug doses that are expressed in mg/kg body weight need to be higher in children than in adults (see BNF, p. 11).

Breast-feeding mothers

Most drugs that enter the maternal circulation are distributed into breast milk. Toxicity can occur only if sufficient quantities are present. Thus **aspirin** is likely to cause bleeding and yet **warfarin** appears to be safe. For many drugs there is insufficient evidence to be certain of safety, thus it is prudent only to expose the infant to such risks if it is absolutely essential (see *BNF*, Appendix 5).

Legal aspects of prescribing

Under the provisions of the Medicines Act (1968), drugs are classified as:

(1) General Sales List medicines (GSL) – considered suitable for unsupervised sale in shops or supermarkets (e.g. household remedies).
(2) Pharmacy only medicines (P) – which can only be sold or supplied in a pharmacy, under the direct supervision of a pharmacist (e.g. **acyclovir, cimetidine, sodium cromoglycate, terfenedine**).
(3) Prescription Only Medicines (POM) – which can only be sold or supplied in accordance with a prescription of a registered practitioner (e.g. **digoxin**).

Certain drugs and combinations of drugs (indicated by ~~NHS~~ in the BNF) are not available on any NHS prescription, but may be prescribed on a private prescription (e.g. Orovite multivitamins).

An NHS prescription for a Prescription Only Medicine, to be dispensed in a community pharmacy, legally must include:

(1) The name and address of the patient.
(2) The age of the patient, if under 12 years.
(3) A description of the item to be dispensed.
(4) The name and address of the prescriber.
(5) The signature, in ink, of the prescriber.
(6) The date.

This information must be written in indelible ink or computer-generated, but computer-generated signatures are not acceptable. Such a prescription is valid for 26 weeks or, in the case of a prescription for a Controlled Drug (see below), for 13 weeks.

These requirements do not apply to hospital prescriptions, but each hospital or Trust has a drug policy, outlining its internal regulations, for example, the name and/or address of the patient can be replaced by a unique patient number. The regulations for prescriptions of Controlled Drugs (see below) always apply whether dispensing is to occur in the community or in hospitals.

Prescriptions for controlled drugs

Under the provisions of the Misuse of Drugs Act (1971) and the Misuse of Drugs Regulations (1985), Controlled Drugs are classified into five Schedules. Schedule 2 contains the opioids, the major stimulant agents and quinalbarbitone.

In addition to the above requirements of the Medicines Act (1968), prescriptions for Schedule 2 Controlled Drugs are subject to a further set of Regulations. They must state *in the prescriber's own handwriting*:

(1) The name and address of the patient (in hospital, the address may be replaced by a unique patient number).

(2) The form and strength of the preparation requested (e.g. morphine sulphate *injection* 10 mg).
(3) The total quantity required, in *both* words and figures, e.g. 20 tabs (twenty tabs), or 30 mg (thirty mg).
(4) The dose.

Computer-generated prescriptions are not acceptable. Under the Misuse of Drugs Act (1971) and the Misuse of Drugs Regulations (1985), it is an offence for a doctor to issue an incomplete prescription and/or for a pharmacist to dispense a prescription for a Controlled Drug that does not fulfil these requirements. Such prescriptions will be returned to the prescriber for correction, an inconvenience to doctor, pharmacist and patient.

Some guidelines for good prescription writing

(1) Write clearly and legibly, or use a computer prescribing program.
(2) Where available, use the generic title of the preparation, but not at the expense of clarity. Do not make up generic names for combination preparations.
(3) Do not use unofficial abbreviations.
(4) Write the dose required, not 'as directed' – patients may forget what they have been told.
(5) Where practicable, prescribe the dose as an amount of drug, not a number of tablets, as several strengths may exist, e.g. frusemide 40 mg daily *not* frusemide 1 tablet daily.
(6) It is better to rewrite a prescription than to change it, but if change is essential, it must be initialled by the original prescriber.

Summary

(1) Write all prescriptions legibly and include instructions to the patient – these will then appear on the medication label.
(2) The format for prescriptions for Controlled Drugs and Prescription only medicines is proscribed by law – if they are written incorrectly, they *must* be changed only by the prescriber.
(3) Patients can buy a wide range of medications, which they may take in addition to prescribed drugs.

Practical problems of compliance with the prescription

The most carefully chosen drug prescribed for a patient may be rendered totally useless if the patient does not take it correctly. Non-compliance is very common – 50% of patients do not take their medication in the manner intended by the doctor. It is important to realize that age, by itself, does not increase non-compliance and that there is simply a greater chance of the factors below occurring.

Not all of these factors are due to the patient. The way that drugs are prescribed can create an environment in which non-compliance is almost inevitable. Some ways to improve compliance are suggested and these are best carried out in partnership with the patient as part of a therapeutic contract.

Factors affecting compliance

(1) *Prescribed medication regimen*. The more complex the regimen that has been prescribed for the patient, the less chance he/she has of understanding it and following the instructions. A large number of drugs given at varying frequencies, and vague instructions ('take as directed'), all contribute.

(2) *Choice of preparation or container*. Unacceptable or unpleasant side-effects may mean that the patient stops taking the medication. The formulation or route may be unacceptable to the patient or he/she may not wish to abide by the required restrictions. Many patients cannot open child-resistant tops – thus they may be unable to comply, no matter how willing they are.

(3) *Patient education*. Lack of the knowledge required to take medication properly inevitably causes problems. The minimum amount of information that is required by the patient is how to take their medication, how to store it, how it is expected to help and how to recognize and manage its side-effects. Lack of such information is a frequent complaint by patients.

(4) *Poor memory*. Many patients cannot remember to take their medication or are confused as to whether they have already taken it. Compliance aids, which contain a week's supply of tablets or capsules, in sections labelled with the day and time that they should be taken, can be useful for such patients. These aids are not panaceas for all causes of non-compliance and the other factors above must be considered first, to ensure that the regimen is as simple as possible.

Summary

(1) Simplify the medication regimen. Make it as easy as possible for the patient to comply.

(2) Write unambiguous instructions on the prescription – the pharmacist can only put on the label those instructions that are on the prescription.

(3) Encourage destruction of medication that is no longer required, to avoid confusion and hoarding.

Unwanted effects of drugs

Because no drug is specific in its therapeutic action, the risk of unwanted effects is inseparable from its therapeutic use.

Definitions

Adverse drug reaction

An adverse drug reaction is a harmful, or seriously unpleasant, effect that occurs at a dose intended for therapeutic (prophylactic or diagnostic) effect and that calls for reduction of dose or withdrawal of the drug and/or forecasts hazard from future administration.

Secondary adverse effect

An adverse drug reaction that has an indirect causation (a subset of the above).

Examples:
Superinfection (antibiotic-associated colitis – AAC) under the conditions of altered bowel flora due to a broad-spectrum antibacterial drug.
Vitamin K deficiency due to an altered bowel flora after a broad-spectrum antibacterial drug.
　　Intolerance to **digoxin** in hypokalaemia due to a diuretic drug.

Intolerance

Intolerance implies an individual patient's small dose threshold for (or great sensitivity to) the production of the normal pharmacodynamic action of the drug (Figure 8.1).

Side-effect

A side-effect is an unwanted but unavoidable consequence of drug administration (less harmful or unpleasant than an adverse drug reaction) arising because the unwanted action is just as integral as the therapeutic effect to the properties of the drug. It is an inherent pharmacodynamic property of the drug that parallels the therapeutic effect (Figure 8.1).

Examples:
Sedation due to *phenobarbitone* in the treatment of epilepsy.
Vomiting due to **digoxin** in the treatment of atrial fibrillation.
Vomiting due to **morphine** in the treatment of pain.
Hypokalaemia due to a diuretic drug in the treatment of oedema.
Effects of muscarinic acetylcholine receptor blockade with a tricyclic antidepressant agent.

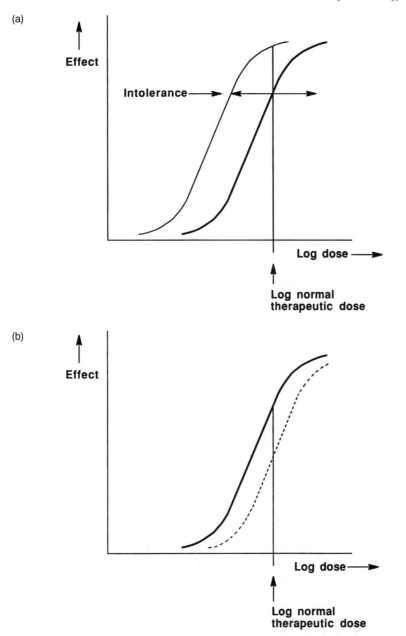

Figure 8.1 Mechanisms of predictable acute unwanted effects of drugs. (a) Log dose/effect curves are shown for the desired therapeutic effect of a drug. Patients vary in their sensitivity (horizontal bar). Intolerance (left-hand, thinner line) leads to the unwanted effect of an augmented therapeutic response to a normal therapeutic dose (compare effects where vertical line intersects the curves represented by thick and thin lines). (b) Log dose/effect curves are shown for the desired therapeutic effect (solid line) of a drug, and a parallel curve for a side-effect (dashed line) of the drug seen at lower potency. The side-effect will be more prominent the less the separation between the curves (compare effects where vertical line intersects the solid and dashed lines)

Toxicity

Toxicity implies direct chemically induced injury to cells by the drug or a reactive metabolite that occurs at large dosage and produces tissue damage.

Examples:
Paracetamol overdosage kills liver cells.
Gentamicin overdosage kills cochlear hair cells.

Hypersensitivity

Hypersensitivity implies an individual patient's inherent qualitatively abnormal but characteristic reaction to a drug (usually due to allergy).

Idiosyncrasy

Idiosyncrasy implies an individual patient's inherent qualitatively abnormal reaction to a drug (usually due to genetic abnormality).

In some cases the adverse effects of drug treatment arise when there is an inappropriate combination of drugs (see Adverse drug interactions, p. 438).

Epidemiology

In hospital practice, adverse effects of drugs (not including acute poisoning qv.) are responsible for approximately 4% of admissions to acute care beds (0.3% to all beds), occur in 10–20% of patients, prolong hospital stay in 2–10% of patients in acute medical beds and may be responsible for approximately 0.1% of deaths in medical wards.

In general practice, adverse effects of drugs are responsible for 2–3% of consultations and may occur in up to 5% of patients.

Predisposing factors

Adverse effects of drugs occur most often in female patients, those aged over 60 years or under 1 month, those with a previous history of adverse drug reaction, or with hepatic or renal disease.

Systems affected

The bodily systems or functions most often adversely affected by a drug reaction are the gut, skin, mental alertness and plasma K^+-concentration.

Drugs responsible

The drugs most commonly responsible for adverse drug reactions vary with the practical setting (occurring in hospital, causing admission, or appearing on death certificates), but include: antibacterial drugs, anticoagulant drugs, antihypertensive drugs, *chloramphenicol*, **digoxin**, diuretic

drugs, glucocorticosteroids, insulin, K⁺ salts, NSAIDs, opioids, tranquilliz-
ing drugs and **warfarin**.

Classification

Two kinds of acute adverse drug reaction are recognizable (Table 8.3).
Predictability refers to that arising from both:

(1) The doctor's knowledge of the pharmacology and toxicology of a drug.
(2) The results of preclinical animal testing during drug development.

Table 8.3 Distinction between the two kinds of acute adverse drug reaction

Label	Type A Augmented Anticipatable	Type B Bizarre
Predictability	Good	Poor
Dose dependency	Usual	Uncommon
Potential reactors	Every recipient	Only a fraction of recipients
Morbidity	High	Low
Mortality	Low	High
Relative incidence	75–80%	20–25%
Usual management	Dosage reduction	Withdrawal of drug

Type A: predictable acute adverse effects

The adverse effect is anticipatable; that is predictable from the known
pharmacological properties of the drug, the size of the dose and the pathophysiological state of the patient.

Examples:
Postural hypotension caused by the loop diuretic agents is a manifestation
of salt and water depletion arising from an excess of the desired or therapeutic effect.
AV blockade caused by **digoxin** may imperil a patient with disease of the
conducting pathways of the heart, yet it is the basis of the therapeutic
action in atrial fibrillation.

Recognizing the cause

The features of an acute augmented adverse drug reaction that suggest a
cause and effect relationship between the drug administration and the
adverse reaction are:

(1) The time sequence between drug taking and occurrence of the adverse
     reaction corresponds with the pharmacokinetic properties of the drug.
(2) The reaction corresponds to the known pharmacodynamic properties
     of the drug.
(3) The reaction ceases on stopping the drug.
(4) The reaction returns on restarting the drug.

Mechanisms

The adverse effect is an augmentation of the normal effects of the drug. A common reason for augmentation is overdosage. This may be caused by the administration of an excessive amount by accident or design. In other circumstances, the dose is standard but the elimination processes are impaired or the patient is particularly intolerant.

Overdosage

This may be accidental, as when a child receives tablets intended for an adult, or when a doctor, pharmacist or nurse makes an error in prescribing, dispensing or administration. The consequences for the recipient and for the professional reputations of those responsible may be very serious.

Intolerance due to impaired elimination

Standard doses produce an excessive concentration at the site of action. The renal or hepatic elimination of drugs may be impaired.

Renal
The GFR is disproportionately small in the newborn baby, particularly when delivered very early preterm (before 28 weeks in gestational age or below 1 kg in weight). The GFR is reduced by advanced cardiac failure, hypothyroidism, old age and shock. All these states predispose to accidental overdosage with water-soluble drugs if the prescriber does not anticipate the problem.

Examples:
Drugs predominantly eliminated by the kidney (aminoglycoside antibiotic agents, **digoxin**).
Drugs that produce pharmacologically active metabolites (**carbamazepine**, **diazepam**, *hydralazine, isosorbide dinitrate,* **metronidazole**).
Shock reduces s/c perfusion with blood with the inevitable distortions of drug absorption after s/c administration.

Hepatic
Impaired hepatic perfusion (congestive heart failure) or advanced hepatocellular disease (cells lost, sick or by-passed) can also lead to accidental overdosage because of impaired drug metabolizing capacity for lipid-soluble drugs. Hypoalbuminaemia impairs the drug-binding capacity of plasma. In thyroid disease the metabolic drug clearance parallels the BMR.

Examples:
Drugs susceptible to extensive first-pass metabolism (see p. 356) show an increased bioavailability (**lignocaine**, **morphine**, **propranolol**).
More slowly metabolized drugs show an increased $t_{1/2}$ (**diazepam**, *phenobarbitone, theophylline*).

Intolerance due to small efficiency of disposal occurs under 1 month of age to *chloramphenicol* (grey baby syndrome) and over 65 years of age to *chlorpropamide*, and tricyclic antidepressant agents.

Intolerance due to increased sensitivity

A standard dose produces a standard concentration at the site of action but this produces an excessive response. This arises when the pathophysiological state of a patient confers special sensitivity to adverse drug effects.

Examples:

Propranolol at conventional dosage seriously aggravates airway obstruction in asthma, which is also characterized by hyperreactivity to direct or indirect agonists at muscarinic acetylcholine receptors.

Morphine causes a life-threatening retention of secretions in severe chronic bronchitis.

Potassium depletion confers excessive sensitivity to **digoxin**.

In encephalopathy all CNS-depressant agents produce coma.

A malfunctioning respiratory centre (increased intracranial pressure, severe pulmonary insufficiency) produces intolerance to all CNS-depressant drugs.

Myocardial infarction predisposes to dysrhythmias with **digoxin** and direct or indirect agonists at β-adrenoceptors.

Infectious mononucleosis predisposes to rash with **ampicillin**.

Prostatic enlargement predisposes to urinary retention with diuretic agents, direct or indirect agonists at α-adrenoceptors or antagonists at muscarinic acetylcholine receptors.

Pain predisposes to confusion when a sedative is administered without an analgesic agent.

Type B: unpredictable acute adverse effects

The patient may be intolerant because he/she is hypersensitive (allergic) or may have a genetically determined abnormal response (idiosyncrasy).

Hypersensitivity

The allergic patient may have received the drug before without the prescriber's knowledge and may have produced tissue sensitizing immunoglobulin E (IgE) antibodies (see Allergically determined hypersensitivity to drugs, p. 423). Even a single subsequent dose of the drug can then result in an adverse effect, ranging from mild urticaria to bronchospasm and to acute circulatory collapse (anaphylactic shock). There may be cross-hypersensitivity to closely related drugs (different penicillins) or more distantly related drugs (cephalosporins and penicillins).

Hypersensitivity may have a cellular basis, as in the systemic lupus erythematosus-like syndrome that sometimes develops after exposure to *hydralazine*. Although not a predictable consequence of excessive dosage, the risk is dose related and there is also a genetic predisposition (slow acetylator status).

Recognizing the cause

The features of an adverse drug reaction that suggest an allergic cause are:

(1) The symptomatology does not correlate with the known pharmacodynamic properties of the drug.

(2) There is no graded dose/effect relationship.
(3) The symptomatology resembles one of the patterns of classical protein allergy.
(4) An induction period is required on primary exposure but not on re-exposure.
(5) The reaction disappears on cessation of drug exposure; it reappears on re-exposure to a small dose.
(6) It occurs in only a minority of recipients.
(7) Desensitization may be possible.

Prescriber's further actions

Avoid further use of the causative drug and its congeners. Make an appropriate and obvious entry on the patient's case folder. Tell the patient to tell other prescribers of his hypersensitivity.

Idiosyncrasy

Genetically determined adverse effects (see Pharmacogenetics, p. 426) vary in frequency with different racial groups. The possibility of detection of the patient's idiosyncrasy by a screening test sometimes exists (atypical cholinesterase, induction of aminolaevulinic acid synthetase, slow acetylator status), but the cost and delay in treatment are unacceptable except in patients believed to be particularly at risk.

Delayed and long-term adverse drug effects

The adverse effect may be delayed in its appearance, in spite of brief exposure, when that is one factor only in a causal sequence, as in teratogenesis, or the cause/effect link may be obscured by a long time lapse from the start of long-term exposure, as in carcinogenesis.

Teratogenesis

Adverse effects on the embryo (see Developmental toxicity, p. 433) are seldom so characteristic or so frequent as they were with thalidomide. More typical is an increase in the incidence of common congenital abnormalities, as reported with anticonvulsant drugs. Dietary deficiency, other drugs and genetic factors probably all contribute to the outcome.

Carcinogenesis

The incidence of many malignant tumours is influenced by reproductive history. Carcinoma of breast, for example, is more common in women who married late, bore no children and had a late menopause. It is very likely therefore that drugs that modify reproductive function (the contraceptive steroids) also alter the incidence of tumours of the reproductive organs. History gives one glaring example – carcinoma of the vagina in the teenage offspring of mothers given large doses of exogenous oestrogens in early pregnancy. Long-term epidemiological studies will no doubt reveal less dramatic changes in the incidence of tumours.

Antineoplastic drugs and immunosuppressant drugs used to prevent transplant rejection increase the risk of developing malignant tumours. The detection of adverse effects that can be greatly delayed demands prolonged surveillance of patients at risk.

Prescribing advice

Safe prescribing stems from knowledge of both the drug and the disease, and an awareness of the possibilities. The incidence and severity of adverse drug reactions can be dramatically reduced by the exercise of skill in the choice and use of drugs by knowledgeable prescribers.

Summary

(1) A general framework is provided for consideration of the unwanted effects of drugs.
(2) These may require long-term drug exposure, or be delayed or acute in appearance after onset of brief drug exposure.
(3) They may be due to intolerance, toxicity, allergy or genetically determined idiosyncrasy.
(4) Fortunately, the predictable kind of adverse drug effect is also the common kind.

Allergically determined hypersensitivity to drugs

Allergy is characterized by a group of qualitatively similar unusual responses involving an antigen/antibody reaction, after a previous uneventful exposure of which the patient may be unaware. Allergy commonly affects the skin, respiratory tract, gut, blood cells and blood vessels as target organs.

Examples:
Anaphylactic reaction to a penicillin.
Haemolytic anaemia due to *methyldopa*.

Patients with a history of allergic disease (see below) develop drug allergy more readily than others. Patients with one allergically based adverse drug reaction are approximately four times more likely to have another than those with none.

STAFFS UNIVERSITY LIBRARY

Production of the sensitized state of the patient

In most cases the drug molecules themselves are too small to induce antibody formation. However, these small molecules or their reactive metabolites behave as haptens, that is they bind covalently to body proteins and these complexes then function as antigens inducing the formation of antibodies directed against the particular hapten and its close chemical relatives.

The sensitization involves the engulfing and detection of the hapten/protein complex by mononuclear cells located in the lymphoreticular organs (thymus, spleen, bone marrow, lymphoid tissue) close to the site of exposure to the antigen. The antigen is presented to, and is recognized as foreign, by a T-lymphocyte that multiplies to produce a memory clone of T-helper lymphocytes and that programmes the proliferation and differentiation of B-lymphocytes into plasma cells committed to the production of an antibody specific for the hapten.

Classification

Allergy-based diseases are classified mechanistically into four kinds, of which three commonly underlie allergic drug reactions.

Type I – immediate/anaphylactic

The antibody responsible for immediate hypersensitivity is an IgE (or reagin). Atopy is an inherited predisposition to exaggerated development of IgE antibody in response to various antigens (allergens), such as the large MW constituents of house-dust mite, dandruff, liquorice, tomato, cow's milk and egg white. A previous medical history of allergic diseases (seasonal rhinitis, eczema, food allergy, asthma of early onset) and a family history of any of these disorders suggest atopy.

The Fc region of IgE has a high affinity for cell surface receptors on tissue mast cells or circulating basophil leucocytes. Hence IgE molecules are cleared from the circulation by being bound to these cells. This results in cellular sensitization that shows itself when subsequent exposure to the antigen results in the antigen becoming bound to the IgE, initiating the release of chemical mediators of tissue anaphylaxis from the mast cells or basophils (Figure 8.2).

The release of chemical mediators from storage granules (degranulation) is a consequence of the allergen/IgE combination making the membrane more permeable to Ca^{2+}. This triggers the release of intracellular Ca^{2+} (modulated by cAMP concentrations) and the aggregation of microtubules results in the movement of granules to the membrane and extrusion of preformed mediators (histamine, chemotactic factors, lysosomal enzymes) and the synthesis of other mediators (kinins, arachidonic acid-derived PGs and especially LTs). These mediators produce tissue anaphylaxis by evoking:

(1) Local arteriolar vasodilatation.
(2) Increased protein permeability of postcapillary venules and oedema.
(3) Contraction of smooth muscle (other than vascular).
(4) Secretion from mucosal glands.

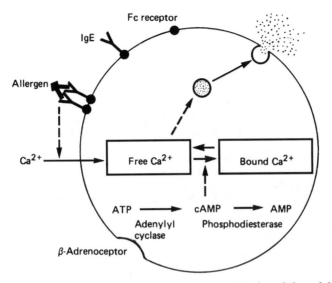

Figure 8.2 Influences upon the mast cell in tissue anaphylaxis and sites of drug action

(5) Leucocyte infiltration.
(6) Sensitization and irritation of afferent nerves.

Because the antibody is bound, the localization of the tissue anaphylaxis developing in response to an initially free antigen depends upon the route of administration of the hapten. Localized reactions produce urticaria in the skin and extrinsic asthma in the lungs. Systemic administration results in anaphylactic shock. This commonly develops within minutes and lasts approximately 2 h.

Penicillins and cephalosporins are common haptens but a huge variety of other drugs produce these reactions.

Treatment of anaphylactic shock

Reduction of the action of some mediators:

(1) By functional antagonism with *adrenaline* 0.5–1 mg i/m (0.5–1 mL of 1 mg/mL or 1 in 1000), repeated at 3 min then every 10 min – this combats, especially, the increased protein permeability of postcapillary venules.
(2) By competitive antagonism of histamine with *chlorpheniramine* 10 mg i/v.

Prevention of the formation of some mediators is best achieved with *hydrocortisone sodium succinate* 100 mg i/m or i/v.

Type II – cytolytic/autoallergy

Hapten binds to a cellular surface protein so the allergen is tissue bound and the IgG and IgM antibodies circulate. When antibodies attach to cell-bound drug, complement is fixed and lysis occurs.

Examples:

Granulocytopenia – *chloramphenicol*, sulphonamides, thioamides, gold compounds.

Thrombocytopenia – *quinidine* and *quinine*, gold compounds, sulphonamides.

Haemolysis – *methyldopa*, penicillins, cephalosporins.

Aplastic anaemia – gold compounds.

Hepatitis and cholestatic jaundice – **carbimazole, chlorpromazine**.

Collagen disease-like lupus erythematosus – *hydralazine, procainamide*.

Some of these examples of depletion of circulating cells may be more related to the type III mechanism; immune complexes become adsorbed on the surface of the cell, cells agglutinate and are removed from the circulation by the reticulo-endothelial system.

Type III – immune complex mediated

Large complexes form from the binding of soluble antigen to circulating IgG antibodies. These deposit in vascular endothelium, activate complement and produce a vasculitis resembling serum sickness. This is a mechanism in sulphonamide and penicillin allergies.

Type IV – delayed/cell mediated

Both the allergen and the antibody are tissue bound. Killer T-cells are activated and tissue cell death is induced. This mechanism is probably responsible for some adverse skin reactions to drugs (general toxic erythema, fixed drug eruption), a common reaction to penicillins, aminoglycosides, local anaesthetic or antihistamine agents applied to the skin.

Summary

(1) Adverse reactions to drugs may have an allergic basis. This is the commonest cause of unpredictable adverse drug reactions.
(2) The four kinds of allergic reaction to drugs resemble the four kinds of allergically mediated disease in their mechanisms and expressions.

Genetically determined adverse effects of drugs – pharmacogenetics

When the adverse effect is part of the normal (but not necessarily main) action of the drug, its size, and therefore severity, depends on the dose. However, the response is neither qualitatively nor quantitatively unusual. Consequently the treated population displays a unimodal frequency

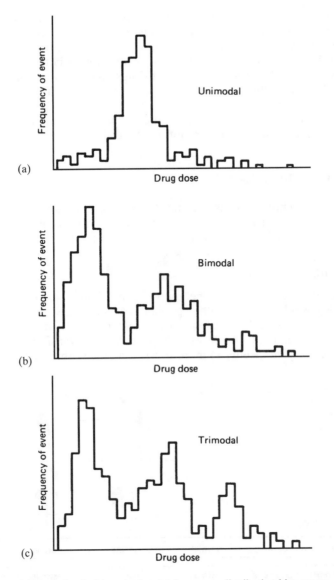

Figure 8.3 Typical uni-, bi- and trimodal frequency distribution histograms

distribution of the toxic response. All individuals show the response if given enough of the drug, so that when the number of individuals showing toxicity (frequency) is plotted against the minimum toxic dose, a smooth, continuous, bell-shaped curve, with a single peak (mode) is obtained (Figure 8.3a). This kind of distribution arises because sensitivity to the drug is the result of the expression of many genes (multifactorial).

When an abnormal reaction to a drug is determined by the expression of a single allele (a single gene, e.g. the synthesis of an atypical enzyme), the frequency distribution curve is discontinuous, that is, multimodal (Figure 8.3b,c), the phenotype (outward expression) of each individual depending upon the genotype (genetic contributions from the parents).

Variation in genotype contributes to variation in both pharmacokinetic and pharmacodynamic properties of drugs among populations of individuals. A genetically determined abnormality may produce a large concentration of drug in plasma on a normal dosage regimen (a form of intolerance due to a slowed drug metabolism) or an abnormal response to a normal plasma concentration of the drug (idiosyncrasy).

Autosomal recessive

Autosomal chromosomes are the 22 pairs of chromosomes that are not sex (X and Y) chromosomes. The inheritance patterns of genes on autosomal chromosomes therefore show no sex linkage (Figure 8.4).

Isoniazid acetylation

In North America and Europe approximately half of the population inactivate **isoniazid** slowly. In other populations the figure may be as small as 20% or as large as 90%. This is due to heterogeneity in the gene responsible for directing the synthesis of hepatic N-acetyltransferase. The atypical enzyme acetylates **isoniazid** more slowly than the normal enzyme. There are

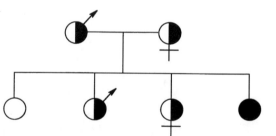

Autosomal recessive	Normal	Normal	Normal	Affected
Autosomal autonomous	Normal	Partially affected	Partially affected	Affected
Autosomal dominant	Normal	Affected	Affected	Affected
X-linked autonomous	Normal	Affected (inherited from mother)	Partially affected (inherited from father)	Affected

Figure 8.4 Typical distribution of phenotype with genotype under various modes of inheritance. Genotypes: ○ = normal + normal (homozygous for the normal gene); ● = affected + affected (homozygous for the affected gene); ◑ = normal + affected (heterozygous for the affected gene)

three possible genotypes – those homozygous (rapid/rapid), those heterozygous (slow/rapid) and those homozygous (slow/slow). These genotypes give rise to two phenotypes – rapid acetylators and slow acctylators (Figure 8.4). When given to slow acetylators at dose rates suitable for rapid acetylators, **isoniazid** accumulates to toxic concentrations, often resulting in peripheral neuropathy. Other drugs that are acetylated, and therefore accumulate in patients with the atypical acetylation enzyme, include *dapsone, hydralazine, nitrazepam*, **phenelzine**, *procainamide* and *sulphasalazine*.

Hereditary methaemoglobinaemia

In hereditary methaemoglobinaemia, NADH methaemoglobin reductase is deficient. This enzyme does not of itself inactivate any drugs but it is the main route for regenerating haemoglobin from methaemoglobin (Figure 8.5). Consequently the methaemoglobinaemia produced by certain oxidizing drugs (nitrites, nitrates, *prilocaine*, sulphonamides, **primaquine**) is severe and prolonged in individuals with this condition. Methylene blue is useful as a reducing agent to regenerate haemoglobin.

Impaired drug hydroxylation

The hydroxylation of debrisoquine (an antihypertensive agent similar to *guanethidine*) is impaired in approximately 9% of people in the UK (20–90% in some other populations). One member of the hepatic cytochrome P_{450} MFO superfamily is deficient or defective. Adverse effects may arise from the loss of metabolizing capacity or the altered profile of metabolites. Other drugs affected include *metoprolol, nortriptyline*, **phenytoin** and **tolbutamide**.

Autosomal autonomous

Autonomous genes are of penetrance intermediate between dominant and recessive ones, so the phenotype is determined by the contributions of each of the genes singly (Figure 8.4).

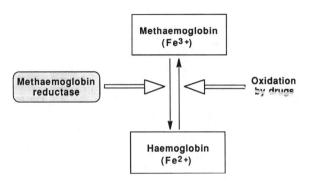

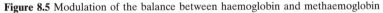

Figure 8.5 Modulation of the balance between haemoglobin and methaemoglobin

Suxamethonium apnoea

Suxamethonium occasionally (1 : 2500) produces unduly prolonged respiratory muscle paralysis, necessitating artificial ventilation, as there are atypical forms of the enzyme cholinesterase. Atypical cholinesterase is due to an abnormality in a single gene. In heterozygotes the trait is partially expressed so that there are individuals with intermediate cholinesterase activities (tri-modal frequency distribution curve, Figure 8.3c). The dibucaine test (see p. 73) identifies individuals with the atypical form of cholinesterase – the enzyme in blood from normal subjects is more easily inhibited by cinchocaine than is the atypical enzyme.

Glucocorticosteroid glaucoma

Topical ophthalmic glucocorticosteroids produce an abnormally large increase in intraocular pressure in 1 : 75 of patients, who have a high incidence of family history of open-angle glaucoma.

Autosomal dominant (Figure 8.4)

Malignant hyperthermia

In the rare condition of malignant hyperthermia the ability of skeletal muscle to sequester Ca^{2+} in the sarcoplasmic reticulum is impaired. **Halothane** and **suxamethonium** depolarize skeletal muscle cells and trigger the intracellular release of Ca^{2+}, which persists too long in the cytosol producing contracture, greatly increased metabolic heat production and lactic acidosis. *Dantrolene* interferes with the Ca^{2+} release from the sarcoplasmic reticulum and reduces the mortality in malignant hyperthermia.

Acute intermittent porphyria

The normal biosynthetic pathway for haem in the liver is shown in Figure 8.6. Haem is required for both haemoglobin and the cytochromes, including cytochrome P_{450} mixed function oxidase enzymes. The rate-limiting step in the pathway is the activity of δ-aminolaevulinic acid synthetase, which is controlled by product feedback inhibition by haem.

Approximately 1 in 10 000 people in the UK suffer an inborn error of metabolism known as acute intermittent porphyria and carry a gene that codes for a defective enzyme (porphobilinogen deaminase) in the haem synthesis pathway. Patients with this condition are usually free from symptoms but acute attacks can be triggered by drugs, especially the barbiturates, but also by benzodiazepines, cephalosporins, gonadal steroids, thiazide diuretics, sulphonamides and sulphonylureas. A common step in drug-induced attacks is a sudden increase in the activity of δ-aminolaevulinic acid synthetase. The drug either directly induces this enzyme or induces cytochrome P_{450} mixed function oxidase which utilizes haem, decreasing its concentration and causing disinhibition of δ-aminolaevulinic acid synthetase. There is a consequent marked increase in formation of δ-aminolaevulinic acid and porphobilinogen, which can be

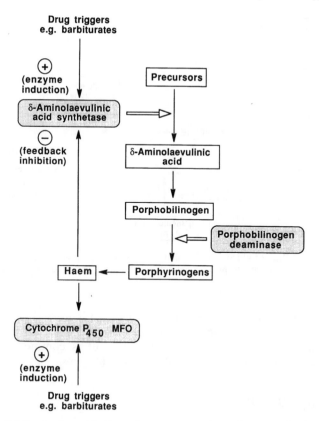

Figure 8.6 Porphyrin metabolism relevant to acute intermittent porphyria

detected in urine. These chemicals give rise to symptoms of abdominal pain, motor neuritis, anxiety and psychosis. An attack can be fatal. Other precipitating factors are ethanol and infections, and one of these could have been responsible for triggering King George III's episodes.

Resistance to warfarin

A small number of patients need a very much larger dose than normal of **warfarin** to produce adequate control of blood clotting. The reason is probably an altered structure of the vitamin K epoxide reducing enzyme, at which **warfarin** is a competitive inhibitor, to induce its anticoagulant action.

X-chromosome linked autonomous (Figure 8.4)

Glucose-6-phosphate dehydrogenase deficiency

People with glucose-6-phosphate dehydrogenase deficiency respond idiosyncratically with haemolysis to the oxidizing (electrophilic) drugs

STAFFS UNIVERSITY LIBRARY

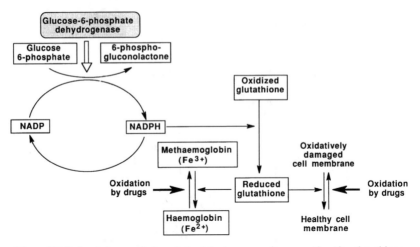

Figure 8.7 Role of glucose-6-phosphate dehydrogenase in generating the glutathione necessary to protect red cells from damage by oxidizing drugs

nalidixic acid, salicylates and sulphonamides (Figure 8.7), as well as to the antimalarial agents **chloroquine** and **primaquine**. The deficiency occurs in approximately 3% of people in the UK but is commoner in African, Mediterranean and South East Asian populations.

Multifactorial

Another example of a drug triggering an attack in a susceptible person is the precipitation of an acute attack of gout by thiazide diuretic agents in individuals with a genetic predisposition to the disease. There is clear evidence of an hereditary component in gout but it is not a simple trait carried by a single gene (that is, it is multifactorial).

Idiosyncrasy of unknown origin

Aplastic anaemia

Approximately 1 in 100 000 patients treated with *chloramphenicol* develops fatal aplastic anaemia. Individuals who are at risk cannot be identified in advance. For a list of other drugs that produce aplastic anaemia, see Table 8.4.

Table 8.4 Potential to produce aplastic anaemia

Definite	Probable
Chloramphenicol	Sulphonamides
Sodium aurothiomalate	**Phenytoin**
Organic arsenicals	**Tolbutamide**
	Chlorpropamide

Mydriatic agents produce an attack of glaucoma in patients with a closed-angle (1 : 500).

Summary

(1) Abnormalities of single genes that control the production of enzymes that provide means of drug inactivation lead to subpopulations of people with unusual rates of drug inactivation.
(2) Four characteristic patterns of inheritance are seen, which depend on the autosomal or sex chromosome location of the abnormal gene and on the dominant, autonomous or recessive penetrance of the gene.
(3) Altered drug inactivation is one cause of augmented unwanted drug effects.
(4) Some bizarre adverse effects occur when enzymes or transporters that promote repair of drug-induced damage are affected or an inborn error of metabolism occurs in a pathway modulated by drug activity.

Developmental toxicity

Drug treatment during pregnancy and lactation is unique in that a second individual receives some of the drug. It can be more difficult to determine the toxicity of drugs on these individuals than on the mother. Drugs taken at the end of pregnancy can exert their predictable reversible effects on the newborn (e.g. respiratory depression with *pethidine*, sedation with benzodiazepines). These effects are likely to last longer in the newborn than the mother due to the slower elimination of drugs by the former, particularly when liver metabolism is the predominant route.

Many drugs have been shown to be toxic to the developing fetus in animal studies, but some human teratogenic agents are not. Therefore drug treatment during pregnancy should be avoided if possible.

A knowledge of the stages of development in utero can provide a logical basis for understanding the permanent adverse effects of drugs on such development.

Human development

Development in utero can be conveniently separated into three stages (Figure 8.8):

(1) Pre-implantation.
(2) Embryonic.
(3) Fetal.

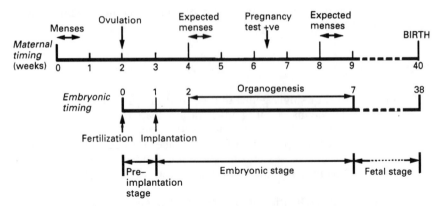

Figure 8.8 Relative timings of maternal and embryonic events from conception to birth

Pre-implantation stage

Fertilization (fusion of haploid oocyte and spermatozoon) occurs in the oviduct to form a zygote. This progressively divides to form a ball of cells. A blastocyst, formed soon after this ball has passed into the uterus, embeds in the endometrium.

Embryonic stage

Implantation occurs 1 week after fertilization or approximately 3 weeks after the commencement of the last menstrual period and pregnancy is not usually confirmed until some 4 weeks after implantation (Figure 8.8). Any restriction of the use of a drug during pregnancy should, therefore, apply to all women of reproductive age. In the human embryo, organogenesis starts soon after implantation. During this stage differentiation of cells is occurring and primordia of organ systems are being formed.

Fetal stage

By approximately 9 weeks after conception, the major organ systems have been formed. Fetal development consists of growth in size, finer differentiation and functional maturation. Some development of major organ systems occurs during this stage – major brain growth occurs around birth in people. Obviously, much human development takes place after birth.

Drug effects on development

Developmental toxicity is the study of factors and mechanisms producing abnormalities of development. It can be assumed that virtually all drugs distribute to the fetus. The physicochemical properties of drugs dictate their rate of distribution but at a steady state fetal plasma and tissue concentrations are likely to be similar to those of the mother (see p. 342). Possible adverse effects of drugs on development include:

(1) Embryonic or fetal death.
(2) Major structural malformation.
(3) Growth retardation.
(4) Functional defects.

The nature of any adverse effect principally depends on the drug and on the time of administration in relation to the stage of development. For example, thalidomide produced limb deformities (phocomelia) and internal organ deformities. The critical period was 3–5 weeks after conception, that is during the period of organogenesis. Thalidomide used towards the end of pregnancy had no effect on development. A comparison of maternal and embryonic timings is shown in Figure 8.8. It should be recognized that there is a spontaneous occurrence of altered embryonic/fetal development – in the absence of drugs natural abortion occurs in 1 in 5 pregnancies.

Drugs affecting development

Anticonvulsant drugs

The incidence of malformations is increased in babies born to mothers who have received anticonvulsant drugs. Some of the malformations are minor or self correcting (hypoplasia of the nails). Cleft lip and palate have been associated with **phenytoin** and neural tube defects with **sodium valproate** and, to a slightly lesser extent, **carbamazepine**, but no anticonvulsant drug can be exonerated. The issues are more fully discussed on page 521.

Cytotoxic drugs

Present cytotoxic drugs show only a small degree of selective toxicity towards neoplasms relative to normal cells. These drugs act particularly on rapidly proliferating cells and could be expected to produce embryo- and fetotoxicity. The group includes antimetabolites (**methotrexate**, *mercaptopurine*) and alkylating agents (**cyclophosphamide**, *busulphan*). If used during the first trimester (one-third) of pregnancy miscarriages or malformations frequently, but not inevitably, result. Following their use in the second and third trimester growth retardation often occurs.

Despite these observations there have been many successful pregnancies in renal transplant and other patients receiving immunosuppressant drugs including *azathioprine*, which is converted to mercaptopurine in vivo, and *cyclosporin*. Exposure of either parent to cytotoxic drugs before fertilization does not seems to increase the incidence of mutations in their children.

Vitamin A analogues

Vitamin A analogues are used for the systemic treatment of some severe skin diseases, *isotretinoin* for disfiguring acne and *acitretin* for psoriasis.

These compounds produce a high incidence of ear, eye and cardiac defects, cleft lip and palate and craniofacial dysmorphology. Contraceptive measures must be taken for at least 1 month before, during and 1 month (*isotretinoin*) or 2 years (*acitretin*) after treatment with these compounds.

Antithyroid drugs

Neonatal hypothyroidism and even cretinism is possible but is rarely seen following the use of antithyroid drugs (**carbimazole**). Thyroid gland enlargement present at delivery is usually temporary.

Tetracyclines

Tetracyclines are readily deposited, by calcium chelation, in developing teeth and bone in the third trimester and postnatally, leading to discoloration and occasionally hypoplasia. Therefore, other antibiotic agents should be used when possible.

Warfarin

There may be an association between **warfarin** use in the first trimester and a variety of structural malformations, including facial deformities and optic nerve atrophy and perhaps mental retardation. Patients are therefore generally advised to avoid conception until it is practicable to withdraw **warfarin** or to use s/c **heparin** in the first trimester. Excessive 'moulding' of the skull during delivery produces intracranial bleeding. Oral anticoagulant drugs are therefore withdrawn in late pregnancy and replaced by s/c **heparin**, which does not cross the placenta.

Antimalarial agents

The seriousness of malaria justifies prophylaxis and treatment. However, many drugs useful against malaria interfere with the folic acid pathway in the malarial parasite (see p. 295) and can affect the same pathway in the developing embryo and fetus. **Chloroquine** or *proguanil* may be used prophylactically and with the latter folate supplements should be taken. Pyrimethamine should be avoided in the first trimester and used only with folate supplements later. *Mefloquine* should not be used.

Chloroquine or *quinine* may be used for treatment but pyrimethamine and *halofantrine* should not be used. Radical cure with **primaquine** should be postponed until after pregnancy is over.

General anaesthetic agents

A higher incidence of spontaneous abortions and deformities in the offspring of females who work in operating theatres was presumed to be due to inhalation of general anaesthetic gases in the atmosphere.

Nowadays scavenging systems to remove these gases from theatres are commonly employed.

Ethanol

There are several reports of a higher incidence of growth retardation, craniofacial abnormalities and mental deficiency in the offspring of chronic alcoholic mothers. Deficiency of maternal diet probably contributes. A withdrawal syndrome may occur in babies born to alcoholic mothers.

Tobacco smoking

This is associated with smaller neonates and a higher incidence of perinatal complications.

The justifiability of treating a pregnant woman with a drug having one of these adverse effects depends on:

(1) The nature and incidence of the effect.
(2) The severity of the disease.
(3) The therapeutic value of the drug to the mother.

As an example, the use of anticonvulsant drugs is generally justified as, despite evidence of an increased incidence of fetal malformations associated with their use, their therapeutic benefit is high. In contrast, the use of antagonists at H_1 histamine receptors (*cyclizine*) or antagonists at muscarinic acetylcholine receptors (**hyoscine**) to treat vomiting in early pregnancy is generally not justified. There is little evidence of any serious adverse effects of these drugs on development but the condition can usually be treated by non-drug methods.

Summary

(1) Drugs can adversely affect development in utero at the pre-implantation, embryonic and fetal stages.
(2) The difficulty of predicting these adverse effects places an important restriction on the use of new drugs in women who are or may be pregnant.
(3) Drugs taken by a woman during pregnancy and acting on the uterine contents can cause the following adverse effects: embryonic or fetal death, major structural malformation, growth retardation or functional defects.
(4) The justifiability of treating a pregnant woman with a drug having one of these adverse effects depends on: the nature and incidence of the effect, the severity of the disease, the therapeutic value of the drug to the mother.

Adverse drug interactions

Many patients take more than one drug simultaneously, and one drug may modify the activity of another, either enhancing or reducing it. Such an interaction may be beneficial, for example, some antibacterial or antihypertensive drugs in combination, but this chapter is concerned with the situation where the interaction is harmful.

Definitions

An adverse drug interaction is an adverse drug reaction (qv.) that arises specifically from the interplay between two or more drugs. An interacting drug modulates the activity of a target drug. The effects of the target drug may be augmented/enhanced/increased, or diminished/impaired/reduced. The mechanisms that underlie these modulations may be summation (see p. 26) or potentiation (see p. 27), or antagonism (see p. 22) or functional opposition (see p. 26).

Epidemiology

In UK hospital practice more than 40% of patients receiving any drugs at all are taking six or more. In them the incidence of unwanted effects is seven times higher than in those taking fewer than six drugs. Table 8.5 shows the relationship between the number of drugs received and number of pairings among drugs. The factors that lead to multiple drug prescriptions are also those that predispose to adverse drug interactions – old age and severe illness.

The total number of known or predicted adverse drug interactions is huge. Discussion here is limited to the more clinically relevant – those that have important repercussions for the patient. These involve modulation of the activity of a target drug having a:

(1) Steep dose/effect relationship.
(2) Small therapeutic index.

Table 8.5 Relationship between the number of drugs prescribed and the number of potential interactions (pairs)

Drugs prescribed	Potential interactions
1	0
2	1
3	3
4	6
5	10
6	15
7	21

Then small degrees of antagonism of the target drug cause loss of therapeutic effectiveness, and small degrees of potentiation produce an augmented adverse effect.

Commonest drugs responsible

Oral anticoagulant drugs, cardiac glycosides, antidysrhythmic drugs, direct or indirect agonists at adrenoceptors, antihypertensive drugs (diuretic agents, antagonists at β-adrenoceptors, blockers of L-type Ca^{2+} channels), anticancer drugs, antiepileptic drugs, oral hypoglycaemic drugs, oral contraceptive agents, alcohol, NSAIDs, Li^+, antidepressant drugs, antipsychotic drugs.

Classification

Adverse drug interactions are of two basic kinds:

(1) Pharmacodynamic interactions can occur between drugs having similar or opposing pharmacological effects and give rise to summation or competitive antagonism or functional opposition. The concentration of each drug, at its site of action, is unaltered by the interaction.
(2) Pharmacokinetic interactions arise because one drug interferes with the disposition of another and give rise to potentiation or antagonism. The concentration of the target drug at its site of action is modified by the presence of the interacting drug.

Pharmacodynamic interactions

Pharmacodynamic interactions are common. They represented the majority of adverse interactions and are, in most instances, predictable.

Pharmacodynamic interactions can be subdivided on the site of action of the interacting drug, which may be:

(1) Near the site of action of the target drug.
(2) Distant from the site of action of the target drug – the interaction depends on a secondary effect exerted through some common necessary link.

Near the site of action of the target drug

Result in summation

Examples:
Ethanol, which is itself sedative, adds to the sedative effect of all CNS-depressant drugs (e.g. antagonists at histamine H_1 receptors that penetrate the blood–brain barrier, benzodiazepines, antipsychotic drugs).
Aminoglycoside antibiotic agents increase the muscle weakness produced by antagonists at nicotinic acetylcholine receptors of skeletal muscle (see p. 58).
Aspirin in large doses reduces the concentration of prothrombin in plasma and so adds to the anticoagulant effect of **warfarin** (see p. 214).

STAFFS UNIVERSITY LIBRARY

Result in antagonism or opposition

Examples:
Simultaneous use of agonists and antagonists at the same receptor.
Antagonists at muscarinic acetylcholine receptors prevent the increase of gastric motility due to *metoclopramide*.

Distant from the site of action of the target drug

Result in summation

Examples:
Antagonists at β-adrenoceptors (e.g. **propranolol**) mask the adrenergically mediated symptoms and homeostatic mechanisms, and add to the severity, of insulin hypoglycaemia (see pp. 191 and 192).
Phenothiazines cause orthostatic hypotension (a reduction in BP on assuming the upright posture) and summate with antihypertensive drugs.
Diuretic agents cause K^+ depletion and so increase the dysrhythmogenicity of **digoxin** (see p. 124).

Result in antagonism or opposition

Examples:
NSAIDs or glucocorticosteroids cause salt and water retention, increasing blood volume and so antagonizing antihypertensive drugs.

Pharmacokinetic or dispositional interactions

This classification of possible sites of such interaction follows the order of their discussion in Chapter 7 on Drug disposition and metabolism.

Outside the body (by chemical reaction)

Examples:
If **suxamethonium** and **thiopentone sodium** solutions are mixed in the same syringe, the former is rapidly hydrolysed by the strong alkalinity of the latter. If **phenytoin sodium** is injected into glucose (5% w/v) solution for i/v infusion, which has a low pH, the phenytoin anion is partly precipitated as the less soluble acid.

At the site of entry before absorption

By forming an insoluble complex

Antacids (calcium, magnesium or aluminium salts) or iron salts with tetracyclines.

By altering gastric emptying

Food has a variable effect on gastric emptying. Opioids and antagonists at muscarinic acetylcholine receptors slow gastric emptying, while *metoclopramide* increases it. The effect of altered gastric emptying on absorption of incompletely absorbed drugs (e.g. **levodopa** or **digoxin**) is seen in altered delay in onset of absorption, rate of absorption and peak blood concentrations. Total absorption (AUC) is usually unchanged. Absorption from liquid formulations is little affected.

By alteration of gut flora

Broad-spectrum antibacterial drugs reduce the size of the colonic bacterial population. A consequent reduction in vitamin K synthesis can lead to potentiation of oral anticoagulant drugs. **Ethinyloestradiol** is normally metabolized to the glucuronide conjugate, which is excreted in bile and then undergoes hydrolysis in the gut resulting in enterohepatic recycling. Thus, reduction in hydrolytic activity, normally produced by gut bacteria, can cause therapeutic failure of the oral contraceptive drugs (see Figure 7.9).

During absorption

Inhibitors of MAO potentiate tyramine by inhibition of the enzyme in the gut wall and in the liver, allowing a greater proportion of the dietary tyramine dose to enter the systemic circulation.

During distribution (by competition for plasma protein binding sites)

Displacement from serum albumin binding occurs at the onset of concomitant exposure to a drug of higher affinity or of equal affinity in larger dose. The effect of this interaction is short-lived because the displaced drug is metabolized, or there is increased tissue binding, and a new steady state is achieved with elimination equal to the dose ingested, that is, the same effect is achieved at a smaller total drug concentration in plasma. The physician must resist the temptation to treat the reduced plasma concentration (total concentration is reported in drug monitoring assays) by dosage increase – it is the concentration free in plasma water and the magnitude of the therapeutic effect that are significant.

This is the basis of a clinically relevant interaction only when the interacting drug has a high affinity for the acid binding site and occupies the majority of the binding sites, and the target drug is extensively bound to the same site (e.g. **warfarin** 99%, **tolbutamide** 98% bound to albumin) and has a small therapeutic index. Free plasma concentration increases a lot only if the volume of distribution is small (e.g. **warfarin** 8 L/70 kg, **tolbutamide** 7 L/70 kg) in relation to plasma volume.

In both of the above cases the displacing drug also interferes with metabolism (see below).

Examples:
Salicylic acid with **warfarin**.
Sulphonamides with **tolbutamide**.

Stimulation of drug metabolism

A number of factors increase the rate at which endogenous (steroid hormones) and exogenous (drugs, foodstuffs) substances are metabolized by hepatic MFO. The capacity for metabolism is greater in smokers, alcoholics (without advanced cirrhosis), in those exposed to hydrocarbons and in patients taking a wide variety of lipid-soluble drugs. This increased rate of drug oxidation is due to enzyme induction (associated with an increase in enzyme activity, cytochrome P_{450} concentration, liver weight and microscopically visible smooth endoplasmic reticulum) and can occur after a few days' or weeks' exposure to the inducing agent. Induction is generally non-specific, so that oxidation of other drugs in addition to that of the inducing agent is promoted.

Table 8.6 lists drugs that induce MFO. Most anticonvulsant drugs (but not **sodium valproate**) and most hypnotic and sedative agents (but not benzodiazepines) are included. Regular consumption of more than 100 mg daily is required for induction to occur. Consequences are more rapid inactivation of target drugs and more rapid activation of target prodrugs.

More rapid inactivation (Table 8.6)

Therapeutic failure of a target drug arises from its greater metabolic clearance.

There are two occurrences that can reveal this interaction: the onset and offset of induction. A patient in steady state with a target drug inactivated by oxidative metabolism commences concurrent treatment with an inducing agent (Figure 8.9). As induced enzyme concentration builds up the steady-state plasma concentration of target drug declines over a few days with associated therapeutic failure.

Compensation for the larger clearance by prescribing a greater dose rate allows therapeutic control to be regained.

Cessation of administration of the inducing agent and declining clearance of the target drug leads to accumulation of the latter over 2–3 weeks and the associated occurrence of toxic effects.

Common settings are the onset and offset of drug treatment of either tuberculosis (with **rifampicin**) or epilepsy (with **carbamazepine**, **phenytoin**, *phenobarbitone*) in a patient under long-term treatment with oral contraceptive agents or **warfarin**.

Table 8.6 Drugs inducing MFO and MFO target drugs

Inducing agents	Target drugs inactivated by oxidative metabolism
Carbamazepine	Glucocorticosteroids
Ethanol	Oral contraceptive steroids
Griseofulvin	*Theophylline*
Phenobarbitone	**Warfarin**
Phenytoin	
Rifampicin	

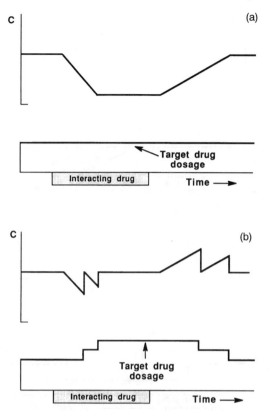

Figure 8.9 Drug interactions based upon induction of enzyme activity. (a) The onset and slower offset of the reduced plasma target drug concentration (C) caused by addition of an interacting inducer of MFO. (b) A response to the anticipated onset of therapeutic failure, increasing the target drug dose rate (D/T) – remember to reduce it again when the interacting drug is withdrawn

More rapid activation

Toxicity of a target prodrug arises from the more rapid production of the active drug. The duration of action is shortened. **Paracetamol** overdosage produces more severe toxic effects when the patient has been taking an inducing agent.

Inhibition of drug metabolism

In general, inhibition of drug metabolism, and the interactions based on it, shows more selectivity than induction. Onset often occurs within 1 or 2 days (Figure 8.10).

Deliberate

The desired therapeutic response to some drugs is mediated by inhibiting the metabolism of endogenous or exogenous substances. The

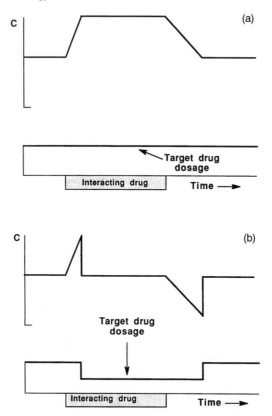

Figure 8.10 Drug interactions based upon inhibition of enzyme activity, (a) The onset and slower offset of the increased plasma target drug concentration (C) caused by addition of an interacting inhibitor of MFO. (*Note*: both onset and offset are faster than in Figure 8.9. (b) A response to the anticipated onset of augmented adverse effects, decreasing the target drug dose rate (D/T) – remember to increase it again when the interacting drug is withdrawn

Table 8.7 Examples of inhibitors of enzymes and drugs whose metabolism is inhibited

Enzyme system	Inhibitor	Metabolism inhibited
Aldehyde dehydrogenase	*Disulfiram*	Ethanol
	Chlorpropamide	
	Metronidazole	
MAO	**Phenelzine**	Tyramine-like agents
	Tranylcypromine	
Xanthine oxidase	**Allopurinol**	*Azathioprine*
		Mercaptopurine
MFO	**Phenelzine**	*Pethidine*
	Cimetidine	**Phenytoin**
	Isoniazid	
	Sodium valproate	
	Sulphonamides	**Tolbutamide**
	Cimetidine	*Theophylline*
	Ciprofloxacin	**Warfarin**
	Erythromycin	
	Sulphonamides	

administration of other drugs, in their presence, can then produce an adverse response. One interacting drug potentiates all alternative substrates.

Incidental

The metabolism of some drugs is inhibited in an unpredictable manner by others. Dosage reduction is usually all that is needed, but changing to a different drug may be desirable. One therapeutically vulnerable substrate may be potentiated by any of several interacting drugs (Table 8.7).

Again, you need to be aware of, and compensate for, the changing interaction at the offset of inhibition as well as that at the onset.

Pharmacokinetic interaction near the site of target drug action

The active transport of released noradrenaline back into the noradrenergic neurone is a site of competitive drug interaction. Tricyclic antidepressant drugs:

(1) Prevent the antihypertensive action of noradrenergic neurone blocking agents (*guanethidine*) (see p. 81).
(2) Potentiate *adrenaline* administered with a local anaesthetic agent (see p. 109).

A part of the potentiation of sympathomimetic amine substrates by inhibitors of MAO arises at the level of the noradrenergic nerve terminal (see p. 85), in addition to the gut mucosa and liver.

Alteration of renal excretion

Diuretic agents (particularly thiazides but also loop diuretic agents) cause Na^+ depletion and the proximal tubules of a patient taking **lithium carbonate** retain more Li^+.

Loop diuretic agents reduce the GFR and therefore the renal clearance of **gentamicin**.

Competition for renal excretory mechanisms

Most drugs are eventually filtered and excreted by the kidney, the 'purpose' of phase I and phase II metabolism being to increase water solubility (polarity). Active tubular secretion of anions and cations is a potential site for interactions of therapeutic relevance (salicylate with **methotrexate**).

Prescribing advice

Every time a physician adds to the number of drugs a patient is taking he may devise a novel combination that has a special risk. (quoted in Laurence and Bennett, 1992, see Suggested further reading and study, p. 548).

Keep the number of drugs you prescribe to a minimum. Select, of the alternatives, the best known to you. When adding a drug to the regimen, consider all the new pairings. Take care when injecting drugs into the giving set of i/v infusion.

Summary

(1) Interactions between two drugs may be beneficial or unwanted.
(2) Most adverse drug interactions are predictable from a basic knowledge of drug properties.
(3) A general framework for considering unwanted drug interactions is offered. This divides them on the basis of their mechanisms into pharmacodynamic and pharmacokinetic kinds.
(4) The possible pharmacokinetic mechanisms are easier to remember if mapped onto the dispositional life history of a drug.

Abuse of drugs

Drug abuse is the taking of a drug or a dose of drug in a manner that deviates from approved medical or generally accepted social patterns within a culture.

In addition to the well-publicized aspects of drug dependence, drug abuse also involves such practices as excessive self-medication with proprietary preparations (analgesic agents, vitamins, cold 'remedies'), the bulk addition of antibiotic agents to animal foodstuffs in factory farming, the use of some drugs in sport in an attempt to improve performance, overprescribing and misprescribing by the medical profession, the unnecessary sale of 'nostrums' by pharmacists, non-compliance by the patient and much else. In this brief coverage so many facets cannot be encompassed. The following points are intended to provide some factual information and to encourage discussion.

Dependence

Dependence is defined in terms of the consequences of stopping drug taking. If the consequences are psychic or mental (craving, behavioural changes), this is psychic or mental dependence (habituation). Drugs that cause psychic dependence include nicotine (as in tobacco), centrally acting sympathomimetic amines (amphetamines, ephedrine), caffeine and cannabis.

If the consequences are physical, this is physical dependence (addiction). Although withdrawal of caffeine or nicotine can give rise to physical effects, these are minor and the drugs are not usually included amongst those that cause physical dependence of concern. Only two groups of drugs cause true physical dependence:

(1) Opioid analgesic agents (see p. 242) – withdrawal syndrome includes diarrhoea, abdominal cramps, sweating, vomiting.
(2) CNS-depressant drugs and anxiolytic agents (see p. 260) – withdrawal syndrome includes confusion, disorientation, convulsions.

The severity of the syndrome depends both on the drug and the frequency of drug taking. **Diazepam** or ethanol require months of regular taking before dependence is detectable, *diamorphine* (heroin) requires a few days. Withdrawal after six consecutive injections of *diamorphine* may produce only a mild syndrome, that after 1 year may be fatal.

The molecular mechanism of dependence is unknown and may vary from one drug to another. Any theory must explain both tolerance (which is a prerequisite of dependence) and the nature of the withdrawal syndrome.

The following should be regarded as a model rather than actual mechanism of action (Figure 8.11). Consider a part of the brain in which there is a balance between the amounts of an excitatory and an inhibitory transmitter (E and I). Assume the drug of dependence (D) acts as a mimic of transmitter I. The balance is altered to a state of inhibition or depression as a result of the primary effect of the drug.

If the drug effect persisted, the body would try to compensate and a method of compensation could be to increase excitatory activity. This could be by an increase in the amount of E (as shown), or by receptor proliferation or other mechanisms of supersensitivity. The balance is restored, although the drug is still present (tolerance). If the drug is

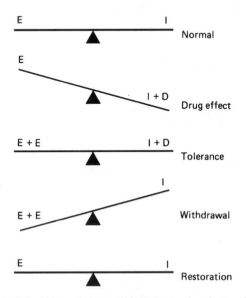

Figure 8.11 A model of the balance between the amounts of excitatory (E) and inhibitory (I) transmitters: tolerance to drug of dependence (D) and its withdrawal

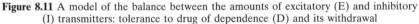
STAFFS UNIVERSITY LIBRARY

withdrawn a new imbalance occurs that produces symptoms opposite to those of the drug (the withdrawal syndrome). It then requires some time (during treatment of the withdrawal syndrome) before the biological adaptation reverts back to normal.

Two other points are pertinent:

(1) There is a grey area between psychic and physical dependence; characteristics are best defined for each drug group.
(2) People are creatures of habit. Dependence can occur to almost anything done habitually. A person accustomed to walking around the block before retiring does not sleep so well (a behavioural response) if deprived of the habit. Linked to this is dependence on an environment (social dependence), which can be a very potent behavioural influence.

Drug-related deaths

Nearly 3000 people die by poisoning each year in England and Wales. Commonly more than one drug appears on the death certificate and it is difficult to list exact poisoning figures. Table 8.8 shows approximate numbers. In 1991 no death was associated with benzodiazepines alone. Appearance in the list is a function of both toxicity and availability.

Major changes that have occurred during the last two and a half decades are a large decrease in barbiturate deaths (previously responsible for approximately two-thirds of all drug deaths) and the virtual disappearance of domestic gas as a cause of death.

In the opposite direction there has been a steady increase in deaths due to ethanol, benzodiazepines and other psychoactive drugs.

If chronic poisoning is considered, tobacco, which causes cardiovascular and lung damage, is more dangerous than any other drug (estimated 75 000 deaths per year).

Incidence of dependence

As with acute fatal poisoning, the incidence of drug dependence is a function of availability. Ethanol is responsible for the greatest incidence of physical dependence (500 000).

Table 8.8 Drug causes of acute fatal poisoning (accidental and deliberate)

Approximate number of acute fatal poisonings in England and Wales (1991)	3000
Carbon monoxide	1508
Analgesic agents total including antirheumatic drugs	854
(salicylates alone)	(51)
Ethanol	152*
Benzodiazepines	28†
Barbiturates	58
Solvents	28

*Excludes deaths from chronic abuse related to liver cirrhosis.
†All cases involved other drugs, often ethanol.

Before 1960 the number of known opioid addicts in the UK had remained constant at approximately 300. During the 1960s there was a large increase to approximately 2000 when the law concerning availability was changed. In the late 1970s there was a sharp increase to a figure of approximately 7500 (in 1984). These are <u>notified</u> addicts – the real figure is probably several-fold greater.

Whatever social reasons may have contributed to the increase in dependence in recent years, a significant contribution is that there are now large supplies of inexpensive diamorphine and cocaine of high purity available illicitly.

The drug laws

An assortment of laws controls the availability, prescribing, storage and labelling of drugs in the UK.

Before 1970 the act that covered the drugs of abuse was the Dangerous Drugs Act, which had little pharmacological basis. It covered the opioids, cannabis and cocaine.

During the 1960s there was an unexpected increase in illicit drug taking and the law was changed progressively in an attempt both to stem this and cope with the changes in drug-taking habits. This culminated in the Misuse of Drugs Act of 1971, which covered the original <u>Dangerous Drugs</u> and those that had become fashionable – the centrally acting sympathomimetic amines (amphetamines and some other anorectic drugs), the hallucinogens (LSD) and the barbiturate-like drug methaqualone. At that time the absence of barbiturates from the Act was a notable anomaly.

Since 1985 the barbiturates too have become <u>Controlled Drugs</u>.

(1) The Controlled Drugs are grouped into four classes (A, B, C and D) dependent on abuse potential; **morphine** is more rigidly controlled than **codeine**.
(2) Control of a drug may vary dependent on its formulation; **morphine** injection is in Class A, kaolin and morphine mixture is exempt.

Some points for discussion

Drugs have always been a part of society. Many primitive societies revolved around (usually hallucinogenic) drug cults (religions). Ethanol was established in Roman and Greek cultures and has remained so in those that succeeded them throughout Europe and the Americas. Cannabis is established in some Asian societies. Because drugs are a part of society drug laws cannot always be rational (some would argue that tobacco should be banned and ethanol put on prescription, or even controlled).

The attitude of society towards drug toxicity changes. Apart from obvious differences between what was deemed acceptable in medieval times and that acceptable now, recent changes have been:

(1) The virtual disappearance of amphetamines and barbiturates compared to their widespread use and acceptance 30 years ago.

(2) Gradual (and unpredictable) changes in the attitude of society to cannabis.
(3) The disappearance of several new NSAIDs from the market, with the re-evaluation of those of similar toxicity that have been on the market for 30 years.

Medication with legally obtained drugs occurs on a vast scale. Sales of antipyretic analgesic agents suggests a national intake of one tablet per person per day. Millions of prescriptions for psychoactive drugs are dispensed each year. It is estimated that half the number of prescription items are unnecessary (overprescribing). The issue of repeat prescriptions for patients who are exempted prescription charges encourages drug hoarding. The likelihood of a patient taking a preparation as instructed can be remote (non-compliance): 5% of all prescriptions are not even handed to a pharmacist to be dispensed. The more complicated the instructions, the greater the non-compliance. This can have serious consequences in certain conditions (notably epilepsy, p. 521). Bacterial resistance can be encouraged by erratic taking of antibiotic agents.

The influence of drug promotion (by advertising and drug company representatives) on prescribing habits in western countries becomes dominant a few years after prescribers qualify, by which time the cost of such promotion roughly equals the cost of medical education. Whilst the volume of medical information (biased and unbiased) is indeed vast, the existence of concise independent assessments of new drugs (*Prescribers' Journal, Drug and Therapeutics Bulletin*) simplifies the problem of keeping up to date.

The cost of prescriptions has increased so much that physicians are now required to restrict the drugs that they prescribe within the NHS to a limited list. The content of that list is essentially that which medical schools have been teaching for years.

Ignorance (not only on the part of the lay public) remains one of the most important contributions to drug abuse. People fail to appreciate that drugs are more or less selective poisons. Lay people commonly categorize strychnine as a poison, penicillin as a medicine, diamorphine as a drug and ethanol as none of these. Cannabis has appeared in all categories. This lack of respect for drugs as poisons contributes much to drug abuse and is also at the root of many well-meant irresponsible habits, such as handing over prescribed drugs to neighbours (irrespective of disorder or drug) or children (parent's anxiolytic agents for child's school examinations). This is the province of health education. Pharmacists are in an ideal position to act as health educators but general practitioners are regrettably seldom involved.

Summary

(1) Abuse of drugs takes many forms including overprescribing and irrational drug selection, addiction and self-poisoning.
(2) Dependence on repeated drug use shows itself as tolerance, followed by the occurrence of mental craving and sometimes also physical symptoms on attempted interruption of use.

(3) Withdrawal only gives serious physical symptoms with opioid agents and non-specific CNS depressants including benzodiazepines.

Drug design, development and testing – clinical phase

Once preliminary toxicity tests in animals show that the compound is unlikely to be toxic in man, short-term, healthy volunteer (phase I) studies are carried out. These are intended to provide quantitative and qualitative information on the absorption, metabolism and excretion of the drug and its pharmacodynamic effects. The volunteers are young and healthy, and able to give their informed consent to participate. They are usually men, as this eliminates the risk of damaging an unrecognized pregnancy (see p. 434). Volunteers are usually paid for their services but it is considered bad practice to offer such large sums that caution is outweighed by financial considerations. The risk of death or serious harm occurring to the volunteer in such studies is comparable to that involved in flying with a commercial airline.

From healthy volunteer studies, likely dosage regimens in clinical practice can often be predicted. Major differences in metabolism between experimental animals and man may also be detected.

When healthy volunteer studies and more detailed pharmacological and toxicological tests have produced favourable results, application can be made to the CSM for a clinical trials certificate. Only when the clinical trials and detailed toxicity tests have been successfully completed and confirm that the drug has the intended therapeutic efficacy and is acceptably safe, can application be made to the CSM for a product licence. Once granted, this enables the manufacturer to promote and sell the new compound under its tradename, for use in certain specified conditions. The CSM attempts to monitor the occurrence of adverse effects and the evidence of therapeutic efficacy for the whole of a product's life on the market. The most critical phase in this postmarketing (that is postproduct licence) surveillance is the first few years, when sales are expected to be highest. Should unacceptable adverse effects be detected, the CSM can modify either the indications for use of the drug, the contraindications to the use of the drug or its recommended dose. It may even recommend withdrawal of the product licence.

Evaluation of new drugs in man

The assessment of new drug action on people is conventionally divided into four phases.

Phase I: volunteer studies

Pharmacological properties (pharmacodynamic and pharmacokinetic) are assessed in a small number of healthy volunteers (often male students). The dose is gradually increased until an effect can be measured. These studies, which require local Ethics Committee but not Regulatory Authority approval, assess immediate responses to the new drug but it is not usually possible to perform long-term studies on these subjects. Sometimes, as with antitumour drugs, the first tests in people are done on patients.

Phase II: patient studies

A few patients, intensively studied in an open uncontrolled manner, are used to see if the desired pharmacodynamic effect is achieved in pathological states. For example, does the drug lower BP in patients with hypertension? These studies are usually carried out within a hospital or a special clinical trials unit.

Phase III: clinical trials

More patients are assessed less intensively. Controlled clinical trials compare the new drug with placebo and/or with established therapy (if any). The indications for the drug and its place in the therapy of a condition are identified, as are dosages and methods of administration. In some therapeutic areas comparison with placebo is considered unethical. Most phase III studies are carried out in many centres simultaneously and may even be international.

Phase IV: post-marketing surveillance

After the drug has been granted a product licence, assessment of its long-term value continues. Does it alter the underlying disease process? Why are some patients non-responsive? What is the potential of the drug for misuse or abuse? Are there any clinically relevant drug interactions? Are there important unusual adverse effects? Are there any novel indications? Is the recommended dose appropriate? In a sense this phase lasts throughout the life of the drug.

Risk versus benefit

At all stages in drug development unwanted effects are searched for and a risk versus benefit analysis is constantly being performed. For example, an effective but toxic agent is unsuitable for treating a minor illness (upper respiratory tract infection) but acceptable if successful against a currently untreatable neoplasm. Increasingly, pharmaco-economic analyses are being used to assess whether newly developed drugs are worth their unavoidably high prices. However, there is still considerable controversy over some of the techniques of pharmaco-economic evaluation.

Clinical trial design

Most trials attempt to disprove the null hypothesis that the new agent is no better than a placebo or the established treatment. Initially the trials are uncontrolled – subjects or patients are identified and the drug administered. This kind of trial is described as an open trial – both the investigator and the subject know a new substance is being given. There is great potential for subjective bias amongst both patients and investigators but it is useful to know that a beneficial response can occur.

To obtain objective data an experiment is performed comparing the drug with either an inert substance (placebo) or conventional therapy. The administration is controlled – the order of giving the two substances is regulated usually by using a random order – and is also double blind – neither the investigators nor the patients know which of the two substances is being administered at any one time.

Aims

These should be as simple and as few as possible. Clear-cut end points must be set before the trial begins. Typical of the questions asked is, after 6 weeks of therapy can drug X (in a specified dose regimen) heal more duodenal ulcers than **cimetidine** (in a specified does regimen)?

Placebo

This is pharmacologically inert (usually starch) but many beneficial and unwanted effects can be demonstrated in a blind subject, possibly mediated through endorphins and enkephalins. Tablet size, shape and colour and the method of administration each influence the response. Placebo formulations should therefore be indistinguishable from the trial drug. Similarly the expectations of the doctor influence both the response of the patient and the assessment by the doctor. For this reason the investigator must also be unable to distinguish the drug from placebo or the novel from the established therapy.

Kinds of trial

The commonest kind of trial design is the parallel groups comparison (Figure 8.12). Patients are randomly allocated to one or other treatment. Large numbers are needed to overcome problems of unsuspected bias (e.g. more smokers in one group than another). If such interfering factors are known or suspected, bias can be minimized by ensuring even distribution of the kinds of patient between the two treatment groups (stratification).

Another problem is that the trial compares populations as a whole rather than individuals. An alternative design is the cross-over trial in which each patient receives courses of treatment with both drugs but in random order. Thus each patient acts as his (or occasionally her) own control. It is necessary to incorporate a washout period to avoid the effects of the initial treatment carrying over into the second period but it does

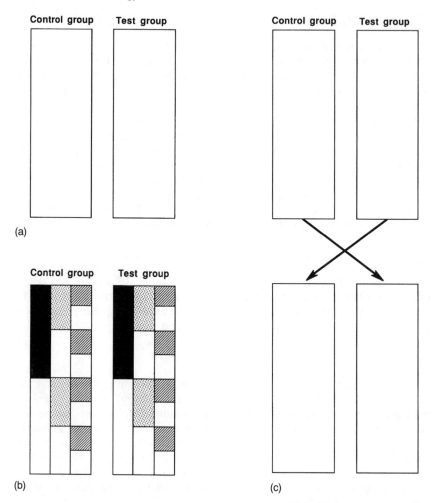

Figure 8.12 Designs of clinical trials. Parallel groups comparison, without (a) and with (b) stratification for three different interfering factors (solid, stippled, cross-hatched) that, if unequally distributed between the groups, might bias the interpretation of the outcome. Such interfering factors might include gender, age, cigarette smoking. In a cross-over design (c) each patient is his/her own control, but test and control periods occur in either order – the separating washout period is crucial

require fewer patients than a parallel groups comparison. The cross-over design is not applicable for diseases in which the first treatment radically alters the disease state (e.g. pneumonia is cured).

Ethical considerations

All trial designs should be scrutinized by a local Ethics Committee of doctors, scientists and lay people not involved in the study. The likely discomfort to the patient and the anticipated risks are discussed. The use of a placebo may be unethical when an effective remedy is available. Prior to a trial a patient must be informed of the possible risks involved and written consent must be obtained (<u>informed consent</u>). The patient must be able to withdraw at any time without detriment to the quality of the medical care provided.

Patient exclusions

Pregnant women, children, the elderly (unless specifically indicated), the acutely ill and patients with an allergic (atopic) history are not included. In volunteer studies those with abnormal findings on initial assessment are also excluded, as are patients with diseases other than that under study.

Dosage

Phase II studies should determine whether the drug has a flat dose/response curve, above a threshold, requiring a fixed dose or whether the dose must be varied according to effect or body weight.

Assessment

Objective measurement is the ideal but is not always feasible. If subjective assessment is unavoidable (e.g. the effect of an analgesic) then use of visual analogue scales reduces observer bias. Alternatively, all the investigators can be given training in the subjective assessment of the condition under study and their performance can be measured statistically until all meet predetermined levels of performance.

Unwanted effects must also be actively sought as they may not be volunteered. Patient compliance in drug taking can be assessed by measurement of blood concentrations. An alternative method is to provide a varied excess of tablets for the known interval between assessments and to count the unused tablets at each visit.

Analysis

Using the null hypothesis, treatment groups or individuals are compared using a number of statistical methods (e.g. χ^2, paired t test, analysis of variance). Further details are beyond the scope of this textbook.

Two common errors in trials are:

(1) Type 1 errors – the two treatments are not different in reality but the trial says they are – the usual reason is poor trial design or analysis.
(2) Type 2 errors – the trial result says that there is no difference between the two treatments when in fact they are different; this fault is usually due to insufficient numbers of patients in the trial, but can also result from small inter-rater reliability, inadequate stratification or inappropriate inclusion or exclusion criteria.

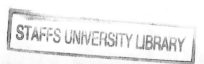
STAFFS UNIVERSITY LIBRARY

Summary

(1) New drugs are developed from preclinical research, through first use in man, to (if successful) an established place in the formulary within a legal framework and through recognizable phases.
(2) Clinical trials are used to answer questions about the effectiveness of medication (or other treatments), not just for drugs in development. They show features intended to avoid biasing the outcome.

9

Pharmacotherapeutics

Aims

- To provide a stimulus to revision of pharmacological actions and their mechanisms.
- To present information on some *BNF* drugs that are missed by the themes chosen for the bulk of the book.
- To provide insight into the pathophysiology of disease and thus a framework for the rational use of drugs in treatment.
- To introduce more of the language of medicine.
- To satisfy the desire of students of pharmacology for an understanding of the uses of drugs as medications.

Introduction

Therapeutics is the craft of the treatment of human disease and pharmacotherapeutics concentrates on the role of drugs in this process. Since this is not a textbook of medicine it is neither possible nor desirable to attempt a general coverage of disease.

The ideal form of therapy would be curative, but therapists are often forced by the lack of effective curative forms of therapy to fall back on symptomatic forms – treatments designed to alleviate symptoms. Hence the chapter headings in this section are either disease states or major symptoms. The criteria adopted for the inclusion of disease states and forms of therapy are:

(1) A disease state should be a chronic condition of relatively common occurrence.
(2) Alternatively or additionally it should be the kind of condition for which GPs and community pharmacists are often asked to advise. Since many proprietary preparations are advertised for self-medication, we have attempted to include some of them so that logical and relevant 'over the counter' advice can be given.

The process of rational therapeutics

The process of rational therapeutics depends on a number of logical sequences of deliberate steps that the prescriber should consider.

Disease process

Before considering therapy, the nature (pathophysiology) of the under-lying condition must be considered. It may be possible to make a firm diagnosis (e.g. pneumonia) that will enable the prescribing of <u>curative</u> therapy (e.g. antibacterial agents). However, in many clinical situations only symptomatic or <u>suppressive</u> treatment is possible (e.g. inhaled for asthma). Patients cannot be cured, yet suppressive therapy can still render the patient asymptomatic. Another possibility is that of <u>preventative</u> therapy on the assumption that a disease process or condition (e.g. pregnancy) can be avoided (e.g. by the use of oral contraception).

Management plan

Once the disease process has been understood and treatment goals have been set, the full range of therapeutic options should be considered. Conditions can often be controlled by the use of <u>non-drug therapy</u> (e.g. essential hypertension with weight reduction, diet modification, reduction in alcohol ingestion), thus avoiding the potential toxicity of drug therapy. Drug treatment involves the concepts of <u>selective toxicity</u> and <u>risk/benefit analysis</u>. The use of antagonists at β-receptors in a patient with hypertension is not acceptable if the patient already suffers from significant asthma, as the risk of adverse effects is too great and there are acceptable alternatives. Prescribing is not only one way, as <u>patient involvement</u> is essential, particularly for long-term therapy. Lifestyle changes may be less acceptable to some hypertensive patients than the relatively low risk of developing adverse effects from low-dose thiazide therapy.

Drug therapy

The scientific basis of rational drug prescribing is that efficacy and safety have been demonstrated by means of the <u>controlled clinical trial</u>. (In fact, less than 25% of all therapeutic interventions have been proven to be of benefit by this technique, although this figure is larger for drug therapy.) Much therapy is <u>experience based</u> or <u>anecdotal</u>, which potentially introduces the possibility of bias of the assessment of efficacy by the prescriber. Nevertheless, this may be the only basis upon which a decision can be made. The influence of the <u>placebo effect</u> should not be underestimated; patients' viral upper respiratory infections often respond rapidly to the administration of a broad-spectrum antibiotic agent despite the drug having no pharmacological effects on the virus, yet producing diarrhoea in up to 15% of patients.

Choice of drug

Factors determining drug choice include the <u>appropriate drug for a given patient</u>. **Gentamicin** is a very useful antibacterial agent in an adult but considerable caution is required for use in patients with immature kidneys (neonates) or those with renal impairment, because of the drug's known renal toxicity. The <u>route</u> of administration may be important; parenteral drug therapy is indicated if a rapid response is required (e.g. i/v **verapamil** can control a supraventricular cardiac dysrhythmia in minutes yet take days if given orally). Other important factors include the target <u>site</u> (e.g. intracerebral disease requires drugs capable of penetrating the blood–brain barrier), and the <u>appropriate dose</u>, <u>dosage form</u> and appropriate <u>duration</u> of therapy.

Response

A realistic target should be set by both the prescriber and the patient. Pain control is achievable in intractable cancer, a cure is not; a reduction in BP can be a useful measure of antihypertensive therapy.

Acute poisoning

The problem

In adults acute poisoning is commonly deliberate and self-inflicted, with the object of harming the patient or manipulating somebody else. It is typically a problem of Western Europe and North America; it is less frequent in countries with a peasant economy and Roman Catholic religion. A small proportion of such patients (less than 20%) have serious psychiatric disease. The annual incidence of hospital admission is approximately 1 : 1000 population and annual deaths (England and Wales) approximately 3000. Eighty per cent of these deaths occur outside hospital – mortality amongst hospital admissions is less than 1%.

In children acute poisoning is an accidental result of oral exploration and is commonest in boys, aged 1.5–2.5 years, social class IV, with several preschool siblings. There is a high incidence of ingestion (probably similar to adult figures), but poisoning (measurable harmful effects) is uncommon and death is rare (less than 50/year). Some poisoning deaths may however be attributed to other causes.

Drugs involved

In adults hypnotic, anxiolytic, minor analgesic, antidepressant and anticonvulsant agents are involved. Medicaments are often combined with each other and with ethanol or carbon monoxide.

STAFFS UNIVERSITY LIBRARY

Children are prone to being poisoned by a random selection of ingestible items in the environment – anything from iron salts to weed killer, contraceptive tablets to antifreeze.

Principles of management

Note the order of priorities carefully.

(1) Establish and maintain a clear airway: remove debris (vomit, mucus, dentures), suck away secretions, consider the need for an oropharyngeal airway or endotracheal tube.

(2) Ensure adequate ventilation: a tidal volume greater than 400 mL and minute volume greater than 4 L/min for adults, by mechanical means if necessary (too little leads to hypoxaemia, too much to alkalosis and hypotension).

(3) Intravenous fluid therapy has two objectives:
(a) Expansion of circulating blood volume, restoration of venous return and cardiac output. *Sodium chloride* (0.9% is isotonic with blood) and *glucose* (5%) i/v infusion are suitable. Plasma expanders (e.g. *dextrans*) may be needed.
(b) Water and salt replacement to replace fluid loss and maintain an adequate urine output (more than 15 mL/h).

(4) Decontamination: removal procedures have a low efficiency (only 20–30% of a recent dose is recovered) and a significant morbidity. Gastric lavage washes out the stomach by means of water entering, and being emptied via a wide-bore rubber tube. It is only of value with most drugs if performed less than 4 h after ingestion. Exceptions are antidepressant drugs (8 h) and salicylates (24 h). *Ipecacuanha* syrup, which directly stimulates both the medulla and the stomach to induce emesis, is still used for children and some adults and probably has comparable efficacy to lavage; however, the risk of aspiration in drowsy or unconscious patients has reduced its popularity. Increasingly, activated charcoal 10–30 g in suspension in 100–200 mL water is being used to bind unabsorbed drug (**digoxin**, *theophylline*, barbiturates, alkaloids). Other binding agents are more suited to other toxic agents – **desferrioxamine** for iron salts and *Fuller's earth* for paraquat.

(5) Convulsions may be provoked by drug overdose (**aspirin**, *theophylline*, antidepressant agents), but usually anticonvulsant drugs are not needed.

(6) Identification. Tablet identification may be difficult with old/white/discoloured preparations. The National Poisons Information Service provides useful data on the content of household cleaners, bleaches, weed killers and solvents. The hospital biochemistry service can assist with assessment of severity of poisoning by **paracetamol, aspirin,** *theophylline*, **lithium** and iron salts; the severity tends to increase with serum drug concentration.

(7) Assisted elimination of the poison is seldom required – if respiration and circulation are adequately supported, hepatic metabolism and renal excretion can eliminate the toxic agent without special assistance.

Table 9.1 Poisons with specific antagonists

Drug	Antagonist	Mechanism
Digoxin	Digoxin-specific antibody fragments	Binding
Iron salts	**Desferrioxamine**	Chelation
Lead salts	Penicillamine	Chelation
Mercury salts	Dimercaprol	Chelation
Opioid analgesic agents	**Naloxone**	Specific competitive antagonism
Organophosphorus	**Atropine** and	Antagonism of acetylcholine
anticholinesterases	**pralidoxime**	Reactivation of cholinesterase
Paracetamol	Acetylcysteine	Reduction of oxidized glutathione

Special cases

Salicylate poisoning in an adult

Alkaline diuresis increases the clearance of salicylate four-fold for each unit increase in pH. High urine pH (above 8.0) may be obtained by i/v infusion of *sodium bicarbonate* (1.4% is isotonic). The major principle is alkalinization of the urine with an adequate urine output rather than a forced diuresis.

Specific antagonists are only available for a few drugs (Table 9.1).

Summary

(1) Progress in the management of acute poisoning has been achieved by the more effective support of vital functions (respiration and circulation). Assisted elimination and drug antagonism have only a limited importance.
(2) Since mortality in hospital is so low, a further reduction of total mortality can only be achieved by removal of social causes of self-poisoning and by more restricted availability of lethal drugs (e.g. barbiturates).
(3) The reduction in the prescribing of benzodiazepines as hypnotic and anxiolytic agents has helped to reduce the frequency of self-poisoning.

Peptic ulceration

Definition

The localized loss of mucosa, submucosa and smooth muscle layers of the oesophagus (oesophageal ulcer), stomach (gastric ulcer) or of the duodenum (duodenal ulcer).

Symptoms and diagnosis

Pain is in the upper part of abdomen, usually the mid-line. Heartburn, nausea and relief of symptoms by food and antacids are common. Poor appetite and weight loss are common in the elderly. Anaemia may be present, as a result of chronic bleeding from the ulcer (see p. 530). Diagnosis requires endoscopy.

Complications

(1) Sudden and severe bleeding.
(2) Perforation with leakage of gastric contents into the abdomen causing peritonitis.
(3) Fibrotic narrowing of the pyloric outlet of the stomach.

Aetiology

Hydrochloric acid (HCl), pepsin and regurgitated bile are potential damaging agents to the mucosa. Mucus and bicarbonate secreted by the epithelial cells overly the mucosa and act as a barrier. Peptic ulceration occurs when the barrier is breached. It is now clear that one of the important factors in the development of ulceration in the duodenum and gastric mucosa is the presence of the organism *Helicobacter pylori*. This spiral bacterium colonizes the gastric antrum and ectopic gastric mucosa in the duodenum, sticking to the surface of the epithelium and surviving in a protected environment between the mucus layer and the epithelium. The presence of *H. pylori* is relatively common throughout the world and its prevalence increases with age.

In most individuals *H. pylori* produces no symptoms and only minor antral gastritis. In other individuals, for reasons that are uncertain, a peptic ulcer develops.

Virtually 100% of patients with classic duodenal ulceration have *H. pylori* in the gastric antrum.

H. pylori is sensitive to **amoxycillin** or **tetracycline** and **metronidazole** and also to *tripotassium dicitratobismuthate*.

Aims of treatment

(1) To relieve symptoms.
(2) To hasten healing.

General therapeutic measures

Determine that a gastric ulcer is not malignant by endoscopic biopsy. Symptoms are reduced by small frequent meals, stopping smoking and avoiding ethanol and any food that makes the symptoms worse. The use of NSAIDs and glucocorticosteroids should be reduced to a minimum. There is a 40% spontaneous cure rate for gastric and duodenal ulcers but both are also highly likely to recur periodically.

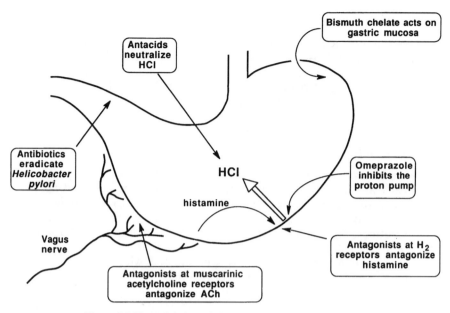

Figure 9.1 Sites of action of drugs useful in peptic ulceration

Symptomatic therapy

Antacids may be used intermittently for the symptomatic management of pain. They are weak bases that neutralize HCl, so the pH of the luminal contents transiently becomes greater than 4 and pepsin is inactive (Figure 9.1). The action of antacids is brief due to their rapid removal from the stomach and duodenum.

Sodium bicarbonate can alter ECF pH to give a metabolic alkalosis and alkaline urine. It is not therefore suitable for prolonged use.

Magnesium hydroxide and aluminium hydroxide are little absorbed. Mg^{2+} is laxative and Al^{3+} causes constipation.

Magnesium trisilicate has a slow onset and relatively prolonged action. On reaction with HCl it forms a hydrated silicic acid that is adsorbent of pepsin.

Therapy that promotes healing

Antagonists at H_2 histamine receptors

Histamine is involved in the final common pathway of stimuli that cause acid and pepsin secretion. **Cimetidine** and *ranitidine* reduce fasting and stimulated acid and pepsin secretion by antagonizing histamine (Figure 9.1).

Inhibitors of acid secretion by the parietal cells

The secretion of acid by the parietal cell requires a specific proton pump enzyme (H^+/K^+-ATPase) located on the luminal membrane of the cell. **Omeprazole** inhibits this pump and virtually abolishes acid secretion. Short-term healing of peptic ulcer is more rapid and effective with this than with other agents. **Omeprazole** has mild to moderate effectiveness against *H. pylori*. Long-term effects are not yet known.

Improvement of mucosal barrier

Tripotassium dicitratobismuthate, a colloidal bismuth chelate, appears to act locally at the site of the ulcer, preventing access by acid and pepsin. The drug is only partially absorbed but this is sufficient to prevent its long-term use; heavy metal poisoning with bismuth may occur. Less serious adverse effects include a bad taste and black discoloration of the mouth and stools.

   Tripotassium dicitratobismuthate is equi-effective with antagonists at H_2 histamine receptors at short-term ulcer healing.

Surgery

Surgery may be used if medical treatment fails or there are dangerous complications (continued or recurrent haemorrhage). It usually involves selective division of the vagal nerve supply to the antrum of the stomach, thus reducing or abolishing the neural component of acid secretion.

Therapy that reduces relapse of ulcer

Although suppression of acid secretion can allow the healing of most peptic ulcers, relapse is common. For patients with frequent symptomatic relapses, regular nocturnal therapy with antagonists at H_2 histamine receptors is effective in providing long-term relief of symptoms.

   Relapses are reduced in patients in whom *H. pylori* has been eliminated. While the precise aetiological role of Helicobacter in ulcer development is yet to be determined, there is now good evidence that eradication of the organism helps to prevent symptomatic relapse. Colloidal bismuth compounds have the ability to kill Helicobacter and, when used in combination with antibiotic agents, particularly **amoxycillin** and **metronidazole**, can achieve eradication of the organism in many patients. Alternative regimens include **omeprazole** in high dose coupled with antibacterial agents as above. Such therapies are likely to become increasingly important in the future.

Summary

(1) Peptic ulcers produce a characteristic clinical presentation, yet diagnosis requires endoscopy (and biopsy for a gastric ulcer). The natural history is of spontaneous healing and recurrence.

(2) Tobacco smoking, alcohol consumption, and use of NSAIDs and glucocorticosteroids make symptoms worse. Antacids relieve symptoms briefly.
(3) Therapy that promotes healing includes antagonists at H$_2$ histamine receptors and inhibitors of the proton pump, that reduce HCl secretion, and *tripotassium dicitratobismuthate.*
(4) Therapy that prevents recurrence includes maintenance treatment with antagonists at H$_2$ histamine receptors and eradication of *H. pylori* with antibacterial agents and either *tripotassium dicitratobismuthate* or **omeprazole**.

Inflammatory bowel disease

Definition

Ulcerative colitis is chronic inflammation of the mucosa of the rectum and colon. Crohn's disease is a patchy chronic inflammation that can affect any part of the gastrointestinal tract. The causes are not known.

Symptoms

Painless bloody diarrhoea is the usual symptom of *ulcerative colitis*. Persistent disease can lead to malnutrition and anaemia. Dilatation and perforation of the colon may occur.

Crohn's disease is associated with similar symptoms to ulcerative colitis but abdominal pain and malnutrition are more frequent, as are mouth ulcers and anal involvement.

General therapeutic measures

Maintain an adequate and balanced diet; artificial feeding may be required.

Symptomatic treatment

Drugs causing constipation

Drugs causing constipation (see below) may be used in mild disease but should be used with extreme care in more severe cases, since they may mask the development of serious complications.

Glucocorticosteroids

Glucocorticosteroids, either by the oral, rectal or i/v route, induce remission by their anti-inflammatory effects but do not remove the underlying cause. Adverse effects limit long-term maintenance therapy.

5-Aminosalicylate (5-ASA) compounds

Sulphasalazine is useful for mild relapses and for maintenance therapy. Its efficacy is due to the 5-ASA moiety of the molecule, which is split from the sulphonamide conjugate by the action of colonic bacteria.

Mesalazine is 5-ASA; the drug is usually employed as a delayed release formulation – it is coated by a resin that delays release until the lower gut is reached.

Olsalazine is a 5-ASA dimer split into two active 5-ASA molecules by colonic bacteria, thus avoiding the use of the sulphonamide component of *sulphasalazine*.

Immunosuppression

More powerful immunosuppressant drugs (*azathioprine*) may be used in patients with severe disease in whom surgery is contraindicated.

Surgery

Ulcerative colitis

Removal of the affected part including the rectum, with the consequent need for an ileostomy (artificial opening of the small intestine through the front of abdomen) or construction of an ileo-anal anastomosis, enables a return to an active life.

Crohn's disease

Resection should be limited to only severely affected areas. In contrast to ulcerative colitis, the disease can recur.

Gastrointestinal motility disorder

Diarrhoea

Aetiology

In the small intestine the contents are liquid. The small bowel, caecum and the proximal colon absorb Na^+, K^+ and Cl^- and the bulk of the water. The distal colon absorbs Na^+ in exchange for K^+, this process being influenced by aldosterone. Water is absorbed, so producing soft but not watery faeces. If the time in the gastrointestinal tract is too short or there is malabsorption of nutrient due to damage to the pancreas or small intestinal mucosa, or if there is inflammation resulting in incomplete water absorption, then diarrhoea results.

Causes

(1) Viruses (gastroenteritis) especially in children.
(2) Bacteria (bacterial food poisoning), usually due to heat-stable toxins (staphylococcal, *E. coli*), but can be infective (Salmonella, bacillary dysentery). Superinfection (Staphylococci, *Cl. difficile*) during treatment with a broad-spectrum antibiotic.
(3) Fungi, usually *Candida albicans*, by superinfection during treatment with an orally administered broad-spectrum antibiotic.
(4) Protozoa or metazoa (amoebic dysentery, worm infestation).
(5) Organic disease of the colon (Crohn's disease, ulcerative colitis).
(6) Malabsorption syndrome due to small intestinal or pancreatic disease.
(7) Consequence of gut resection.
(8) Drugs – **cimetidine**, diuretic agents, cytotoxic drugs, **digoxin**, tetracyclines, **ampicillin**, magnesium salts, abuse of purgative agents, antagonists at β-adrenoceptors.
(9) Emotion.
(10) Disturbance of endocrine control (hyperthyroidism).

Treatment

The underlying disorder should be diagnosed and treated.

General therapeutic measures

Many episodes of diarrhoea, especially viral and bacterial, are short-lived and self-limiting. Severe diarrhoea (especially in infants, elderly people or in tropical climates) may lead to dehydration needing replacement therapy with i/v or oral electrolytes. An orally administered solution containing sugar and NaCl (oral rehydration salts) makes use of the linked sodium/glucose absorption mechanism.

Symptomatic treatment

(1) Opioids (**codeine, morphine, loperamide**, see p. 245). These drugs reduce secretion, decrease the propulsive intestinal contractions and increase the tone of colonic muscles and sphincters, allowing increased water absorption. **Loperamide** displays slight selectivity for peripheral enteric neural versus central actions and may be useful for long-term, non-infective diarrhoea in adults.
(2) Adsorbents (kaolin). These are said to adsorb bacteria and toxins. They are commonly used with **morphine**.
(3) Bulk-forming agents (*bran, methylcellulose*) absorb water so solidifying stools in diarrhoea.
(4) Antibiotic agents have no place in self-limiting viral or bacterial toxin-induced diarrhoea. Their use can be complicated by bacterial or fungal superinfection (see p. 313). However *Cl. difficile* infection, usually induced by broad-spectrum antibiotic agents, can be treated by oral **vancomycin** or **metronidazole**. It is appropriate to treat diarrhoea caused by invasive bacteria that result in more than mild dysentery, for example Shigellae with antibiotic agents (**ciprofloxacin**).

Constipation

Aetiology

If the passage of contents through the colon is unduly prolonged there is greater water absorption therefore constipation.

Causes

(1) Diet containing too little fibre and fermentable carbohydrate.
(2) Prolonged bed rest.
(3) Habitual denial of defaecatory urges.
(4) Organic obstruction of colon (carcinoma, strictures, diverticular disease).
(5) Drugs – opioids (see p. 245), antagonists at muscarinic acetylcholine receptors (see p. 69), aluminium-containing antacids (see p. 463).
(6) Disturbance of endocrine control (hypothyroidism).
(7) Neuropathy or myopathy.

If faeces stagnate and harden, straining may prolapse and thrombose haemorrhoidal veins (piles) or tear the anus. Painfulness of defaecation may make constipation worse.

Specific treatment

The underlying disorder should be diagnosed and treated.

General therapeutic measures

Encourage a well-balanced diet with roughage and exercise. Explain that the frequency of defaecation is very variable. Try to establish a habitual time for defaecation.

Symptomatic treatment

Chronic use of laxative agents may damage the colon and result in an atonic bowel and therefore is contraindicated. Defaecation is promoted by increased colonic or small intestinal propulsive motility and altered electrolyte transport – the exact mechanism of action is unknown for most drugs. One classification is as follows:

Bulk-forming laxative agents

Bran and *methylcellulose* swell in water to form a gel, which maintains hydrated, soft faeces. The bulk promotes peristalsis. The onset of action is slow (approximately 24 h). This group is preferred for long-term use.

Emollient laxative agents

These act by direct softening of the faeces. *Docusate* lowers surface tension, which may explain its action. *Glycerol* [glycerin] suppositories act by softening faeces.

Osmotic laxative agents
Magnesium salts (e.g. sulphate) are poorly absorbed from the digestive tract and so retain water by osmosis; peristalsis is increased indirectly. There is a fairly rapid onset of action (2–3 h). A sodium *phosphates* enema acts as an osmotic laxative.

Stimulant laxative agents
Their action is to alter water and electrolyte transport as well as to stimulate intestinal motility. The effective dose varies considerably from patient to patient. They act approximately 8 h after ingestion. *Bisacodyl* is, in part, absorbed, conjugated in the liver, excreted in the bile and deconjugated by bacteria in the colon to exert its action there. The anthraquinone senna is a prodrug metabolized by bacteria in the colon to the active aglycone.

Congestive heart failure

Definitions

A syndrome resulting from a chronically impaired contractility of the heart (interfering with its efficiency as a pump) and the homeostatic compensations for this.

Pathophysiological

Depression of the (Frank–Starling) curve relating cardiac ventricular performance to the ventricular filling pressure.

Clinical

In clinical practice congestive heart failure is identified by the presence of salt and water retention, an enlarged, tender liver and pulmonary congestion. An inadequate cardiac output causes fatigue, pulmonary congestion causes breathlessness when lying flat or on exertion, and fluid retention causes oedema (ankle swelling).

Aetiology and pathophysiology

Aetiology

There are background causes of impaired contractility on which are usually superimposed precipitating factors, bringing about a further impairment and the development of the syndrome. Hypertension, atrial fibrillation, anaemia, hyperthyroidism and the use of salt-retaining drugs are factors, the effects of which can be reversed. Damage to the heart valves (congenital, rheumatic or infective) and the most common cause, coronary vascular obstruction, are more difficult to influence.

STAFFS UNIVERSITY LIBRARY

Pathophysiology

The slow onset of impaired cardiac pumping allows time for the development of compensatory changes that, to some extent, offset the direct ill effects of low cardiac output but produce their own, different, symptomatology.

The <u>forward features</u> of cardiac failure are those that originate in the insufficiency of cardiac output. They include easy fatiguability (at first on exercise but progressing until present at rest), peripheral cyanosis and salt and water retention – due to underperfusion of muscle, skin and kidney respectively. Patterned vasoconstriction (brain, heart and skeletal muscle are spared at the expense of skin, gut and kidney vascular beds), tachycardia and positive inotropic action are the noradrenergically mediated responses to decreased output (triggered by baroreceptors). (Antagonists at β-adrenoceptors are contraindicated because cardiac performance is supported through activation of β-adrenoceptors.)

Central venous pressure increases (due to expanded ECF volume and constriction of veins) and increased atrial priming adds to increased passive ventricular filling, bringing about the Frank–Starling improvement in ventricular performance. The ventricles may dilate to the point of stretching the AV ring (functional valvular incompetence) and the ventricular muscle hypertrophies.

The <u>backward features</u> of cardiac failure are those that originate in the increased central venous pressure. High pressure within pulmonary veins, backwards (upstream) from the left ventricle, makes for stiff lungs (reduced compliance) and breathlessness (at first on exercise but progressing until present at rest).

High pressure within the venae cavae backwards from the right ventricle, causes the liver to become congested.

Renal underperfusion promotes renin release and hence (via the angiotensins) secondary hyperaldosteronism (see pp. 181, 197) – distal tubular NaCl and water retention with K^+ and H^+ loss. The exaggerated NaCl and water retention increases the circulating blood volume and also the interstitial fluid volume, which makes oedema inevitable. The increased venous pressure and gravity localize it. These are the backward features of failure.

The compensatory processes alleviate the forward features at the expense of aggravating the backward features.

Treatment

General measures include the treatment of any precipitating factors, anaemia (see p. 528), thyrotoxicosis (see p. 177), cardiac dysrhythmia (see p. 113), infection (see p. 302) and fever and avoidance of salt-retaining steroids or NSAIDs.

There are three aims of therapy, which are detailed below.

Reduce cardiac work

The patient should rest from physical activity (but this increases the risk of deep vein thrombosis) and, if obese, restrict calorie intake. Treat hypertension (see p. 475).

Vasodilator agents

Vasodilator agents decrease ventricular end-diastolic pressure. Venular dilatation (nitrates), or mixed venular and arteriolar vasodilatation (**capto-pril**) reduce either the <u>pre-load</u> (ventricular end-diastolic pressure; controlled mainly by the state of the capacitance vessels) or <u>after-load</u> (diastolic BP; controlled mainly by the state of the resistance vessels) upon the ventricles. Venular dilatation improves the backward features of failure. Tachycardia and postural hypotension are unwanted effects with arterial, venular or mixed site dilators but are generally less severe with venular dilators.

Inhibitors of ACE (e.g. **captopril**, *enalapril*, see p. 197) reduce renin secretion and thus arteriolar resistance and also reduce aldosterone production, which decreases sodium and water retention. They are the only drugs in the treatment of heart failure that have been shown to increase longevity and are the mainstay of current therapy.

Arteriolar dilatation allows the ventricles to achieve higher cardiac output at lower working pressures and hence improves the forward features of failure. Tachycardia, postural hypotension and fluid retention (except with **captopril**) are unwanted effects.

Nitrates (see pp. 137, 337, 482) can be given by the oral, sublingual, buccal, i/v or transcutaneous routes.

Decrease pulmonary congestion and peripheral oedema

Diuretic therapy is indicated – start with a thiazide (**bendrofluazide**, see p. 136), which has a shallow dose/response curve. If the response is inadequate change to a loop diuretic. The response is aided by a moderate reduction in dietary salt intake to approximately 80 mmole Na^+ daily.

Potassium supplements (effervescent potassium salts) may be required (especially in elderly patients) when loop or thiazide diuretic agents are prescribed for heart failure; the K^+-losing action of these diuretic agents adds to that of the secondary hyperaldosteronism (contrast with essential hypertension in which potassium salt supplements are rarely needed when a thiazide is prescribed, see p. 475).

K^+-sparing diuretic agents are **amiloride** and *triamterene* (see p.138) and **spironolactone** (an antagonist of aldosterone). They have a relatively low clinical efficacy when used alone. **Amiloride** is best used in combination with a loop diuretic agent in patients in whom it is important to maintain a normal serum K^+ concentration. Stop potassium salt supplements when adding **amiloride** or another K^+-sparing diuretic. Never use **amiloride** together with another K^+-sparing diuretic drug (risk of hyperkalaemia). Patients who are taking these diuretic agents and also an inhibitor of ACE need careful monitoring of serum K^+ concentration.

Increase cardiac output

Low cardiac output is commonly due to myocardial ischaemia (coronary artery disease). The capacity for increasing the cardiac output (contractility) is greatest with valvular heart disease, atrial fibrillation or hypertensive heart disease.

Digoxin

Digoxin increases myocardial contractility (positive inotropic effect, see p. 122), which allows the cardiac output to be maintained at a lower ventricular filling pressure.

It slows the ventricular rate in atrial fibrillation, thus allowing a longer diastolic filling time, which reduces pulmonary congestion. The ventricular rate should not be depressed below 60/min.

It has a small therapeutic index – the toxic dose (nausea, heart block, ectopic ventricular beats) is very close to the therapeutic dose, especially if there is K^+ depletion. This is another indication for potassium salt supplementation. An oral loading dose of **digoxin** may be given, succeeded by a once-daily oral maintenance dose. Dosage reduction is imperative in the elderly and others with renal impairment (see p. 384).

When **digoxin** therapy has been given for 3 months to patients in sinus rhythm, it is doubtful if continuation is either necessary or beneficial. Prescription should certainly be reviewed regularly and not repeated automatically.

Sympathomimetic agents

By virtue of their agonist action at cardiac β_1-adrenoceptors (see p. 96), *dopamine* and *dobutamine* can increase the stroke volume of the failing heart. The associated undesirable tachycardia is limited by the admixed agonist action at vascular α_1-adrenoceptors causing vasoconstriction, increase in BP, baroreceptor activation and reflex restraint on the cardiac pacemaker.

Dopamine is also an agonist at renal vasodilator dopamine receptors. The $t_{1/2}$ of *dopamine* is 2 min and so it can only effectively be given by i/v infusion. A lower dose rate results in an increase in renal perfusion. Higher dose rates increase the cardiac output but the renal effect is lost. *Dopamine* should only be given into a central vein, as peripheral vasoconstriction can become the dominant response otherwise.

Dobutamine, likewise, has a $t_{1/2}$ of only 2 min, hence its administration by i/v infusion. A logical treatment of heart failure associated with hypotension (cardiogenic shock) is a combination of *dobutamine* and low-dose *dopamine*. *Dobutamine* can be given via a standard peripheral venous cannula.

Pulmonary oedema – left ventricular failure

If the left ventricle fails before, or more severely than, the right, the backward features of the failure are localized to the pulmonary vascular circuit.

Pulmonary oedema occurs when the pulmonary capillary pressure exceeds the osmotic pressure exerted by the plasma proteins (principally albumin). Urgent reduction of pulmonary congestion is required. Sit the patient up. Administer 60% oxygen (mask flow rate 6 L/min). Give a loop diuretic agent i/v (**frusemide**, see p. 137) for its rapid onset of action, steep dose/response curve and possible dilatation of pulmonary veins before diuretic action. Unwanted effects include gastrointestinal upsets, bone marrow depression and, rarely, reversible ototoxicity.

The distress and severe dyspnoea of acute pulmonary oedema can be relieved with **morphine** i/v, which also promotes venous pooling and reduction of venous return.

Summary

(1) Congestive heart failure is a syndrome resulting from chronic under-performance of the heart together with, and usually dominated by, the homeostatic changes in physiological state that the body makes in compensation.
(2) Treatment should reverse any precipitating factor, such as anaemia, thyrotoxicosis, cardiac dysrhythmia, infection, fever and use of drugs that promote salt and water retention.
(3) Reduce the cardiac work with rest, reduction of obesity and treatment of hypertension. Vasodilator agents, inhibitors of ACE or nitrates, are effective.
(4) Decrease pulmonary congestion and peripheral oedema with diuretic agents (avoid potassium depletion).
(5) Increase cardiac output by judicious use of positive inotropic agents.
(6) For acute pulmonary oedema a loop diuretic agent and **morphine** are effective.

Hypertension and antihypertensive drugs

General principles

Hypertension (high BP) is the product of many complex physiological and pathological interactions. In normal individuals systolic BP increases with age and is higher on waking than in the afternoon and evening. Long-term hypertension is associated with vascular damage and other complications, to an extent proportional to the prevailing BP. The threshold for treat-ment should be decided on the evidence from controlled clinical trials that have demonstrated the degree of benefit to be gained by groups of patients from intervention at particular BP levels. For adults, benefit has now been shown from treating patients whose systolic BP remains above 160 mmHg after a 6-month period of observation. Sustained diastolic BP above 105 mmHg should also be treated. Because BP usually declines with repeated measurements, at least three measurements of BP over three separate visits are required to obtain readings equivalent to the entry BP used in clinical trials, except for patients with severe hypertension (see below).

Classification

Hypertension can be classified on the basis of the recorded diastolic BP. The hypertension is considered:

(1) Mild with a diastolic BP of 90–105 mmHg (after three or more readings).
(2) Moderate with 105–120 mmHg (after three or more readings).
(3) Severe with greater than 120 mmHg (after two or more readings).

In patients with severe hypertension there is a 50% probability that a first degree relative will also have hypertension. The genetic basis for hypertension is currently being defined using the techniques of molecular biology. High BP in relatively young individuals without a strong family history generally prompts a search for an underlying cause. In 10% of such patients hypertension is secondary to underlying renal disease. Polycystic renal disease should be evident from its autosomal dominant pattern of inheritance (see Figure 8.4). Renal artery stenosis is more commonly found in those patients with extensive atheroma in other vessels. Catecholamine-secreting phaeochromocytoma or aldosterone-secreting adrenal adenoma only account for 1 in every 5000 unselected hypertensive patients.

The current clinical approach is to treat hypertension along with other risk factors for cardiovascular disease. These include smoking, obesity and hypercholesterolaemia. Drugs such as NSAIDs and oestrogens can have an adverse effect on BP control.

Consequences of hypertension

The higher the sustained arterial BP the higher the mortality from coronary artery disease and stroke. Severe hypertension may progress to an accelerated or malignant phase. This is characterized by damage to small arteries in the retina, resulting in haemorrhages and exudates, and to arterioles in the kidney, resulting in albuminuria and impaired renal function.

Antihypertensive treatment

The treatment of accelerated or malignant hypertension is life-saving. (Before treatment was available, 90% of such patients died within 12–18 months.) The beneficial effects of treating moderate hypertension are less dramatic. Reduction of BP to below 161 mmHg systolic and 91 mmHg diastolic reduces the subsequent incidence of stroke by 45% but that of myocardial infarction by only 18%. For patients with mild hypertension large trials have shown a significant reduction in stroke, but for individual patients the change in absolute risk is small.

The underlying haemodynamic abnormality in patients with sustained hypertension is an increase in peripheral resistance. This can be reduced either directly, by modifying the contractile biochemistry of resistance vessels, or indirectly by interfering with their noradrenergic vasoconstrictor supply. Reducing peripheral resistance by either mechanism results in a compensatory increase in cardiac output, which partially restores the BP. Therefore drugs that depress the cardiac output (e.g. by interfering with the cardiac noradrenergic activity) work well in combination with vasodilator agents. In theory an antagonist at both α- and β-adrenoceptors should be effective, but achieving the optimum balance between α- and β-blockade in a single molecule has proved difficult.

Antihypertensive drugs

These came into clinical use in the late 1950s. The first agents included diuretics and antagonists at α-adrenoceptors. In the late 1960s and early 1970s, antagonists at β-adrenoceptors gained prominence. Blockers of L-type Ca^{2+} channels and inhibitors of ACE came into general use in the 1980s.

Diuretic agents

The thiazides (e.g. **bendrofluazide**) constitute the major group of diuretic agents used as antihypertensive agents. These drugs exert an antihypertensive action through increased Na^+ excretion and a reduction in ECF volume in the short term. Na^+ depletion stimulates the renin-angiotensin-aldosterone system, resulting in a compensatory increase in Na^+ reabsorption by the kidney after the first few weeks of therapy. The long-term antihypertensive actions of diuretic agents are the result of vasodilatation produced by the opening of potassium ion channels in vascular smooth muscle, leading to membrane hyperpolarization and relaxation. In the Medical Research Council trial for the treatment of mild hypertension the annual incidence of impotence for patients taking **bendrofluazide** at high dosage was 3%. This side-effect is reversible within 8 weeks of stopping therapy.

Antagonists at β_1-adrenoceptors

Antagonists at β_1-adrenoceptors (beta-blockers, see p. 100) possess antihypertensive properties, yet attempts to define their site of action have yielded no definite answer. Each of three mechanisms has some experimental evidence in its favour and a combination of actions seems likely.
    These mechanisms are:

(1) A reduction in cardiac output.
(2) An inhibition of renin release.
(3) An interference with CNS pathways involved in BP control.

Although antagonists at β_1-adrenoceptors may precipitate cardiac failure in patients with limited cardiac reserve, the majority of hypertensive

STAFFS UNIVERSITY LIBRARY

patients self-evidently have good left ventricular function. They may produce bronchospasm (by blocking β_2-adrenoceptors). They indirectly enhance the vasoconstrictor activity of noradrenaline, which can result in cold hands (Raynaud's phenomenon) and more severe claudication. In insulin-dependent diabetic patients they may mask the sympathetically mediated sweating and tremor that can warn the patient of impending hypoglycaemia. Hepatic glycogenolysis may also be impaired. Lipid-soluble antagonists at β-adrenoceptors (e.g. **propranolol**) may produce sleep disturbance marked by vivid dreams; this is less likely with water-soluble β-blockers (e.g. **atenolol**).

The antagonists at β-adrenoceptors are widely used. They counter symptoms of sympatho-adrenal overactivity, which are common in young hypertensive patients or when vasodilator agents are prescribed. **Atenolol** is excreted by the kidney and has a plasma $t_{1/2}$, which allows once-daily administration. It works effectively in combination with vasodilator or thiazide diuretic agents.

Vasodilator agents

The vasodilator agents form the most diverse group of antihypertensive drugs and all reduce peripheral resistance. With most members of this group this results in an initial tachycardia, mediated by the baroreceptor reflex. This compensatory response can be blocked by using an antagonist at β-adrenoceptors, thereby reducing symptoms associated with noradrenergic activation and enhancing the antihypertensive effect.

The vasodilator agents fall into two groups – directly and indirectly acting.

Directly acting vasodilator agents

These modify the electromechanical properties of the vascular smooth muscle contractile process.

Blockers of L-type Ca^{2+} channels

Nifedipine and **verapamil** reduce the influx of Ca^{2+} (see p. 125) into vascular smooth muscle that occurs during stimulation by vasoconstrictor agents. **Nifedipine** has a greater effect on peripheral vascular smooth muscle, while **verapamil** has a greater effect on cardiac conduction tissue. **Nifedipine** causes a reduction in peripheral resistance and in BP. **Verapamil** slows the heart rate and is also useful as an antidysrhythmic agent. It may cause heart block and concurrent use with antagonists at β-adrenoceptors is best avoided as the combination may cause heart block and/or cardiac failure. *Amlodipine* resembles **nifedipine** but has a longer plasma $t_{1/2}$ and therefore can be given once daily. There are few contraindications to the use of **nifedipine**. Headaches, flushing and palpitations are common initial unwanted effects, which result from vasodilatation; these can be avoided by starting medication at low dosage.

Inhibitors of ACE

Captopril, *enalapril* and other drugs within this group inhibit the ACE in the lungs and the vascular endothelium (see p. 196), thereby blocking the production of the vasoconstrictor agent angiotensin II. ACE also breaks down the vasodilator peptide, bradykinin, and impaired metabolism of this substance may also contribute to the reduction in BP.

Blocking the production of angiotensin II reduces the production of aldosterone, resulting in an increase in plasma potassium concentration. Because diuretic agents stimulate renin, angiotensin and aldosterone production, inhibitors of ACE and diuretic agents, when given together, act synergistically. The inhibition of ACE counters the compensatory response of the renin-angiotensin system to diuretic therapy. This effect is so powerful that inhibitors of ACE should only be introduced at low dosage to patients already taking diuretic agents. There must be careful monitoring for postural hypotension and reduction in renal function.

The –SH group within **captopril** can cause alteration of taste (ageusia) and the short $t_{1/2}$ necessitates multiple daily dosage. The longer-acting inhibitors of ACE (e.g. *enalapril*) have therefore found favour in the treatment of hypertension but all inhibitors of ACE can induce a persistent dry cough and, very rarely, angio-oedema.

Indirectly acting vasodilator agents

These modify the function of noradrenergic mechanisms either in the CNS or in the periphery.

Drugs that act on the cardiovascular control centres
These drugs are thought to act by reducing the frequency of efferent impulses to peripheral noradrenergic nerves. *Methyldopa* is converted to α-methylnoradrenaline, a potent agonist at presynaptic $α_2$-adrenoceptors on noradrenergic neurone terminals.

Tiredness, lethargy, drowsiness and depression are common unwanted effects, probably reflecting reduced noradrenergic transmission elsewhere in the CNS. Although the use of centrally acting drugs is now small, *methyldopa* is still the drug of choice for treating hypertension in pregnancy because of its established safety.

Selective antagonists at postsynaptic $α_1$-adrenoceptors
Prazosin, and the longer-acting *doxazosin*, are selective antagonists at $α_1$-adrenoceptors. They dilate both arteriolar and venous smooth muscle. Postural hypotension is a common initial unwanted effect that can be circumvented by giving a small first dose on retiring to bed. Tachyphylaxis can develop and necessitate frequent alterations in drug dosage. Retrograde ejaculation (into the lumen of the bladder rather than the external urethra) is a possible unwanted effect as antagonism at adrenoceptors causes relaxation of the bladder neck.

Labetalol (and, more recently, carvedilol) combine within one molecule antagonism at β- and α-adrenoceptors. With *labetalol* the effects of antagonism at α-adrenoceptors predominate; a more balanced action is claimed for carvedilol.

Selection of an antihypertensive drug

Antihypertensive drug treatment is often commenced in early middle age and continues thereafter. The long-term safety of diuretic agents and antagonists at β-adrenoceptors has been tested in trials lasting up to 5 years. The results show that these drugs have no adverse effect on all causes of mortality whilst reducing the incidence of stroke by nearly 50%. Although there have been no similar trials for blockers of L-type Ca^{2+} channels or inhibitors of ACE, it appears that lowering BP *per se* rather than the class of drug used is the important factor.

Long-term drug therapy requires confidence by both patient and doctor in the efficacy of drug treatment. Untreated hypertensive patients are usually free of symptoms; any unwanted effects induced by drug treatment are usually resented by the patient and result in failure to continue drug therapy. Patient compliance is improved by using a single drug given once daily rather than a multiple drug regimen requiring divided doses at different times of the day.

In the recent past diuretic agents and antagonists at β-adrenoceptors were recommended as standard first-line therapy for hypertension. However, these agents, together with blockers of L-type Ca^{2+} channels and inhibitors of ACE, are now all regarded as first-line agents.

Treatment of severe hypertension

In severe hypertension it is necessary to lower BP but it is safer if this can be done in a controlled manner with oral therapy because rapid reduction in BP in such cases may lead to reduced cerebral perfusion and subsequent cerebral infarction.

Nifedipine capsules can be readily obtained from ward stocks. Biting the capsules results in rapid absorption of **nifedipine** and a speedy onset of action. The initial dose can be repeated 4-hourly until a satisfactory reduction in BP has been achieved (or 24 h has elapsed). If there has been no reduction in BP after the second dose, then a short-acting antagonist at β-adrenoceptors (e.g. *metoprolol*) can be added. In severe hypertension, not associated with acute renal failure, the circulating blood volume is reduced and diuretics are not of benefit in initial therapy.

Treatment for hypertensive emergencies

General

Hypertensive emergencies are rare. However, if diastolic BP is greater than 130 mmHg, or in the presence of eclampsia, hypertensive encephalopathy, acute aneurysm of the aorta, or acute left ventricular failure, the BP needs to be lowered urgently. A reliable method of reducing BP in these circumstances is by controlled *sodium nitroprusside* infusion.

Sodium nitroprusside

Sodium nitroprusside is a nitrovasodilator agent, which activates soluble guanylyl cyclase in both arteries and veins (see p. 132). Its action is very rapid (1–2 min) and wanes rapidly on cessation of infusion which is usually given via a constant infusion pump. In the blood, the drug is broken down to CN⁻, which is converted to thiocyanate in the liver. It can therefore only be given for up to 12 h before thiocyanate toxicity occurs.

Phaeochromocytoma

This is a tumour of chromaffin cells derived from the sympathetic chain and most commonly found in the adrenal medulla. The tumour contains large quantities of catecholamines, which may be released on an intermittent, paroxysmal basis causing marked surges in BP. Such tumours are slow growing and the circulation partially adapts to the high catecholamine concentrations. If patients are treated with **phenoxybenzamine** (an antagonist at α-adrenoceptors) and **propranolol** (an antagonist at β-adrenoceptors), the circulation responds to this pharmacological blockade by a reduction in BP and an expansion in the circulating blood volume. Drug treatment before surgery reduces the risk from sudden surges in BP when the tumour is handled during surgery, and from a precipitous reduction in BP once the tumour is removed.

Primary aldosteronism

Spironolactone is a specific competitive antagonist of aldosterone. In patients with proven excessive production of aldosterone from an adrenal adenoma, **spironolactone** (over 6–8 weeks) corrects hypokalaemia and reduces BP values to those that could be expected after surgical removal of the adenoma. Unfortunately, if the excessive BP has been sustained for many years, structural narrowing of the resistance vessels may result in a degree of persisting hypertension, even when the primary cause has been removed.

Cost-effective therapy

The annual cost to the NHS of a single antihypertensive drug can range from £2 to £200. Pharmacological therapy for young patients with mild hypertension results in huge expenditure year on year. The benefit in terms of fewer strokes will not be felt for many years. In financial terms this is a poor investment. The cost/benefit ratio can be improved by prescribing the cheapest drugs for patients with mild hypertension. In elderly patients, or those with severe hypertension, the cost/benefit ratio is more favourable as shorter periods of treatment are required before significant reductions in the incidence of stroke are achieved.

The full benefits of drug therapy are only delivered when target BP levels are maintained. The process of clinical audit should be used to monitor the effectiveness of antihypertensive therapy.

Summary

(1) Lifelong treatment of symptomless primary hypertension reduces mortality from its vascular complications, coronary artery disease and stroke. Quantitatively this benefit is greater the higher the BP. Risk factors of cardiovascular disease (smoking, obesity, hypercholesterolaemia) should be minimized.
(2) The drugs of first choice must have minimal unwanted effects, to promote continued compliance, and minimal cost. Compliance is greatest with a single drug given once daily.
(3) Thiazide diuretics are effective in relatively low dosage, probably by initial reduction in circulating blood volume, with later reduction in peripheral resistance due to arteriolar vasodilatation.
(4) Antagonists at β-adrenoceptors are effective, probably by initial reduction in positive cardiac output responses to sympatho-adrenal excitation combined with inhibition of renin release and a CNS action.
(5) Vasodilator agents are effective by reducing peripheral resistance. Blockers of L-type Ca^{2+} channels and inhibitors of ACE are effective.

Angina of effort

Ischaemic heart disease may manifest itself as stable angina pectoris, unstable angina, acute myocardial infarction or sudden death. The basic underlying pathology of these different clinical syndromes is myocardial ischaemia produced by narrowing of the coronary arteries, due to atherosclerosis. This degenerative process can develop in individuals who have a genetic predisposition or who indulge in the modern western lifestyle characterized by:

(1) Cigarette smoking.
(2) Overnutrition.
(3) Sedentary work and leisure pursuits.
(4) Low-fibre diet.
(5) Hyperlipidaemia.

Atherosclerosis is the consequence of the deposition of a lipid material beneath the endothelium of arteries (atheroma), which become thickened, scarred and calcified (sclerotic) and impede the flow of blood (ischaemia). Ischaemia is not an inevitable consequence of coronary atherosclerosis but atheroma is undoubtedly the principal factor underlying myocardial ischaemia. Increased cardiac work or reduced blood O_2 carrying capacity (obesity, hypertension, cardiac dysrhythmias, valvular heart disease and anaemia) are important contributory factors.

Myocardial ischaemia results when the workload of the ventricular myocardium exceeds the metabolic reserve. Cardiac muscle is incapable of operating anaerobically. This concept of supply and demand is demonstrable in atrial pacing experiments. A critical threshold of exercise, and therefore of O_2 consumption, can be established, above which angina is precipitated.

The rapidity of development of the occlusive process determines the mode of presentation of the patient. Those with fixed or slowly progressive occlusions may present with angina, while those with sudden occlusion may present with sudden death or a myocardial infarction. An intermediate stage of unstable angina occurs in the case of haemorrhage, oedema or thromboses on a pre-existing plaque of atheroma.

The characteristic symptom of angina of effort is a sensation of tightness in the chest (retrosternal) precipitated by exertion and relieved by rest. It may radiate to the left arm, neck or jaw. Patients commonly present with pain in atypical sites and may even present to the dentist with an ache in the lower jaw.

There is a rare variant form of angina pectoris (Prinzmetal's angina) in which the ischaemia results from a reflex spasm of a coronary artery in response to such stimuli as a heavy meal or a chill wind on the face and neck; it thus lacks the characteristic association with exercise. Some patients have a combination of the two kinds.

Myocardial work

The work and O_2 consumption of the heart are directly related to:

(1) Heart rate.
(2) Peripheral resistance (and BP).
(3) Ventricular end-diastolic filling pressure ('venous return').
(4) Cardiac contractility.
(5) Plasma free fatty acid concentrations.

Cardiac work may be increased when no external physical work is performed (watching television or arguing). Increased sympathetic activity can increase heart rate and BP separately or together. Such adrenergic (sympatho-adrenal) stress may precipitate angina at rest in susceptible patients, and these attacks last 5–15 min. In contrast, angina of effort rarely lasts longer than 3 min if the exertion is lessened or stopped.

Coronary perfusion

The major resistance to flow through the terminal branches of the coronary arteries as they penetrate the myocardium is provided by the tension in the ventricle walls. This tension is a reflection of the ventricular pressure. Little or no flow occurs during systole and therefore mean flow is reduced if the total time in diastole is reduced (when the heart rate is high). In addition, flow is reduced if left ventricular end-diastolic pressure is increased (increased pre-load).

Treatment

The aim of treatment is to reduce myocardial oxygen demand or improve blood flow.

STAFFS UNIVERSITY LIBRARY

Prevention of coronary atherosclerosis – avoid risk factors

(1) Do not smoke cigarettes.
(2) Nutrition:
    (a) avoid obesity;
    (b) eat a high-fibre diet;
    (c) treat severe hyperlipidaemia.
(3) Maintain physical fitness.

Prophylaxis of angina

(1) Remove contributory factors – anaemia, hypertension, heart failure, obesity, thyrotoxicosis.
(2) Reduce cardiac work.

Three groups of drugs are useful in the treatment of angina pectoris:

(1) Organic nitrates.
(2) Antagonists at β-adrenoceptors.
(3) Blockers of L-type Ca^{2+} channels.

Organic nitrates

Ischaemia is a most potent stimulus for increasing tissue perfusion, and atherosclerotic arteries are not capable of dilatation, so that capillary beds supplied by atherosclerotic arteries are likely to be fully dilated already. Coronary blood flow is unchanged or reduced by **glyceryl trinitrate** given for angina. Vasodilatation of capacitance veins and resistance vessels other than in the coronary circulation accounts for the therapeutic efficacy. Cardiac pre-load and after-load (see p. 471) are decreased by increased venous capacity and reduced peripheral resistance respectively. Cardiac work and myocardial O_2 consumption are decreased despite a reflex increase in heart rate. The reduction in ventricular end-diastolic filling pressure also reduces resistance in the coronary circulation, allowing perfusion to begin earlier in diastole. The smooth muscle relaxation is also helpful in patients with coronary artery spasm.

Peripheral vasodilatation accounts for the principal unwanted effects of nitrate therapy (headache, light headedness, fainting attacks). Nitrates undergo extensive first pass metabolism and are best given by the sublingual route if a rapid onset of action is required.

Glyceryl trinitrate:

(1) Is the drug of choice for treating angina of effort.
(2) Has an onset of action within 2 min if the chewed tablets are kept under the tongue or an aerosol spray is used.
(3) Has a duration of action up to 20 min.

Isosorbide dinitrate and *isosorbide mononitrate* are long-acting formulations, resistant to degradation in the gut and liver. They are useful in the prophylaxis of angina. However, development of tolerance with continuous long-term use occurs to these preparations that can be avoided by ensuring drug-free periods (most conveniently, several hours during the night) in order to regain effectiveness. **Glyceryl trinitrate** can also be administered for longer lasting effect as buccal or oral sustained release tablets, an ointment or a <u>patch</u> for transdermal diffusion.

Antagonists at β-adrenoceptors

Heart rate, cardiac contractility and BP increase during exercise and stress. **Atenolol** and other antagonists at β-adrenoceptors (see p. 100) prevent increases in these determinants of myocardial O_2 consumption and are most effective prophylactic agents in angina, with up to 70% of patients gaining benefit. As the bulk of coronary perfusion occurs during diastole, slowing the heart increases the total time the heart is in diastole and allows increased coronary flow. Therapeutic efficacy is related to antagonism at cardiac β-adrenoceptors and not to the *quinidine*-like activity (see p. 100) or the intrinsic sympathomimetic (partial agonist) activity possessed by some antagonists at β-adrenoceptors. The dose of **atenolol** should be increased until relief is obtained or until the resting heart rate is reduced to 50–60 beats per min. Twice-daily administration has proved satisfactory.

In patients with congestive heart failure, antagonists at β-adrenoceptors can precipitate severe cardiac failure. In patients with asthma **propranolol** can precipitate bronchospasm (see p. 488). This risk is diminished but not abolished if an antagonist selective at $β_1$-adrenoceptors is used (**atenolol**).

Lipid-soluble drugs (**propranolol**) are more likely to cause visual disturbances, vivid dreams and hypnagogic hallucinations as they cross the blood–brain barrier readily. Water-soluble drugs (**atenolol**) have the advantage of once-daily dosage and hence encourage compliance. Sustained release preparations of the shorter-acting preparations are also available but are more expensive.

Blockers of L-type Ca^{2+} channels

This group of drugs interferes with Ca^{2+} movement across muscle cell membranes (see p. 125), reducing the amount of Ca^{2+} available to the contractile mechanism. In the heart, this reduces the force of contraction and therefore reduces the oxygen demand. On peripheral resistance and capacitance vessels, impaired Ca^{2+} entry causes relaxation and consequently vasodilatation that reduces both pre-load and after-load.

Blockers of L-type Ca^{2+} channels are also useful in the treatment of angina due to coronary artery spasm.

Verapamil acts mainly on the heart (see p. 128). **Verapamil** may precipitate bradycardia and cardiac failure, especially if used parenterally in conjunction with an antagonist at β-adrenoceptors.

The principal unwanted effects are headache, flushing and ankle oedema due to vasodilatation in the case of **nifedipine** and bradycardia and heart failure with **verapamil**.

Nifedipine has little action on the heart. It relieves angina primarily by virtue of its vasodilating action. The reduction in after-load considerably reduces the risk of cardiac failure

Openers of K+ channels

The openers of K^+ channels are a new class of anti-anginal agent exemplified by **nicorandil**. As yet their clinical import is incompletely evaluated, but initial studies suggest this class of drug may be a useful addition to the therapeutic approaches to angina pectoris.

Summary

(1) Angina pectoris is transient pain (retrosternal tightness) arising from the heart, the blood supply of which is limited by partial obstruction of the coronary arteries by atherosclerosis.
(2) It arises when the rate of oxygen utilization by a part of the working heart exceeds the rate of supply via its arterial blood.
(3) Factors that increase the work of the heart, such as exercise or sympatho-adrenal excitation, precipitate an attack of angina pectoris and factors that reduce it, such as rest, then relieve the attack.
(4) Drugs that relieve attacks do so by reducing the work of the heart. Sublingual **glyceryl trinitrate** reduces pre-load by dilating veins and after-load by dilating arterioles.
(5) Prophylactic drug treatment reduces the frequency and severity of attacks, again by reducing the work of the heart. Antagonists at β_1-adrenoceptors do this mainly by reducing the heart rate, **verapamil** mainly by reducing the force of cardiac contraction, while other classes of useful drug, longer-acting nitrates, **nifedipine** and openers of K^+ channels do so mainly by relaxing peripheral vascular smooth muscle.

Asthma

Definition

Asthma is characterized by widespread narrowing of peripheral airways in the lungs, varying in severity over short periods of time either spontaneously or as a result of treatment.

A more pragmatic clinical description is a symptom complex of breathlessness, wheeze and/or chest tightness with specifically:

(1) Prominent night-time symptoms.
(2) Early morning symptoms.
(3) Bronchial irritability to a variety of non-specific, bronchoconstrictor stimuli (e.g. exercise, change in temperature of inhaled air, smoke, fumes, perfumes, paint).

The fundamental pathophysiological abnormality is bronchial hyperreactivity, increased airways responsiveness to any bronchoconstrictor stimuli, including inhalation of non-isotonic solutions, allergens and chemicals (histamine, methacholine, PGs). Inhalation of allergen (e.g. pollen, house dust mite) produces an early, immediate bronchoconstrictor response in sensitized asthmatic subjects. In one-half of such subjects, allergen induces a dual response with an early reaction and a late (onset some 8 h after challenge) response. This late response probably correlates most closely pathogenetically with clinical asthma.

Pathologically, asthma is a chronic inflammatory disease of the airways. Mild clinical disease may be accompanied by marked pathological changes with smooth muscle hypertrophy, airways constriction, mucus hypersecretion with formation of luminal plugs, and shedding of the airways epithelium. A chronic inflammatory infiltrate is apparent, comprising neutrophil and eosinophil polymorphonuclear leucocytes and lymphocytes, all of which may play a pathogenetic role.

Epidemiology

Asthma is a common disease, which is increasing in prevalence, and currently affects up to 10% of the adult population.

Asthma is also increasing in severity. Up to 2000 people die from asthma each year in England and Wales, a retrospective analysis of such deaths suggesting avoidable factors in 80% of cases. These included a failure to diagnose asthma and an underestimation of the severity of an attack by patients, their relatives and attending medical practitioners.

Investigation

When asthmatics are wheezy, pulmonary function tests demonstrate airflow obstruction with diminished values of forced expiratory volume in 1 s (FEV_1), the ratio FEV_1/forced vital capacity (FVC) and peak expiratory flow rate (PEFR). Administration of a bronchodilator drug invariably demonstrates acute reversibility of these changes with improvements in all physiological measurements. However, when many asthmatics are seen by their GPs, complaining of episodic breathlessness, PEFR values are normal. A single, normal PEFR value does not exclude the diagnosis of asthma.

Thus, in addition to accurate history taking, a diagnosis of asthma may be confirmed by the use of domiciliary PEFR meter readings, whereby patients record PEFR throughout the 24-h period but particularly when breathless and wheezy. In non-asthmatic subjects PEFR values do not vary by more than 15%.

Domiciliary PEFR monitoring may also give an indication of asthma severity. Patients with 50% variability in PEFR over a 24-h period are at an increased risk of sudden death from asthma. PEFR monitoring can also objectively demonstrate response to any prescribed therapy.

Additional investigation of asthmatic subjects should include a blood eosinophil count and measurement of serum IgE concentration. Very small amounts of antibody to specific allergens (e.g. house dust mite, pollen, cats fur) in the serum can be detected by a radio-allergosorbent test (RAST). This employs a tiny cellulose disc to which an allergen (antigen) is bound. Serum IgE binding to the allergen is detected by the use of radiolabelled anti-IgE antibody. Skin prick testing to common allergens is occasionally performed. Up to 80% of asthmatic subjects are atopic, compared to 40% of a control population.

Basic mechanisms

The mechanism underlying bronchial hyperreactivity, which appears to be fundamental to the pathogenesis of asthma, is not known. Pathophysiological disturbances at various levels may contribute to the development of bronchial hyperreactivity. These include abnormalities of:

(1) The noradrenergic innervation of the airways and/or the sympatho-adrenal release of catecholamines.
(2) The acetylcholinergic control of the airways at the level of muscarinic acetylcholine receptors.
(3) The non-acetylcholinergic, non-noradrenergic inhibitory innervation of the airways.
(4) The permeability of the airway mucosa allowing increased penetration of causal agents.
(5) The synthesis and release of inflammatory mediators and local hormones derived from mast cells, eosinophils, basophils and macrophages.

It is likely that regulation of the airways is not achieved through a single system but rather through an integration of several of these mechanisms. Current research effort is focused on the pathological role and therapeutic antagonism of inflammatory mediators. Antagonists of such mediators have not yet found a niche in clinical practice.

The mast cell

By virtue of its capacity to manufacture and release inflammatory mediators (e.g. histamine, PGs, LTs), the mast cell has classically been thought the pivotal cell in the pathogenesis of asthma.

The mast cell is, however, not unique in its production of inflammatory mediators. Sputum eosinophilia has long been recognized as a hallmark of asthma, but a putative pathogenetic role of the eosinophil has only recently been recognized. The eosinophil, upon activation, releases platelet activating factor (PAF) from its membrane. This is an extremely potent bronchoconstrictor substance that increases non-specific bronchial hyperreactivity. PAF is also an eosinophil chemotactic factor and causes eosinophil activation, producing a positive feedback loop. Eosinophils also release major basic protein, which causes shedding of the airway epithelium.

Anti-asthma drugs

Sodium cromoglycate

Sodium cromoglycate is inhaled either as a finely divided powder using an insufflator (Spinhaler^R) or as an aerosol. Its mechanism of action is unclear but may involve inhibition of neurotransmitter release from non-acetylcholinergic, non-noradrenergic nerves or suppression of the release of mediators from sensitized mast cells. It is of no value when administered after the stimulus to release but is useful when given 30 min before exercise to prevent bronchoconstriction. Unwanted effects are minor and seen only with the cheaper powder formulation – cough, transient bronchoconstriction and throat irritation.

Anti-inflammatory glucocorticosteroids

Oral **prednisolone** or inhaled glucocorticosteroids (e.g. *beclomethasone*) provide very effective asthma prophylaxis. Oral glucocorticosteroids are particularly prone to produce serious, systemic, adverse effects (see p. 183). These are largely circumvented by the use of inhaled glucocorticosteroids. Concerns that inhaled glucocorticosteroids cause growth retardation in children and osteoporosis in adults are probably largely unfounded.

Selective agonists at β$_2$-adrenoceptors

Salbutamol (see p. 96) and *terbutaline* are relaxants of airways smooth muscle that are more effective against the early, rather than the late, phase of airway narrowing in an attack of asthma. Unwanted effects (tremor, nervous tension, tachycardia) are rare with low doses administered by aerosol but more prevalent with the larger doses used orally and by nebulization. A novel member of the group, *salmeterol*, has an airway $t_{1/2}$ of 12 h and is a useful prophylactic agent when used once or twice daily.

Methylxanthines

Theophylline (see p. 130), in a sustained-release formulation, may be given once or twice daily and both absorption and metabolism vary with age, smoking and dietary habits, with concomitant liver and heart disease and in the presence of other therapeutic agents (e.g. **ciprofloxacin**). The therapeutic window is 5–15 mg/L and plasma or saliva assay is advisable to develop a dosage regimen.

Theophylline is complexed to increase water solubility as *aminophylline* for i/v injection. Unwanted effects (nausea, vomiting, headache, faintness, tachycardia, cardiac dysrhythmias, convulsions) are related to blood concentration and dose.

Quaternary ammonium antagonists at muscarinic acetylcholine receptors

Ipratropium inhibits reflex bronchoconstriction (see p. 69). It is inhaled as an aerosol. Therefore, it has a local action with delayed onset (30–60 min).

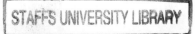
STAFFS UNIVERSITY LIBRARY

Preferred route of administration of anti-asthma drugs

The inhaled route of administration confers many advantages over the oral route. Administration of a drug by the inhaled route results in the production of a large concentration of drug locally in the airways, thereby minimizing unwanted systemic effects. In addition, the inhaled route of administration results in rapid bronchodilatation when using an agonist at β_2-adrenoceptors.

The major objection to inhaled therapy, observed particularly in children and the elderly, is difficulty in synchronizing inhalation with activation of the pressurized metered dose inhaler (50% of asthmatic patients fail to derive maximum benefit from their inhalers). However, the introduction of new inhaler devices has largely circumvented this problem. There are various such devices available:

(1) Dry powder inhalers (e.g. the Diskhaler^R and Rotahaler^R for inhalation of **salbutamol** and *beclomethasone*).
(2) Spacing devices (e.g. the Volumatic^R for **salbutamol** and *beclomethasone*)

It is desirable that inhaler technique be checked in each asthmatic patient at all consultations to ensure adequate technique and thus effective drug delivery to the airways.

Management of chronic, persistent asthma

Avoidance of triggering factors

Where certain drug triggers (e.g. antagonists at β-adrenoceptors, **aspirin**, NSAIDs) or particular allergens (e.g. pets, bedding material, moulds, food) are identified, or occupational asthma is diagnosed, such triggers should be avoided if possible. If severe allergy to house dust mite occurs, protective Intervent^R bedding may reduce allergen concentrations and reduce symptom severity. Antagonists at β-adrenoceptors are dangerous (including eye-drop formulations) and extreme caution must guide the use even of antagonists selective at β_1-adrenoceptors (see p. 100) in patients with asthma. There is no role for immunotherapy in the form of desensitization of asthmatic patients to specific allergens (e.g. pollen).

The British Thoracic Society introduced guidelines (1993) for management of chronic asthma, suggesting a stepwise approach to treatment. Treatment is to advance from one step to the next if asthma persists in limiting the patient's quality of life. Conversely, consider every 3–6 months whether steps can be descended if control has been achieved.

Bronchodilators only – step 1

A selective agonist at β_2-adrenoceptors (e.g. **salbutamol**, *terbutaline*) should be used as required rather than in a regular regimen (historically, four times daily). In this way, patients monitor the frequency of inhalation of agonist at β_2-adrenoceptors as an indication of severity of asthma by using it as a rescue inhaler. The exclusive use of an agonist at β_2-adrenoceptors in the management of asthma should be reserved for patients who have no sleep disturbance, normal lung function and infrequent symptoms.

Inhaled anti-inflammatory agents – steps 2 and 3

Patients who require to use their bronchodilator (agonist at β_2-adrenoceptors) inhaler more than once daily and/or awake at night with symptoms, require regular, inhaled anti-inflammatory drug treatment. The treatment options include:

(1) Inhaled glucocorticosteroids.
(2) Inhaled **sodium cromoglycate**.

Inhaled glucocorticosteroids are the treatment of choice and should be instituted at a small dose twice daily every day (low-dose inhaled glucocorticosteroid: step 2). In patients who fail to respond symptomatically with persistent variability in PEFR values, inhaler technique should be re-checked and, if satisfactory, the inhaled glucocorticosteroid can be used in higher doses (step 3). Rinsing the mouth immediately after inhalation of glucocorticosteroid helps to prevent oral thrush and hoarseness (dysphonia). Spitting out after rinsing limits systemic absorption. Once symptoms are controlled, the dose of inhaled glucocorticosteroid should be reduced to the minimum required to maintain this control.

For patients with persistent, nocturnal asthma, despite inhaled glucocorticosteroid treatment, the addition of a long-acting agonist at β_2-adrenoceptors (*salmeterol*) or modified-release *theophylline* taken on retiring is often helpful.

There is recent evidence, in asthma of varying severity, that extra benefit may be conferred by the addition of *salmeterol* to low-dose inhaled glucocorticosteroid rather than increasing the dose of the inhaled glucocorticosteroid.

Inhaled **sodium cromoglycate** is used (step 2) infrequently in adults with limited benefit. In children, **sodium cromoglycate** has historically been the treatment of choice. Recent evidence has suggested that substituting a small dose of an inhaled glucocorticosteroid invariably improves symptom control further, decreases hospital admissions with acute asthma and results in improved pulmonary function with no significant unwanted effects. Thus, there is an increasing trend to prescribing inhaled glucocorticosteroid early in asthmatic children.

Additional agents – step 4

Therapeutic trial might be made, in the specified order, of the addition of one or more of inhaled *salmeterol*, modified-release oral *theophylline*, inhaled *ipratropium*, modified-release oral agonist at β_2-adrenoceptors, high-dose inhaled bronchodilator agents and **sodium cromoglycate**.

High-dose inhaled bronchodilator therapy

In patients with chronic severe asthma, with persistent poor pulmonary function, further benefit may be derived by administering larger doses of bronchodilator and anti-inflammatory agents, either via spacer devices, e.g. Nebuhaler^R, Volumatic^R (preferred by 30% of patients), or via a nebulizer (preferred by 70%). Large doses of agonists at β_2-adrenoceptors or antagonists at muscarinic acetylcholine receptors can be delivered from prediluted vials through a nebulizer (e.g. **salbutamol**, *terbutaline*, *ipratropium*), but ideally this should be supervised through a hospital. In addition, *beclomethasone* can be administered as a nebulizer solution in high dosage. Rarely, patients who do not derive benefit from nebulizer therapy do respond to parenteral administration of an agonist at β_2-adrenoceptors, either i/m injection, 6 hourly, or via continuous s/c infusion.

Oral glucocorticosteroids – step 5

Maintenance, long-term, oral **prednisolone** should only be added to the treatment regimen if adequate control cannot be achieved on maximal doses of inhaled glucocorticosteroids and an adequate trial of the additional agents that comprise step 4. Large doses of inhaled glucocorticosteroids should always be continued in patients receiving oral glucocorticosteroid treatment, to minimize the dose of oral glucocorticosteroid required.

Long-term treatment with oral glucocorticosteroids is used very infrequently in the management of chronic asthma. However, oral glucocorticosteroids have an important role used in short courses to regain symptom control in deteriorating/acute severe asthma (see below).

The commonest cause for poor asthma control is non-compliance with prescribed treatment. It is essential that patients are educated about the difference between agonists at β_2-adrenoceptors (rescue therapy) and inhaled glucocorticosteroid (preventer therapy). Otherwise, the preventer is often used as required only. Compliance with glucocorticosteroid inhalation is often poor because such explanation is not given and patients find that inhalation of an agonist at β_2-adrenoceptors, rather than the inhaled glucocorticosteroid, works best at times when they are wheezy.

Indications for oral glucocorticosteroids (short course)

The purpose of this treatment is to gain control over asthma in its more stubborn forms:

(1) Deteriorating asthma with recent onset of sleep disturbance and diminishing PEFR (to prevent deteriorating asthma from becoming acute severe asthma).
(2) Whenever emergency nebulized or injected bronchodilators are necessary.
(3) Acute severe asthma.
(4) As a trial of reversibility in chronic severe airflow obstruction.

Management of acute severe asthma

Acute severe asthma is a misnomer. One-half of admissions so labelled have been waking every night for the previous 2 weeks. One-half have previously sought medical help prior to admission. In many, a short, sharp course of oral glucocorticosteroid would have prevented admission with a potentially life-threatening condition. Patients presenting to an Accident and Emergency department need to be seen quickly by an experienced doctor.

Patients should ideally always be admitted to hospital, even if there is an apparent 'good response' in the Accident and Emergency room to nebulized bronchodilator therapy.

The three cardinal physical signs of severe asthma that should be rapidly assessed are:

(1) Tachycardia greater than 120 beats/min (take into account any previous administration of bronchodilator drugs with positive chronotropic effects).
(2) Pulsus paradoxus (an exaggeration of the normal swings in systolic BP with respiration) measured using a sphygmomanometer.
(3) Cyanosis.

The objective assessment must at least include:

(1) Chest X-ray (to exclude other causes of severe breathlessness – pulmonary oedema or pneumothorax). All that wheezes is not asthma!
(2) Arterial blood gas analysis. During an attack of acute severe asthma, low arterial Pao_2 (hypoxaemia) and low $Paco_2$ (hypocapnoea) usually occur. A normal or high $Paco_2$ in a patient with acute severe asthma indicates an extremely severe attack.
(3) PEFR. This can be judged against the patient's usual best value.

Oxygen

Oxygen should be administered in high concentration (e.g. 60%) using either an Edinburgh or MC mask. This contrasts sharply with the controlled oxygen therapy (less than 28%) delivered to patients with chronic airflow obstruction, who may be reliant on hypoxaemic drive.

Bronchodilator agents

Agonists at β_2-adrenoceptors should be administered, ideally by the nebulized route, which permits high doses to be administered locally to the airways. **Salbutamol** and *terbutaline* are both available as nebulizer solutions in break-off nebule form. If bronchoconstriction is severe, with no response to nebulized bronchodilator agent, a parenteral agonist at β_2-adrenoceptors is often helpful.

Glucocorticosteroids

Glucocorticosteroids should be administered both orally and by the i/v route. For the first 24 h, the patient should receive *hydrocortisone* 6 hourly i/v and a suggested oral regimen would be **prednisolone** daily for one week. There is no need to reduce the dose over several days. In patients taking maintenance glucocorticosteroids, relatively large daily doses are advised.

Intravenous fluids

Patients with acute severe asthma are dehydrated at the time of admission and may benefit from *sodium chloride*, 0.9% i/v for the first 24 h (e.g. 4 L).

Antibacterial agents

These should not be routinely administered, since acute severe asthma is not usually triggered by bacterial infection. Green sputum during an exacerbation usually indicates sputum eosinophilia rather than bacterial infection. However, if the patient is febrile, or the circulating white blood cell count is elevated, or pathogens are cultured from sputum, then the appropriate antibiotic agent should be administered.

Assisted ventilation

Rarely, nowadays, is it necessary to ventilate patients with acute severe asthma. However, the decision whether or not to ventilate must be made by a doctor experienced in the management of such patients. The indications may be purely the appearance of the patient from the end of the bed on the grounds of impaired speech and gross exhaustion. Deteriorating partial pressures of blood gases are an obvious indication but in many cases the indication to ventilate may be present prior to obvious worsening of hypoxaemia or hypercapnia. Close cooperation with anaesthetists providing intensive care facilities is vital.

Only in exceptional cases should i/v *aminophylline* or nebulized *ipratropium* be instituted. Although i/v *aminophylline* is a bronchodilator agent of similar efficacy to a nebulized agonist at β_2-adrenoceptors, it is a relatively toxic agent and, in patients being managed in the manner suggested, *aminophylline* confers no extra advantage but does produce many adverse effects. Intravenous *aminophylline* is to some extent contraindicated in patients currently receiving an oral *theophylline* preparation. If *aminophylline* is administered, plasma concentrations should be monitored.

Response to treatment is best monitored by regular PEFR measurements (e.g. four times daily) and special attention must be paid to any patient who persists in early morning dipping or with marked variability in readings (more than 30% variability in PEFR over 24-h periods).

All patients, having been admitted to hospital with acute severe asthma, should be discharged on an inhaled glucocorticosteroid via a device they have been taught to use effectively, and one which they like. Asthma education should have been given by either the doctor or asthma nurse.

Drugs that are contra-indicated

Respiratory depressant, opioids and sedative agents (benzodiazepines) can kill asthmatic patients if administered during an acute attack, and they should be avoided.

Sudden-onset, life-threatening asthma

Rarely, asthma may become severe within minutes in spite of little instability of asthma in the preceding days. Such patients are at great risk of sudden death. Although loan of a domiciliary nebulizer for inhalation of a high dose of an agonist at β_2-adrenoceptors may help, many physicians educate such patients in the self-administration i/m of a pre-loaded syringe (Min-I-Jet) containing *adrenaline*.

Summary

(1) Asthma is a chronic inflammatory disease of the airways characterized by breathlessness, wheeze, chest tightness and variability in PEFR values greater than 15% that are due to reversible airway obstruction, and bronchial hyperreactivity.

(2) Of the classes of drugs available for treatment (**sodium cromoglycate**, glucocorticosteroids, selective agonists at β_2-adrenoceptors, methylxanthines and quaternary ammonium antagonists at muscarinic acetylcholine receptors), all but methylxanthines can be administered by the preferred inhaled route.

(3) Chronic persistent asthma is managed in a stepwise fashion, seeking to control the asthma so that it does not limit the patient's quality of life. Step 1 is the use of inhaled bronchodilators (selective agonists at β_2-adrenoceptors) only. Patients who use their inhaled bronchodilator agent for relief more often than once daily, or who are awakened at night by their symptoms, require regular inhaled anti-inflammatory drug prophylaxis – glucocorticosteroids, initially in low dosage (step 2), are the most reliably effective preventers.

(4) More difficult cases might require increase dosage of inhaled glucocorticosteroid (step 3), additional agents (step 4), of which a long-acting agonist at β_2-adrenoceptors and modified-release methylxanthine are the most helpful, and higher doses of inhaled bronchodilators. Step 5 is the therapy of last resort with oral glucocorticosteroids.

(5) A short course of oral glucocorticosteroid therapy at high dosage is invaluable for preventing deteriorating asthma from evolving into acute severe asthma.

(6) Acute severe asthma is a medical emergency suggested by tachycardia, pulsus paradoxus and cyanosis. Oxygen at high concentration, nebulized bronchodilator agents at high dosage and glucocorticosteroids both i/v and orally are the mainstay of treatment.

Coughs and colds

Cough

This is a powerful reflex initiated through irritation of receptors in the mucosa of the upper respiratory tract. These receptors are sensitive to stimulation by the mediators of inflammation associated with allergy or infection, by chemicals (sulphur dioxide, cigarette smoke) or by particles, foreign bodies and secretions. They are also responsive to distortions, or changes in the calibre, of the airways. Stimulation of these receptors discharges afferent impulses to the cough centre in the brain stem. From here, efferent impulses are carried along somatic motor pathways to the diaphragm and the intercostal and abdominal muscles. Convulsive contraction of these muscles causes a rapid expulsion of air from the lungs in an attempt to remove any irritating particles or mucus from the respiratory tract. The secretion of mucus by the goblet cells is increased by the reflex.

A cough may be one of two kinds:

(1) Productive cough – the act of coughing removes mucus from the lungs and respiratory tract that might otherwise act as a site of infection and disturb gaseous exchange.
(2) Non-productive cough – this is usually a dry, irritating or tickly cough that does not produce mucus. It may be present after the common cold and in chronic bronchitis. Such a cough may be initiated by the dripping of mucus from the postnasal space onto the pharynx and trachea, or by oedema of the pharyngeal mucosa after a sore throat.

If the cough is the main complaint of the patient, the rational treatment is to suppress a non-productive cough. A productive cough should not be suppressed (it is attempting to clear the airways) but the clearance may be improved by altering the consistency of the mucus. A cough that persists may indicate a more serious disease (bronchitis, tuberculosis, cancer) and should be investigated accordingly.

Expectorant agents

Normal bronchial mucosa has ciliated columnar cells with few goblet cells. Mucus is also secreted by submucous glands, which receive vagal innervation. The cilia beat rhythmically and move upwards a layer of fluid on which the mucus floats. This is then usually swallowed. (The bronchial mucosa of smokers has many more goblet cells and fewer ciliated cells than normal. The daily coughing up of mucus is indicative of chronic bronchitis).

The aim of using expectorant agents is to aid the clearance of mucus from the lungs. This is achieved by increased bronchial secretions and the production of mucus that is less viscous and therefore coughed up more easily. Clearance of mucus can be assessed, in the laboratory, by measuring the rate of removal of inhaled radioactive microspheres from the lungs.

Expectorant agents are claimed to act by irritation of the gastric mucosa, which reflexly stimulates bronchial mucus secretion. There is doubt as to their effectiveness. Unfortunately many preparations containing expectorant agents also contain a cough suppressant (see below): these preparations should be avoided.

Inhalation of steam aids expectoration. The warm water vapour hydrates the bronchial tree and increases the secretion of mucus that is less viscous and can more easily be removed by coughing. Additions (menthol, eucalyptus oil) probably exert no additional effect on secretion but may encourage deep inhalation of the steam.

Mucolytic agents

These reduce the viscosity of the mucus by changing the structure of its components. Acetylcysteine breaks disulphide bonds in proteins in the mucus. Despite these effects on the viscosity of mucus (which can be assessed by measuring sputum viscosity at different shear rates), there is no clear evidence that the majority of patients experience any beneficial effects from the use of mucolytic agents. Fragmentation of the mucus may interfere with ciliary movement and therefore clearance of the airways.

Cough suppressant agents

A non-productive cough causing sleep loss may be suppressed by drugs acting at some stage of the cough reflex. Cough-suppressant agents can be assessed by their ability to suppress cough induced by a citric acid aerosol. The most effective cough-suppressant agents are the opioids (see p. 244), which act at the cough centre and reduce impulses in the efferent pathways to the muscles involved in the act of coughing. *Diamorphine* is the most potent but because of abuse potential both it and *methadone* are used only in painful cough associated with terminal illness. In other situations opiate derivatives showing cough suppression at subanalgesic doses (**codeine**, pholcodine) or selective antitussive agents (**dextromethorphan**) are used. **Codeine** linctus is liable to abuse. Preparations offered for the treatment of cough that contain the irrational combination of a cough suppressant and an expectorant should not be used.

Antagonists at H_1 histamine receptors may suppress coughing by acting at receptors in the bronchial mucosa that are involved in initiating the reflex. The antagonistic activity at muscarinic acetylcholine receptors also possessed by many of these compounds reduces the secretion of mucus; however, such antihistamines are offered inappropriately combined with expectorant agents.

Coryza – the common cold

The common cold is a viral infection resulting in an inflammatory reaction of the lining of the upper respiratory tract, particularly the nasal mucosa.

This is manifested as local vasodilatation, increased blood flow, oedema and a watery discharge from the nose. As the infection is viral, only symptomatic treatment is available. An antipyretic analgesic (**aspirin**, **paracetamol**) relieves any associated fever or headache (see p. 253) and a decongestant reduces the nasal symptoms.

Production of mucus by the nasal mucosa may be reduced by antagonists at muscarinic acetylcholine receptors, most often as antagonists at H_1 histamine receptors with antimuscarinic activity (**chlorpheniramine**). These are liable to cause sedation and antimuscarinic side-effects, including dry mouth, disturbed accommodation and mydriasis (a danger in patients predisposed to closed angle glaucoma).

Decongestant agents

Decongestant agents directly or indirectly activate α_1-adrenoceptors, resulting in constriction of the blood vessels in the nasal mucous membranes. Both oral and topical preparations are used. With oral preparations (pseudoephedrine) the possibility of serious systemic unwanted effects or interaction with other drugs (inhibitors of MAO, tricyclic antidepressant agents, see p. 83) exists. They are best avoided at night or their stimulant effect on the CNS may prevent sleep. Oral decongestant agents are usually formulated with other components (cough suppressant and analgesic agents, and antagonists at histamine H_1 receptors).

Local application of decongestant agents to the nasal mucosa is made by sprays or drops containing *ephedrine* or phenylephrine. The risks of systemic effects are small. The most common problem with these drugs is local reactive hyperaemia through overenthusiastic and prolonged use.

Sinusitis

The air sinuses within the facial bones and communicating with the nasal passages may become inflamed in coryza and constant nose blowing forces nasal discharge into them. Decongestant agents shrink the mucosa and aid drainage from here. If the sinuses become blocked with infected material antibiotic treatment may be necessary.

Allergic rhinitis

This occurs as a result of exposure to allergens. It can be seasonal (pollen) or perennial (house dust mite). Symptoms are similar to a cold but the conjunctivae may also be involved.

Antagonists at H_1 histamine receptors (see p. 201) administered systemically are of doubtful value, may produce sedation and are often associated with adverse effects due to blockade of muscarinic acetylcholine receptors. Newer compounds (*terfenadine*) that do not readily cross the blood–brain barrier are claimed to cause very little sedation, psychomotor impairment or antimuscarinic effects.

Prophylactic intranasal and eye-drop use of **sodium cromoglycate** (see p. 200) may prevent attacks and nasal application of a glucocorticosteroid (*beclomethasone*, see p. 183) is also helpful.

Some patients may benefit from a course of hyposensitizing injections of allergen extracts if the responsible allergen can be identified.

Summary

(1) Coughs may be:
(a) productive, treated with expectorants or mucolytic agents to aid mucus clearance;
(b) non-productive, suppressed with centrally acting opioid analgesic drugs (**codeine**) or selective antitussive opioid derivatives (**dextromethorphan**).
(2) Common cold may be treated symptomatically with:
(a) antagonists at both H_1 histamine and muscarinic acetylcholine receptors (**chlorpheniramine**) to reduce nasal mucus production;
(b) decongestants, agonists (direct or indirect) at α_1-adrenoceptors, topically (*ephedrine*) or systemically (pseudoephedrine) to constrict nasal mucosal blood vessels.
(3) Sinusitis may be treated with decongestants, or antibacterial agents if infection is present.
(4) Allergic rhinitis may be treated with:
(a) systemic antagonist at H_1 histamine receptors (*terfenadine*);
(b) intranasal **sodium cromoglycate** to prevent attacks;
(c) intranasal glucocorticosteroid (*beclomethasone*).

Analgesia

Revise the physiological mechanisms of pain.

Adverse effects of pain

Pain is a mode of sensation essential for the protection of the body from damaging stimuli. If however the stimulus/damage continues, pain persists and can lead to a number of adverse effects including agitation/anxiety, nausea and vomiting, increased secretion of catecholamines, vasoconstriction, hypotension, decreased cerebral function.

Thus analgesia not only relieves discomfort but also improves physiological function. Acute pain is most efficiently managed by logical analgesia:

(1) Determine the cause of the pain.
(2) Target drug therapy to the cause (e.g. nitrates for angina).

(3) Remember both patient and pharmacokinetic factors (e.g. after severe trauma, analgesic agents must be given i/v for a rapid response in a shocked hypovolaemic patient).

(4) The earlier the intervention, the less analgesic agent is required.

Non-specific analgesia

The step-wise approach, starting with agents of low analgesic effect (e.g. **paracetamol**) (see Figure 1.2), progressing to opioids of moderate analgesic effect (like *dihydrocodeine*) and finally to those with high analgesic effect (**morphine**, *diamorphine*), is widely used. This strategy has the virtue of simplicity, but fails to take into consideration the multi-factorial nature of pain (Table 9.2). These differing interventions may need to be combined to achieve maximal effect.

Special situations

Postoperative pain

An assessment should be made as to the likely severity of the pain, in order to determine the appropriate analgesia (e.g. skin suturing only – minor; tooth extraction – moderate; laparotomy – severe). There is wide interpersonal variation. In severe pain, analgesia is frequently inadequate due to insufficient dosage, too long an interval between doses and the mistaken belief that opioid dependence is likely to develop. Repeated patient-controlled, but carefully regulated, i/v boluses of opioids is a useful method that deserves to be more widely practised.

Intractable pain from cancer

Patients may be in pain because of bony secondary tumours (NSAIDs and opioids), visceral involvement of the tumour growth (opioids) or neural involvement (tricyclic antidepressant and anticonvulsant agents). The opioid of choice is oral, slow-release **morphine** which will need to be progressively increased in dose with time as the patient develops pharmacological tolerance (see p. 246). Repeated adequate dosage should ensure a pain-controlled terminal existence.

Table 9.2 Matching analgesia to the nature of the pain

Nature of pain	Treatment
Minor pain	**Paracetamol** (see p. 254)
Movement-dependent and inflammatory pain	NSAIDs (see p. 213)
Visceral pain	Opioids (see p. 243)
Neuropathic pain	Tricyclic antidepressant agents; **carbamazepine**
Chronic pain	Physical techniques; behaviour modification

Chronic pain in non-terminal conditions

Chronic pain may be unresponsive to classical analgesic agents and can be helped by pain management techniques, which include improving general fitness, relaxation techniques and improving mood and confidence. In some patients electrical stimulation of nerves may be beneficial (e.g. transcutaneous electrical nerve stimulation (TENS)).

Headache and migraine

Headache

Headache is a common symptom and is usually due to:

(1) Muscular spasm – the tension headache.
(2) Referred pain – from arthritis in the cervical spine, sinusitis, glaucoma or errors of refraction. Within the cranium, only large blood vessels and the lining of the inside of the skull have receptors for pain, the brain itself has none. The tissues of the scalp (e.g. blood vessels) are sensitive to pain.
(3) Vasodilatation – responsible for the headache associated with migraine, endogenous histamine release, **glyceryl trinitrate** and systemic infections.

Contrary to popular belief, headache is not a feature of essential hypertension.

Treatment

Wherever possible the underlying cause should be identified so that specific and effective therapy can be instituted (for meningitis, cerebral tumour, depression). If intracranial pathology is suspected opioid analgesic agents should not be given because the associated respiratory depression increases intracranial pressure via hypercapnia. They may also disturb consciousness. Antipyretic analgesic agents (see p. 253) should be the first treatment for headache. Proprietary, over-the-counter preparations usually contain **aspirin**, **paracetamol** or **codeine**. Singly or in combination, these drugs are adequate for all kinds of moderate headache. Double-blind controlled trials have shown that 500–1000 mg of **paracetamol** and **aspirin** are equipotent as antipyretic and analgesic agents and are as effective, as analgesic agents, as **codeine** (30 mg), *dihydrocodeine* (30 mg) and *dextropropoxyphene* (65 mg). Increasing the dose of analgesic drugs does not provide further analgesia but should prolong the duration of action at the expense of increased toxicity – gastric irritation with **aspirin**, constipation and drowsiness with opioids. The short-term use of an anxiolytic (**diazepam**) may occasionally be warranted if stress is an important causative factor. Which analgesic a doctor or a patient chooses is usually based on habit rather than on recognized prescribing considerations (apart from the risk of gastric mucosal ulceration with salicylates, although modern formulations of dispersible **aspirin** are much less hazardous, and avoidance of **aspirin** in children under 12 years of age, see p. 254). In the UK frequently prescribed compound analgesic preparations are co-proxamol (paracetamol and dextropropoxyphene) and co-dydramol (paracetamol and dihydrocodeine), although such preparations rarely have any advantage and can complicate the treatment of overdosage.

Migraine

Migraine is a familial disorder characterized by recurrent attacks of headache, which is widely variable in intensity, frequency and duration and is often associated with neurological disturbances. The classical syndrome comprises:

(1) A prodromal phase, in which visual disturbances are common – blind spot (scotoma), hemianopia, scintillating lines – accompanied by drowsiness, nausea and vomiting, thought to be due to intracerebral vasoconstriction.
(2) The headache, which is usually unilateral and throbbing, due to vasodilatation of extracerebral vessels.

All the above characteristics are not present in each attack or in each patient.

The mechanism of the instability of intracranial and extracranial blood vessels is unknown. This abnormality of vasomotor control is of pharmacological interest because 5-hydroxytryptamine has been implicated in its pathogenesis and drugs that mimic or antagonize 5-hydroxytryptamine are of value in the prophylaxis of migraine. The effects of 5-hydroxytryptamine on the cardiovascular system are complex but intracarotid infusion causes constriction of the temporal artery and scalp pallor, both of which occur in the prodromal phase of migraine.

Normally, 5-hydroxytryptamine is confined to platelets but during an attack a factor in the plasma activates the release of 5-hydroxytryptamine from platelets. Tyramine-containing foods precipitate attacks in susceptible patients and the headache associated with ingestion of these foods by patients on inhibitors of MAO shows features of migraine. A higher premenstrual incidence of migraine may be related to a decrease in platelet MAO activity after ovulation. PGs released from activated platelets promote aggregation, the further release of 5-hydroxytryptamine and a lowering of the pain threshold in vessel walls. The lateralization of many migrainous headaches is unexplained.

Therapy

Based on the above considerations, a number of approaches might prove of value in the prophylaxis of migraine and in the treatment of an acute attack.

Prophylaxis

(1) Remove factors triggering the disorder, for example, avoid stressful situations – psychotherapy, anxiolysis (**diazepam** or better **propranolol**, which can also reduce the effects of increased sympathetic activity); withdraw offending foodstuffs and ethanol. Inhibit ovulation.
(2) *Pizotifen* [pizotyline] is an antagonist at 5-HT$_2$, H$_1$ histamine and muscarinic acetylcholine receptors. Whilst effective, the predictable side-effects are impairment of motor coordination, increased sedation with ethanol and dry mouth.
(3) Tricyclic antidepressant agents (**amitriptyline**) at night.
(4) Inhibition of PG synthesis with **aspirin** (600 mg twice daily) has been shown to reduce the frequency of headache in migrainous patients by more than 75%.

Treatment of the acute attack

It would appear rational to use agents that can cause vasoconstriction of scalp vessels to treat the headache.

(1) **Sumatriptan**, an agonist at 5-HT$_1$ receptors, is the most effective agent for relief and the only drug proven to abort an established attack. Subcutaneous administration is more effective than oral therapy and can be repeated once after a lapse of at least 1 h, but is less convenient and more expensive.

   5-HT$_1$ receptors are found predominantly in extracranial blood vessels and the drug produces a dose-related vasoconstriction in mainly cranial arterioles but a small degree of constriction occurs in other vessels (e.g. cardiac) – caution in ischaemic heart disease and hypertension. The major unwanted effect is localized pain at the injection site. **Sumatriptan** is expensive, and should not be used with *ergotamine* (see (5) below).
(2) Analgesic agents (**paracetamol**, **aspirin**, **codeine**) have useful palliative effect if taken early in the vasoconstrictor phase.
(3) For nausea and vomiting an antiemetic agent (by suppository to ensure its absorption) – *prochlorperazine, metoclopramide* (see p. 241). If nausea and vomiting are frequent features of recurrent attacks, their oral use together with antipyretic analgesic agents during the vasoconstrictor phase may be effective.
(4) If drowsiness is a problem *caffeine* is a weak cerebral stimulant and is a constituent of some compound analgesic preparations. In excessive doses or on withdrawal, *caffeine* may itself cause headache.
(5) *Ergotamine* is a useful agent for relief but to be maximally effective it must be given parenterally (i/m or s/c) before the vasodilator phase. *Ergotamine* suppositories are also used (formulated with *caffeine*, which may enhance absorption). To overcome the erratic absorption from the gut a pressurized aerosol delivering a metered dose of micronized *ergotamine* is available. A maximum of six doses in 1 day has been recommended. The drug is highly toxic, causing vomiting and diarrhoea, convulsions and severe vasoconstriction, leading to paraesthesiae and gangrene (cf. St Anthony's fire of ergot poisoning

STAFFS UNIVERSITY LIBRARY

due to fungal contamination of rye). For this reason a treatment course is restricted to 12 doses in a week, with a break of at least 4 days between courses. It is contraindicated in patients with vascular disease, thrombophlebitis, hepatic or renal disease and during pregnancy.

Trigeminal neuralgia

This consists of excruciating pain that shoots across the cheek, chin and lips. Attacks last for a few seconds but can recur frequently. Attacks can be precipitated by the lightest of touches to a defined trigger zone.

The electrophysiological defect of trigeminal neuralgia must be related to that in epilepsy since anticonvulsant drugs are effective. Amongst these **carbamazepine** is the drug of choice. **Carbamazepine** has no other analgesic activity.

Drugs and mental disease

Aims

For each of anxiety neurosis, depressive illness and schizophrenia to elucidate the:

(1) Nature of the disease.
(2) Rational selection and use of drugs.
(3) Role of drug therapy in the context of other therapies.

Anxiety neurosis

Anxiety states are neuroses – deviations from normal experience, but insight is preserved. There is no clear separation from the normal experience of anxiety in response to the worries and stresses of life. The diagnosis is made if the symptoms are prolonged and persistent (more than 2 weeks) and if they are incapacitating.

Neurosis is the result of the action of stressful events on the personality – enough to be regarded as a 'disease' by the doctor, patient or the patient's social contacts. Different forms of anxiety neurosis include panic disorder, agoraphobia, social phobia, obsessional-compulsive disorder and cardiac hypochondriasis. Environmental factors are often causative, and patterns of neurotic behaviour are easily learned in childhood. Stress can push each of us into these behaviour patterns (e.g. examination anxiety, bereavement depression). The neurotic patient has a lower threshold for, and a longer persistence of, this behaviour. However, some patients experience spontaneous panic attacks in the absence of obvious stress or neurotic traits.

Symptoms

Psychological

These symptoms are a sense of fearful anticipation, dread and sense of imminent death. Associated symptoms include: irritability, sensitivity to noise, feeling of restlessness, impaired concentration and disturbed sleep. Depressed mood may often co-exist and should not be missed.

Physical

(1) *Resulting in part from autonomic overactivity* – palpitations, dry mouth, sweating, diarrhoea, frequency of micturition and impotence or frigidity.
(2) *Caused by overactive skeletal muscles* – headaches and aching in the back or neck.
(3) *Caused by hyperventilation* – dizziness, paraesthesiae, faintness and palpitations.

Natural history and prognosis

There is a high rate of spontaneous resolution, especially in a sound personality with a short-lived stress. However, in many cases the condition is relapsing and remitting.

Objectives of treatment

The treatment objectives are to remove the symptoms and to promote mechanisms for coping with stress. In mild cases, psychological methods suffice. In more severe cases, drugs may be used for short-term relief while learning psychological techniques.

Treatment

A combination of treatments is aimed at changing aetiological factors amenable to change.

Psychological

Simple psychotherapy sometimes suffices. Listen carefully to the patient's account of his/her symptoms and anxieties. Demonstrate that you recognize these as part of a common illness. Explain the nature of the illness and its likely causes. Reassure the patient that a more feared illness is not present and that treatment, which the doctor will supervise, will be effective. Provide relaxation training and teach behavioural and cognitive procedures for controlling anxious thoughts. Specialist psychodynamic psychotherapy may be needed.

Anxiolytic agents

Today antidepressant drugs are replacing the benzodiazepines as the principal anxiolytic drugs (see p. 260) in use. In the 1960s the advertising strategy of the pharmaceutical industry promoted a syndrome to the medical profession and to the public. The typical patient was an over-anxious housewife with young children, unable to cope with her lot, exhibiting physical manifestations of sympatho-adrenal overactivity. This syndrome was alleged to respond dramatically to the first benzodiazepine, chlordiazepoxide – 'a sedative anticonvulsant with marked taming effects in vicious animals'. Anxiety neurosis became respectable, chlordiazepoxide fashionable, and more potent analogues were introduced (**diazepam**, *lorazepam*). Controlled trials reveal a high rate of spontaneous remission in anxiety neuroses with only small additional effects of benzodiazepines. These additional benefits are short-lived. Physical dependence and withdrawal anxiety develop rapidly.

It is increasingly recognized that antidepressant drugs, particularly those active in inhibition of 5-hydroxytryptamine re-uptake (clomipramine, **fluoxetine**; see p. 234), are effective in anxiety states with significant symptoms of depression, severe obsessional–compulsive disorder and panic disorder.

Selection of a benzodiazepine

Each benzodiazepine possesses all the properties of the group; they differ only in relative potency. Some effects are readily demonstrable in people – sedation, suppression of paradoxical sleep, safety in overdosage and anterograde amnesia. Others (appetite stimulation and relaxation of voluntary muscle – an effect mediated by depression of spinal synaptic transmission) are less so. The clinical use of individual drugs is determined to some extent by the marketing strategy of the manufacturers – *nitrazepam* is promoted as a sedative, *clonazepam* as an anticonvulsant.

Most benzodiazepines have an active metabolite with a prolonged elimination phase ($t_{1/2}$ more than 24 h). Administration once daily is therefore appropriate, preferably at night to prevent insomnia due to anxiety, but they are often given thrice daily. In the elderly, elimination is less efficient ($t_{1/2}$ up to 90 h) with cumulation leading to confusion, ataxia, drowsiness and incontinence. A few (*lorazepam, oxazepam*, **temazepam**) show a shorter elimination $t_{1/2}$ and this may promote dependence because of withdrawal symptoms between doses.

Benzodiazepine drug therapy should not be continued for more than 1 month. There are however many patients who have received benzodiazepines daily for many years. Withdrawal then becomes very difficult and requires strong motivation and support. Strangely, there is little tendency to escalate the dose and the costs of withdrawal may sometimes outweigh the benefits.

CSM advice on the use of benzodiazepines

'Benzodiazepines are indicated for the short-term relief (2–4 weeks only) of anxiety that is severe, disabling or subjecting the individual to unacceptable distress, occurring alone or in association with insomnia or short-term psychosomatic, organic or psychotic illness.

The use of benzodiazepines to treat short-term 'mild' anxiety is inappropriate and unsuitable.'

Disadvantages of benzodiazepines

Delay psychological adjustment
Their use diverts attention from the provision of more effective aid directed at causes.

Unwanted effects
Sedation – drowsiness, ataxia, impaired judgement, prolonged reaction time, interference with the ability to drive or operate machinery safely, hostility, aggression, antisocial acts, confusion and summation with alcohol.

Drugs of dependence
Tolerance, with psychological and physical dependence, that is worse in alcoholism, drug abuse or personality disorder can occur after long, high-dose exposure. Withdrawal gives insomnia, apprehension, anorexia, tremor, sweating, disordered perception, confusion and convulsions after an onset time of approximately 24 h after short-acting drugs and 3–10 days after long-acting ones. This withdrawal syndrome lasts 8–10 days.

Managing withdrawal from benzodiazepines

In 75% of patients a tapering regimen (reduce dose by one-quarter weekly) is successful if agreed with the patient. If sleep is disrupted, advise against catnapping.

In 25% of patients withdrawal symptoms are unavoidable; transfer from a short- to a long-acting benzodiazepine, substitute **propranolol** and again taper the dose of benzodiazepine. Interpret the occurrence of the problem as a signal to use an alternative strategy in managing anxiety.

Other anxiolytic agents

Antagonists at β-adrenoceptors (**propranolol**) leave untouched the primary psychological symptoms of worry, tension and fear. They reduce the somatic adrenergic symptoms of palpitations, sweating and tremor and the secondary psychological symptoms that arise from them.

The anxiolytic effect of *buspirone* shows a slow (2 weeks) onset. It does not substitute for benzodiazepines in their withdrawal syndrome.

Summary

(1) Anxiety states may require treatment if severe, disabling or subjecting the patient to unacceptable distress. Drugs may provide short-term relief while psychological techniques are being learned.

(2) Benzodiazepines (especially the shorter-acting kind), if used continuously for more than 1 month, are liable to induce physical dependence

STAFFS UNIVERSITY LIBRARY

and withdrawal anxiety. **Propranolol** is useful during withdrawal from benzodiazepine dependence. Antidepressant drugs, especially those inhibiting 5-hydroxytryptamine re-uptake, may be effective if the anxiety neurosis contains significant symptoms of depression, severe obsessional-compulsive disorder and panic disorder.

Depressive illness

Symptoms of depressive illness

Mood changes

Depressed mood is the core feature. Persistence for more than 2 weeks, crying and a distinct quality differentiate morbid depressed mood from normal.

Anxiety symptoms

These include worrying and/or nervous tension, hypochondriasis, headache and other tension pains, restlessness and/or agitation, panic attacks and phobias and/or obsessional symptoms.

Cognitive symptoms

Self-deprecation, loss of self-confidence, ideas of guilt and/or worthlessness come under this heading. It is essential to enquire of hopelessness and suicidal ideas and/or plans.

Biological symptoms

Disturbed sleep pattern, loss of libido, loss of energy and/or fatigue, appetite/weight loss, diurnal variation of mood and psychomotor retardation (mental and physical slowing), impaired concentration, inefficient thinking and loss of interest are biological symptoms.

Psychotic symptoms

These comprise depressive delusions and depressive hallucinations.

Natural history

Depressive illness is common. It represents 3.5% of all male and 7.5% of all female patients presenting to GPs. In one-quarter it shows a rapid recovery, in one-half it fluctuates over a period of approximately 1 year and in the remaining quarter it becomes a chronic problem.

Treatment

If there is persistent depressed mood with four or more biological symptoms, physical treatment outperforms placebo. A combination of treatments is aimed at changing the aetiological factors amenable to change. Determining aetiology should be kept distinct from making the diagnosis; a common fallacy is that understandable depression is not amenable to drug treatment. Psychological and social causes (marital difficulties, difficult children) may be intractable. Nevertheless, social and psychological treatments are crucially important in the treatment of depression.

Psychological

An opportunity to explore difficulties may be of more benefit than drugs in mild depression. Cognitive therapy. Help in dealing with the problems of social isolation, employment, money and children.

Physical

Physical forms of treatment are needed in moderate and severe depressive illness:

(1) *Drugs* – tricyclic antidepressant and related drugs, 70% respond (20–35% respond to placebo; the placebo response is less in moderate and severe depression than in mild depression); inhibitors of MAO or, where depression is part of manic-depressive illness, **lithium** salts.
(2) *Electroconvulsive therapy* (ECT) is indicated when the delay in the onset of drug action is undesirable.

Antidepressant drug selection

The biochemical basis of depression may be related to a loss of functional monoamine neurotransmission in the brain due to diminished release (see p. 220) or to disturbance of presynaptic receptor function. Early treatment used amphetamine-like agents for mild depression and ECT for severe depression. Important developments in treatment stemmed from observations of mood elevation in patients receiving drugs for other illnesses:

(1) with the antitubercular drug **isoniazid**, which was shown to be due to inhibition of MAO. The dietary restrictions and adverse drug interactions of the inhibitors of MAO (see p. 86) are disadvantages. **Phenelzine** is most used because of acute stimulant effects and least tendency amongst inhibitors of MAO to cause serious unwanted effects.
(2) with **imipramine**, a tricyclic compound that was on trial as an antipsychotic drug in schizophrenia, was later shown to inhibit re-uptake of noradrenaline (see p. 88) and 5-hydroxytryptamine.

More selective blockers of re-uptake have been developed that selectively inhibit the uptake of either noradrenaline (dothiepin, maprotiline, *lofepramine*) or 5-hydroxytryptamine (**fluoxetine**, *fluvoxamine*). Drugs of the latter kind are known as selective serotonin re-uptake inhibitors (SSRIs).

   Mianserin and *trazodone* have minimal effects on amine uptake and their mechanism of action is obscure. They may enhance noradrenaline release by blocking presynaptic α_2-adrenoceptors that inhibit noradrenaline release. They also block postsynaptic 5-hydroxytryptamine receptors. Evidence for superior efficacy is not compelling and they account for little of the market. Patients treated with *mianserin* require regular blood counts because of the small risk of dyscrasia.

Selection is based on considerations of safety in use, unwanted effects, length of experience and cost. More sedative drugs (**amitriptyline**, *trazodone*) are prescribed at night for the more agitated or anxious patient. Less sedative drugs (**imipramine**) are preferred for the withdrawn, apathetic patient.

Safety in overdosage is an important consideration given the hazard of a suicide attempt. Tricyclic antidepressant drugs are less safe than selective inhibitors of re-uptake. SSRIs appear safer on overdosing. Patients should be provided with only a small supply of the drug. A relative should be made aware of the dangers associated with the drug. However, significant risk of suicide should result in referral to a psychiatrist before prescribing.

Unwanted effects (see below) will deter the patient from taking the drug. Patient compliance can be improved by building up the dose over 1 week and informing the patient of unwanted effects. This is important, because the onset of antidepressive effect is delayed for some 1–2 weeks after the start of treatment.

Suicidal tendencies necessitate admission to hospital because of the delay in therapeutic effect.

Imipramine is commonly used in severe depression but electroconvulsive therapy may occasionally be needed for a rapid effect. **Amitriptyline** is more sedative and is suitable if agitation or insomnia are problems. Recent pharmacokinetic studies have shown that once-daily administration is adequate. The sedative effect is turned to advantage by taking the drug at night and dose-related antimuscarinic adverse effects (dry mouth, blurred vision) do not obtrude during sleep.

SSRIs have fewer peripheral antimuscarinic unwanted effects and are less likely to affect the cardiovascular system (see p. 234). They are useful in treating depression in patients suffering from heart disease. They are less sedative than non-selective blockers of re-uptake. The selective blockers of 5-hydroxytryptamine uptake are the only antidepressant drugs that do not cause weight gain.

The atypical antidepressant drugs *mianserin* and *trazodone* are strongly sedative but reasonably safe because of their lack of cardiotoxicity and antimuscarinic effects.

Unwanted effects and cautions with antidepressant drugs

(1) *Sedation* (**amitriptyline**) and respiratory depression in overdose.
(2) *Cardiotoxicity* (tricyclic antidepressant drugs), including dysrhythmias and conduction defects, are especially dangerous after a recent myocardial infarction and in the elderly. The mechanism is not known.
(3) *Antagonism at muscarinic acetylcholine receptors* (tricyclic antidepressant drugs more than SSRIs) produces dry mouth, impaired vision, constipation, difficulty of micturition, glaucoma and urinary retention.

These effects are worst in the elderly.
(4) *Antagonism at α-adrenoceptors.* Postural hypotension occurs.
(5) There is a reduction in convulsive threshold.
(6) Blood dyscrasia occurs in approximately 1 : 10 000 with *mianserin.*

Life events on the prescribing of tricyclic antidepressant drugs
In pregnancy there is some danger of neonatal toxicity. Too little is secreted in milk to be harmful to the breast-fed child. Dosage reduction is required in renal and liver impairment.

In elderly patients halve the dose. The prescribing problem is greater because: depressive illness is commoner, other disease is often present, including heart disease and glaucoma, and an interacting drug is likely to be in use. Most antidepressant agents may cause confusional states (delirium) in the elderly.

Response to tricyclic antidepressant drugs and relatives

Improvement occurs early in insomnia and anxiety and after 10–14 days in other symptoms, but can take up to 6 weeks.

If no improvement occurs (15% of patients) increase the dose or change to another form of physical treatment. In patients successfully treated, withdrawal of the drugs produces relapse in less than 6 months in 50%, while 50% remain symptom free. Maintenance therapy improves these figures to 20% and 80% respectively. Treatment should be maintained for 4 months after recovery and then tailed off over 6 weeks.

Lithium salts

Severe depression (so-called <u>unipolar</u> illness) may be one pole of the bipolar manic-depressive psychosis and recovery from depression may be followed by pathological elevation of mood with acute mania. Suppression of such swings of mood can be achieved with a **lithium** salt. Its acute toxicity can be avoided by regular monitoring of blood concentrations and by the use of slow-release preparations. It always causes a degree of polyuria and dry mouth. The mechanism of action is not known but it inhibits both Na^+/K^+-ATPase and inositol-1-phosphatase.

Serum concentration should be 0.6–1.2 mmole/L at 12 h after dosage. Dosage adjustment is aided by further serum lithium concentration assays at 3–4 days, 1 week and then at 4-weekly intervals. At concentrations within the therapeutic window, **lithium**:

(1) Regulates the mood in mania.
(2) Reduces the incidence and severity of recurrent bipolar or unipolar depressive illness. (So do prophylactic antidepressant drugs but in bipolar disease they may increase the risk of mania.) **Lithium** can significantly enhance the antidepressant effect of inhibitors of re-uptake.

Toxicity of lithium salts
Toxicity in the CNS may lead to tremor, ataxia, dysarthria, nystagmus and convulsions; in the kidney to impaired function. Toxicity is treated by

withdrawal of **lithium** salts and administration of salt and water.

Summary

(1) Depressive illness is common, with psychological and biological symptoms, and amenable to social, psychological and physical forms of treatment. With all drug treatments there is a delayed (1–2 weeks) onset of antidepressant effect; full benefit may take 6 weeks. ECT relieves suicidal depression more rapidly than does drug treatment.
(2) The tricyclic and related group of antidepressant drugs comprises agents that inhibit the re-uptake of one or both of noradrenaline and 5-hydroxytryptamine, and some atypical agents. Inhibitors of MAO are effective but impose dietary restrictions and cause adverse drug interactions. Lithium salts regulate mood in mania and reduce the incidence and severity of recurrent bipolar or unipolar depressive illness. Selection between these is based on safety in use, unwanted effects, length of experience and cost.

Schizophrenia

Psychosis involves qualitative abnormalities of mental functions, including thought disorder, delusions and hallucinations. A <u>delusion</u> is an unshakeable false belief, such as the conviction that newscasters are referring to the patient. <u>Hallucinations</u> are false perceptions, e.g. hearing completely realistic voices discussing the patient.

First rank symptoms of schizophrenia

These symptoms are: thought insertion (experience of thoughts being put into one's mind); thought broadcasting (experience of one's thoughts being known to others); feelings of passivity (experience of emotions, or specific bodily movements or specific sensations being caused by an external agency or being under some external control); voices discussing one's thoughts or behaviour, as they occur, sometimes forming a running commentary; voices discussing or arguing about one, referring to 'he/she'; voices repeating one's thoughts out loud or anticipating one's thoughts.

In primary delusions, <u>primary</u> means arising inexplicably from perceptions that in themselves are normal (e.g. the traffic lights change and this is taken to mean that a message is being conveyed by the colours to the patient).

Treatment

Admission to hospital is often required, to protect both the patient and their family. Usually this is voluntary but compulsory admission is sometimes necessary. Antipsychotic drugs reverse or reduce the thought disorder, hallucinations and delusions (though the memory of these events is unaffected) and prevent relapse.

Acute phase (first month)

Table 9.3 Selection of antipsychotic drugs

	Sedation	Antimuscarinic effects	Extrapyramidal effects
Short-acting preparations			
Phenothiazines			
Group 1 (**chlorpromazine**)	+++	++	++
Group 2 (*thioridazine*)	++	+++	+
Group 3 (*trifluoperazine*)	+	+	+++
Butyrophenones (*haloperidol*)	++	+	+++(+)
Diphenylbutylpiperidines (*pimozide*)	+	+	+++
Substituted benzamides (*sulpiride*)	+	+	++
Clozapine	++	+	+
Risperidone	+	0	+
Long-acting depot preparations			
Thioxanthenes (*flupenthixol decanoate*)	+	+	+++(+)
Phenothiazines (fluphenazine decanoate)	+	+	+++(+)
Butyrophenones (haloperidol decanoate)	++	+	++++

For the florid, acute, positive and disturbed patient a sedative antipsychotic drug is indicated (Table 9.3). For the withdrawn, negative and inactive patient a less sedative drug (low dose *sulpiride*) is better.

Medium term (1–3 months)
Exert effort to avoid the rejection of the patient by his/her family, workmates and employer. Depot i/m antipsychotic drug (every 2 weeks at first, then monthly) can return patient behaviour nearly back to normal.

Long term
Continue with maintenance antipsychotic drug treatment. Rehabilitation involves finding the optimum balance between patient initiative and planned help. The patient may need to seek less ambitious work than he/she held down before the onset of illness.

Antipsychotic drug selection

On first administration of a depot formulation of antipsychotic drug it is wise to administer a test dose. The route is deep i/m injection and extrapyramidal reactions are usually present a few hours to 2 days after each dose.

Clozapine has a broader range of efficacy, often being effective where other agents have failed. However, weekly full blood counts are monitored by a central agency because of the tendency to induce aplastic anaemia. The drug is dispensed weekly, conditional upon receipt of samples and a stable cell count.

Risperidone has fewer extrapyramidal side-effects than conventional antipsychotic agents.

Adverse effects of antipsychotic drugs

Antagonism at muscarinic acetylcholine receptors, gives dry mouth, constipation, difficult micturition and blurred vision.

Antagonism at α-adrenoceptors leads to hypotension and tachycardia, and erectile failure.

Antagonism at D_2 dopamine receptors, causes movement disorders, collectively known as extrapyramidal adverse effects:

(1) Parkinsonism (hypokinesia, rigidity, tremor) is dose related and more common with the potent antipsychotic drugs (*haloperidol, pimozide*). Patients who need high doses and show these effects also require treatment with centrally acting antagonists at the muscarinic acetylcholine receptors *procyclidine* or *benzhexol* (note peripheral antimuscarinic unwanted effects).

(2) Acute dystonic responses occur in the young on first exposure to the drug and may be mistaken for tetanus. They require treatment with oral or i/v antimuscarinic agents (*procyclidine, benzhexol*).

(3) <u>Akathisia</u> is inner turmoil and restlessness of the legs and may cause continuous pacing and an inability to sit still. Antimuscarinic agents sometimes help; **propranolol** may also help.

(4) Tardive dyskinesia occurs in patients chronically taking antipsychotic drugs. It is of delayed onset (<u>tardive</u>) and may be irreversible. The disorder involves buccolingual masticatory movements and less commonly jerky and bizarre movements (dyskinesia) of the limbs, trunk or head and neck. The cause is not understood, although proliferation of dopamine receptors following prolonged blockade (upregulation) has been suggested.

Tardive dyskinesia occurs after many months of treatment in 15–20% of patients (long duration of treatment, high dose and old age of patient seem to be risk factors). It is difficult to manage – the best policy seems to be gradual reduction of antipsychotic drug over 1–2 years, perhaps with drug holidays.

Neuroleptic malignant syndrome comprises pyrexia, muscle rigidity and CNS depression. The plasma concentration of creatine phosphokinase is markedly increased. The syndrome occurs in any stage of therapy. The outcome may be fatal and intensive care may be needed.

Temperature regulation is disturbed, leading to hypothermia (occasionally pyrexia).

Sedation occurs, giving feelings of uneasiness, mental fatigue and lethargy.

Hypersensitivity leads to skin rashes, photosensitivity, jaundice (intrahepatic obstruction), agranulocytosis, aplastic anaemia.

Purplish pigmentation of the skin, cornea, conjunctiva and retina occurs and corneal and lens opacities.

Life events on the prescribing of antipsychotic drugs

Do not stop the drugs in pregnancy. Too little is secreted in milk to be harmful to the breast-fed child. Dosage reduction is required in renal and liver impairment.

In elderly patients lower the dose. Select drugs showing less sedation, extrapyramidal symptoms and hypothermia (e.g. Group 2 phenothiazines – *thioridazine*).

Prognosis

In patients successfully treated for a first attack of acute schizophrenia, withdrawal of the drugs produces relapse in 75%, while 25% remain symptom free. Maintenance therapy improves these figures to 33% and 67% respectively. Treatment should be maintained for 1–2 years after overt symptoms have disappeared and then tailed off over 6 weeks.

Duration of treatment

Maintenance treatment is effective but associated with adverse effects. The danger of relapse (present over several weeks) with its social consequences makes continuation a preferable strategy to withdrawal. Withdrawal should only occur with specialist approval, when the patient is in a stable social environment, when there have been no psychotic symptoms for 6 months and the patient has the insight to recognize early signs of relapse and respond by returning for resumption of therapy. Abrupt withdrawal produces a syndrome lasting a few weeks, resembling acetylcholinergic overactivity plus insomnia and dyskinesias. Dosage should instead be reduced over several months.

Summary

(1) Schizophrenia is a psychosis involving thought disorder, delusions and hallucinations. Antipsychotic drugs treatments reverse or reduce these features and prevents relapse.
(2) Selection among the drugs available is based on duration of action, other properties and unwanted effects.

Epilepsy

The characteristic feature is a sudden and brief interruption of consciousness or <u>seizure</u>. Approximately 1 person in 50 experiences a seizure at sometime during their life and the prevalence of people who experience repeated seizures or who need drugs to prevent them is almost 1 in 100. Thus epilepsy is the commonest serious neurological disorder.

During the seizure there is a rapid and synchronous discharge from cerebral neurones. This can arise in the normal brain if the destabilizing stimulus (e.g. hypocalcaemia or hypoglycaemia) is sufficient but in epilepsy either the threshold for starting a seizure is low throughout the brain (primary generalized epilepsy) or there is a locally damaged area from which the seizure starts (localization-related epilepsy).

Classification of seizures

Generalized seizures

The abnormal neuronal discharge involves the whole of the cerebrum. It is primary when it arises simultaneously in all parts.

(1) Generalized tonic-clonic (grand mal): consciousness is lost suddenly and all skeletal muscle contracts, first continuously (tonic) and then rhythmically (clonic). Falls and injury are common. Recovery is slow and often requires sleep.
(2) Myoclonic jerks: brief muscle contractions without loss of consciousness. They often affect the shoulders and upper limbs. Minor accidents and spillages may be reported. Less commonly the whole body is affected and falls are caused.
(3) Absences (petit mal): the patient (usually a child) is vacant for a few seconds whilst the electroencephalogram (EEG) typically shows a generalized 3 Hz spike and wave discharge. There may be flickering eye movements but the patient docs not fall and recovers instantly.
(4) Atonic: postural tone in skeletal muscle is suddenly lost. The resulting falls can cause acute injury and cumulative brain injury (subcortical dementia).

Partial seizures

Only a part of the cerebrum is involved, but consciousness can be lost (complex).

(1) Simple: depending on the part affected these may be autonomic (skin pallor, pilo-erection), sensory (abnormal smell or sound; tingling or feeling of swelling), motor (twitching of face or limb) or psychic (déjà vu or fear).
(2) Complex (temporal lobe): stereotyped movements often involving hands or mouth. There may be fumbling with clothing or objects. The patient may wander into danger or do familiar tasks without purpose or recall (automatism).

The seizure may start simple ('warning') and become complex. A motor seizure may spread from hand or face to the whole of one side (Jacksonian progression). Similarly, any partial seizure may progress to a tonic-clonic one (secondary generalization). Conversely, drug treatment that suppresses tonic-clonic events may reveal previously unrecognized partial seizures.

Serial seizures

A series of seizures can arise particularly if administration of CNS-depressant drugs (antiepileptic agents, alcohol) is suddenly stopped. Status epilepticus arises when consciousness is not recovered between seizures. Convulsive status can cause lasting brain damage if not treated promptly.

Classification of syndromes

The chief distinction is between primary generalized and localization-related epilepsy but each of these broad groups includes several distinct syndromes, which differ in prognosis and treatment.

In Childhood Absence Epilepsy typical absence seizures arise early in life. They respond to **sodium valproate**, *ethosuximide* or *lamotrigine*. Absences often cease in adulthood, enabling treatment to be withdrawn. Another primary generalized epilepsy (Juvenile Myoclonic) often begins in the teens with myoclonic jerks on awakening. There may also be absences and tonic-clonic seizures. **Sodium valproate** is effective and may be needed throughout life. **Carbamazepine** makes the jerks worse.

Localization-related epilepsies generally respond well to **carbamazepine** but when drugs are not effective, surgery should be considered. Partial seizures may start in areas of cortical dysplasia (abnormal development) or gliosis, which are so sited that excision does not endanger function.

Causes of epilepsy

Every pathology that affects the brain (vascular malformation, abscess, injury, tumour, haemorrhage, ischaemia or infarction) can be manifest as localization-related epilepsy. Gliosis of the anteromedial part of a temporal lobe, which can arise after prolonged febrile convulsions in infancy, is an important cause of temporal lobe epilepsy. Primary generalized epilepsy can have a genetic basis, e.g. juvenile myoclonic epilepsy is associated with an abnormality in the HLA region of chromosome 6.

Precipitating factors

In a predisposed person, a seizure can be precipitated by a variety of stimuli (alcohol excess, drug withdrawal, excitement, fever, flashing lights (photoconvulsive epilepsy), overbreathing, sleep lack). It is not uncommon, however, for a seizure to occur without any obvious precipitant.

Epileptiform activity in the EEG is accentuated during sleep and by i/v drugs used for anaesthesia. Antidepressant, corticosteroid and antipsychotic drugs can increase the likelihood of seizures when used at conventional doses in predisposed patients.

Seizures can occur when organ failure (kidney or liver) causes serious metabolic disturbance and when disease states (eclampsia, severe hypertension) cause cerebral oedema.

Electrophysiology

Hughlings Jackson (born 1835) defined a seizure as 'a sudden, excessive, rapid and local discharge in the grey matter of the brain'.

Recording from the neurones of an epileptic focus in an experimental animal (Figure 9.2) reveals spontaneous depolarization (a paroxysmal depolarization shift) that initiates a train of action potentials (synchronized burst discharge). Usually this burst is terminated by hyperpolarization as shown, but if it continues and spreads to involve sufficient surrounding neurones a seizure is generated.

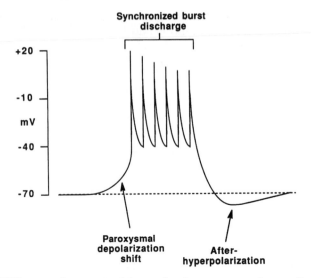

Figure 9.2 Transmembrane potential recording from a neurone in an epileptic focus

The onset of spontaneous temporal lobe seizures has been studied in patients with indwelling recording electrodes and microdialysis probes, which were introduced before surgery for epilepsy. The first detectable change was the release of the excitatory neurotransmitter glutamate, which preceded the EEG seizure discharge and was quickly followed by release of the inhibitory transmitter, GABA.

Antiepileptic drugs

The most widely used are **carbamazepine**, **sodium valproate** and **phenytoin**; comparative trials show equal efficacy against generalized tonic-clonic and complex partial seizures. *Phenobarbitone* and *primidone* (active metabolites include phenobarbitone) are more sedative at equi-effective doses and their use in the developed world has therefore waned. *Ethosuximide* and **sodium valproate** prevent absence seizures.

Carbamazepine is chemically related to tricyclic antidepressant agents. It is effective against tonic-clonic and partial seizures but patients with absence or myoclonic seizures are not helped. It is also useful in trigeminal neuralgia and bipolar affective disorder. Dose-related unwanted effects include double vision and unsteadiness. The drug induces hepatic MFO, thereby shortening its own $t_{1/2}$ and interacting with other drugs as described under Adverse drug interactions (see p. 442). Inappropriate ADH secretion shows itself as hyponatraemia; recurrent cough or sore throat suggests white cell suppression (leucopenia); an allergic skin rash is produced in approximately 5% of patients but despite these problems **carbamazepine** is generally well tolerated and is now the most popular antiepileptic drug in the UK.

Sodium valproate is effective against primary generalized seizures

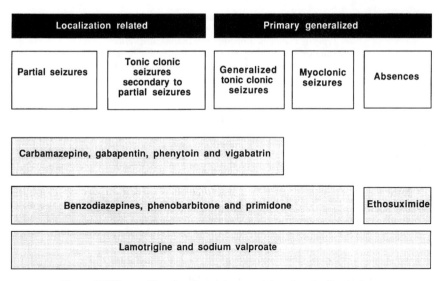

Figure 9.3 The profile of anticonvulsant activity of antiepileptic drugs

including absences and myoclonic jerks; it is the drug of choice in juvenile myoclonic epilepsy. It is also effective against partial and secondarily generalized seizures, thus having a broad spectrum of efficacy (Figure 9.3). Unwanted effects include weight gain, hair loss and tremor but they are generally mild. Nausea and heartburn have been overcome by enteric coating of the tablets (see p. 333). A biochemical abnormality may underlie the rare but life-threatening liver toxicity that is almost confined to children aged below 3 years or patients with metabolic or degenerative disorders. In contrast to **carbamazepine** and **phenytoin**, **sodium valproate** does not induce, but rather inhibits, MFO and tends to increase the plasma concentrations of other antiepileptic drugs, particularly *lamotrigine* (see below).

Phenytoin, once the most popular of these drugs, is now less used. It is no less effective than **carbamazepine** against tonic-clonic and partial seizures but unwanted effects and awkward pharmacokinetic properties (see p. 388) discourage its use. Gum overgrowth, acne and increased facial hair can be disfiguring. Headache, double vision, slurred speech and unsteadiness are symptoms of excessive plasma concentration and can be corrected without loss of effectiveness by dosage adjustment that follows the pharmacokinetic principles described earlier. Excessive concentrations are sometimes caused not by increase in dose but by concurrent treatment with a drug that inhibits MFO (e.g. **cimetidine, erythromycin**).

Gabapentin was the third of the new antiepileptic drugs to receive a produce licence in the UK. Clinical trials in which the drug was added to established medication, showed halving of seizure frequency in 20–30% of patients with localization-related epilepsy. Although a structural analogue of GABA, it does not bind to $GABA_A$ receptors and its mode of action is not yet known. In add-on studies it shares the type A adverse effects that are common to many antiepileptic drugs (Table 9.4) but it seems

STAFFS UNIVERSITY LIBRARY

Table 9.4 Unwanted effects of antiepileptic drugs

Type A, augmented or predictable unwanted effects
(Common (active drug 50–60%, but placebo 30–40%)
and reversible (fade with time or dosage reduction))

Non-specific		
drowsiness	diplopia	mood change
tiredness	ataxia	confusion
headache	gut disturbance	
Drug specific		
hyponatraemia	**carbamazepine**	
weight gain	**sodium valproate**	
gum hyperplasia	**phenytoin**	
disinhibition	benzodiazepines	
skin rash	*lamotrigine*	
agitation	*vigabatrin*	

Type B, bizarre or idiosyncratic adverse effects
(These are infrequent and may persist despite dosage reduction)

Drug specific	
agranulocytosis	**carbamazepine**
acute pancreatitis	**sodium valproate**
neuropathy	**phenytoin**
psychosis	*vigabatrin*
Stevens–Johnson syndrome	*lamotrigine*

relatively free from serious, unpredictable (type B) effects. It is eliminated by renal excretion of unchanged drug and is not involved in pharmacokinetic interactions. The relatively short plasma $t_{1/2}$ means that the dosage interval is also short (approximately 8 h). The daily dose can be increased at short intervals so that its efficacy in the individual patient can be judged after treatment for a couple of months; when there is no benefit, withdrawal also seems to be generally trouble free.

Lamotrigine is unusual amongst antiepileptic drugs in that it reduces interictal EEG spike activity and, like **sodium valproate**, it has a broad spectrum of antiepileptic efficacy (Figure 9.3). Unlike **carbamazepine** and **phenytoin** it is effective against absences, atonic seizures and myoclonic jerks. Apart from the common type A unwanted effects (Table 9.4), its most important adverse effect is skin rash which is occasionally severe and associated with systemic illness. The likelihood of this is greatly increased in the presence of **sodium valproate**, which inhibits the major route of *lamotrigine* elimination (glucuronidation); the clearance is halved and the plasma concentration on a given dose is doubled. Since the risk of rash appears to be dose related, it is important to build up the dose slowly over a period of months. The recommended starting dose and the maximum are both halved in the presence of **sodium valproate**. When *lamotrigine* is added to **carbamazepine**, treatment symptoms of **carbamazepine** intoxication (double vision and unsteadiness) can appear. The interaction seems to be pharmacodynamic since there is no slowing of **carbamazepine** elimination.

Vigabatrin (see Figure 5.4), in combination with one of the established drugs, can further reduce the frequency of partial and generalized tonic-clonic seizures. Unwanted effects include drowsiness, dizziness, confusion and rarely psychosis. There is no evidence in human brain tissue removed during surgery or post-mortem of the oedema in myelin observed in the white matter of rat and dog brain. If current clinical trials confirm the efficacy of single drug treatment with *vigabatrin*, and postmarketing surveillance (see p. 452) detects no long-term neurotoxicity, it is likely to be used in the treatment of newly diagnosed epilepsy.

Ethosuximide is used primarily for the treatment of absence seizures particularly in early childhood, where the risk of hepatotoxicity with **sodium valproate** is greatest. Unwanted effects include nausea, vomiting, tiredness and unsteadiness. They can usually be prevented by dosage reduction.

Benzodiazepines suppress myoclonic jerks, partial seizures and generalized tonic-clonic seizures. Entry into brain is rapid with immediate onset of antiepileptic action but effectiveness wanes with continued use (tolerance, see p. 265). CNS depression is manifest as drowsiness and lack of concentration but seldom as depression of respiration. These properties make benzodiazepines very suitable for emergency use and for intermittent use. A series of tonic-clonic seizures can often be stopped by **diazepam** as rectal solution; this acts more quickly than tablet or suppository and can be given by relatives or carers not able to give i/v injections. For intermittent use, the 1–5 benzodiazepine *clobazam* is preferred to the other more sedative (1–4) members of the group (e.g. *clonazepam*). It may be taken orally by the patient to prevent seizures during a special social occasion, over a high risk time (e.g. the week before the menstrual period) or whilst experiencing a cluster of partial seizures. Once the special indication has passed the drug is stopped and held in reserve until the next time.

Paraldehyde is a cyclic trimer of acetaldehyde. It is used in solution as an alternative to rectal **diazepam**. Unlike **diazepam** it is also effective by i/m injection. It becomes oxidized if stored too long, is incompatible with plastic syringes on more than brief contact, and gives an unpleasant smell to the expired air. Despite these drawbacks, it is safe and effective.

Acetazolamide may increase the threshold to seizures by reducing salt and water retention (e.g. premenstrually) and by increasing brain P_{CO_2}. Tolerance develops within a few weeks, making the drug more suited to intermittent treatment.

Development of new drugs

There is need for more effective drugs with less toxicity. Antiepileptic activity is demonstrated by prevention of experimental (electrical or drug-induced) seizures in animals and freedom from short-term adverse effects is demonstrated in healthy volunteers. Therapeutic efficacy can, however, only be established in patients with epilepsy. It would not be ethical to expose new patients to an unproven agent, nor to alter treatment when an established drug had given complete control of seizures. Early clinical trials must therefore rely on volunteers from that small proportion of patients whose epilepsy responds poorly to established drugs. This gives an inevitable bias against the new drug.

Management of epilepsy

The history from the patient and a description of the supposed epileptic events from an observer often gives the diagnosis. Cardiovascular causes for syncope must be excluded and the search for an underlying cause pursued.

With drug treatment 70–80% of newly diagnosed patients become free from seizures. If only one seizure has occurred and there was a clear precipitant (e.g. severe sleep deprivation), it may be proper to give no drug but the likelihood of chronic epilepsy is increased in proportion to the number of seizures experienced before drug treatment is started.

Choice of drug

Since **carbamazepine**, **sodium valproate** and **phenytoin** are broadly equi-effective the choice is often based on the relevance to the individual patient of the common unwanted effects described earlier. With any of the drugs, drowsiness, dizziness and lack of concentration are often experienced at the start of treatment but these fade as tolerance develops; the drug is therefore best started at a low dose, which is increased slowly according to the clinical response.

A diary of epileptic events kept by the patient or relatives is essential. Benefit means fewer seizures per month, reduced duration or severity of seizures (less secondary generalization) or an increase in seizure-free days. This is weighed against cost in unwanted effects; the aim is not freedom from seizures at any price but preservation of function with maximum realization of individual potential.

Guided by the response and, in some instances, by the plasma drug concentration, the daily dose is adjusted until the optimum for the individual is found. In this process the recommended plasma concentration ranges (Table 9.5) are interpreted flexibly. A big variation in plasma concentration without a change in dose indicates poor compliance. This should be discussed with the patient who may be troubled by unwanted effects or simply forgetful. Reduction of dose or simplification of treatment may give more consistent plasma concentrations.

Pharmacokinetic factors

Most of the antiepileptic drugs listed above remain effective when given as two spaced doses per day. The necessary persistence of effect is based

Table 9.5 Recommended antiepileptic drug concentration in plasma

Drug	mg/L
Carbamazepine	6–12
Sodium valproate	50–100
Phenytoin	10–20
Ethosuximide	40–100
Phenobarbitone	10–30

on slow decay of plasma drug concentration (**phenytoin**, *phenobarbitone*), active metabolites (carbamazepine epoxide, *N*-desmethyl clobazam) and long-lasting inhibition of enzymes (carbonic anhydrase, GABA amino-transferase). This removes the need to take medicines to school or work for a mid-day dose. Young children have a shorter $t_{1/2}$ and may sometimes need three spaced doses each day. Similarly, *gabapentin* has a relatively short $t_{1/2}$ and is routinely prescribed three times daily.

The saturable nature of **phenytoin** metabolism demands small dosage increments when approaching the recommended plasma concentration range. Failure to appreciate this can cause the plasma concentration to overshoot into the toxic range.

Drug combinations

Treatment with one drug alone is the ideal. If the first drug does not work well, a second is introduced and the dose built up until it is safe to withdraw the first; the response to the second drug in isolation is then assessed. When strict monotherapy fails, a satisfactory result may still be obtained by adding a second drug (*clobazam* or less commonly *acetazolamide*) on an intermittent basis as described for benzodi-azepines above. In more severe cases with multiple kinds of seizure, combinations of two or even three major antiepileptic drugs are sometimes unavoidable.

Drug withdrawal

When a patient on drug treatment has been free from epileptic events for 2 years it is right to question whether the drug is still needed. One option is to withdraw the drug by small reductions in dosage at intervals of a month or more, to avoid precipitating withdrawal seizures. In the case of **phenytoin**, the early reductions must correspond with the smallest avail-able dosage form (25 mg capsule). Before recommending any dosage reduction, the question of driving must be fully discussed.

Driving

UK law permits someone with epilepsy to drive a private vehicle when they have been free from all epileptic events (including simple partial seizures or myoclonic jerks) for 12 months. Driving is also permissible if epileptic events arise exclusively during sleep.

For many people, gaining a driving licence is the hallmark of therapeutic success in epilepsy and the fear of losing it deters many drivers from contemplating the withdrawal of antiepileptic medication. There is however a greater fear – that of having a child with a drug-induced congenital abnormality.

Pregnancy

Congenital malformations have been reported in association with each of the major drugs and none can be considered entirely safe; on the other hand, falls caused by seizures can also harm the fetus. The aetiology of congenital malformations is multifactorial (see p. 435), thus avoidance of alcohol and smoking, provision of a balanced diet and prevention of folate deficiency are all relevant.

The overall population risk of major congenital malformation (2–4% of pregnancies) is doubled when the mother is receiving one antiepileptic drug. Since the damage generally occurs within 8–10 weeks of conception, any preventive steps must be taken before conception. When the seizures are absences or simple partial seizures, the prospective mother often chooses to stop all medication, but when they are tonic-clonic, it is usual to continue treatment with one drug at modest dosage.

In the case of **sodium valproate** there is a special risk of spina bifida (1–2% of pregnancies: higher in one recent series), which may be minimized by prescribing no more than 1000 mg/day and dividing this into three or four doses. **Folic acid** supplementation may also reduce the risk. Although neural tube defects can be diagnosed in utero (alphafetoprotein assay, ultrasound scan), this only prevents the birth of a handicapped child if the parents can contemplate termination.

In mid and late pregnancy it may be necessary to increase daily dosage to offset the tendency for increased liver metabolism to lower the plasma drug concentration. Allowance must however be made for the reduction in plasma albumin concentration, which increases the proportion of drug in the free state. After delivery, antiepileptic drug therapy does not prevent breast feeding except when high plasma concentrations of *phenobarbitone* are present. It may be necessary, however, to reduce dosage gradually to the prepregnant rate as liver metabolism returns to normal.

Summary

(1) Epileptic seizures arise from a variety of causes and adversely affect the lives of many people.
(2) When the seizures are classified and the syndrome identified, it is usually possible to give a valid prognosis and select an effective antiepileptic drug.
(3) Understanding of the pathophysiology of seizure generation and the mechanisms of antiepileptic drug action has increased recently.
(4) The drugs differ in spectrum of efficacy. **Carbamazepine** is widely used in localization-related epilepsy and **sodium valproate** in primary generalized. Newer drugs may be added (e.g. *gabapentin* in the former, *lamotrigine* in the latter) when the response to the first choice is not adequate.
(5) Patients must understand the need for strict adherence to the daily treatment schedule, which should be kept as simple as possible. Similarly they must be aware of possible adverse effects.
(6) When treatment is effective driving becomes an attainable target.

(7) Pregnancy and parenthood provide special challenges, particularly when it is the mother who has epilepsy. With forward planning the adverse effects of the antiepileptic drug on the baby can be reduced to a minimum.

Drugs and fertility

Choice of family planning method

Reasons for family planning include the desire to:

(1) Temporarily prevent pregnancy.
(2) Increase the interval between births.
(3) Permanently prevent pregnancy when the required family size is achieved.

The decision on whether to use family planning and which method is influenced by the above and:

(1) Political, cultural and religious background, including whether family planning is accepted as a male or female prerogative.
(2) Efficacy (Table 9.6) – less efficient methods may become acceptable as fertility declines with age.
(3) Acceptability.
(4) Availability.
(5) Cost.

Family planning has had a major influence on individual families but none on the populations of countries unless accompanied by socioeconomic development.

'Natural' methods of contraception

Lactational amenorrhoea

During lactation, suckling reflexly induces prolactin secretion (and reduces that of LH and FSH), which acts upon the ovary to inhibit follicular development. Consequently, the first ovulation postpartum is delayed (by approximately 30 weeks) and subsequent ovulations are less frequent. Therefore, the interval between births is on average increased. This method has a major influence on family size in developing countries. Its reliability for individual women is unpredictable.

Withdrawal

Coitus interruptus describes withdrawal of the penis from the vagina before ejaculation. This method is widely used but of doubtful reliability.

Rhythm methods

The knowledge that ovulation occurs approximately 14 days before the next menstrual period and that sperm can survive up to 3 days and ova 1 day in the female reproductive tract allows the prediction of 'safe' times for intercourse. The time of ovulation may be calculated from the date of onset of the last menstrual period or identified by keeping a daily early morning temperature record, as body temperature increases following ovulation. Alternatively, the cervical mucus can be sampled, as the mucus changes from a watery consistency to thick and extendable at ovulation. A disadvantage of these methods is the difficulty in predicting the time of ovulation with any accuracy. Domestic urinary hormone assay methods can detect the surge of LH 24–36 h before ovulation.

Mechanical methods of contraception

Condom

Both male and female versions are available. The male condom is widely used and with correct use family size, on average, may be reduced to two to three children. The <u>method</u> failure rate is low but the <u>user</u> failure rate is higher. There are no adverse effects and no medical involvement. Male condoms may be impregnated with spermicide and both versions also offer protection from sexually transmitted diseases.

Diaphragm and cap

These block the entry of sperm into the cervix. Supplementation with spermicidal preparations makes them moderately effective. There are no adverse effects and, following a preliminary training session, no medical involvement. These methods were widely used until oral contraceptive agents and intrauterine devices (IUDs) became available.

Intrauterine devices

Fertilization may be prevented with an IUD (a plastic loop or coil) in place. If a blastocyst develops, implantation does not occur. An intrauterine immune response to the IUD probably contributes to the mechanism of action. An IUD does not prevent ectopic pregnancies. An IUD is also effective if inserted within 72 h after coitus. Once fitted it usually remains in the uterus for several years. Occasional problems are expulsion, perforation, prolonged uterine bleeding and pelvic inflammatory disease. The efficacy is slightly improved and unwanted effects reduced if copper wire is wound around the IUD; the mechanism of action of the copper is unknown. This method is generally undesirable for nulliparous women, but it is effective and safe in older women.

Chemical methods of contraception

Spermicides

Spermicides promote the solution of lipids from cells and so kill sperm by destroying their membranes. They are formulated as creams, gels, foams and pessaries, but are not very effective by themselves. They lose activity after 2–4 h in situ. Evidence suggests that spermicides kill the biological vectors of sexually transmitted diseases, including the AIDS virus.

Hormonal methods

For mechanisms of action, see page 170.

Combined oral contraceptive preparations

This is the most popular systemic contraceptive method, and is widely used in developed countries. It has a negligible failure rate; any reported failures are likely to be due to missed tablets. Epidemiological studies suggest caution in their use in women over 35 or in heavy smokers and obese women due to a higher incidence of cardiovascular disease compared with non-users. The existence of numerous preparations permits the less severe unwanted effects to be controlled by changing the dose and/or the steroid analogue content.

Progestogen-only contraception

This may be achieved by depot injection, s/c implantations of silastic capsules containing progestogen or tablets. Depot injection of *medroxy-progesterone acetate* lasts 3–6 months. Regular injection causes disturbance and eventually absence of menstrual cycles and a delay in the return to fertility on cessation. Consequently it is a very effective contraceptive. The method is popular in developing countries, especially as it does not affect lactation and rigid compliance is not required. In developed countries it is mainly used after rubella vaccination or before vasectomy becomes effective. An association with breast tumours has been claimed.

Tablets of a 19-nortestosterone derivative, **norethisterone**, are administered continuously. The efficacy is lower than that of combined oral contraceptive preparations. It is useful in women during breast feeding or where the combined oral contraceptive preparations are contraindicated due to high cardiovascular risk (older patients). Full compliance is important, as efficacy is lost even if the tablet is taken late by as little as 3 h.

High-dose combined oral contraceptive preparations

These are effective postcoitally if given within 72 h of intercourse but are not recommended for routine use. Two tablets containing the maximum oestrogen dose (50 µg) are given, followed by another two 12 h later. Contraception is achieved by effects upon the fallopian tube, endometrium and ovary. Considerable nausea and vomiting occurs at this oestrogen dose.

Table 9.6 Approximate failure rates of contraceptive methods

Method	Pregnancy rate per 100 woman years*
Oviductal occlusion	Approximately 0.02
Vasectomy	Approximately 0.02
Combined oral contraceptive tablets	0.03–0.10
Progestogen-only depot injection	Approximately 0.5
Progestogen-only contraceptive tablets	1.5–3.0
Intrauterine device	1.5–3.0
Lactational amenorrhoea	3–5
Condom	4–28
Diaphragm	4–35
Spermicides	4–38
Rhythm	8–40
No contraception	Approximately 80

*100 women treated for 1 year.

The long-term use of oestrogens is associated with cardiovascular disease, therefore this method should serve only as an occasional measure.

Surgical methods of contraception

These methods are sought by 20–30% of couples after completion of their families. They are essentially permanent.

Vasectomy

The vas deferens is divided and the ends occluded. This is minor surgical procedure usually done as an outpatient under local anaesthesia. Sperm continue to be produced in the testis but do not reach the ejaculate. Fertility may be restored in a small proportion of cases using micro-surgery.

Oviductal occlusion

Access to the oviducts may be gained by abdominal, transvaginal or transcervical routes. They are either tied or sealed by cautery, clips or bands. Usually it is performed as an inpatient procedure. Very occasional recanalizations and subsequent pregnancies occur. The operation is expensive in medical resources.

Abortion

The distinction between a method of contraception (requiring precoital action) and a method of abortion (requiring postcoital action) is not always clear (see pp. 170, 524 and 525).

It is estimated there are 125 million live births, 40 million spontaneous abortions and 30 million induced abortions annually in the world. In some countries abortion on demand is available as a contraceptive measure. The hazards of abortion increase with gestational and maternal age.

Surgical methods

Vacuum aspiration

Up to approximately 4 weeks of gestation it is possible to remove the uterine contents by suction with a syringe using a plastic cannula. At this time it will not be certain that the woman is pregnant. After 6 weeks of gestation cervical dilatation is usually required first. These are outpatient procedures.

Dilatation and curettage

Following cervical dilatation, the uterine contents can be removed by scraping (curettage) and suction. This method is used at 9–12 weeks of gestation. There is evidence that forced cervical dilatation is followed by a higher subsequent spontaneous miscarriage rate, so cervical softening should be produced first by local application of *dinoprostone* (PGE$_2$).

Other non-surgical methods

Chemical methods are used in the second trimester (13–26 weeks of gestation). Prostaglandins induce abortion when administered vaginally or by extra-amniotic injection (*dinoprostone*). They probably act by a combination of a direct contractile action on the myometrium and a reduction in the placental endocrine support of pregnancy. Vomiting and diarrhoea are frequent unwanted effects.

Oral **mifepristone** can terminate pregnancy up to 9 weeks of gestation. Withdrawal of hormonal support to the uterus is brought about by this antagonist at progesterone receptors. Evacuation of the uterine contents by curettage or prostaglandins is needed to ensure efficacy.

Summary

(1) The wide variety of contraceptive methods available accommodates variation in personal, cultural and medical requirements.
(2) Hormonal changes underlie the mechanisms of the natural methods, which include lactational amenorrhoea (the suppression of follicular growth by prolactin) and the prediction of ovulation from changes in either ovarian steroid secretion detected by secondary physiological changes or urinary gonadotrophin measurement.
(3) Physical barriers that restrict the access of spermatozoa to the ovum include the condom, diaphragm and cap, and are usually supplemented with a spermicide. Their efficiency is limited by discontinuity of user compliance.
(4) Intrauterine devices inhibit implantation and possibly fertilization. They are particularly useful in multiparous women and those in whom

the systemic contraceptives are contraindicated.

(5) Combined oral contraceptive preparations are widely acceptable, relatively safe and have a negligible failure rate. However their use is restricted by a risk of cardiovascular disease. In high doses as a short course of treatment they are used for emergency contraception.

(6) Progestogens are contraceptives given either orally each day or as a depot injection or implant, which can last for several years. Injections and implants are popular as the need for continuous patient compliance is removed. Inhibition of ovulation is unreliable, and consequently the efficacy of progestogens is lower than that of the combined oral contraceptive preparations. Menstrual irregularities are common.

(7) Access of the gametes to the site of fertilization is denied by vasectomy and oviductal occlusion, which require minor surgical intervention. Both are highly effective and permanent.

(8) Abortion is the most hazardous contraceptive technique. Uterine contents can be removed physically by aspiration or dilatation and curettage. Termination of pregnancy can also be achieved by PGs with (up to 9 weeks) or without (13-25 weeks) the antagonist at progestogen receptors, **mifepristone**.

Haematinic drugs and the cellular elements of blood

Anaemia

Anaemia (lit. lack of blood) means deficiency of haemoglobin. It usually has an insidious onset and is asymptomatic. If very severe or of a more rapid onset the anaemic patient may have some of the following symptoms: listlessness, tiring easily, palpitations, muscle aches and pains, 'blackouts'; angina pectoris, intermittent claudication, breathlessness on exertion (high output cardiac failure).

The major clinical feature is pallor. This may be more evident in the mucous membranes than in the skin. However, pallor is unreliable as a diagnostic aid because it correlates poorly with blood haemoglobin content. Definitive recognition requires measurement of blood haemoglobin content (normally 14 g/dL men; 12 g/dL women). The haemoglobin content and red cell (erythrocyte) count of blood are closely linked.

There are two general ways in which erythrocytes are reduced in number. Formation may be impaired or destruction accelerated.

Impaired formation of erythrocytes arises from defects of:

(1) Haemoglobin synthesis – the functional erythrocyte mass is selectively reduced in iron-deficiency anaemia.

(2) DNA synthesis – erythrocytes, granulocytes and platelets are all

affected in megaloblastic anaemias (large peripheral blood cell parent cells in the bone marrow).

(3) Cell synthesis – erythrocytes, granulocytes and platelets are all reduced in numbers in aplastic anaemia.

Accelerated destruction or loss of erythrocytes arises from:

(1) Chronic blood loss, which leads to iron-deficiency anaemia.
(2) Haemolysis, which leads to a macrocytic anaemia (abnormally large erythrocytes in the peripheral blood).

Drugs used to correct these disorders are known as haematinic agents.

Iron-deficiency anaemia

Normal iron balance

In western countries the average daily intake of iron amounts to 20 mg. Most dietary iron is in the ferric (Fe^{3+}) form. Gastric secretions dissolve the dietary iron and facilitate its reduction to the ferrous (Fe^{2+}) form. This is an important physiological process, for iron can only be absorbed in the ferrous form. Normally only approximately 5% of the daily iron intake is absorbed and this occurs largely in the proximal duodenum.

Since no excretion mechanism for iron exists, the efficiency of iron absorption is modulated to maintain iron balance. It is the mucosal cells of the proximal duodenum that regulate the efficiency of iron absorption. When body iron stores are low, a large proportion of the iron taken up by the mucosal cell is transported by a carrier mechanism into the plasma, where it binds to the plasma transport protein, transferrin. A relatively small proportion of the iron taken up by the mucosal cell is stored there

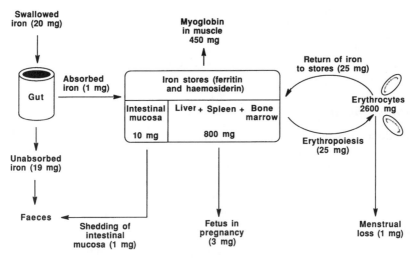

Figure 9.4 The amounts of iron in key locations and the average daily movements between locations

in the form of ferritin. In contrast, when body iron stores are replete, the mucosal cell transports relatively little iron into the plasma and greater amounts of iron are stored within the cell as ferritin.

The serum iron transport protein, transferrin, is synthesized in the liver at a rate inversely proportional to the state of the iron stores. It is measured as <u>total iron binding capacity</u>. In iron deficiency anaemia the serum iron concentration is smaller but the total iron binding capacity of the serum is greater than normal.

Ferritin is the tissue storage form of iron and is found not only in the gut mucosa but also in the liver, spleen and bone marrow. Serum ferritin concentration provides a more accurate index of tissue iron stores than relative saturation (serum iron concentration/total iron binding capacity) of the serum iron binding capacity.

Figure 9.4 shows the pools of iron and their turnover. Iron is essential for haem synthesis.

Causes

It is essential to find an underlying cause, as specific therapy is curative.

(1) Inadequate intake:
  (a) absolute – the elderly poor living alone, infants over 6 months of age fed exclusively on milk;
  (b) relative to a high need – pregnant women, premature or twin babies and infants delivered by caesarean section.
(2) Inadequate absorption – partial gastrectomy, resection of small bowel, malabsorption syndrome.
(3) Excessive loss – apparent or occult bleeding:
  (a) gastric damage from irritant drugs – NSAIDs (10–15% of patients with rheumatoid arthritis taking 900 mg of **aspirin** four times daily lose more than 10 mL of blood a day from gastric erosions), ethanol;
  (b) peptic ulceration;
  (c) gastrointestinal neoplasm;
  (d) heavy menstrual bleeding;
  (e) hookworm infestation (the commonest cause of iron-deficiency anaemia world wide).

Clinical features

Iron deficiency produces anaemia, inflamed corners of the mouth (angular stomatitis), a smooth shiny tongue that is sore when eating (atrophic glossitis) and longitudinally ridged, flat (even concave) nails (koilonychia). The angular stomatitis, atrophic glossitis and koilonychia are consequences of iron deficiency that are independent of impaired haemopoiesis.

Tests

The blood film shows hypochromic (paler red), microcytic (smaller) red cells that vary in size and shape. Evidence is sought for depletion of iron stores (serum ferritin concentration is low, bone marrow cellular iron is absent and serum total iron binding capacity is increased) and for lack of iron immediately available for haemoglobin synthesis (serum iron concentration and total iron binding capacity saturation is low).

Treatment

The cause, the iron deficiency and the anaemia may need treatment.

Oral iron

Ferrous sulphate dried 200 mg supplies 65 mg of iron.
Ferrous fumarate 200 mg supplies 65 mg of iron.
Ferrous glycine sulphate 225 mg supplies 40 mg of iron.
Approximately 5% of swallowed iron is absorbed from a normal diet. This increases in iron deficiency to approximately 25%. Swallowing more iron increases the amount but reduces the proportion of the dose absorbed. An erythrocyte has a life-span of approximately 100 days, so the proportion (1%) of erythrocytes replaced each day creates a daily requirement for 25 mg of iron. In severe deficiency at least 100 mg of iron must be swallowed daily for approximately 5 months for restitution of haemoglobin and stores.

Gastrointestinal unwanted effects of the therapeutic dose are common. Nausea and epigastric pain are dose related, diarrhoea and constipation are less so. If gastrointestinal unwanted effects are troublesome, the following manoeuvres may alleviate them and aid continued compliance: take the dose after a meal, try other salts and add ascorbic acid, which increases absorption.

Parenteral iron

The indications for parenteral iron are non-compliance or malabsorption. *Iron sorbitol*, by deep i/m injection, may cause pain and local staining. A significant incidence of hypersensitivity reactions occurs with i/m injections of *iron sorbitol*. Guard against severe reactions by a test dose experiment.

Response to treatment

A brisk reticulocytosis (appearance of newly formed erythrocytes in the peripheral blood) occurs within a week. Haemoglobin concentration should then increase by approximately 0.15 g/dL daily. Failure to respond suggests a wrong diagnosis, continuing blood loss or that the prescribed iron is not being taken.

Prophylaxis

The high requirement for iron in pregnancy is commonly met by the prescription of 100 mg daily of oral iron as a salt.

Vitamin B$_{12}$ deficiency megaloblastic anaemia

Normal vitamin B$_{12}$ balance

Dietary (meat, eggs, milk) vitamin B$_{12}$ combines with a glycoprotein, intrinsic factor, secreted into the lumen by the parietal cells of the gastric mucosa. The intrinsic factor/vitamin B$_{12}$ complex combines with receptors located on the surface of mucosal cells in the terminal ileum. Perhaps by triggering the process of endocytosis, the intrinsic factor promotes the absorption of vitamin B$_{12}$ at this site. Sufficient stores of vitamin B$_{12}$ are maintained in the liver for approximately 3 years supply of the daily requirement of approximately 3 µg.

Vitamin B$_{12}$ is essential for the conversion of methylmalonate to succinate. When the former accumulates, abnormal fatty acids are formed and are incorporated into neuronal cell membranes. This process results in the neurological disorders of neuropathy and subacute degeneration of the spinal cord. Vitamin B$_{12}$ is also essential for the formation of THF from the stored form, methyl THF. Therefore deficiency of vitamin B$_{12}$ resembles that of folate in so far that both cause megaloblastic anaemia. However, it is essential to distinguish between them, as an attempt to treat vitamin B$_{12}$ deficiency with folate could result in neurological defects being precipitated or aggravated and these may become irreversible.

Causes

(1) Low intake occurs rarely – vegans.
(2) Impaired absorption:
   (a) Cessation of intrinsic factor secretion occurs with gastrectomy and in pernicious anaemia. The latter represents an autoimmune gastritis, which typically begins at over 40 years of age and has an annual incidence of 9 per 10^5. Other gastric mucosal secretory functions are also lost – achlorhydria.
   (b) Damage to, or bypass of, the terminal ileum – ileal surgery, fistula, inflammatory disease or stasis in a blind loop.

Clinical features

Vitamin B$_{12}$ deficiency produces anaemia, pallor with a lemon-yellow tinge, sore mouth and tongue (glossitis), sterility and neuropathy and spinal cord degeneration. The neurological problems are often manifested as paraesthesiae (pins and needles) of the hands and feet, impairment of vibration sense and ataxia.

Tests

The blood film shows large oval erythrocytes, hypersegmented nuclei in polymorphonuclear leucocytes and large platelets. The bone marrow shows large stem cells of these three peripheral blood cells. There is a high unconjugated bilirubin (due to shortened cell life) and low vitamin B$_{12}$ concentration in serum. Patients with pernicious anaemia have circulating antibodies to gastric parietal cells. Approximately 50% of such patients also have circulating antibodies to intrinsic factor. Gastric biopsy reveals atrophy of the gastric mucosa with infiltration of lymphocytes and loss of parietal and chief cells.

The absorption of vitamin B_{12} can be assessed by the Schilling test, in which ^{57}Co-labelled cyanocobalamin is given orally to the fasting patient. A large dose of unlabelled cyanocobalamin is administered by i/m injection to saturate systemic binding sites and to promote the renal excretion of the radiolabelled cyanocobalamin. Urine is collected for 24 h. A normal subject excretes more than 10% of the radioactive dose in the urine. If significantly less appears, malabsorption of vitamin B_{12} is indicated. The mechanism of any malabsorption can be clarified by repeating the test after the oral administration of porcine intrinsic factor. If the renal excretion of the radioactive cyanocobalamin is still below normal, the lesion may lie in the terminal ileum. If, instead, renal excretion of the radioactive material now assumes a near-normal value, pernicious anaemia is indicated.

In recent years the Schilling test has tended to be replaced by whole-body counting. The whole-body count of radioactivity is made no less than 7 days after the oral administration of radiolabelled cyanocobalamin.

Treatment

Whenever vitamin B_{12} deficiency is suspected it is important to institute replacement therapy as soon as possible in order to arrest/prevent the development of serious neurological disorders. Such treatment should be instituted before the results of the diagnostic test are known.

Hydroxocobalamin is the form of vitamin B_{12} with the best retention characteristics after injection. The dose is 1 mg i/m five times over 2 weeks to replenish stores; approximately 30% is retained. In patients with impaired absorption (see Causes above) treatment needs to be life long. One milligram every 3 months is adequate. Potassium salt supplements may be needed at first because new cell formation occurs so very quickly.

Response to treatment

The bone marrow becomes normal in 2 days. Reticulocytosis is obvious within a week and there is complete correction of the anaemia within 2 months. **Hydroxocobalamin** therapy may reverse the early neurological changes in pernicious anaemia. It may also arrest (but not reverse) the progression of late neurological changes.

Folic acid-deficiency megaloblastic anaemia

Normal folate balance

Dietary folate complexes (yeast, liver, green vegetables) are hydrolysed to folic acid in the brush border of the mucosa of the proximal jejunum and then absorbed there. Body stores are limited. Most body folate is in metabolic use. Folate is needed for the production of an essential co-factor in the biosynthetic processes, involving single carbon units that occur in purine and deoxythymidylate synthesis. Purines and deoxythymidylate are both essential to DNA synthesis.

Causes

(1) Inadequate intake – commonest (alcoholic, food faddist, psychotic, mentally defective, old poor living alone).
(2) Increased utilization combined with poor diet. This occurs during pregnancy (incidence 1 : 200) particularly in the last trimester.
(3) Malabsorption – rare (gluten-sensitive enteropathy).
(4) Drugs:
    (a) anticonvulsant agents (**phenytoin**, *phenobarbitone*, *primidone*) interfere with absorption;
    (b) **methotrexate** (folinic acid is needed to overcome inhibition), *pyrimethamine*, *proguanil* and **trimethoprim** interfere with utilization.

Clinical features

Folate deficiency shows similar clinical features and blood picture to that of vitamin B_{12}, except there is no neurological disturbance. It must be distinguished by history and tests from vitamin B_{12} deficiency, as an attempt to treat vitamin B_{12} deficiency with folate can precipitate neuropathy.

Tests

There is a low erythrocyte folate concentration.

Treatment

Folic acid 5 mg daily by mouth for 4 months.

Prophylaxis

In pregnancy routine prophylaxis employs iron and folic acid tablets that contain 100 mg and 350 μg respectively.

Anaemia associated with chronic renal failure

Erythropoietin is a glycoprotein hormone. It stimulates the production of erythrocytes (erythropoiesis) in the bone marrow. In adults, 85% of the circulating erythropoietin is synthesized in the endothelial cells of the peritubular capillaries in the renal cortex; the remainder is synthesized in the liver. The normal stimulus for erythropoietin synthesis is hypoxia. When the plasma concentration of erythropoietin is low, erythroid stem cells in the bone marrow exhibit DNA cleavage followed by apoptosis (programmed cell death). Erythropoietin prevents this process. It increases the number of committed stem cells that are converted to red blood cell precursors and subsequently to mature erythrocytes.

In chronic renal failure the ability of the kidney to produce an adequate supply of erythropoietin is lost and the deficiency cannot be made good by synthesis in the liver. The erythropoietin deficiency results in the development of a normocytic, hypochromic anaemia though this may sometimes be complicated by other factors such as deficiency of iron or folate.

The anaemia associated with erythropoietin deficiency in chronic renal failure may be treated by the s/c or i/v injection of *epoetin* (recombinant human erythropoietin).

Transfusion – iron overload

If any anaemia needs correction more urgently than can be achieved with haematinic agents, packed red cells may be slowly transfused. The danger is of circulatory overload and precipitation of cardiac failure.

If many transfusions are needed in treating any anaemia, surplus Fe^{2+} (iron overload) can be chelated with **desferrioxamine**.

Summary

(1) The haemoglobin deficiency that underlies anaemia may result from impaired formation, accelerated destruction or excessive loss of erythrocytes.

(2) The absorption of Fe^{2+} is regulated by the mucosal cells of the proximal duodenum and is stimulated when body iron stores are low.

(3) Iron-deficiency anaemia is characterized by hypochromic, microcytic red blood cells, and a reduced iron concentration and increased total iron binding capacity of the serum.

(4) Iron-deficiency anaemia may result from inadequate intake, inadequate absorption or excessive loss of iron. Treatment involves both attention to the cause of the iron deficiency and replacement therapy by the oral administration of ferrous salts (e.g. **ferrous sulphate**).

(5) After combining with intrinsic factor secreted by the gastric mucosa, dietary vitamin B_{12} is actively absorbed in the terminal ileum.

(6) Vitamin B_{12} deficiency results in megaloblastic anaemia and serious neurological disorders.

(7) Vitamin B_{12} deficiency usually results from impaired absorption due to failure of the stomach to produce intrinsic factor (pernicious

STAFFS UNIVERSITY LIBRARY

anaemia) or malfunction of the terminal ileum.
(8)   When vitamin B_{12} deficiency is suspected, replacement therapy (with **hydroxocobalamin**) is instituted as soon as possible to arrest/prevent the development of neurological disorders.
(9)   Folate deficiency results in megaloblastic anaemia.
(10) Folate deficiency may result from inadequate intake, increased requirement, or drug-induced impaired absorption or interference with folate utilization.
(11) Folate deficiency may be corrected by oral therapy with **folic acid**.
(12) Erythropoietin deficiency may result from chronic renal failure and can result in a normocytic hypochromic anaemia. This may be corrected by *epoetin*.
(13) Iron overload can be corrected by the iron-chelating agent, **desferrioxamine**.

Drugs in joint disease

<u>Arthritis</u> means joint inflammation and occurs in a variety of diseases such as rheumatoid arthritis, juvenile chronic arthritis, septic arthritis and gout. Septic (pyogenic) arthritis is relatively uncommon but very important to diagnose, requiring prompt treatment with appropriate antibacterial drugs.

<u>Rheumatism</u> is an ill-defined term covering a variety of painful musculoskeletal disorders, both non-articular and articular.

<u>Rheumatic fever</u> is an inflammatory disease of autoimmune origin. It can follow a pharyngeal infection with group A β-haemolytic streptococci. The heart, joints, skin and CNS can be involved. Bed-rest, **aspirin** and a penicillin (for both eradication of the throat infection and prophylaxis against further episodes) are the mainstays of treatment.

Arthritis

Two common forms of arthritis are osteoarthritis and rheumatoid arthritis.

Osteoarthritis (sometimes referred to as osteoarthrosis) is often regarded as a degenerative disease, although it is now recognized that its pathogenesis is very much more complex than simple 'wear and tear'. Traditionally osteoarthritis has been classified into primary (idiopathic) and secondary forms (occurring as a late result of a number of joint problems, e.g. injury). It particularly affects those over the age of 50 years: hips, knees, hands and spine are most commonly involved. Movement may be limited with loss of function. Pain is variable but can be severe. Weight loss, physiotherapy and other measures to protect the joints from excessive loading (e.g. walking stick) are often helpful. It is important to maintain joint mobility. The simple analgesic **paracetamol** may relieve pain and only if this is inadequately effective should an NSAID (*ibuprofen*) be additionally prescribed. Surgery may be indicated for severe disease.

Rheumatoid arthritis is an inflammatory disease, which has a higher incidence in women than men (ratio 2–3 : 1) and a usual age of onset of 35–65 years. The cause of the disease is unknown but it is associated with the production of abnormal antibodies. Usually joint involvement is symmetrical, with early involvement of the small joints of the hands and feet. Morning stiffness is a common complaint. The disease course is variable, often with acute exacerbations followed by quiescent periods. In severe cases irreversible joint damage occurs, with deformity. All synovial joints can be affected.

Treatment of rheumatoid arthritis

The main aspects of management are:

(1) Rest affected joints, with splinting, during acute exacerbations.
(2) Physiotherapy.
(3) Occupational therapy.
(4) Chiropody.
(5) Patient education and encouragement to come to terms with a disease likely to be chronic.
(6) Drug treatment – to control pain and suppress disease (see below).
(7) Surgery – to relieve pain or improve function.

The NSAID group of drugs

These drugs (**aspirin**, *ibuprofen*, *naproxen*, *indomethacin*) inhibit cyclo-oxygenase activity, and thereby PG synthesis and the inflammatory response, in a variety of tissues (see p. 213). They are the first line of treatment in rheumatoid arthritis, though they are of value principally for providing symptomatic relief. This can be obtained from any of these drugs, although the response to each varies between individuals. The toxicity, as well as the beneficial effect, is dose related and determines the largest dose of an individual drug that can be used. Most unwanted effects are probably related to loss of PGs and include gastric mucosal damage (erosions, ulcers, gastrointestinal bleeding), decreased platelet aggregation, nephrotoxicity, salt and water retention and asthma (diversion of PG substrate to LT synthesis may contribute).

A large number of NSAIDs is now available but all share similar unwanted effects. Suppository preparations may be helpful in minimizing (but not eliminating) gastrointestinal side-effects.

Disease-modifying drugs

These drugs modify disease activity in rheumatoid arthritis and are useful in progressive disease not controlled by NSAIDs. Their mechanisms of action are not fully understood. Onset of action is slow and a beneficial effect of treatment may not be apparent for several months. The patient should therefore continue on NSAID treatment in addition to disease-modifying therapy as long as symptoms are troublesome. All disease-modifying drugs can have potentially serious unwanted effects.

(1) *Penicillamine* (see p. 215) can cause renal and bone marrow toxicity (leucopenia, thrombocytopenia, occasionally aplastic anaemia), rashes and other unwanted effects. The blood haemoglobin concentration, white cell and platelet counts and urinalysis (presence of protein and blood) must be monitored throughout treatment. The maintenance dosage should be as low as is compatible with control of disease activity.

(2) Gold compounds (see p. 215) are usually administered by i/m injection (*sodium aurothiomalate*) but an oral preparation (*auranofin*) is available. Adverse effects include those on the kidney, bone marrow and skin, and a full blood count and urinalysis must be performed before each gold injection and also monitored regularly with oral treatment.

(3) *Chloroquine* (see p. 215) and *hydroxychloroquine* can cause retinal damage and regular (3–6 monthly) ophthalmic monitoring is essential.

(4) *Sulphasalazine* (the beneficial effect is presumed to be associated with the 5-ASA moiety, see p. 466) is often associated with gastrointestinal side-effects, malaise and headache. Serious unwanted effects are unusual, although leucopenia and hepatotoxicity can occur.

(5) Immunosuppressant drugs (*azathioprine*, **cyclophosphamide, methotrexate, cyclosporin**) may be indicated in patients with severe, aggressive articular disease who have not responded to, or who do not tolerate, other disease-modifying treatment, or in patients with life-threatening disease. Unwanted effects (see p. 321) are relatively frequent and can be serious.

(6) Glucocorticosteroids (see p. 214). Although very effective in reducing inflammation and providing symptomatic relief, systemic glucocorticosteroids should be avoided if possible because of the unwanted effects (see p. 183) associated with the long-term use of doses needed to suppress symptoms. Exacerbation of symptoms on withdrawal makes dosage reduction difficult. Nevertheless, patients with severe systemic disease may require high-dose systemic glucocorticosteroids. Intra-articular injection of a glucocorticosteroid is useful is suppressing inflammation in a severely inflamed joint provided there is no infection.

Gout

Gout is caused by the inflammatory response to crystals of monosodium urate monohydrate, which are formed as a result of hyperuricaemia. Crystal deposition in and around the joints can cause arthritis, and in the kidney renal damage. The plasma urate concentration is increased (more than 0.4 mmole/L). Either overproduction or underexcretion of uric acid (or a combination of both) may be responsible.

Usually gout initially affects a single joint (typically the metatarsophalangeal joint of the big toe), and then recurrent attacks occur in which other joints may be involved. If left untreated, a patient may develop chronic tophaceous gout (tophi are macroscopic nodules of deposited urate crystals bounded by fibrous tissue).

Gout may result from:

(1) Hereditary predisposition.
(2) Drugs – some diuretic agents, low-dose salicylate, alcohol.
(3) Excessive cell break-down (e.g. myeloproliferative and lymphoprolif-
    erative disorders).
(4) Renal failure.
(5) Ketoacidosis and starvation.

Renal handling of urate is complex, and net urate excretion depends on
the balance of the following processes:

(1) Glomerular filtration.
(2) Proximal tubule reabsorption.
(3) Active tubular secretion.
(4) Postsecretory reabsorption.

Drugs used to enhance urate excretion (uricosuric agents – *probenecid,
sulphinpyrazone*) disturb this balance.

An alternative way to lower uric acid concentration in blood is to inhibit
xanthine oxidase, which catalyses the metabolism of purines to urate (via
hypoxanthine and xanthine) with **allopurinol**.

Treatment of acute attacks of gout

Symptomatic treatment is with an NSAID (*indomethacin, naproxen,* but
not **aspirin**, which is contraindicated), initially at high dose, which can then
be quickly reduced as symptoms permit.

An alternative, now seldom used except for patients in whom NSAIDs
are contraindicated, is *colchicine*, an antimitotic agent, which often causes
diarrhoea.

Prophylaxis of acute attacks

General therapeutic measures include:

(1) Avoidance of excessive consumption of ethanol and foods that contain
    purines.
(2) Reduction of weight.
(3) Withdraw or replacement of any drug (e.g. diuretic) that precipitates
    the attacks.

Prophylactic drug therapy, if considered necessary, should be initiated only
once the acute attack has settled. Treatment should be continued indefinitely.

Inhibition of uric acid synthesis

Allopurinol is particularly useful in patients in whom uric acid is overpro-
duced.

Uricosuric agents

These agents (*probenecid, sulphinpyrazone*) should not be used if there is renal impairment or a history of renal stones. Fluid intake should be increased to prevent crystallization of urate in the urine.

During the first weeks of treatment with either **allopurinol** or a uricosuric agent, an NSAID or *colchicine* should be prescribed concomitantly, as an acute attack may be precipitated.

Summary

(1) Osteoarthritis is most appropriately treated with an antipyretic analgesic agent (**paracetamol**).
(2) Rheumatoid arthritis, being an inflammatory disease, is more appropriately treated by NSAIDs to suppress symptoms. Disease-modifying drugs are also available but may produce severe unwanted effects.
(3) Gout features an inflammatory response to crystals deposited around joints from an excessive blood concentration of uric acid. Drugs that reduce renal clearance of uric acid may precipitate gout. The acute attack is treated by a high dose of an NSAID (but not **aspirin**). Prophylaxis involves drugs that inhibit the synthesis of uric acid or ones that increase its renal clearance.

Drugs and the skin

Infections

Infestations have been dealt with on page 287 and fungal infections on page 299.

Bacterial infections

Many formulations of antibacterial drugs are available for topical application to the skin but their use is often not necessary. Washing and other hygienic practices are usually adequate to combat bacterial skin infections. Not all skin complaints are manifestations of infection. Antibiotic agents can themselves cause sensitivity reactions in the skin (see p. 542).

Staphylococcus aureus

A carbuncle is a coalescence of deep boils and needs to be treated systemically with an antibacterial agent because the infection is too deeply sited for topical formulations to be effective.

Impetigo is a spreading superficial infection of the skin. Because it is superficial, topical antiseptic agents are effective (*cetrimide, chlorhexidine, hexachlorophane, povidone-iodine*). *Fusidic acid* or *mupirocin* can be applied topically.

If impetigo is widespread on the body then a systemic antibiotic (**flucloxacillin** or **erythromycin**) should be used. To minimize the development of resistant micro-organisms the drugs used topically and systemically should be different.

Streptococcus pyogenes

Erysipelas is differentiated from impetigo by an advancing, raised, sharply demarcated edge, thin seropurulent discharge from ruptured vesicles and lymphatic spread. One per cent of cases suffer allergic acute glomerulonephritis 1–3 weeks later. Treat erysipelas promptly with systemic **phenoxymethylpenicillin**.

Viral infections

Herpes simplex (cold sore) – local **acyclovir** or *idoxuridine* treat the cause but treatment needs to be started at the onset of sore development (see p. 315).

Herpes zoster (shingles) appears when immunity wanes and latent chickenpox virus in the posterior root ganglia spreads down the sensory nerves to invade the dermal segment supplied. It should be managed by early treatment with systemic **acyclovir**, and analgesic agents.

Human papilloma virus (warts) is self-limiting – 5–20% regress spontaneously within 6 months therefore treatments that are painful or leave scars are not appropriate. *Salicylic acid*, with or without lactic acid in a collodion paint, local soaking with *formaldehyde* or *glutaraldehyde*, or *podophyllum resin* paint are chemical alternatives to curettage under local anaesthesia or cryotherapy. The preparations, which are keratolytic, act slowly to remove the hyperkeratotic layers. They are all irritant to normal skin.

Acne

Cause

The hair follicle sebaceous glands produce too much sebum and their necks too much keratin that is too cohesive. The incidence is 90% in teenagers, declining to 15% at approximately 25 years of age; there is a familial tendency. Local sensitivity to androgens determines the pathophysiology. In females the functional antagonism of androgens by oestrogens is revealed by the exacerbation of acne premenstrually when plasma oestrogen concentration is minimal (see p. 159).

Clinical features

The pilosebaceous canal is obstructed by a comedone (blackhead). Sebum excessively secreted behind this obstruction blows up the gland. Bacterial colonization by the commensal anaerobe *Propionobacterium acnes* and breakdown by its lipases lead to a further increase in volume. Rupture into the dermis initiates an inflammatory response.

Self-management

Sunlight (short of burning) is beneficial in increasing keratin turnover. The commensal skin flora are reduced by skin cleaning with antiseptic detergents (*cetrimide*).

Treatments

Local

(1) UV irradiation.
(2) Keratolytic agents (benzoyl peroxide, salicylic acid, *tretinoin*) produce a plug of loosely packed horny cells that unseats the existing comedone. The effectiveness of abrasive agents (aluminium oxide) is uncertain.
(3) Topical antibiotics (erythromycin, tetracycline, clindamycin) are beneficial in many patients with mild acne. They may cause mild irritation of the skin and allow the appearance of resistant strains of micro-organisms.

Systemic

Antibacterial agents (tetracyclines, **erythromycin**) in small doses for weeks, or even months, are accumulated in sebum.

In females severe acne may respond to **ethinyloestradiol** with **cyproterone** – the antagonist at testosterone receptors; this preparation is also contraceptive.

Seborrhoeic dermatitis

Cause

Excessive sebum secretion (greasy skin), fungal infection with the yeast form of *Pityrosporum ovale* plus low-grade bacterial infection.

Clinical features

This is a recurrent dermatitis with characteristic distribution on the scalp, which shows scaling and hair loss (cradle cap in a baby), in and behind the external ears, eyebrows, nasolabial fold, over the sternum, between the shoulder blades, axillae, pubis and groins.

Management

Regular cleaning with antiseptic detergent shampoo (*cetrimide, hexachlorophane*) is carried out. The imidazoles (*ketoconazole* shampoo) are very effective in clearing the fungal infection. Inflammation may be severe enough to warrant glucocorticosteroids.

Contact dermatitis

Two very different causes operate – irritation and sensitization.

Irritant contact dermatitis

The causes of this dermatitis are alkali cleaners, abrasive agents and solvents. Nappy rash is an irritant dermatitis to the ammonia formed by bacterial breakdown of urea. Ensure adequate frequency of nappy changing and cleaning of the nappy, if not the disposable kind, and use a barrier cream.

Sensitization contact dermatitis

Causes

A delayed (type IV) hypersensitivity reaction to cutaneous allergens or haptens:

(1) Vehicles – lanolin (wool fat, wax and alcohol used in ointments, creams and cosmetics) and parabens (alkylhydroxy-benzoates used as preservative agents in creams, lotions and cosmetics).
(2) Antibacterial drugs topically applied – penicillins (especially **ampicillin**), aminoglycosides, *chloramphenicol* and sulphonamides are all common causes; *fusidic acid* is an infrequent cause and *chlortetracycline* a rare cause.
(3) Antiseptic agents – *iodine* and *hexachlorophane*; occasionally hydroxyquinolines, rarely *chlorhexidine* and *benzoyl peroxide*.
(4) Local anaesthetic agents – all are liable to sensitize the skin when locally applied but **lignocaine** is least so.
(5) Antagonists at H_1 histamine receptors – all are liable to sensitize the skin when locally applied.
(6) Adhesive agents – colophony and rubber chemicals but not acrylate monomer.
(7) Miscellaneous – including elastic, nickel, rubber, plants.

Incidence

Up to 10% of all patients with dermatitis have allergic contact dermatitis; 1–2% of those with eczema are allergic to lanolin (rare in those with normal skin).

Clinical features

Previous contact with skin is essential for the development of sensitization. Once developed, the whole skin is abnormally reactive, both to skin contact and blood-borne allergens. The condition persists for years and is specific to close chemical analogues of the sensitizer. It occurs more commonly in adults than children and more commonly with damaged skin. The rash is symmetrically distributed. A detailed history of temporal associations suggests the agent, which may then be identifiable by patch testing.

Treatment

To treat specifically, identify the cause and exclude it. However, this is not always a practical option for the patient. For symptomatic treatment, see page 545.

Atopic eczema

Eczema means little more than dermatitis of unknown cause. It is one of the diseases of atopy (see p. 424). There is (incidence 1–3%) a heritable tendency to low itch threshold, deficient sweat and sebum secretion and ready cutaneous vasodilatation. Scratching produces most of the damage to skin (excoriation, thickening, reddening, exudation, soreness).

Clinical features

In infants eczema begins (at 2–3 months) on the face then becomes generalized. A dietary origin is relatively common. In childhood (1.5–7 years) flexures are most affected and inhaled allergen is commoner. It tends to decline in steps, at the onset of puberty and at 18 years.

Treatment

Avoid any demonstrable cause. For symptomatic treatment, see page 545.

Psoriasis

This is a genetically transmitted tendency to a ten-times faster than normal epithelial cell proliferation rate. Cell life becomes four, instead of 28 days. The surface layer shows poor differentiation towards a keratinized corneum.

Incidence

Between 2% and 3% of the population show psoriasis, beginning in the age range 25–60 years. It fluctuates, is triggered by normal stimuli to cell multiplication and is commonly subject to spontaneous remissions and recurrences.

Clinical features

Well-defined plaques of red thickened skin covered with loose silvery scales. Commonest sites – scalp, elbows, knees and knuckles.

Management

Local

Sunlight (the 280–310 nm band, UVB) is beneficial in mild to moderate psoriasis.

Various irritant agents have been found empirically to hasten remission: *coal tar* (0.5–5%) is effective but messy. Irritant preparations for addition to the bath water have little effect. The standard treatment in this irritant group is the application to the lesion of **dithranol** [anthralin] 0.1-2% (combined with *coal tar* and/or *salicylic acid* in some preparations). It is applied daily (to thick plaques) or twice a week (to thin ones) and accurately, in an amount just sufficient to cause a feeling of local warmth. The area is covered for 1 h and then the application is washed off; a red-brown staining of the skin occurs. Treatment is continued until the skin is clear as judged by appearance, feel and lack of scale on scratching. Applications should cease if soreness or weeping develops.

Calcipotriol (a vitamin D derivative) is useful for topical application for mild to moderate psoriasis of the skin and scalp.

Glucocorticosteroids should be avoided, as tachyphylaxis may occur and local pustules emerge.

Systemic

Some dermatology clinics offer PUVA – the combination of long-wave ultra-violet irradiation (310–400 nm, UVA) with an oral psoralen (methoxsalen; chemicals occurring naturally in some plant saps that interact with skin and sunlight to produce phototoxic dermatitis) which, when activated by UV, binds to DNA. Hazards of PUVA treatment in the short (severe burning) and long term (cataracts, skin cancer) require its careful regulation.

Severe resistant cases may be treated orally with **methotrexate** in low dosage or the retinoid *acitretin*.

Symptomatic management of dermatitis

The symptomatic treatment of dermatitides depends less on the cause of the dermatitis or the distribution of or name given to the rash and more on the stage of skin inflammation and patient complaints.

Acute weeping stage

Dressings are wetted (replaced so area never dries) with lotions of aluminium acetate or *potassium permanganate*, which are both astringent (precipitate proteins and reduce the serous oozing) and soothing to sore skin. *Potassium permanganate* is also antiseptic.

Local anti-inflammatory glucocorticosteroids (see below) may be necessary if such wet dressings are unbearable. Antibacterial drugs may be required if the lesion is secondarily infected.

Subacute stage

When weeping stops the lesions can be protected by a thickly spread paste (*zinc compound paste*) twice daily.

Dry fissured and scaly stage

Washing the lesions with soap irritates and defats the skin, emulsifying ointment is useful as a soap substitute. An emollient (*aqueous cream*) soothes, smooths and hydrates the epidermis, thus relieving irritation. The incorporation of astringent (zinc oxide) and antipruritic (*calamine*) agents can enhance the relief afforded by an emollient.

Chronic stage

This is characterized by marked thickening of the skin and pronounced scaling. Keratolytic agents (*salicylic acid, coal tar* – the look and smell of which make it unpopular) increase the rate of loss of surface scale. They are irritant and must be avoided or discontinued on broken or acutely inflamed skin.

Topical glucocorticosteroids

These are non-specifically anti-inflammatory and patients with dermatitis, eczema and psoriasis frequently demand them, having heard of their efficacy from other patients. *Hydrocortisone* cream (0.1 and 1%) and ointment (1%) are available from retail pharmacists without prescription for short-term (maximum 7 days) use in irritant dermatitis, allergic contact dermatitis and insect bite reactions.

Between 3 and 10% of an applied dose can enter the skin, depending on the vehicle and diluent. For maximal effect a soft white paraffin-based ointment is the simplest satisfactory base; creams, lotions and propylene glycol diluents all interfere with activity.

The intensity of the anti-inflammatory effect obtained depends on the potency and efficacy of the glucocorticosteroid drug used and the dose rate of application to the skin. To avoid unwanted effects the least intensity that controls the disease should be used. Preparations producing four intensities of effect are recognized:

I   The highest: preparations are available but their use is usually ill-advised.
II   High: *betamethasone valerate* 0.1% and *hydrocortisone butyrate* 0.1% are equi-effective.
III Moderate: *clobetasone butyrate* 0.05%.
IV   Mild: *hydrocortisone* 1%

Florid inflammatory skin lesions can be brought under control by systemic **prednisolone** or a high intensity local glucocorticosteroid. As soon as control is achieved continued treatment should be local and with the minimum intensity of glucocorticosteroid that retains control of the lesions.

The topical glucocorticosteroids are so effective (though only providing symptomatic relief) and so widely used that an appreciation of their limitations is essential.

Local complications

Glucocorticosteroids are contraindicated in any infected condition (whether fungal or bacterial) because they mask the inflammatory response to, and therefore the signs of, infection. They also predispose to infection.

Glucocorticosteroids cause skin atrophy (both dermal and epidermal), telangiectasia (groups of visible dilated small blood vessels), purpura and striae. These effects are maximal with more intensely active preparations, used on the face, in younger patients and for long treatment times.

Systemic complications

Toxicity identical to that of systemic glucocorticosteroids (see p. 183), due to systemic absorption, is uncommon but is seen when application is extensive, is to permeable skin and/or is under occlusive dressings.

Sunlight

Sunscreens

Medium wavelength UV (280–310 nm, UVB) burns normal skin and, with longer wavelength UV (310–400 nm, UVA), contributes to long-term skin changes (cancer, ageing). Sensitive skins may react to the same wavelengths as normal skins, or to longer wavelengths. Lotions or creams that contain sun screens (aminobenzoic acid, padimate O) protect against UVB and sunburn, if generously and frequently applied. The inclusion of reflective substances (titanium dioxide) also protects to some extent against UVA, but the thick, greasy preparation may not be acceptable to the patient.

Summary

The skin:

(1) Is the largest and most accessible bodily organ.
(2) May be the target organ of drug action and/or a route of drug administration.
(3) Has many pharmaceutical preparations manufactured for its use.

Some pharmaceutical preparations applied topically to the skin:

(1) Have beneficial effects but do not contain a pharmacologically active drug.
(2) Contain a pharmacologically active drug but are not recommended;
(3) Can cause local unwanted effects.
(4) Can be absorbed and produce undesirable or desirable systemic effects.

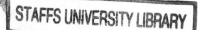
STAFFS UNIVERSITY LIBRARY

Suggested further reading and study

Alberts, B., Bray, D., Lewis, J., Raff, M., Roberts, K. and Watson, J.D. (1994). *Molecular Biology of the Cell*, 3rd edition. Garland, New York

Amdur, M.O. (1993). *Casarett and Doull's Toxicology: the basic science of poisons*, 5th edition. McGraw Hill

Aronson, J.K., Hardman, M. and Reynolds, D.J.M. (1993). *ABC of Monitoring Drug Therapy*. BMJ Publishing Group, London

Association of British Pharmaceutical Companies. *ABPI Data Sheet Compendium*, latest edition. Datapharm Publications

British National Formulary, latest edition. British Medical Association and Royal Pharmaceutical Society of Great Britain, London

Brody, T.M., Larner, J., Minneman, K.P. and Neu, H.C. (1994). *Human Pharmacology: molecular to clinical*, 2nd edition. Mosby-Year Book Inc, London

Carpenter, J. (1988). *Pharmacology from A to Z*. Manchester University Press, Manchester

Cooper, J.R., Bloom, F.E. and Roth, R.H. (1991). *The Biochemical Basis of Neuropharmacology*, 6th edition. Oxford University Press

Coulson, C.J. (1993). *Molecular Mechanisms of Drug Action*, 2nd edition. Taylor and Francis, Basingstoke

Dale, M.M. and Dickenson, A.H. (1993). *Companion to 'Pharmacology': a study for self-assessment and revision*. Churchill Livingstone, Edinburgh

Drug and Therapeutic Bulletin. Consumer's Association, Hereford

Franklin, T.J. and Snow, G.A. (1989). *Biochemistry of Antimicrobial Action*, 4th edition. Chapman and Hall, London

Garrod, L.P., Lambert, H.P. and O'Grady, F. (1991). *Antibiotic and Chemotherapy*, 6th edition. Churchill Livingstone, London

Gibson, G.G. and Skett, P. (1994). *Introduction to Drug Metabolism*, 2nd edition. Blackie Academic and Professional

Gilman, A.G., Rall, T.W., Nies A.S. and Taylor P. (1992). *Goodman and Gilman's The Pharmacological Basis of Therapeutics*, 8th edition. McGraw-Hill

Goldzieher, J.W. and Fotherby, K. (1994). *Pharmacology of the Contraceptive Steroids*. Raven Press, New York

Grahame-Smith, D.G. and Aronson, J.K. (1992). *Oxford Textbook of Clinical Pharmacology and Drug Therapy*, 2nd edition. Oxford University Press, Oxford

Greenspan, F.S. and Baxter, J.D. (1994). *Basic and Clinical Endocrinology*, 4th edition. Prentice-Hall, New York

Katzung, B.G. (1995). *Basic and Clinical Pharmacology*, 6th edition. Appleton and Lange

Kenakin, T. (1993). *Pharmacologic Analysis of Drug-Receptor Interaction*, 2nd edition. Raven Press, New York

Kruk, Z.L. and Pycock, C.J. (1991). *Neurotransmitters and Drugs*, 3rd edition. Chapman and Hall, London

Laurence, D.R. and Bennett, P.N. (1992). *Clinical Pharmacology*, 7th edition. Churchill Livingstone, Edinburgh

Laurence, D.R. and Carpenter, J.R. (1994). *A Dictionary of Pharmacology and Clinical Drug Evaluation*. University College London Press

Neal, M.J. (1992). *Medical Pharmacology at a Glance*, 2nd edition. Blackwell Science, Oxford

Prescriber's Journal, Hannibal House, Elephant and Castle, London

Nogrady, T. (1988). *Medicinal Chemistry: a biochemical approach*, 2nd edition. Oxford University Press, Oxford

Pharma-CAL-ogy Consortium. Computer Assisted Learning packages developed under the auspices of the Teaching and Learning Technology Programme.

Pratt, W.B. and Taylor, P. (1990). *Principles of Drug Action: The Basis of Pharmacology*, 3rd edition. Churchill Livingstone, Edinburgh

Rang, H.P., Dale, M.M. and Ritter, J.M. (1995). *Pharmacology*, 3rd edition. Churchill Livingstone, Edinburgh

Rees, J. and Price, J. (1995). *ABC of Asthma*. BMJ Publishing Group, London

Ritter, J.M., Lewis, L.D. and Mant, T.G.K. (1995). *A Textbook of Clinical Pharmacology*, 3rd edition. Edward Arnold, London

Rowland, M. and Tozer, T. (1995). *Clinical Pharmacokinetics: concepts and applications*, 3rd edition. Williams and Wilkins, Baltimore

Ryall, R.W. (1989). *Mechanisms of Drug Action on the Nervous System*, 2nd edition. Cambridge University Press, Cambridge

Taylor, J.B. and Kennewell, P.D. (1993). *Modern Medicinal Chemistry*. Ellis Horwood

Trends in Pharmacological Science. Elsevier, Amsterdam

Trevor, A.J. (1993). *Pharmacology: examination and board review*, 3rd edition. Appleton and Lange, New York

Webster, R.A. and Jordan, C.C. (1989). *Neurotransmitters, Drugs and Disease*. Blackwell Science, Oxford

World Health Organisation Expert Committee on the Use of Essential Drugs. (1992). WHO Technical Report Series; 825, *The Use of Essential Drugs*, 5th report. HMSO, London

Index

STAFFS UNIVERSITY LIBRARY

CARDIFF UNIVERSITY LIBRARY